Saunders Review *of* Practical Nursing *for* NCLEX-PN

Saunders
Review *of*
Practical
Nursing *for*
NCLEX-PN

3RD EDITION

Esther Matassarin-Jacobs, R.N., Ph.D., O.C.N.
Associate Professor and Associate Dean
Director, Undergraduate Program
Niehoff School of Nursing
Loyola University
Chicago, Illinois

Consulting Editor
Maureen B. Barrett, R.N., M.S.N.,C

W.B. SAUNDERS COMPANY
A Division of Harcourt Brace & Company
Philadelphia London Toronto Montreal Sydney Tokyo

W.B. SAUNDERS COMPANY
A Division of Harcourt Brace & Company

The Curtis Center
Independence Square West
Philadelphia, Pennsylvania 19106

Library of Congress Cataloging-in-Publication Data

Matassarin-Jacobs, Esther.

Saunders review of practical nursing for NCLEX-PN /
Esther Matassarin-Jacobs. -- 3rd ed. /
consulting editor, Maureen B. Barrott.

p.   cm.

Includes bibliographical references and index.

ISBN 0–7216–5872–5

1. Practical nursing—Examinations, questions, etc.   2. Practical nursing—
   Outlines, syllabi, etc.   I. Barrett, Maureen B.   II. Title.

[DNLM: 1. Nursing, Practical—examination questions.   2. Nursing, Practical—
outlines.   3. Licensure, Nursing—United States—examination questions.
WY 18.2 M425s   1997]

RT62.M38   1997
610.73'069'3076—dc20   96–4869

Saunders Review of Practical Nursing for NCLEX-PN
Third Edition   ISBN 0–7216–5872–5

Printed in the United States of America.

Last digit is the print number: 9   8   7   6   5   4   3   2   1

To my dear husband,
Philip B. Jacobs.
You continue to be the reason.

To the memory of my beloved mother,
Grace Matassarin, R.N.,
always my favorite nurse!

To my father,
F. W. Matassarin, M.D.,
for all his strength and courage.

Contributors

Carol Barbarich, R.N., B.S.N.
Practical Nursing Department,
    Danville Area School District,
    Washingtonville, Pennsylvania

Joan Darden, R.N., Ph.D.
Nursing Department, Darton College,
    Albany, Georgia

N. Jayne Denham, R.N.C.
University of Texas at Brownsville,
    and Texas Southmost College,
    Vocational Nursing Program at
    Weslaco, Weslaco, Texas

Denise F. Fowler, M.S.A., B.S.N.
Practical Nursing Department,
    Augusta Technical Institute,
    Augusta, Georgia

Jeanette Kamp
Nursing Department,
    Delta College,
    University Center, Michigan

Cindi Papendick, R.N., M.S.
Adjunct Faculty, School of Nursing,
    Lake Michigan College, Benton
    Harbor, Michigan. Community
    Mental Health Nurse, Home Health
    Services of Indiana, Michigan City,
    Indiana

Sally Roach, M.S.N.
School of Nursing, University of
    Texas at Brownsville, Weslaco,
    Texas

Alicia Rodriguez, R.N., B.S.N.
School of Nursing, University of
    Texas at Brownsville, Weslaco,
    Texas

Patricia R. Schultz, R.N., Ed.D.
Nursing Faculty, University of
    Tampa, Tampa, Florida

Reviewers

Carol Barbarich, R.N., B.S.N.
Practical Nursing Department,
   Danville Area School District,
   Washingtonville, Pennsylvania

Nancy K. Buttry, R.N., M.S.N.
Director, Practical Nursing
   Department, Southeastern Illinois
   College, Harrisburg, Illinois

Veronica K. Casey, R.N.C., B.S.N., M.A.
J.M. Wright Technical School,
   Stamford, Connecticut

Beth Ann Cook, R.N., B.S.N., M.S.N.
Ivy Tech Community College,
   Evansville, Indiana

Joan Darden, R.N., Ph.D.
Associate Professor, Nursing, Darton
   College, Albany, Georgia

JoAnn Dever, R.N., M.S.N.Ed.
Director, Practical Nursing
   Department, Indiana Vocational
   Technical College, Fort Wayne,
   Indiana

Janet M. Dicke, R.N., M.S.N.
Practical Nursing Department,
   Minnesota Riverland Technical
   College, Rochester, Minnesota

Jewel K. Diller, R.N., M.S.Ed.
Practical Nursing Department, Ivy
   Tech State College, Fort Wayne,
   Indiana

Donna C. Henry, R.N., B.S.N., M.S.N.
Practial Nursing Department, Wabash
   Valley College, Mount Carmel,
   Illinois

Judith Ingrasin, M.S., R.N.
Professor, Practical Nursing, Iona
   College, New Rochelle, New York

Bethany Jagers, R.N., M.S.
Instructor, Practical Nursing, School
   of Nursing, Hocking College,
   Nelsonville, Ohio

Prescilla LaHann, R.N., B.S.N.
Instructor, Practical Nursing
   Department, School of Applied
   Technology, Idaho State University,
   Pocatello, Idaho

Denise Marshall, R.N., B.S.N., M.Ed.
Practical Nursing Department, Wor-
   Wic Community College, Salisbury,
   Maryland

Gail Miller, R.N., B.S.N.
Northeast Iowa Community College,
   Peosta, Iowa

Marion E. Monahan, R.N., B.S.E.,
   M.A.Ed.
Practical Nursing Coordinator, Jeff
   Tech, Reynoldsville, Pennsylvania

Kathleen M. Nelson, R.N., M.S.N.
Practical Nursing Department,
   Wabash Valley College, Mount
   Carmel, Illinois

Annie Opuda, B.S.N., R.N.C.
Santa Fe Community College,
   Gainesville, Florida

Paula Ott, R.N., B.S.N., M.Ed.
Delta Ouachita Regional Technical
   Institute, West Monroe, Louisiana

Linda Parrish, R.N., B.S.N., M.S.N., Ed.D.
Chair, School of Nursing, George C.
   Wallace State Community College,
   Dothan, Alabama

Alice Rasmussen, R.N., B.S.N., M.S.N.
School of Nursing, Lake Michigan
   College, Benton Harbor, Michigan

Preface

This is the third edition of a review book that has helped many practical and vocational nurses through their programs and to pass the NCLEX-PN and become licensed. The text reflects changes in the licensure process, the introduction of computer adaptive testing (CAT), and a revised text blueprint.

I designed this review book to help you through this sometimes confusing and always stressful time in your life. The review content has been expanded for this edition, and test-taking hints are incorporated into the first practice test. You will also find many practice test questions following the review outlines so that you can test your level of knowledge as you go through the text. The questions are designed to look just like those you will find on the NCLEX-PN. Although no book can replace your education, this text can help you tie it all together so that you can be successful in taking the NCLEX-PN.

The book includes a computerized version of the practice test questions so that you can gain valuable experience in test taking on the computer. The software screen simulates that of the actual NCLEX-PN test in both appearance and procedures. You will have the option to take a ten-question quiz in adult health, child health, maternity, or mental health, or you may select a comprehensive examination of 100 questions. You may also choose the study mode, which allows you to review the rationales for each question immediately upon selecting your answer. All questions are randomly generated from a pool of more than 1000 questions taken from the book. So every test is different, allowing you to use the software again and again!

As with other editions, I have drawn considerably from nursing faculties throughout the United States. These faculty members helped me identify the needs of the PN graduates and determine how a review text could help them.

The National Council of State Boards of Nursing sets the standards, puts the examination together after it is written by PN faculty and supervisors, and validates the examination. The Council is actively involved in researching and constantly updating the examination. Because nursing and health care are in a state of constant flux, so is the examination. Even though the examination is now computerized, this does not change the content or what you need to to pass. You must demonstrate that you have the minimal competency to practice vocational or practical nursing.

I wish you all the best as you work toward your goal, licensure as a practical or vocational nurse. With hard work and proper preparation, you will be successful.

ESTHER MATASSARIN-JACOBS

Acknowledgments

I want to thank Maureen Barrett, R.N., M.S.N., for all her help with manuscript preparation and Franklin Hicks, R.N., Ph.D.(c), C.C.R.N., for all his help with proofreading. It is good to have friends you can depend on.

I would like to acknowledge the following item writers for their work on the Second Edition of *Saunders Review of Practical Nursing for NCLEX-PN*: Sandra Benson, B.S.N., M.S.; Beulah Bloodworth, R.N.; Diane M. Chudomelka, R.N., B.S.N., M.S.Ed.; Jody A. Eckler, R.N., B.S.N.; Judy M. Fair, R.N., M.Ed.; Sally J. Winckler Flesch, B.S.N., M.A., Ed.S.; and T. Jan Woods, R.N., B.S.N., M.S.N., F.N.P.

Contents

1 Preparing for the NCLEX-PN 1

Part One: Preparing for the Test, 1
Part Two: Using This Text, 2
Part Three: Format of the NCLEX-PN, 3
General Description, 3
Test Plan, 4

2 Improving Your Ability to Pass the Examination 7

Part One: Test-Taking Strategies, 7
Phases of the Nursing Process, 8
Categories of Client Needs, 8
Part Two: Hints for Retaking the Examination, 10
Practice Test 1, 11
Questions, 11
Answers and Rationales, 31

3 The Nursing Process and Basic Skills 47

I. THE NURSING PROCESS, 47
II. BASIC SKILLS, 47
Questions, 59
Answers and Rationales, 63

4 Medication Administration 65

I. OVERVIEW OF PHARMACOLOGY, 65
II. COMMON CATEGORIES OF DRUGS, 67
III. PRINCIPLES OF MEDICATION ADMINISTRATION, 77
Questions, 81
Answers and Rationales, 85

5 Diet Therapy 87

I. PRINCIPLES OF NORMAL NUTRITION, 87
II. THERAPEUTIC DIET MODIFICATIONS, 91
Questions, 97
Answers and Rationales, 101

6 Special Needs of Older Adults 103
  I.   PHYSIOLOGIC ALTERATIONS RELATED TO AGING, 103
  II. PSYCHOLOGIC ALTERATIONS RELATED TO AGING, 105
  III. LEGAL CONCERNS OF OLDER ADULTS, 106
  IV. COMMON HEALTH PROBLEMS OF OLDER ADULTS, 106
  V.   MEDICATIONS AND OLDER ADULTS, 106
  VI. NURSING PROCESS APPLIED TO THE SPECIAL NEEDS OF
         OLDER ADULTS, 107
           Questions, 111
           Answers and Rationales, 115

7 The Adult Client 117
  GROWTH AND DEVELOPMENT, 117
  Life Stages
  I.   MIDDLE-AGED ADULT, 117
  II. THE OLDER ADULT, 118
  Reproductive System in Women
  I.   NORMAL FUNCTION, 119
  Reproductive Changes and Disorders in Women
  I.   BREAST, 119
  II. UTERINE TUMORS: BENIGN, 120
  III. CERVICAL CANCER, 120
  IV. ENDOMETRIOSIS, 121
  V.   MENOPAUSE, 121
  Reproductive Disorders in Men
  I.   BENIGN PROSTATIC HYPERPLASIA, 122
  II. CANCER OF THE PROSTATE, 123
           Questions, 125
           Answers and Rationales, 129
  OXYGENATION AND CARDIOPULMONARY DISORDERS, 130
  Cardiovascular Disorders
  I.   ARTERIOSCLEROSIS/ATHEROSCLEROSIS, 130
  II. HYPERTENSION, 131
  III. CORONARY ARTERY DISEASE, 132
  IV. ANGINA PECTORIS, 135
  V.   MYOCARDIAL INFARCTION, 136
  VI. CONGESTIVE HEART FAILURE, 137
  VII. PERIPHERAL VASCULAR DISORDERS, 138
  Diseases of the Blood
  I.   LEUKEMIA, 142
  II. LYMPHOMA, 143
  III. SICKLE CELL DISEASE, 145
  IV. SHOCK, 145
  Pulmonary Disorders
  I.   PNEUMONIA, 146
  II. TUBERCULOSIS, 147
  III. CHRONIC OBSTRUCTIVE PULMONARY DISEASE OR
         CHRONIC OBSTRUCTIVE LUNG DISEASE, 148
  IV. LUNG CANCER, 149
  V.   CHEST SURGERY, 150
  VI. LARYNGEAL CANCER, 150

Cardiopulmonary Resuscitation
I. ASSESSMENT: A, B, C, 152
II. IMPLEMENTATION, 152
III. EVALUATION, 152

Fluid and Electrolyte Balance
I. NORMAL FLUID BALANCE, 153

Fluid Imbalances
I. EDEMA—EXTRACELLULAR FLUID EXCESS, 154
II. DEHYDRATION—EXTRACELLULAR FLUID DEFICIT, 154

Electrolyte Imbalances
I. HYPERNATREMIA, 155
II. HYPONATREMIA, 156
III. HYPERKALEMIA, 156
IV. HYPOKALEMIA, 157
V. HYPERCALCEMIA, 157
VI. HYPOCALCEMIA, 158

Acid-Base Imbalances
I. NORMAL VALUES, 158
II. IMBALANCES, 158
III. RESPIRATORY ACIDOSIS, 158
IV. RESPIRATORY ALKALOSIS, 159
V. METABOLIC ACIDOSIS, 160
VI. METABOLIC ALKALOSIS, 161
Questions, 163
Answers and Rationales, 167

SENSORY/PERCEPTUAL ALTERATIONS, 169
I. NORMAL FUNCTION, 169

Disorders of the Cerebral and Central Nervous System
I. INCREASED INTRACRANIAL PRESSURE, 169
II. INFECTIOUS CONDITIONS, 170
III. ACUTE DISORDERS, 171
IV. CHRONIC DISORDERS, 175

Eye: Normal Function
I. LOCATION, 179
II. COMPOSITION, 179
III. CHAMBERS, 180
IV. CONJUNCTIVA, 180
V. LENS, 180
VI. LACRIMAL APPARATUS, 180

Visual Disorders
I. CONJUNCTIVITIS, 180
II. CATARACT, 180
III. GLAUCOMA, 181
IV. DETACHED RETINA, 181

Hearing: Normal Auditory Function
I. OUTER EAR, 182
II. MIDDLE EAR, 182
III. INNER EAR, 182

Auditory Disorders
I. OTOSCLEROSIS, 182
II. ACUTE OTITIS MEDIA, 183
Questions, 185
Answers and Rationales, 189

PROTECTIVE FUNCTIONS, 190

Sexually Transmitted Diseases
- I. CHLAMYDIAL INFECTIONS, 190
- II. GONORRHEA, 190
- III. SYPHILIS, 192
- IV. ACQUIRED IMMUNODEFICIENCY SYNDROME (AIDS), 193

Skin Disorders
- I. BURNS, 194

Perioperative Care
- I. PREOPERATIVE PERIOD, 195
- II. INTRAOPERATIVE PERIOD, 197
- III. POSTOPERATIVE PERIOD, 197

Immune/Autoimmune Disorders
- I. CANCER, 199
- II. SYSTEMIC LUPUS ERYTHEMATOSUS, 200
  - Questions, 205
  - Answers and Rationales, 207

MOBILITY, ACTIVITY, COMFORT, 208

Hazards of Immobility
- I. GENERALIZED, 208
- II. CARDIOVASCULAR SYSTEM, 208
- III. RESPIRATORY SYSTEM, 208
- IV. GASTROINTESTINAL SYSTEM, 208
- V. MUSCULOSKELETAL SYSTEM, 209
- VI. INTEGUMENTARY SYSTEM, 209
- VII. URINARY SYSTEM, 210
- VIII. PSYCHOLOGICAL ASPECTS, 210

Musculoskeletal Disorders
- I. TRAUMATIC DISORDERS, 211
- II. CHRONIC DISORDERS, 214
  - Questions, 219
  - Answers and Rationales, 221

METABOLISM AND ELIMINATION, 221

Endocrine Disorders
- I. THYROID, 221
- II. PARATHYROID, 226
- III. ADRENALS, 227
- IV. DIABETES MELLITUS, 229

Digestive Disorders
- I. PEPTIC ULCER DISEASE, 231
- II. HIATAL HERNIA, 235
- III. GASTRIC CANCER, 237

Lower Intestinal Disorders
- I. DIVERTICULOSIS/DIVERTICULITIS, 239
- II. ULCERATIVE COLITIS, 241
- III. REGIONAL ENTERITIS (CROHN'S DISEASE), 243
- IV. HERNIA, 244
- V. HEMORRHOIDS, 245
- VI. COLON/RECTAL CANCER, 246

Liver and Biliary Disorders
- I. HEPATITIS, 248
- II. CIRRHOSIS, 250
- III. CHOLELITHIASIS/CHOLECYSTITIS, 253
- IV. PANCREATITIS, 255

Renal/Urinary Disorders
    I.   URINARY TRACT DISORDERS, 256
    II. URINARY CALCULI (NEPHROLITHIASIS), 260
    III. HYDRONEPHROSIS, 261
    IV. RENAL FAILURE: ACUTE AND CHRONIC, 262
    V. KIDNEY TUMORS, 265
    VI. BLADDER TUMORS, 266
        Questions, 269
        Answers and Rationales, 275

8 The Pediatric Patient 279

GROWTH AND DEVELOPMENT: LIFE STAGES, 279
    I.   THE INFANT (1 MONTH TO 1 YEAR), 279
    II. THE TODDLER (1 TO 3 YEARS), 281
    III. THE PRESCHOOLER (3 TO 5 YEARS), 284
    IV. THE SCHOOL-AGED CHILD (5 TO 12 YEARS), 284
    V. THE ADOLESCENT (12 TO 19 YEARS), 288
        Questions, 291
        Answers and Rationales, 293

OXYGENATION, 294

Cardiovascular Disorders
    I.   CONGENITAL; ACYANOTIC HEART DEFECTS, 294
    II. CONGENITAL; CYANOTIC HEART DEFECTS, 297
    III. CARDIAC SURGERY, 298
    IV. CHRONIC CONDITIONS, 299
    V. CARDIOPULMONARY RESUSCITATION (CPR), 300

Diseases of the Blood
    I.   SICKLE CELL ANEMIA, 300
    II. LEUKEMIA, 301
    III. HODGKIN'S DISEASE, 302
    IV. HEMOPHILIA, 302
    V. INFECTIOUS MONONUCLEOSIS, 303

Pulmonary Disorders
    I.   ACUTE DISORDERS, 304
    II. CHRONIC DISORDERS, 306

Fluid and Electrolyte Balance
    I.   NORMAL FLUID AND ELECTROLYTE BALANCE, 308
    II. FAILURE TO THRIVE, 308
        Questions, 309
        Answers and Rationales, 311

SENSORY/PERCEPTUAL ALTERATIONS, 312

Disorders of the Cerebral or Central Nervous System, 312
    I.   SEIZURE DISORDERS, 312
    II. CONGENITAL DISORDERS, 313
    III. INFECTIOUS DISORDERS, 315
    IV. BRAIN TUMORS, 316
    V. DEGENERATIVE DISORDERS, 317

Vision/Hearing/Speech
    I.   AMBLYOPIA, 317
    II. STRABISMUS, 317
        Questions, 319
        Answers and Rationales, 321

PROTECTIVE FUNCTIONS, 322

Immunization/Trauma/Accidents
I.   ACCIDENTS, 322

Communicable Disease
I.   VIRAL DISEASES, 322
II. BACTERIAL DISEASES, 326

Abuse
I.   ABUSE OF CHILDREN, 327

Poisoning
I.   POISONING IN CHILDREN, 328

Skin Disorders
I.   BURNS, 328
II.   INFANTILE ECZEMA, 329
III. IMPETIGO, 329
IV.   RINGWORM, 330
V.   PEDICULOSIS, 330
VI.   HIVES (URTICARIA), 330
VII. ACNE VULGARIS, 331

Perioperative Period
I.   PREOPERATIVE PREPARATION, 331
II. POSTOPERATIVE PERIOD, 332

Immune Disorders
I.   HUMAN IMMUNODEFICIENCY VIRUS AND ACQUIRED
     IMMUNODEFICIENCY SYNDROME, 333
         Questions, 335
         Answers and Rationales, 337

MOBILITY, 338
I.   CONGENITAL MUSCULOSKELETAL DISORDERS, 338
II.   TRAUMA, 338
III. OTHER DISORDERS, 340
         Questions, 343
         Answers and Rationales, 345

METABOLISM/ELIMINATION, 345

Metabolic/Endocrine Disorders
I.   CONGENITAL DISORDERS, 345
II. CHRONIC DISORDERS, 346

Upper Gastrointestinal Disorders
I.   CONGENITAL DISORDERS, 347
II.   ACUTE DISORDERS, 349
III. CHRONIC DISORDERS, 349

Lower Intestinal Disorders
I.   CONGENITAL DISORDERS, 350
II.   ACUTE DISORDERS, 351
III. CHRONIC DISORDERS, 352

Renal/Urinary Disorders
I.   CONGENITAL DISORDERS, 354
II.   ACUTE DISORDERS, 354
III. CHRONIC DISORDERS, 355
         Questions, 357
         Answers and Rationales, 359

9   The Childbearing Family 361

YOUNG ADULT DEVELOPMENT, 361
I.   PHYSIOLOGIC DEVELOPMENT, 361
II. PSYCHOLOGIC DEVELOPMENT, 362

PSYCHOLOGIC AND PHYSICAL CHANGES DURING PREGNANCY, 362
  I. MATERNAL DEVELOPMENTAL TASKS OF PREGNANCY, 362
  II. EFFECTS ON BODILY SYSTEMS, 362
  III. SIGNS OF PREGNANCY, 363

PREGNANCY, 364
  I. PRENATAL DEVELOPMENT, 364
  II. PRENATAL PERIOD, 365
      Questions, 373
      Answers and Rationales, 375

LABOR AND DELIVERY, 376
  I. NORMAL LABOR AND DELIVERY, 376
  II. DEVIATIONS IN NORMAL LABOR PROCESS, 381
  III. OPERATIVE PROCEDURES, 383
  IV. SPECIAL CONCERNS, 383
      Questions, 385
      Answers and Rationales, 389

POSTPARTUM PERIOD, 390
  I. NORMAL POSTPARTUM PERIOD, 390
  II. COMPLICATIONS OF POSTPARTUM, 391
      Questions, 395
      Answers and Rationales, 397

NEONATE, 397
First 4 Weeks of Life
  I. PHYSIOLOGIC DEVELOPMENT, 397
  II. SENSORY DEVELOPMENT, 398
  III. CARE OF NEONATE, 399
      Questions, 401
      Answers and Rationales, 403

10 The Mental Health Client 405
COMMUNICATION, INTERACTION, AND BEHAVIOR, 405
Communication Process
  I. PROCESS, 405
Interpersonal Relationships
  I. INTERACTIONS, 406
  II. THERAPEUTIC INTERPERSONAL RELATIONSHIPS, 406
Patterns of Behavior
  I. WITHDRAWAL PATTERN OF BEHAVIOR, 407
  II. OVERLY SUSPICIOUS PATTERN OF BEHAVIOR, 408
  III. PATTERNS OF BEHAVIOR INVOLVING MOOD AND AFFECT, 409
  IV. SUICIDAL PATTERN OF BEHAVIOR, 411
  V. BEHAVIOR PATTERNS OF YOUNG, CHRONICALLY MENTALLY ILL, 411
  VI. ANXIOUS PATTERNS OF BEHAVIOR, 412
  VII. BEHAVIOR PATTERN RELATED TO ORGANIC MENTAL DISORDERS, 414
      Questions, 417
      Answers and Rationales, 421

EMOTIONS, BEHAVIOR, AND MENTAL HEALTH, 423
Coping or Mental Mechanisms
  I. DEFENSE MECHANISMS, 423
Crisis Intervention
  I. DEALING WITH LOSS (GRIEF AND GRIEVING), 424

II. CRISIS/CRISIS INTERVENTION, 425
III. PERSON ABUSE (TRAUMA), 425

Substance Abuse and Dependence
I. ABUSE AND DEPENDENCE, 427
II. CESSATION OF USE, 428

Eating Disorders
I. BULIMIA, 429
II. ANOREXIA NERVOSA, 430
    Questions, 431
    Answers and Rationales, 433
    Practice Test 2, 435
    Questions, 435
    Answers and Rationales, 455

Appendix...471
Index..475

Preparing for the NCLEX-PN

Preparing for the Test

The NCLEX-PN is a computerized examination that can last a maximum of 5 hours. The number of questions on the examination ranges from a minimum of 85 to a maximum of 205. The examination is described as computer-adaptive testing. This means that the computer selects your next question based on your answer to the current question. If you answered incorrectly, the next question may be at the same difficulty level or slightly easier. If you answered correctly, the computer gives you a question that is of the same difficulty or slightly higher. This process continues until the computer is able to establish that your answers are either consistently above or consistently below the passing standard; the maximum number of questions, 205, has been reached, or the 5-hour time limit has been reached. You may have to answer anywhere from 85 to 205 questions to establish your score. You have only about 1 1/3 minutes to answer each question. The time constraints can be one of the most difficult things for you to handle in the testing situation. Suggestions on how to handle this potential problem are given in Chapter 2.

Prior to the beginning of the test, a short computer tutorial is provided to ensure your understanding of the process of testing. There are only two live keys on the computer, the space bar and the enter key. The space bar allows you to move from answer to answer within the question. Once you have found the correct answer, you should highlight it by using the space bar and then pressing the enter key. The computer then asks you to confirm that you are choosing the one you have picked, and you must hit the enter key a second time. Your answer is not recorded until you confirm it the second time. You must answer each question because the computer does not allow you to leave a question blank. Also, because you cannot go back once you have finally entered your answer, be sure before you press the enter key a second time (Figure 1–1).

The examination is composed of a maximum of 205 single, multiple-choice items. "Single" means that for each question, there are only four single choices. This type of question tests your knowledge without unnecessarily confusing you as the older multiple, multiple-choice questions often did. You can get practice reading these types of questions and answering them in the practice tests at the beginning and end of this review text. A computer disk is also included so that you can practice answering questions on the computer. The form of the questions is shown in Figure 1–2.

There is no penalty for guessing on this examination, but be careful not to start "wild guessing." If you guess, make it an educated guess by eliminating one or two of the possible responses. This can double your chances of being correct. Remember, you must answer each question, or the computer does not allow you to proceed. Also, remember that you cannot go back once you have answered a question.

The passing score for this test is set at the level of minimal competency for a safe, effective practical nurse. The score is referred to as criterion-referenced. The National Council of State Boards of Nursing (NCSBN) sets this passing score, and each state is given the option of either accepting this score or choosing one of its own. At the present time, all states have chosen to use the National Council score. After you have taken the examination and it has been scored, you will receive a letter stating either Pass or Fail from your State Board of Nursing about 1 month after the test. If you do not pass, you will receive feedback on your areas of weakness. This should help you to prepare if you have to retake the examination. Hints for retaking the examination are included in Part 2 of Chapter 2.

You should begin to prepare for the examination well in advance of the test date (see Appendix). The best preparation is the course of study you have

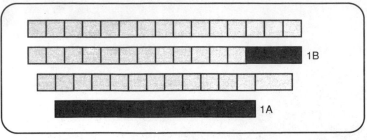

Only two keys needed

FIGURE 1-1 Functional keys. *1A*, Spacebar. *1B*, Enter key (return ↵).

taken to prepare you as a practical nurse; nothing can replace that. If you were successful in your course of study, with proper and adequate preparation you should be able to complete the NCLEX-PN success-fully. Your notes and your textbook can provide you with a great deal of material for your preparation. This review text can help you to organize and focus your study.

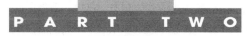

PART TWO

Using This Text

This text is designed to help you approach your preparation in a systematic and logical manner. By carefully identifying the specific areas you know less about, you can target them for more review and improve your chances for success on the NCLEX-PN.

How should you use this text to help you prepare for the NCLEX-PN? One of the first steps you should take is to read the next section of this chapter. Part 3 tells you about the NCLEX-PN itself, how it is organized, the number of questions it contains, and the type of material included in this examination. This knowledge should improve your self-confidence when you finally see the examination.

Of course, a simple list of the material to be covered is not the only thing you will need. Chapter 2 is directed at helping you improve your test-taking skills. By learning better ways of taking multiple-choice tests, you can improve your testing ability. Many people needlessly lose points because they are not "test-wise." Application of the information in Chapter 2 can help you avoid such pitfalls.

With proper use, this review text can help you prepare for the examination. There are at least two ways to use the review material. First, you can simply review the sections containing material with which you feel uncomfortable. In this way, if you have already identified your own learning deficits, you can progress quickly through the material. The problem with this method is that most people either try to go through everything or spend unnecessary time reviewing material they have already mastered. Sometimes, it is difficult to identify what you do not know.

The other way to use this text is to start by taking one of the practice examinations at the beginning of the text. You don't even have to take the whole test at once. Start with about 10 questions or two situations. Look up the answers and rationales, and identify the content included in any of the questions you missed and those that you answered correctly. Write this down, and do another 10 or so questions following the

---

JUN 7, 1996   1

Following a modified radical mastectomy with axillary lymph node dissection, to decrease the postoperative lymphedema of the affected arm, the client should:

▶ (1) Elevate her arm on pillows above the heart
(2) Keep the arm fixed at her side
(3) Apply a warm pad over the affected arm
(4) Use only the unaffected arm for all activities

FIGURE 1-2 Examples of how test questions look on the computer screen.

same pattern. By the time you have taken the practice test of about 100 to 105 questions, you should have a good list of the areas that you know and those that require more study. You should then spend your time on the areas that you do not know, saving the areas you are familiar with until the end for a quick review. Four practice tests are included in this book, so that you can use the two at the beginning of the book in this way and still have two to practice with, simulating an actual test situation.

Each section of content also has questions following it. You can use these as either pretests or post-tests. When you answer these questions, go back and review the material covered in the questions you missed. Always focus on the areas you do not know, and briefly review the areas of content with which you are most familiar.

When you feel that you are prepared, you can take one of the practice tests as though it were the actual test. Set an alarm clock for 5 hours and try to take the test within the time limit. When you are finished, check your answers carefully, read all the rationales, and write down those areas that are still giving you trouble. Go back and study those areas. You have four practice tests with questions similar to the actual test, and you have practice questions at the end of each chapter to help you study. Success in the practice tests can also be a great confidence builder. When you see how much you know, you will feel better able to handle the material that you do not know as well.

No review text can teach you everything you should have learned in your practical nursing program. If you find an area that you really do not understand and if the review book does not provide enough information, go back to your textbooks or class notes to study that area in greater detail. Remember, this is just a review text; if used as such, it can help you be successful on the NCLEX-PN.

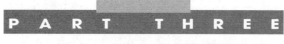

Format of the NCLEX-PN

GENERAL DESCRIPTION

The NCLEX-PN is a 5-hour examination designed by the National Council of State Boards of Nursing to test the graduate's ability to practice practical nursing in a safe, effective manner. The graduate's knowledge of practical nursing is tested through the application of that knowledge to health care situations requiring practical nursing interventions. The contents of the examination are based on a study that analyzed the activities performed by practical nurses. This study produced a competency model of entry-level practical nursing. The test plan was then derived from this competency model. Your course in practical nursing should have adequately prepared you to succeed in the examination and in the role of the practical nurse.

The examination is graded on a Pass–Fail basis. A Pass level is set by the NCSBN using criteria of minimal competence. Your goal should be to do as well as possible to demonstrate your mastery of the required knowledge. You may arrange to take this examination anytime after 30 days after you complete your program. The process for registering for the examination is detailed in the *NCLEX Candidate Bulletin* available at your school.

TEST PLAN

The test plan is composed of two main areas: (1) phases of the nursing process and (2) categories of client needs. Different percentages of the questions apply to these areas. To help you prepare for these questions, it is useful to know what is included in these areas.

Phases of the Nursing Process

The practical nurse assists in client assessments, contributes to the planning of care, performs basic and therapeutic nursing interventions, and helps evaluate the outcomes of this nursing care. The beginning practitioner may assume a more dependent role in the planning and evaluation phases but should be fairly independent in assessing clients and implementing care.

Assess (Collecting Data—25%–30% of the Questions)—Code I

The practical nurse contributes to the development of a data base about clients by (1) observing physiologic, psychosocial, health, and safety needs of clients; (2) collecting information from the client, significant others, health team members, and records; (3) determining the need for more information; and (4) communicating findings of the data collected. The practical nurse also participates in the formulation of nursing diagnoses.

Planning (15%–25% of the Questions)—Code II

The practical nurse contributes to the development of nursing care plans by (1) assisting in formulation of goals; (2) participating in identification of clients' needs and nursing measures required to achieve goals; (3) communicating needs that may require alteration of the care plan; and (4) communicating with the client, significant others, or health team members in planning nursing care.

Implementation (25%–35% of the Questions)—Code III

The practical nurse implements care by (1) performing basic therapeutic and preventive nursing measures by following a prescribed plan of care to achieve established client goals; (2) providing a safe, effective environment; (3) assisting the client, significant others, and health team members to understand client's plan of care; and (4) recording client information and reporting it to other health team members.

Evaluation (15%–25% of the Questions)—Code IV

The practical nurse evaluates care by (1) participating in evaluating the effectiveness of the client's nursing care; (2) assisting in evaluating the client's response to nursing care and in making appropriate alterations; (3) evaluating the extent to which identified outcomes of the care plan are achieved; and (4) recording and describing the client's response to therapy or care.

Categories of Client Needs

To structure the health needs of individuals, the NCSBN, based on the results of its job analysis survey, has identified four categories of client needs that the practical nurse addresses. These categories, rather than traditional subject matter areas, are the means by which the test is divided. Under each of these areas, specific nursing content is identified (NCSBN, 1989).

Safe, Effective Care Environment (24%–30% of the Questions)—Code I

A safe, effective care environment includes the *basic* knowledge, skills, and abilities that include, but are not limited to, data-gathering techniques; interpersonal communication skills; alternative methods of communication for clients with special needs; prepara-

tion for prescribed treatments and procedures; providing safe, effective treatments and procedures for the client; environmental and client safety; infection control, including signs and symptoms of infection; client rights, both legal and ethical; confidentiality; individualization of care, including religious, cultural, and developmental influences; team participation in care planning and evaluation; and general knowledge of community planning.

Physiologic Integrity (42%–48% of the Questions)—Code 2

Physiologic integrity includes the *basic* knowledge, skills, and abilities that include, but are not limited to, providing for physiologic adaptation of the client; therapeutic and life-saving procedures; specialized equipment; principles of administering medications, including both expected and unexpected effects of medication; maintenance of optimal body functioning and prevention of complications; principles of body mechanics and assistive devices; comfort measures; reduction of risk potential; basic physical assessment skills; side effects of chemotherapy and radiation therapy; maintaining intact skin; providing for mobility and preventing its hazards; performing basic nursing measures; and reporting changes in a client's condition.

Psychosocial Integrity (7%–13% of the Questions)—Code 3

Psychosocial integrity includes the *basic* knowledge, skills, and abilities that include, but are not limited to, obvious signs of emotional and mental health problems; self-concept; life crises; chemical dependency; coping and adaptation; self-destructive behavior; sensory deprivation and overload; adaptive and maladaptive behavior; therapeutic communication; common therapies; and general knowledge of community resources.

Health Promotion and Maintenance (15%–21% of the Questions)—Code 4

Health promotion and maintenance includes the *basic* knowledge, skills, and abilities that include, but are not limited to, family interactions; concepts of wellness; adaptations to altered health states; reproduction and human sexuality; birthing and parenting; continued growth and development, including normal maternity nursing care; encouraging self-care; diet modification; death and dying; integrity of support systems; prevention and early treatment of disease; immunization; health teaching that is appropriate to the scope of practice; and general knowledge of community resources.

Although this test plan may seem somewhat complicated, it is important for the practical nurse candidate to be familiar with it so that preparation for the examination can be systematic and complete. By becoming familiar with the areas tested, the graduate can be ready for the examination.

Categories of Human Functioning

These content divisions are not imposed by the NCSBN but are given so that you can group the content into functional areas. This is how the content is divided within most chapters of this text, and the test items are labeled this way so that you can find the content areas of your weakness more easily.

Growth and Development—Code A

This category includes content and development of children and adults, sexuality, reproductive disorders in both men and women, maturation throughout the life span, childbearing, and child rearing.

Oxygenation—Code B

Oxygenation includes the body's ability to maintain fluid balance and to transport oxygen and other gases; fluid and electrolyte balance; acid-base balance; cardiopulmonary disorders; cardiopulmonary resuscitation (CPR); anemias; hemorrhagic disorders; and leukemia and lymphomas.

Sensory/Perceptual Alterations—Code C

This category includes the ability to perceive, interpret, and respond to sensory and cognitive data; hearing, vision, and speech disorders; sensory deprivation or overload; cerebral and central nervous system disorders; brain tumors; seizures; laryngectomy; organic brain syndrome; degenerative neurologic disorders; and learning disabilities.

Protective Functions—Code D

Protective functions include physiologic defenses; prevention of trauma, infection, and threats to health; communicable diseases; sexually transmitted diseases; immunity; basic cancer and therapies; trauma; physical abuse; skin disorders; asepsis; safety hazards; poisoning; and surgical intervention.

Mobility/Activity/Comfort—Code E

Mobility/activity/comfort includes hazards of immobility, musculoskeletal disorders, fractures, and degenerative disorders.

Metabolism/Elimination—Code F

Metabolism/elimination includes the intake and utilization of essential nutrients, normal and therapeutic nutrition, diet in pregnancy and lactation, obesity, diabetes, gastric and metabolic disorders, the body's ability to remove waste products, endocrine disorders, gastrointestinal disorders, ulcers, hernias, neoplasms, liver disease, renal disorders, and prostatic disorders.

Psychosocial-Cultural Functions—Code G

This category includes the ability to function in intrapersonal, interpersonal, group and sociocultural relationships; loss and grieving; psychotic and neurotic behaviors; therapeutic communication; group dynamics; ethical-legal aspects; community resources; spiritual needs; situational crises; and substance abuse.

BIBLIOGRAPHY

National Council of State Boards of Nursing. (1989). *NCLEX-PN: Test plan for the National Council licensure examination for practical nurses.* Chicago: Author.

Improving Your Ability to Pass the Examination

PART ONE

Test-Taking Strategies

How do you successfully take a multiple-choice examination? The answer to this question is fairly long, but as your understanding of multiple-choice test items increases, so do your chances for answering them successfully. Hints and strategies can be learned to improve your ability to answer multiple-choice questions.

First, the most important point is to focus on *reading* and understanding the question. Reading may seem like a simple matter, but most mistakes are made because the test taker does not read the question carefully and completely. Along with reading the question, it is vital that you carefully read each response that follows the "stem" of the question. Test takers often read quickly and choose the first response that looks good; sometimes they do not even read all the possible responses.

When you read the question, pay close attention to any specific information within the question that can direct you to the correct answer. Sometimes the stem contains statements such as, "your first action," "which would be appropriate," "an inappropriate intervention for this client," "all except," "an important assessment," "the best goal," and "the most appropriate response." Phrases such as these can focus the area of your response. If the question asks for a priority action, it means that all the responses might be correct but you have to choose the first priority.

For example:

Unsuccessful adaptation to the middle years would be characterized by:
1. Reassessment of role within the home
2. Achievement of career goals
3. Increased involvement in community activities
4. Acceptance of retirement

A question such as this, which looks for the one thing that does not fit, can be easy to answer. The best way to approach it is to treat each response as a "true-false" question. In this question, look at each response. #1 is true: Middle years is a time to reassess the roles within the family. #2 is true: It is a time when most adults achieve their career goals. #3 is true: It is a time when adults focus more on their role in the community. #4 in this case is false and the correct answer for this question: The middle years is not a time of accepting retirement, only the beginning preparation for it. By focusing on the important part of the question—"unsuccessful"—and treating each response as a separate question, you should be able to find the one false response. This method is appropriate when the question contains a negative such as "least" or "inappropriate." Even if you can narrow down the possibilities to two responses, you have doubled your chances of guessing correctly.

Time control is another important factor. You have only about 1 1/3 minutes per question. Answering in this time is another skill that can be learned. Take one of the practice tests and block out 10 items. Set an alarm clock for 12 minutes and begin. Doing this several times helps to improve your speed. During the actual test situation, you can do two important things to help improve your speed. First, take a watch and set limits and checks for yourself, such as deciding that by 1/2 hour you should be on at least question #30. If you are not, you must speed up. Do not wait until the end to notice that you are behind. The other thing to do is to omit the difficult items and come back to them at the end, or simply guess at the answer. If an item is taking you more than 1 minute, go on.

Understanding the focus of the question can also help direct your response to it. The focus of the question can be the phases of the nursing process. For instance, a question that asks for an assessment requires an answer that provides more data. One that asks for a plan requires you to focus on the specific problem addressed and find a measurable, realistic goal. Another major area of focus is the categories of client functioning. To give you some ideas on questions from both these categories, an example of each along with an analysis follows.

To assist with your understanding of your learning needs, a code is included after each answer. The code is as follows:

I, II, III, or IV for the phase of the nursing process.

1, 2, 3, or 4 for the category of client needs.

A, B, C, D, E, F, or G for the category of human functioning.

Specific content category by name; i.e., cholecystectomy.

PHASES OF THE NURSING PROCESS

Assessment (Collecting Data) (I)

Which of the following observations should the practical nurse make when the client returns from having a long leg cast applied to a newly broken tibia?
1. *Circulation and sensation proximal to the cast*
2. *Temperature of the cast*
3. *Capillary refill of the toes*
4. *Presence of Homans' sign in the opposite leg*

This item focuses on assessment. The correct answer is #3; the most important assessment for the nurse to make is the circulation and sensation distal to the cast. #1 is incorrect because it states "proximal." #2 is not important on a fresh cast because "hot" spots of infection would not appear this soon and because casts become warm with drying. #4 is an important assessment at any time, but a fresh-fracture client would probably not have developed thrombophlebitis yet. At the end of the rationales in this text, you will see the following code: *I, 2, E, Fractures/casts.* This tells you exactly what was tested, so you can refer to those areas when studying.

Planning (II)

Which of the following is an appropriate goal for a primipara on her first postpartum day?
Mother will be able to:
1. *Bathe infant without help*
2. *Provide complete care of newborn*
3. *Hold and interact with newborn*
4. *Feed newborn without assistance*

This question asks the nurse to set an achievable goal for a new mother with her first baby. #1, #2, and #4 are probably unrealistic goals for a new mother on the first day after birth. #3 is not only realistic but

also the most desirable goal, because mother-infant bonding is one of the most important goals to achieve. *II, 4, A, Postpartal care.*

Implementation (III)

You have difficulty inserting the rectal catheter for an enema. Your best action is to:
1. *Wait a few minutes for the lubricant to take effect*
2. *Tell the client to calm down*
3. *Wait a few seconds until the sphincter relaxes, then proceed*
4. *Chart that you were unable to give the enema*

The best answer for this is #3. The nurse knows that temporarily waiting often allows the sphincter to relax. The other answers are not appropriate actions. *III, 2, F, Lower gastrointestinal.*

Evaluation (IV)

Which of the following would indicate successful learning by your client, to whom you have been teaching an 1800-calorie diabetic diet?
1. *Client eats all food on tray*
2. *Client states understanding of diet*
3. *Client's partner understands dietary restrictions*
4. *Client correctly marks menu for 1800-calorie ADA diet*

To evaluate learning, the practical nurse must have measurable data. The only answer that provides this is #4. #1 does not reflect learning. #2 is not measurable; how do you know that the client understands? #3 is also not measurable and does not address the client directly. *IV, 4, F, Diabetes mellitus.*

CATEGORIES OF CLIENT NEEDS

Safe, Effective Care Environment (1)

The client at greatest risk for postoperative bleeding would be an arthritic who has been taking:
1. *Aspirin*
2. *Maalox*
3. *Prednisone*
4. *Acetaminophen*

This item focuses on client safety and expected outcomes of treatment. In order to answer it, you need some knowledge of drug side effects. #1 is the answer, because aspirin has an anticoagulant effect on the blood and may predispose to postoperative bleeding. A question such as this could be followed with one or two related questions, such as "Precautions to take to decrease the risk of bleeding include," or "To prevent the bleeding risk in the previous question, the nurse should." Questions often come in a series, so it is important to be sure of your first answer and then follow along that same line to answer them all correctly. *I, 1, D, Surgery.*

Physiologic Integrity (2)

Mr. Wilson is admitted with chronic obstructive pulmonary disease (COPD). He tells you that his breathing treatments leave him unable to eat because of all the mucus he brings up. To decrease his anorexia and improve his nutritional intake, the practical nurse should:
  1. Suggest he have the treatments right after meals
  2. Administer frequent mouth care, especially before meals
  3. Request a change to a liquid diet
  4. Ask the physician about starting hyperalimentation

This item focuses on a physiologic need for adequate nutrition and an expected result of treatment. #1 makes no sense, because it is likely to increase vomiting. #3 and #4 take away the normal diet, an important part of preventing debilitation in the chronically ill client. Only #2 would be appropriate for this client. This question offers an example of a situation in which the test taker often wants another answer: *5. Schedule the treatments between meals.*

This can be frustrating, because the answer you want isn't there. Forget it and go with the best answer there. You are not allowed to write in your choice. *IV, 2, B, COPD.*

Psychosocial Integrity (3)

Mary had a bad day at work and is angry with her supervisor. When she comes home from work, she punishes her daughter by grounding her for a week for not taking out the trash. This is an example of what defense mechanism?
  1. Projection
  2. Denial
  3. Displacement
  4. Sublimation

This is a fairly simple, comprehension-level question. You should be able to recognize the description of #3, displacement. The items from this section test your knowledge of the mental health concepts, which make up the smallest percentage of questions on the test. The other responses are other defense mechanisms. *I, 3, G, Defense mechanisms.*

Health Promotion and Maintenance (4)

Discharge instructions for Mr. Wilson, who has COPD, should not include which of the following?
  1. Smoking cessation
  2. Avoidance of temperature extremes
  3. Avoidance of industrial air pollution
  4. Avoidance of humidified air

This item asks for the one thing you would *not* teach Mr. Wilson about health promotion. Using the true-false approach, #1 and #3 are easily apparent as being true. Again, if you do not know at this point, guess. Looking at the other two, we know that the COPD client has thick tenacious sputum, so humidity should help, making #4 the false answer that is the correct answer in this case. Do not make the mistake of reading too fast and missing "avoidance." *III, 4, D, COPD.*

Another common mistake that test takers often make is changing their first answer. Many people continue to mentally rehash a question and convince themselves that there is a hidden meaning or some trick. There are no "trick" questions on this examination, and the items have been examined closely to make sure that there are no hidden meanings. It is rarely correct to change an answer. The odds of changing it to a correct response are low, and your first instinct is usually correct. Change an answer *only* if you have truly seen some missed information or suddenly remembered an important fact. Otherwise, leave that eraser alone. Also, changing answers undermines your confidence, and you start to change more and more as you panic. You should stop, take a deep breath, and go on without changing answers.

Your state of mind is another important factor. Many people have "test anxiety." This means that the simple thought of the test makes you tense and you are liable to freeze up or become nervous during a test. If you have test anxiety, there are a number of things you can do ahead of time to prepare. First, practice some sort of relaxation exercises, such as those you teach mothers during childbirth. Practice those slow, deep breaths and imagine yourself blowing away all your tension. If you become comfortable with this technique before the test, it can be useful during the test. Practice this technique when you take the practice tests in this book.

People also tend to experience anger and frustration over certain test items, a feeling guaranteed to break their concentration. If you find this happening because you think an item is "dumb" or that the situation is unlikely to happen in nursing, laugh, but do not get angry. Put the emotion away until after the test. Anger and frustration occur when the response you want is not listed. Don't let them. Your only choices are those listed, so choose the best one.

Another tension breaker is *not* studying the night before the examination or between your morning and afternoon sessions. It is a terrible temptation to do so, but it does not help. It only increases your anxiety. Also, avoid talking about the questions with other test takers between tests. This also increases your tension and fears. Put the first test out of your mind, and focus your thoughts on doing well on the second test. Keep imagining yourself as having successfully completed the test and as a successful practical nurse.

Should you guess at answers? Yes, but make educated guesses, which means first try to decrease the number of possible responses. With four responses, you have a one in four, or 25%, chance at a correct answer. With three responses, you have a one in three, or 33%, chance; reducing the possible responses to two gives you a 50% chance of guessing correctly. Even on difficult items, taking a little time to eliminate even one answer improves your odds. Do not just guess recklessly. This can decrease your confidence. When you reach a dilemma—is it #1 or #3—guess and go on. Do not spend time going back and forth between the two. Simply choose one, go on, and forget it.

These tips should improve your test-taking skills; combined with a proper planned review, they should help you do better on the licensure examination and achieve your goal.

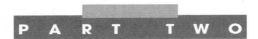

PART TWO

Hints for Retaking the Examination

If you are not taking the test for the first time, the advice in this chapter applies to you especially. You must first decide why you did not pass the first time. Some of the previous suggestions may help you if it was anxiety or lack of time that contributed to your failure. You need to look at your performance as honestly as you can. You must identify your areas of weakness so that you can change them and be successful at the next testing.

When you fail the examination, the National Council sends you a diagnostic profile showing you what your weaknesses were. This profile first tells you approximately how close you were to passing. The ranges given are 12 or fewer items; 13–24 items; 25–36 items; or 37 or more items. If you were close, a little more effort should lead to success. The other information given is your proximity to the reference point in the "Phases of the Nursing Process" and the "Categories of Client Needs." If you do well in all but one area, focus on that area for your next attempt. An index in the front of each practice test divides the questions by categories to help you practice to retake the examination.

You need to be honest with yourself about your reasons for not passing. Ask yourself whether you truly studied for the examination. If you did not have a regular program of preparation, that is exactly what you need to establish now. Prepare, and you stand a much better chance of passing.

If you had a weakness in school, such as maternity nursing, and your lowest performance seemed to be in the area of "Health Promotion and Maintenance," focus heavily on maternity nursing for the next examination. If you are a poor test taker, use the suggestions in this book and practice your test-taking skills.

If you are lost as to what your weaknesses were, take the first two practice tests in this text. When you have finished, look up the answers and write down exactly what you were missing. This then becomes the focus of your study.

You can also use some of the questions at the end of each chapter as pretests. That means that you answer these questions before studying the chapter to see if you already know the material. If you do well on this test, that content is less important to study; focus first on the areas on which you cannot answer questions.

Will these suggestions help you pass next time? If you follow the guidelines in this text and study hard for the examination, you should be successful. Do not give up on yourself. With hard work and preparation, you can achieve your goal of becoming a licensed practical nurse.

PRACTICE TEST 1

QUESTIONS

1. Jill Cohen, a 64-year-old factory worker, is admitted through the emergency department. She is diaphoretic and nauseated and complains of severe chest pain. She weighs 180 pounds and is 64 inches tall. She is an insulin-dependent diabetic patient with a history of hypertension. Her vital signs are blood pressure, 80/60 mm Hg; temperature, 97° F; pulse, 120; and respiration, 36. Her diagnosis is myocardial infarction. What usual immediate complication of a myocardial infarction do Jill's signs and symptoms indicate?

   ① Pulmonary edema
   ② Angina pectoris
   ③ Congestive heart failure
   ④ Cardiogenic shock

2. Jill Cohen, a 64-year-old factory worker, is admitted through the emergency department. She is diaphoretic and nauseated and complains of severe chest pain. She weighs 180 pounds and is 64 inches tall. She is an insulin-dependent diabetic patient with a history of hypertension. Her vital signs are blood pressure, 80/60 mm Hg; temperature, 97° F; pulse, 120; and respiration, 36. Her diagnosis is myocardial infarction. Jill finds breathing more difficult unless she is in high Fowler's position. She has also begun to have a cough with blood-tinged, frothy sputum. Your assessment leads you to believe that the following has developed:

   ① Atrial fibrillation
   ② Right-sided heart failure
   ③ Left-sided heart failure
   ④ Mitral valve prolapse

3. Jill Cohen, a 64-year-old factory worker, is admitted through the emergency department. She is diaphoretic and nauseated and complains of severe chest pain. Jill weighs 180 pounds and is 64 inches tall. She is an insulin-dependent diabetic patient with a history of hypertension. Her vital signs are blood pressure, 80/60 mm Hg; temperature, 97° F; pulse, 120; and respiration, 36. Her diagnosis is myocardial infarction. Jill finds breathing more difficult unless she is in high Fowler's position. She has also begun to have a cough with blood-tinged, frothy sputum. Her respiratory status is recorded as:

   ① Stertorous
   ② Apneic
   ③ Orthopneic
   ④ Cheyne-Stokes

4. Propranolol (Inderal) has been ordered for an atrial arrhythmia. A note should be made on the nursing care plan to assess the client frequently for:

   ① Increased blood pressure
   ② Restlessness and anxiety
   ③ Bradycardia
   ④ Decreased level of consciousness

5. A client who has had a myocardial infarction is placed on intravenous heparin sodium. Considering the side effects of this drug, nursing care should include monitoring the client for:

   ① Diarrhea
   ② Hematuria
   ③ Increased white blood count
   ④ Shortness of breath

6. A client has been receiving intravenous heparin. The heparin has been changed to subcutaneous injections. Injections should be:

   ① Massaged to promote absorption
   ② Limited to upper arms and anterior thigh
   ③ Given in the lower abdomen
   ④ Rotated between the arms, thighs, gluteal area, and abdomen

7. Jill becomes depressed 2 days after admission for an acute myocardial infarction. The nurse should:

   ① Remind her that she is fortunate to be alive after her heart attack
   ② Show her a tape of what happens during a myocardial infarction
   ③ Encourage her to get more exercise to take her mind off her problems
   ④ Encourage her to express her fears and answer her questions

8. In teaching a client how to plan a nutritious diet, the nurse would inform the client that according to the Food Guide Pyramid which of the following should be included in the daily diet?

    ① 6 to 11 servings from the bread, cereal, and pasta group
    ② 4 to 6 servings from the meat and egg group
    ③ No more than 3 servings from each group
    ④ At least 2 servings of foods high in fat

9. Which of the following foods would the nurse include in planning the daily diet of a lacto-ovo-vegetarian?

    ① Cottage cheese and beef broth
    ② Vegetables and veal
    ③ Eggs and milk
    ④ Grains and liver

10. In discussing the function of carbohydrates, which of the following statements is the *most* appropriate?

    ① Carbohydrates are used in the body to form hemoglobin.
    ② Carbohydrates are the body's most important source of energy.
    ③ Carbohydrates supply the essential component for tissue building.
    ④ Carbohydrates promote the absorption of fat-soluble vitamins.

11. Ms. Jones asks the nurse which foods to avoid on a cholesterol-restricted diet. The *best* response by the nurse is:

    ① Fresh fruits
    ② Green leafy vegetables
    ③ Egg yolks and whole milk
    ④ Rice and pasta

12. To develop a care plan for a client with diverticulosis, which of the following diets would the nurse expect the physician to prescribe?

    ① Gluten-free diet
    ② High-protein diet
    ③ Low-fat diet
    ④ High-fiber diet

13. Which of the following foods would the nurse instruct a client on a high-fiber diet to include in the daily meal plan?

    ① Eggs, milk, and cheese
    ② Whole grain breads and cereals

    ③ Fish and poultry
    ④ Unsaturated vegetable oils

14. In discussing fast foods with a teenager, the nurse would inform the teen that fast foods:

    ① Are considered "junk foods"
    ② Have no part in a healthy diet
    ③ Can be eaten if selections are made wisely
    ④ Are excellent sources of vitamins

15. An 80-year-old man was admitted for cataract surgery. An important element of his postoperative plan of care is to:

    ① Increase cardiac output
    ② Promote safety
    ③ Have a quiet, dark environment
    ④ Prevent excess fluid volume

16. Your 82-year-old client, with a diagnosis of congestive heart failure, will be discharged soon. Which of the following instructions would be *inappropriate?*

    ① Store digitalis in a tightly closed container away from light.
    ② Check your weight periodically.
    ③ Follow a low-sodium diet.
    ④ Spend as much time as possible in bed.

17. Which of the following is an *inappropriate* intervention for a client with chronic obstructive pulmonary disease?

    ① Prevent respiratory infection
    ② Reduce or stop smoking tobacco products
    ③ Perform breathing exercises several times a day
    ④ Limit the amount of information taught about the disease

18. A 73-year-old client, recovering from hip surgery, complains to the nurse, caring for her, "It seems I'm falling apart. Is there any part of me that I won't keep losing?" The best response would be:

    ① "Your basic intelligence remains unchanged, but remembering things may take a little longer."
    ② "Your hair will remain thick for your entire life."
    ③ "Your appetite will remain the same since the number of taste buds remain the same."
    ④ "Your sense of smell remains the same."

19. The incidence of falls is higher in the older adult. An age-related change that contributes to this higher incidence is:

① Increase in leaner body mass
② Increase in bone mass
③ Reduced visual acuity
④ Reduction in fat tissue

20. Which of the following statements about depression in the elderly is *false*?

① Depression often goes undetected by family members.
② Elderly frequently describe psychologic, not physical, symptoms.
③ Depression not treated results in suicide, a major health concern for this age population.
④ Symptoms of depression are often different from those seen in younger people.

21. A 16-year-old primigravida is in for her first prenatal visit at 8 weeks' gestation. She asks, "What does my baby look like?" The nurse replies:

① "Although your baby is still very small, he or she is recognizably human, has a large head compared to the body, and will now begin to grow and mature inside your uterus."
② "Babies who have been developing for 8 weeks are almost 12 inches long and are covered with fine, downy hair."
③ "We can usually tell with an ultrasound test if the baby is a boy or a girl at 8 weeks."
④ "Your baby is still too small to see, but he or she will be getting bigger very soon."

22. A 25-year-old primigravida has been in labor for 15 hours. The fetus is in an occiput posterior position, and the client has been complaining of severe back discomfort. Which of the following nursing actions is *most likely* to hasten the birth of the baby?

① Assist the physician to switch to internal fetal monitoring techniques.
② Assist the client to a hands-and-knees position.
③ Increase the rate of the intravenous solution and administer oxygen by nasal cannula.
④ Place a cool cloth on the client's forehead, and rub her back.

23. A gravida 4 who has been laboring for several hours suddenly yells out, "The baby is coming!" You call for assistance while controlling the delivery of the infant's head. After the head has been delivered, the *next* step you should take when assisting in a precipitous delivery is to:

① Quickly pull the baby upward to deliver the posterior shoulder
② Dry the baby's face and suction the nose and mouth
③ Instruct the client to bear down once more
④ Instruct the client to pant and wait for the physician to arrive to complete the delivery

24. The nurse wishes to facilitate bonding between the parents and the infant. Which activity is *least likely* to promote early bonding?

① Allowing the client to breast-feed immediately after delivery, if desired
② Encouraging the father to be present during the birth process and actively involving him in the care of the infant
③ Performing necessary eye prophylaxis immediately after birth
④ Providing for the mother and father to spend time together with the baby shortly after birth

25. The anesthesiologist has just begun to administer lumbar epidural anesthesia for pain relief on a primigravida in active labor. The client is alert and conversant in the supine position. The nurse notes that the blood pressure has dropped to 80/40. What nursing intervention should be done *first*?

① Give oxygen by tight face mask at 10 L/minute.
② Notify the charge nurse of the event.
③ Recheck the blood pressure.
④ Reposition the client to a side-lying position.

26. Your client is 3 days post–cesarean section delivery and is bottle-feeding her infant. During the morning assessment, breast engorgement is noted. The *most appropriate* intervention to add to the care plan is:

① Apply ice packs to the breasts intermittently
② Apply a warm, wet washcloth to the nipples three times daily
③ Assist the client to pump her breasts whenever painful engorgement is noted
④ Instruct the client to massage the breast to relieve engorgement

27. Which medication would put the postoperative client at a higher risk for dehiscence?

① Dexamethasone (Decadron)
② Heparin sodium, heparin
③ Morphine sodium, morphine
④ Aminophylline

28. Which signs or symptoms would the client exhibit if the digoxin level was 2.2 ng/mL? *Normal level is between 0.5 and 2.0 ng/mL.*

① Hypertension, fluid and electrolyte imbalances, edema
② Nervousness, tremors, anxiety, tachycardia
③ Arrhythmias, anorexia, blurred vision with yellow-green halos
④ Hyperkalemia and hypocalcemia

29. The client is receiving 300 mg theophylline (Theo-Dur) b.i.d. The theophylline level is 24 μg/mL. Which of the following nursing interventions is *incorrect* for this client? *Normal level is between 10 and 20 μg/mL.*

① Assessing for tachycardia and palpitations
② Assessing for nervousness, tremors, and anxiety
③ Give half the dose and call the physician
④ Hold the A.M. dose and call the physician

30. Aminophylline would *not* be administered for which disease process?

① Chronic obstructive pulmonary disease
② Asthma
③ Emphysema
④ Upper respiratory infection

31. Which intervention is *inappropriate* when administering a Z-tract medication?

① Placing 0.2 cc of air in the syringe
② Bunching the skin
③ Aspirating for blood
④ Waiting 5 to 10 seconds while needle is still in the skin

32. Spironolactone (Aldactone) is administered with furosemide (Lasix) in clients with congestive heart failure to:

① Prevent dehydration or fluid deficit
② Prevent hypokalemia
③ Prevent hyperkalemia
④ Prevent thrombophlebitis

33. A client arrived in the emergency department with third-degree burns and hypovolemic shock. Which of the following assessment data does not indicate early shock?

① Tachypnea
② Bradycardia
③ Cool clammy skin
④ Restlessness

34. A possible complication of third-degree burns related to the gastrointestinal system is:

① Metabolic alkalosis
② Aspiration
③ Infection
④ Diarrhea

35. A client has just returned to the surgical unit after open reduction surgery for fractures. How would you most accurately evaluate adequate pain relief for this client?

① Monitor amount of pain medication used
② Ask the client to tell you when he or she has pain
③ Monitor physical and verbal cues
④ Place the self-administered medication system close to the client

36. You are taking care of a client who is receiving intravenous morphine. You notice 10 minutes after the first dose that the client's respirations have dropped from 28 to 8. You should:

① Call the physician
② Administer naloxone (Narcan)
③ Notify the RN
④ Check the client in 1 hour

37. Your client has just had major surgery. He refuses to reposition or deep breathe because of fear of pain. He also refuses to take pain medication for fear of addiction. Your best response to this client is to:

① Praise him for wanting to be drug-free
② Inform him that he has to take the pain medication
③ Educate him about the benefits of pain relief and risk of addiction
④ Inform him that the physician is ordering him to take the pain medication

38. A noninvasive nursing intervention for pain management is to:

① Increase fluids
② Administer oral pain medications
③ Alter environmental stimuli
④ Tell the client that pain is only an imagined experience

39. Clients receiving chemotherapy for cancer treatment should:

① Decrease fluids
② Increase fluids
③ Decrease calories
④ Increase social interactions and outings

40. Your client is a 32-year-old woman who has had a mastectomy 3 days ago. As you are changing her incisional dressing, you notice that she refuses to look at the wound. Your *best* nursing response would be to:

① Tell her that she is lucky they found the cancer early
② Continue changing the dressing and allow her to express her feelings
③ Change the dressing quickly and allow her to have time alone
④ Inform her that by tomorrow she has to change her own dressing

41. A 78-year-old woman is recovering well after total hip replacement and has regained activities-of-daily-living function after surgery. She tells you that she is afraid her family will not let her live alone anymore. You know that when working with the elderly it is important to:

① Do what the family wants done
② Provide the client reasonable choices
③ Place the client in a restrictive environment to prevent future injuries
④ Always allow the client to do what he or she wants

42. A client who has been in the intensive care unit for 3 days is *most* likely to be at risk for which of the following alterations in psychosocial integrity?

① Sensory overload
② Boredom
③ Sensory deprivation
④ Addiction to narcotics

43. You are caring for a client who is confined to bed in a private room in a skilled extended-care facility. As you assess this client, you realize that he or she is at *highest* psychosocial risk for:

① Sensory overload
② Falls
③ Sensory deprivation
④ Altered communication patterns

44. The client you are caring for has been in the intensive care unit for 5 days. You notice that he is staring at the corner of the room and is picking at the air. He is probably suffering from which of the following psychosocial alterations?

① Cerebrovascular accident
② Diversional activity deficit
③ Sensory deprivation
④ Sensory overload

45. Your client begins to experience tremors and becomes increasingly anxious. You notice on the admission assessment that this client admitted to drinking "a few beers" every evening. Your *best* nursing intervention would be to do which of the following?

① Tell the client he has to calm down.
② Ask the client to have his family bring beer in for him.
③ Call the physician.
④ Report your assessment and findings to the RN.

46. According to the American Heart Association, the first step in performing CPR is to:

① Establish an airway
② Establish unresponsiveness
③ Check the pulse
④ Check for respirations

47. The most common airway obstruction in sudden death is caused by the:

① Absence of nerve stimuli to the brain
② Inability to swallow secretions
③ Swelling of the epiglottis
④ Tongue falling backward

48. The ratio of compressions to breaths by one rescuer on an adult is:

① 2 breaths to 15 compressions
② 4 breaths to 12 compressions
③ 1 breath to 5 compressions
④ 1 breath to 15 compressions

49. Which of the following is an appropriate reason to discontinue CPR?

① Resuscitation efforts have been unsuccessful after 15 minutes.
② You are too tired to continue.
③ The pupils are dilated.
④ The victim has vomited.

50. The primary goal in shock management is to:

① Raise the systolic blood pressure to 90 mm Hg or above
② Restore and maintain tissue oxygenation
③ Maintain heart rate between 70 and 90
④ Increase urine output

51. The emergency management of a hemorrhagic shock victim requires that an airway is established, blood loss is stopped, and then:

① An intravenous infusion is established
② An indwelling catheter is inserted
③ Blood is drawn for arterial blood gases
④ An electrocardiogram is done

52. When assessing the client in hypovolemic shock, which of the following findings would be evident?

① Warm, dry skin and tachycardia
② Pale skin and a slow pulse
③ Decreasing level of consciousness and increased urine output
④ Cold, clammy skin and hypotension

53. Mrs. Potts is admitted to the emergency department in anaphylactic shock following an insect bite. Initially, nursing care should focus on:

① Assessing level of consciousness
② Maintaining an open airway
③ Providing fluid replacement
④ Maintaining body temperature

54. Lucy, a widow age 85 years, is admitted to the hospital and scheduled for extraction of a cataract of her left eye and insertion of an intraocular lens. Her right eye also has a cataract but has better vision. Her general health is good. She lives alone in a small apartment, but her daughter and son-in-law live nearby and check on her daily. Admission procedures have been completed, and Lucy has been oriented to her surroundings. In contributing to her care plan, the nurse added the diagnosis of potential for injury related to impaired vision. An important intervention to include in Lucy's care plan is to:

① Maintain all four side rails at all times
② Restrain her with a vest restraint when in bed to ensure that she does not climb out
③ Maintain the location of items at her bedside, furnishings, and other items in her immediate environment
④ Encourage a family member to stay with her at all times

55. Lucy, a widow age 85 years, is admitted to the hospital and scheduled for extraction of a cataract of her left eye and insertion of an intraocular lens. Her right eye also has a cataract but has better vision. Her general health is good. She lives alone in a small apartment, but her daughter and son-in-law live nearby and check on her daily. When Lucy returns to her room after surgery, the nurse should observe for:

① Sudden or severe pain in the eye
② Diplopia
③ Equality of carotid pulses
④ Equality of pupil reactions to light and accommodation

56. Lucy, a widow age 85 years, is admitted to the hospital and scheduled for extraction of a cataract of her left eye and insertion of an intraocular lens. Her right eye also has a cataract, but has better vision. Her general health is good. She lives alone in a small apartment, but her daughter and son-in-law live nearby and check on her daily. A postoperative nursing diagnosis for Lucy is risk for injury related to hemorrhage. An important nursing intervention is to:

① Maintain Lucy on complete bed rest for 24 hours
② Remind Lucy not to cough or sneeze
③ Reinforce loose dressing to maintain pressure
④ Maintain Lucy on her operative side

57. Which of the following statements is *most* helpful when planning a diet low in fats?

① Fats contain 4 calories per gram.
② Fruits are a good source of fats.
③ Essential fatty acids must be supplied in the diet.
④ Saturated fats come from plant sources.

58. Because Ms. Smith is placed on a diuretic, her physician instructs her to include foods high in potassium in her daily diet. Which of the following foods would the nurse tell Ms. Smith to include in her diet?

① Citrus fruits, bananas, and tomatoes
② Liver, organ meats, and fish
③ Seafood, coffee, and nuts
④ Whole grains, cereals, and pasta

59. A client asks the nurse to explain saturated fat. The *best* response by the nurse is:

① "A saturated fat is a solid fat from an animal source."
② "A saturated fat is an oil from a plant source."
③ "A saturated fat is a fat obtained from fish."
④ "A saturated fat is a type of fat that contains essential fatty acids."

60. Which of the following foods would the nurse tell a client on a sodium-restricted diet to *avoid*?

① Broccoli
② Pretzels
③ Bananas
④ Fresh meat

61. Which of the following statements is true related to Medicare (Title XVIII)?

① It is a state-administered health plan for people over the age of 65.
② It has three parts: "A" for hospital, "B" for outpatient care, and "C" for nursing home care.
③ It is free to all people who have worked.
④ Its original intent was to provide medical coverage to all elderly.

62. The nurse is caring for a 79-year-old man who is dying. The nurse who is most effective in helping the family cope with his death is one who:

① Views dying people as a specific group of people in need of help
② Attends classes on death and dying
③ Has contemplated his or her own mortality and death
④ Can keep his or her emotions distant while providing care for the patient

63. An 84-year-old client begins talking about all his losses and the fact that all his friends are dead. He starts to cry. What would be the nurse's *best* response?

① Give the patient a tissue and tell him it is okay to cry
② Change the subject
③ Tell him to stop crying and everything will be okay
④ Begin to make the bed and ignore his comments

64. A 76-year-old man is admitted with a fractured hip. Which of the following assessments would be *least* important when the nurse evaluates the client for peripheral nerve damage?

① Pain
② Sensation
③ Bleeding
④ Pulselessness

65. When caring for an elderly immobile client, the nurse wants to prevent external rotation of the client's leg. Which piece or pieces of equipment should the nurse use to prevent external rotation?

① Sandbags
② High footboard
③ Abductor splint
④ Bed cradle

66. A client who delivered 24 hours ago is preparing for discharge. Which of the following statements made by the client indicates a need for further teaching?

① "I asked my mother to bring some tampons so I will feel fresh when I go home."
② "I'm looking forward to relaxing in my recliner at home while the baby sleeps."
③ "I plan to go back to work in 3 months if the doctor approves."
④ "I will take sitz baths in the morning, after lunch, and just before I go to bed."

67. Which of the following nursing interventions is *inappropriate* to include on the care plan of a client who delivered by cesarean section?

① Encourage frequent maternal-infant contact
② Massage fundus every 4 hours
③ Monitor intake and output every 8 hours
④ Observe and assist with breast-feeding techniques

68. Your client is on intravenous magnesium sulfate for the treatment of pregnancy-induced hypertension (PIH). Nursing assessment reveals absent deep tendon reflexes and a respiratory rate of 10. The action that should be taken *first* is to:

① Continue close monitoring of the client
② Discontinue the infusion of magnesium sulfate
③ Give oxygen by nasal cannula
④ Observe for seizure activity

69. An initial assessment is performed on a newborn. Which of the following assessment findings should be brought to the physician's attention?

① Apical pulse rate of 150.
② Engorged breast tissue.
③ Passage of dark green, tarry fecal material.
④ Two umbilical vessels, one vein and one artery.

70. A new mother asks the nurse about a large bluish-black discoloration on her baby's back. The nurse's *most appropriate* response is:

① "I will report this to the doctor."
② "Many babies have this marking. Frequently these marks fade as the child grows."
③ "Your baby was bruised as he passed through the birth canal. The bruising will disappear in a few days."
④ "This mark is called a mongolian spot and often is associated with mental retardation."

71. A 9 pound, 5 ounce term neonate born 1 hour ago is jittery, startles easily, and has tremors. He remains under the radiant warmer. The *priority* nursing action is to:

① Bathe the infant in tepid water
② Perform a heel stick to determine blood glucose level
③ Take the baby to the mother for breast-feeding
④ Wrap the baby snugly in a blanket, and soothe him with cuddling and rocking

72. A client who has had a myocardial infarction is placed on intravenous heparin sodium. Considering the side effects of this drug, nursing care should include monitoring the client for:

① Diarrhea
② Hematuria
③ Increased white blood cell count
④ Shortness of breath

73. Mr. James, a 40-year-old sedentary executive, has a positive family history of heart disease. He asks you about changes that could prevent a heart attack. You should counsel him that:

① Relaxation techniques are the best means of prevention
② A low-sodium, low-cholesterol diet will dramatically lower his risk

③ Gender, age, and family history are non-modifiable risk factors
④ If he stops alcohol and nicotine consumption, he will not have a heart attack

74. Ms. Hays, 69 years old, has undergone a cardiac catheterization procedure. After the examination, you must carefully monitor the catheter site for:

① Hematoma formation
② Local reaction to the dye
③ Circulatory collapse
④ Heparin effects

75. Mary is seen in the clinic with a diagnosis of urinary tract infection. Mary reports the following symptoms. Which one is unrelated to her primary diagnosis?

① Nausea and vomiting
② Frequency of urination
③ Nocturia
④ Burning on urination

76. How would the PN report client's complaint of painful voiding, using medical terminology?

① Enuresis
② Anuresis
③ Dysuria
④ Urinary colic

77. Cranberry juice is frequently recommended for patients with urinary tract infections because cranberry juice tends to:

① Promote diuresis
② Increase acidity of urine
③ Decrease urinary tract spasms
④ Relax the bladder

78. Mary, a young woman with a urinary tract infection, is seen in the clinic and sent home on sulfisoxazole (Gantrisin). Discharge instructions should include:

① Take your temperature twice a day
② Limit food with high salt content
③ Set alarm to take fluids hourly
④ Take fluids hourly while awake

79. A young woman comes to the clinic because she thinks she may have a venereal disease. The appropriate action for the PN to take initially is to:

① Determine whether she is promiscuous
② Ask her for a list of all sexual partners

③ Explore the reasons she thinks she has a venereal disease

④ Determine whether she is a minor

80. A young woman comes to the clinic because she thinks she may have a venereal disease. She says that her boyfriend has venereal disease, that about a month ago she had a painless sore on her genitals that disappeared, and that she is afraid. Given her description, which of the following venereal diseases may be the likely diagnosis?

① Syphilis
② Gonorrhea
③ Herpes
④ Chlamydial infection

81. The routine test for syphilis involves a:

① Urine test
② Blood test
③ Vaginal smear
④ Wound culture

82. The physician orders probenecid and penicillin for a client with a diagnosis of syphilis. The rationale for administering probenecid with penicillin is that it:

① Inhibits renal secretion of penicillin
② Prevents allergic reactions
③ Decreases side effects of penicillin
④ Prevents hepatic damage

83. Olivia, 4 months old, is brought to the hospital by her mother. The mother reports that Olivia has been ill for several days with a cold and that today she awakened with a cough and problems breathing. Which of the assessment findings would indicate that Olivia is in acute respiratory distress?

① Respiratory rate of 35 at rest
② Flaring of the nares
③ Bronchial breath sounds
④ Experiencing diaphragmatic respirations

84. The RN charge nurse reports to you that Olivia, age 4 months, has a diagnosis of viral bronchiolitis and that she is to be placed in a mist tent. In which of the following positions would you expect Olivia to be most comfortable?

① Left side
② Abdomen
③ Semi-Fowler's
④ High Fowler's

85. Olivia, age 4 months, has a diagnosis of viral bronchiolitis and is placed in a mist tent. Which of the following actions would be most important for the nurse to implement while Olivia is in the mist tent?

① To maintain hydration, feed Olivia every 3 hours
② To keep her dry, change her clothing frequently
③ Observe for cyanosis by turning off the mist frequently
④ Take her out of the mist test hourly for cuddling

86. Olivia, age 4 months, has a diagnosis of viral bronchiolitis and is placed in a mist tent. How should the PN plan to take Olivia's temperature?

① Orally
② Axillary
③ Rectally
④ Skin-heat sensor

87. Olivia, age 4 months, has a diagnosis of viral bronchiolitis and is placed in a mist tent. Which urine specific gravity would indicate that Olivia is in good fluid balance?

① 1.002
② 1.015
③ 1.030
④ 1.035

88. Olivia, age 4 months, has a diagnosis of viral bronchiolitis and is placed in a mist tent. Which of the following would be correct information to be given to Olivia's mother?

① A vaccine will prevent future attacks.
② She should be placed on prophylactic antibiotics.
③ Repeated attacks may be associated with asthmatic allergic reactions.
④ She will most likely be placed on bronchodilators.

89. Olivia, age 4 months, has a diagnosis of bilateral otitis media. Her physician has ordered ear drops and an intramuscular antibiotic. When administering the ear drops to Olivia, the PN should pull her ear:

① Up and back
② Down and back
③ Straight up
④ Straight down

90. Which of the following injection sites should be used for the injection of antibiotics in a 4-month-old infant?

① Ventrogluteal
② Deltoid
③ Dorsogluteal
④ Laterofemoral

91. Olivia, age 4 months, has a diagnosis of bilateral otitis media. In observing Olivia for pain, which of the following would be an unexpected physiologic response to pain?

① Flushing
② Restlessness
③ Constriction of pupils
④ Increase in pulse rate

92. Olivia, age 4 months, has a diagnosis of bilateral otitis media. Olivia's mother tells you that she is due for her immunization. The PN should know that:

① This should be Olivia's first immunization
② Olivia's appointment is out of sequence for the normal immunization series
③ Olivia should be due for her second DPT
④ Olivia should have completed her DPT immunizations

93. Your client has bone cancer and is experiencing constant pain. The most appropriate pain management/intervention for this client is to:

① Administer the pain medication only when the client asks for it
② Administer pain medications when the client's pain increases
③ Assess the client's pain on a scale of 0 to 10
④ Administer pain medication on a routine schedule

94. The client you are caring for has blood in his stool. Your first action should be to:

① Call the physician
② Apply pressure to the client's rectal area
③ Educate the client not to strain with defecation
④ Notify the RN

95. The client you are caring for is taking iron. You would expect:

① Fatty stools
② Darker stools
③ Tan-colored stools
④ Diarrhea

96. Jason is 5 years old. He has had several hospitalizations for recurrent ear infections and myringotomy. He is being admitted to the hospital for a tonsillectomy and adenoidectomy. In preparing Jason for his admission, the PN should initially:

① Meet Jason and his parents at their home
② Supply him with a book about going to the hospital
③ Because of his past experience, nothing is necessary
④ Explore Jason's concept of hospitalization

97. Jason is 5 years old. He has been hospitalized several times for recurrent ear infections and myringotomy. He is being admitted to the hospital for a tonsillectomy and adenoidectomy. Considering Jason's age, his dominant fear during hospitalization will be that of:

① Body mutilation
② Abandonment
③ Death
④ Stranger anxiety

98. Jason is 5 years old. He has been hospitalized several times for recurrent ear infections and myringotomy. He is being admitted to the hospital for a tonsillectomy and adenoidectomy. Jason is to receive an injection preoperatively. He is most concerned and asks you, the PN, "Will it hurt?" Your best reply is:

① "Yes, it will hurt a little, but not for long."
② "Big boys are not afraid."
③ "I can't believe that you are afraid."
④ "You may watch television as soon as this is over."

99. Jason is 5 years old. He has been hospitalized several times for recurrent ear infections and myringotomy. He is being admitted to the hospital for a tonsillectomy and adenoidectomy. Jason's preoperative orders are: meperidine (Demerol) 35 mg and hydroxyzine pamoate (Vistaril) 12.5 mg. The Demerol available is 50 mg/mL. Which of the following is the appropriate amount of Demerol that Jason should receive?

① 1.7 mL
② 0.7 mL
③ 0.8 mL
④ 0.5 mL

100. Jason is 5 years old. He has been hospitalized several times for recurrent ear infections and myringotomy. He is being admitted to the hospital for a tonsillectomy and adenoidectomy. He is to receive hydroxyzine pamoate (Vistaril) 12.5 mg. The hydroxyzine available is 100 mg per 2 mL. Which of the following is the appropriate amount of Vistaril that Jason should receive?

① 1 mL
② 0.5 mL
③ 0.25 mL
④ 0.1 mL

101. The PN is unsure if meperidine (Demerol) and hydroxyzine pamoate (Vistaril) are compatible when mixed in the same syringe. Which of the following options would be best for her to choose?

① Mix the medications but discard if clouding occurs
② Assume that they are not compatible and give the medications in two syringes
③ Ask another nurse
④ Check the compatibility chart in the medication room

102. Jason is 5 years old. He has been hospitalized several times for recurrent ear infections and myringotomy. He is being admitted to the hospital for a tonsillectomy and adenoidectomy. As you come into the room to give Jason his preoperative injection, he starts to cry and scream "I hate you. Get out of my room." Which of the following actions would be most appropriate for the nurse to take?

① Ask another nurse to give Jason his injection because he does not like you
② Explain to Jason in a calm voice what you are going to do and then do it
③ Ask Jason's parents to leave the room, as you will then be able to calm him
④ Tell Jason that he is acting like a baby and that big boys do not act like that

103. Jason, age 5, has just returned from a tonsillectomy and adenoidectomy. Which of the following would be an appropriate liquid to give Jason postoperatively?

① Orange juice
② Tepid water
③ Hot tea
④ Milk

104. Jason, age 5, has just returned from a tonsillectomy and adenoidectomy. Jason's parents ask you why Jason is susceptible to hemorrhage in about 5 days. The most likely reason for this is:

① Decreased platelet count
② Sloughing of the membrane from the throat
③ An anticoagulative effect of aspirin
④ Eating rough foods

105. Ann is a 3-year-old who has a tentative diagnosis of pinworm infestation. Ann's physician has ordered a cellophane tape test to be performed at home. The PN should explain to Ann's mother that the most effective time to perform this test is:

① At bedtime before bathing
② Following a bowel movement
③ Immediately after lunch
④ Early morning before arising

106. Ann is a 3-year-old who has a diagnosis of pinworm infestation. Which of the following should the nurse include in the teaching plan for Ann and her family?

① Good hand-washing technique
② Proper food preparation
③ Proper isolation techniques
④ Sterilization techniques

107. Ann is a 3-year-old who has a diagnosis of pinworm infestation. Pyrvinium pamoate (Povan) has been ordered to treat it. It is important to note on Ann's care plan that a side effect of pyrvinium pamoate is that it makes the stool:

① Black
② Green
③ Red
④ Blue

108. Terri, age 3 years, is admitted to the pediatric unit with a diagnosis of Wilms' tumor. The PN should be aware that the most important aspect of Terri's care preoperatively is to:

① Avoid palpating the abdomen
② Maintain a high-protein and low-salt diet
③ Obtain daily weights
④ Enforce strict bed rest

109. Terri, age 3 years, is admitted to the pediatric unit with a diagnosis of Wilms' tumor. When it is time for Terri's parents to leave, the nurse should encourage the parents to:

① Wait until the child is asleep to leave
② Tell Terri truthfully that they are leaving
③ Wait until Terri is distracted in play
④ Tell the child that the nurse said that they must go

110. Terri, age 3 years, is admitted to the pediatric unit with a diagnosis of Wilms' tumor. Which type of behavior would you expect from Terri the first time that her parents leave?

① Wave goodbye to them
② Cry
③ Hide under the bed
④ Ask to go to the playroom

111. Terri, age 3 years, was admitted with a diagnosis of Wilms' tumor. Terri has returned from surgery. When Terri's blood pressure is taken, the blood pressure cuff:

① Will produce a higher reading if too wide
② Should cover about two thirds of the upper arm
③ Should be applied only to the thigh
④ Will produce a low reading if it is too narrow

112. Terri, age 3 years, was admitted with a diagnosis of Wilms' tumor. Terri has returned from surgery. In assessing Terri for pain, the PN should know that the *first* observable behavioral change is usually:

① Irritability
② Lethargy
③ Loss of appetite
④ Disturbed sleep patterns

113. Nine-year-old Paul has been admitted to the pediatric unit with the diagnosis of Legg-Calvé-Perthes disease. In completing your nursing assessment of Paul, you should expect him to complain of pain in which of the following areas?

① Hip
② Calf
③ Lower abdomen
④ Lumbar spine

114. Nine-year-old Paul has been admitted to the pediatric unit with the diagnosis of Legg-Calvé-Perthes disease. Treatment for Paul is aimed at:

① Preventing deformity of the femur
② Preventing degeneration of the knee joint
③ Reducing muscle spasms of the back
④ Preventing pressure on the head of the femur

115. Nine-year-old Paul has been admitted to the pediatric unit with the diagnosis of Legg-

Calvé-Perthes disease. In dealing with Paul, one of the most difficult aspects of his care is expected to be the:

① Compliance with the prescribed diet
② Overwhelming feeling of fatigue
③ Overconcern for missing school
④ Necessity of prolonged immobility

116. Nine-year-old Paul has a diagnosis of Legg-Calvé-Perthes disease. He is now being discharged with braces. His teaching for home care of the braces should include which of the following instructions?

① Apply alcohol to bony prominences
② Check skin weekly for signs of irritation
③ Clean plastic molds weekly with soap and water
④ Use crutches if braces need repair

117. Nine-year-old Paul has a diagnosis of Legg-Calvé-Perthes disease. He is now being discharged with braces. Which of the following activities might Paul be able to participate in following discharge?

① Swimming
② Tennis
③ Football
④ Horseback riding

118. Nine-year-old Paul has a diagnosis of Legg-Calvé-Perthes disease. He is now being discharged with braces. Paul should be mastering Erikson's stage of:

① Industry versus inferiority
② Intimacy versus isolation
③ Trust versus mistrust
④ Autonomy versus shame

119. Shannon, a 17-year-old, has been admitted to the hospital with infectious mononucleosis. Her symptoms are fever, sore throat, muscle soreness, and general malaise. The PN should expect to find which of the following during her initial nursing assessment?

① Abdominal distention
② Productive cough
③ Lesions of the lips
④ Enlarged lymph nodes

120. Shannon, a 17-year-old, has been admitted to the hospital with infectious mononucleosis.

The PN should plan to prevent the spread of the disease by adhering to which of the following precautions?

① Good hand-washing technique
② Respiratory isolation
③ Enteric isolation
④ Complete isolation

121. The diagnosis of infectious mononucleosis is confirmed by which of the following?

① Chest radiograph
② Urinalysis
③ Blood test
④ Skin test

122. Shannon, a 17-year-old, has been admitted to the hospital with infectious mononucleosis. In the plan to meet Shannon's dietary needs, which of the following items should be excluded?

① Orange juice
② Puddings
③ Milk shakes
④ Warm tea

123. Shannon, a 17-year-old, has been admitted to the hospital with infectious mononucleosis. Which of the following is a potential complication that might occur with infectious mononucleosis?

① Cystitis
② Diarrhea
③ Weight gain
④ Hepatomegaly

124. Shannon, a 17-year-old, has been admitted to the hospital with infectious mononucleosis. Which of the following statements indicates that Shannon understands the teaching about her convalescence?

① "I must have complete bed rest to prevent relapse."
② "Bed rest is not necessary, but I can have only quiet activities."
③ "Additional rest periods will be necessary, but I must avoid only strenuous activities."
④ "Activity limitations are not necessary, but I must avoid crowds."

125. Shannon, a 17-year-old, has been admitted to the hospital with infectious mononucleosis. During Shannon's hospitalization, it is most important for the nurse to recall that adolescents are most likely to be fearful of:

① Separation from family and school
② Falling behind in academic studies
③ Loss of body integrity
④ Loss of self-control in front of others

126. Shannon, a 17-year-old, has been admitted to the hospital with infectious mononucleosis. In response to Shannon's parents' questions about the spread of her disease, it is correct to tell them that mononucleosis is spread by:

① Contact with oral secretions
② Contact with the stools
③ The respiratory system
④ Contact with blood

127. Yolanda, age 3 years, has a pink rash, and the diagnosis is rubella. Identify the correct statement regarding Yolanda's condition:

① Yolanda should have Koplik spots in her mouth.
② She should not be visited by her aunt, who is 2 months pregnant.
③ Yolanda's treatment should consist of antibiotics.
④ Encephalitis is a frequent complication of this condition.

128. The PN learns that Mike in room 400 has Koplik spots. Koplik spots are considered diagnostic of:

① Rubella
② Roseola
③ Rubeola
④ Chicken pox

129. Which of the following statements regarding rubeola is *false*?

① The duration of symptoms is about 3 days.
② The disease is highly contagious.
③ The incubation period is 10 to 14 days.
④ Photophobia is a frequent symptom.

130. Tony, age 3 years, has been admitted to the pediatric unit with the diagnosis of nephrotic syndrome. Which assessment finding would the PN most likely find, given Tony's diagnosis?

① Edema
② Hypernatremia
③ Hematuria
④ Increased urinary output

131. Tony, age 3 years, has been admitted to the pediatric unit with the diagnosis of nephrotic syndrome. In response to Tony's parents' questions about the cause of Tony's disease, the PN could reply that the etiologic agent is:

① Unknown
② Hyperimmune response
③ Acute glomerulonephritis
④ An allergic response

132. Tony, age 3 years, has been admitted to the pediatric unit with the diagnosis of nephrotic syndrome. Tony is given steroid therapy. The aim of this therapy is to prevent:

① Diuresis
② Hematuria
③ Proteinuria
④ Potassium loss

133. Tony, age 3 years, has been admitted to the pediatric unit with the diagnosis of nephrotic syndrome. The diet for Tony during the acute stage will most likely be:

① Normal for age
② High in protein, low in sodium
③ Low in protein, low in sodium
④ High in protein, high in sodium

134. Which of the following nurse actions will help to ensure an accurate urinalysis?

① Force fluids to 1000 mL before collection
② Take the urine specimen to the laboratory as soon as it is obtained
③ Collect all of the urine
④ Cleanse the container with povidone-iodine (Betadine) before collecting the specimen

135. Cathy is admitted to the hospital with acute glomerulonephritis. Many infections commonly precede glomerulonephritis. Which of the following is *not* known to precede the disease?

① Tonsillitis
② Mononucleosis
③ Scarlet fever
④ Impetigo

136. Cathy is admitted to the hospital with acute glomerulonephritis. The PN should expect that Cathy's urinalysis would reflect the presence of:

① A specific gravity of 1.045
② Blood

③ Glucose
④ Bacteria

137. Carl, age 6 years, fell from his bicycle, and the result was a fracture to his lower leg. He has been admitted to the hospital for casting. When obtaining the admission history, the PN should first:

① Assess Carl's reaction to the hospital
② Inquire about health insurance
③ Review Carl's development with his mother
④ Establish a rapport with Carl and his parents

138. The nurse should use the palms of her hands when handling the wet cast to:

① Assess dryness of the cast
② Facilitate easy turning
③ Keep the limbs balanced
④ Prevent indenting the cast

139. Which of the following assessment findings would cause the PN to suspect that an infection has developed under a long leg cast?

① Complaint of numbness
② Cold toes
③ Increased respirations
④ Foul smell

140. Carl suffered a broken leg following a fall from a bicycle. He is being discharged with a long leg cast in place. In planning for Carl's discharge, the nurse may use which intervention to relieve itching?

① Blow cool air under the cast with a fan
② Squeeze lotion beneath the cast
③ Use a straightened coat hanger to scratch the area
④ Sprinkle powder beneath the cast

141. Your neighbor, Mrs. Smith, tells you that her baby has impetigo. She has many questions. Which of the following statements regarding impetigo is false?

① Impetigo is caused by a bacterium.
② Scarring rarely occurs.
③ Impetigo commonly occurs on the face.
④ Impetigo is usually not contagious.

142. Which of the following is a potentially dangerous complication of impetigo?

① Reye's syndrome
② Erythema multiforme

③ Pyelonephritis
④ Glomerulonephritis

143. In which of the following situations would a PN be most likely to suspect the incidence of child abuse?

① A child who cries during the physical examination
② A broken arm in a 6-year-old child
③ Bruises on a child's forehead and knees
④ A 4-year-old with a broken nose

144. Which of the following would be inappropriate in the case of suspected child abuse?

① Document all bruises and cuts
② Chart interactions between the child and parent
③ Document staff perceptions of the family relationships
④ Report to the state child welfare agency or law enforcement agency

145. Which of the following would not be a common cause of anxiety?

① Nonspecific threats to self
② Poorly functioning defenses
③ Aggressive behavior
④ Threat to biologic integrity

146. When administering a major tranquilizer such as a phenothiazine, the nurse should report which of the following signs or symptoms to the physician immediately?

① Dry mouth
② Drowsiness
③ Orthostatic hypotension
④ Abnormal facial grimaces

147. If your client is given diazepam (Valium) to treat anxiety, which of the following should be included in your client teaching?

① Take the drug with milk or food to decrease nausea.
② If you are drowsy, stop taking the drug.
③ Do not drink alcohol while taking the drug.
④ Food and drink with caffeine should be eliminated.

148. Your recovery room client is positive for human immunodeficiency virus (HIV). In keeping with the guidelines set up by the Centers for Disease Control and Prevention, the nurse caring for postpartum clients should wear:

① Gloves when handling soiled materials
② Gloves and a mask
③ Gloves, mask, and a special gown
④ No special precautions are necessary after delivery

149. A postpartum patient who is HIV-positive should:

① Not handle her infant
② Room-in if possible
③ Be in complete isolation
④ Wear gloves and a mask when handling her infant

150. The single most important precaution in preventing any type of infection is:

① Wearing gloves at all times
② Wearing a gown and mask
③ Hand washing
④ Wearing scrub uniforms

151. The nurse caring for the HIV-positive mother understands:

① Breast-feeding is not allowed
② The infant is always infected
③ The mother is an intravenous drug user
④ The mother should breast-feed and care for her infant as usual

152. Which of the following actions indicates successful postpartum teaching for the HIV-positive mother?

① Client washes her hands after handling the infant
② Client wears gloves when holding the infant
③ Client demonstrates appropriate care and feeding of infant
④ Client verbalizes understanding as to why she should not care for the infant

153. The progressive increase in function and the acquisition of new functions best describes:

① Maturation
② Development
③ Growth
④ Learning

154. Based on the principles of cephalocaudal development, which of the following would the child gain control of last?

① Neck
② Arms
③ Feet
④ Back

155. The type of play most characteristic of toddlers is:

① Cooperative
② Solitary
③ Competitive
④ Parallel

156. By what age should infants double their birth weight?

① 4 months
② 6 months
③ 8 months
④ 12 months

157. The feeling of guilt that the child "caused" his or her disability is especially critical in which of the following age groups?

① Toddler
② Preschooler
③ School-age
④ Adolescent

158. At what period do children have the most difficulty coping with death, particularly if it is their own?

① Toddlers
② Preschooler
③ School-age
④ Adolescence

159. Which age group is most likely to personify death as a devil or monster?

① Toddler
② Preschooler
③ School-age
④ Adolescence

160. A social smile can be elicited from most infants by:

① 2 weeks
② 1 month
③ 2 months
④ 4 months

161. According to Erikson, if a mother is inconsistent and neglectful in the care of her infant, the infant can develop:

① A sense of shame and doubt
② A feeling of inferiority
③ A sense of mistrust
④ Identity confusion

162. The age at which stranger anxiety appears is:

① Birth to 2 months
② 2 to 4 months
③ 6 to 9 months
④ After 12 months

163. According to Erikson, the developmental task of adolescence is the acquisition of a sense of:

① Autonomy
② Industry
③ Initiative
④ Identity

164. Which of the following is an unusual characteristic in an adolescent?

① Predictability
② Tendency toward idealism
③ Rebellion
④ Moodiness

165. Which of the following is *not* a risk factor for uterine cancer?

① Postmenopausal bleeding
② History of genital herpes
③ Obesity
④ History of infertility

166. The major diagnostic test to confirm the presence of uterine cancer is a:

① Papanicolaou (Pap) smear
② Colposcopic examination
③ Fractional dilatation and curettage (D&C)
④ Ultrasonography

167. The leading cause of death in adults in the United States is:

① Diabetes mellitus
② Cancer
③ Chronic obstructive pulmonary disease
④ Cardiovascular disease

168. The physician orders nitroglycerin sublingually to relieve chest pain. When Mr. Jones asks how this drug affects his heart, the nurse tells him that it:

① Relieves the muscle spasms
② Increases the blood flow through the chambers
③ Increases the diameter of the coronary arteries
④ Has a sedative effect that relieves the chest pain

169. Which of the following side effects is common with coronary vasodilators and should be explained to Mr. Jones?

①　Loss of appetite
②　Increased urine output
③　Headache
④　Increased blood pressure

170. Oxygen is taken to the myocardial cells by the:

①　Pulmonary arteries
②　Subclavian arteries
③　Aorta
④　Coronary arteries

171. Which of the following is not classified as coronary artery disease?

①　Congestive heart failure
②　Myocardial infarction
③　Coronary occlusion
④　Angina pectoris

172. The nurse explains to Mr. Jones that isoenzyme blood levels are checked to determine:

①　Whether there is myocardial damage
②　Whether he has an arrhythmia
③　The strength of his myocardium
④　Whether the heart valves are effective

173. Mr. Jones is to have a Holter monitor. He is instructed that he will be required to:

①　Wear the monitor 24 hours, keeping a log of activity
②　Have a special electrocardiogram (ECG) while walking on a treadmill
③　Be on bed rest during this period
④　Not take any medication during this test

174. Mr. Jones is on a 2-g sodium, low-fat diet. He should be instructed:

①　To use salt substitutes as desired
②　That cheese may be substituted freely for meat
③　That canned soups are low in sodium
④　To use alternative condiments for salt

175. Mr. Jones is to have an arteriogram; immediately following this procedure, the nurse should assess for bleeding at the insertion site and the:

①　Pulses below the dressing
②　Urinary output
③　Level of consciousness
④　Ability to move the affected limb

176. Mr. Bynum is seen in the health clinic with a diagnosis of peripheral vascular disease. Teaching for Mr. Bynum should include:

①　Massaging feet and legs briskly twice a day to promote circulation
②　Wearing open-toed sandals only
③　Cutting his nails at least weekly
④　Inspecting feet daily for any injuries

177. Mr. Bynum is seen in the health clinic with a diagnosis of peripheral vascular disease. Mr. Bynum has intermittent claudication. This is:

①　Burning and tingling of the extremities
②　Periodic severe pain not associated with activity
③　Cramping pain brought on by exercise and relieved by rest
④　Dull aching calf pain brought on by activity, not relieved by rest

178. Mr. Burns has a stasis ulcer on his left ankle. This ulcer will probably:

①　Heal slowly with periods of exacerbation
②　Require debridement often to promote healing
③　Not heal without surgery such as sympathectomy
④　Heal quickly if protected from injury

179. Thrombophlebitis is most accurately described as:

①　Venostasis
②　A blood clot occurring in the legs or pelvis
③　Inflammation of a vein associated with clot formation
④　Infection resulting from injury to a superficial blood vessel

180. Assessment of the client with thrombophlebitis would reveal:

①　A positive Homans' sign in the affected leg
②　Cold, pale extremities
③　Vasoconstriction of the surrounding veins
④　Cyanosis of the entire affected limb

181. Clients with deep vein thrombosis should be instructed to:

①　Elevate legs when sitting
②　Check peripheral pulses often
③　Perform Berger-Allen exercises daily
④　Keep knees flexed with a pillow when in bed

182. The most serious complication of deep vein thrombosis is a:

① Stasis ulcer
② Pulmonary embolus
③ Phlebitis
④ Varicose veins

183. Mrs. Jan Smith has bilateral varicose veins. Which of the following would *not* be discussed with her prior to discharge?

① Putting support stockings on before getting out of bed
② Maintaining proper weight
③ Avoiding exercises such as walking or jogging
④ Elevating the foot of the bed for sleeping

184. Mrs. Jan Smith has bilateral varicose veins. Mrs. Smith is to have a ligation and stripping of the saphenous vein. An appropriate priority in postoperative nursing care includes:

① Maintaining knee-level pressure bandages on both legs
② Assessing for pain related to inadequate circulation
③ Encouraging dangling of legs for 5 to 10 minutes before getting up to ambulate
④ Keeping legs flat and providing sand bags to prevent external rotation

185. George Ellis is admitted to the hospital with a diagnosis of pulmonary tuberculosis. The persons most susceptible to tuberculosis are:

① Middle-aged, white women
② People who work in high-pollution conditions
③ Elderly, non-white men
④ Obese, multiparous women

186. The most accurate diagnostic test for tuberculosis is a:

① Magnetic resonance imaging (MRI) scan
② Purified protein derivative (PPD) skin test
③ Chest radiograph
④ Sputum for acid-fast bacillus

187. George Ellis is admitted to the hospital with a diagnosis of pulmonary tuberculosis. Mr. Ellis asks how long he will need to continue his antitubercular medicines. He is instructed that treatment is usually:

① 3 months
② 6 months

③ 1 to 2 years
④ 4 to 5 years

188. George Ellis is admitted to the hospital with a diagnosis of pulmonary tuberculosis. Mr. Ellis's wife was given a tine test; she is instructed to return to have it read in:

① 24 hours
② 72 hours
③ 1 week
④ 2 weeks

189. George Ellis is admitted to the hospital with a diagnosis of pulmonary tuberculosis. Mrs. Ellis's skin test was positive. This means that she:

① Has inactive tuberculosis
② Has active tuberculosis
③ Is immune to tuberculosis
④ Has antibodies against tuberculosis

190. George Ellis is admitted to the hospital with a diagnosis of pulmonary tuberculosis. Mrs. Ellis also has a positive skin test. Prophylactic treatment for Mrs. Ellis will probably last for:

① 6 weeks
② 6 months
③ 1 year
④ 2 years

191. Characteristics of *Mycobacterium tuberculosis* infection are that it:

① Affects only the lungs
② Is an acid-fast bacillus
③ Is an anaerobic organism
④ Multiplies rapidly

192. Charles Brown, age 55 years, is admitted to the oncology ward. Mr. Brown has a history of weight loss, has a persistent cough that has increased, and has had blood-tinged sputum for 2 weeks. He has smoked up to two packs of cigarettes a day for 20 years. He is an accountant and had delayed seeking medical attention until his work load was lighter. His chest radiograph revealed a mass in the right lung. He is being admitted for further evaluation and treatment. An early sign or symptom of lung cancer seen in Mr. Brown's history is:

① Persistent cough
② Hemoptysis

③ Weight loss
④ Dyspnea

193. Charles Brown, age 55 years, is admitted to the oncology ward. Mr. Brown has a history of weight loss, has a persistent cough that has increased, and has had blood-tinged sputum for 2 weeks. He has smoked up to two packs of cigarettes a day for 20 years. He is an accountant and had delayed seeking medical attention until his work load was lighter. His chest radiograph revealed a mass in the right lung. He is being admitted for further evaluation and treatment. An MRI evaluation is scheduled. You prepare Mr. Brown for this study by telling him that:

① He will have to take laxatives before the study
② A dye will be injected into his veins just before the test
③ No physical preparation is needed before the test
④ A nuclear medication is administered by the radiology department 24 hours before the test

194. Charles Brown, age 55 years, is admitted to the oncology ward. Mr. Brown has a history of weight loss, has a persistent cough that has increased, and has had blood-tinged sputum for 2 weeks. He has smoked up to two packs of cigarettes a day for 20 years. He is an accountant and had delayed seeking medical attention until his work load was lighter. His chest radiograph revealed a mass in the right lung. He is being admitted for further evaluation and treatment. Mr. Brown is scheduled for a bronchoscopy so that the lesion can be evaluated for biopsy. Mr. Brown's preoperative teaching will include an explanation that following the biopsy he will:

① Be unable to talk for several days
② Have nothing by mouth until his gag reflex returns
③ Will be unable to swallow for 12 hours
④ Experience no soreness of the throat

195. Which of the following would not be a common method of obtaining a specimen to diagnose lung cancer?

① Thoracentesis
② Needle biopsy
③ Mediastinoscopy
④ Wedge resection

196. Charles Brown, age 55 years, is admitted to the oncology ward. Mr. Brown has a history of weight loss, has a persistent cough that has increased, and has had blood-tinged sputum for 2 weeks. He has smoked up to two packs of cigarettes a day for 20 years. He is an accountant and had delayed seeking medical attention until his work load was lighter. His chest radiograph revealed a mass in the right lung. He is being admitted for further evaluation and treatment. The risk factor for lung cancer demonstrated by Mr. Brown is:

① A sedentary occupation
② Stress
③ Cigarette smoking
④ Weight loss

197. Charles Brown, age 55 years, is admitted to the oncology ward. Mr. Brown has a history of weight loss, has a persistent cough that has increased, and has had blood-tinged sputum for 2 weeks. He has smoked up to two packs of cigarettes a day for 20 years. He is an accountant and had delayed seeking medical attention until his work load was lighter. His chest radiograph revealed a mass in the right lung. He is being admitted for further evaluation and treatment. To assist Mr. Brown and his family to cope with his diagnosis, the nurse should:

① Explain procedures and their purposes before they are carried out
② Tell him the physician will have to tell him about the tests
③ Limit the number of visitors for a few days
④ Provide extensive teaching regarding his illness

198. Following a thoracotomy, the nurse positions the client:

① Only on the affected side
② On his back or affected side
③ On his back or unaffected side
④ On either side or his back

199. Which of the following surgical procedures would not require the insertion of chest tubes?

① Pneumonectomy
② Lobectomy
③ Wedge resection
④ Open biopsy

200. The main purpose of a chest tube is to:

　① Remove drainage from the alveoli
　② Remove air and fluid from the pleural space
　③ Supply oxygen to the lung
　④ Provide an easy access for chemotherapy

201. The PN is caring for a client with a chest tube connected to a three-bottle drainage system connected to suction. Which of the following observations concerning the drainage system should be reported to the physician immediately?

　① Fluctuation of fluid in the water-seal tube during ventilatory movements
　② Intermittent bubbling in the water-seal bottle
　③ Bubbling in the suction control bottle
　④ Continuous bubbling in the water-seal bottle

202. If a chest tube becomes disconnected from the drainage system, the nurse should first:

　① Reconnect and tape the tube
　② Remove the tube and apply a dressing
　③ Clamp the tube close to the disconnected area
　④ Clamp the tube near the chest wall

203. Which of the following clients, scheduled for surgery, would be most likely to experience dehydration postoperatively?

　① Adolescent clients
　② Clients with a history of cancer
　③ Clients with a history of gout
　④ Elderly clients

204. Preoperative medications ordered for your client were meperidine (Demerol) 100 mg and atropine 0.3 mg. Doses available were Demerol, 50 mg/mL, and atropine, 0.4 mg/mL. You should prepare:

　① Demerol, 0.75 mL; atropine, 1.2 mL
　② Demerol, 1.5 mL; atropine, 0.5 mL
　③ Demerol, 2 mL; atropine, 1 mL
　④ Demerol, 2 mL; atropine, 0.75 mL

205. Atropine is given to the client preoperatively to:

　① Provide general muscle relaxation
　② Cause a decrease in pulse and respiration
　③ Produce a decrease in oral and respiratory secretions
　④ Enhance the effectiveness of meperidine (Demerol)

! ANSWERS AND RATIONALES

Includes test-taking hints for the first 100 questions.

The important terms here are "usual" and "immediate complication." Although all of the answers represent possible complications, you are looking for the usual and immediate one, cardiogenic shock.

1.
④ Cardiogenic shock is characterized by the more acute symptoms the client is exhibiting. Although CHF and pulmonary edema are possible complications, they are not indicated by the symptoms.
I, 2, Myocardial infarction

You must know what "blood-tinged sputum" means to answer this question. If you realize it has to do with the lung, the only logical answer is left-sided failure, which predisposes pulmonary edema, the cause of the blood-tinged sputum.

2.
③ Left-sided heart failure is characterized by a backup of pressure and fluid in the lungs. Jill's symptoms indicate that this has occurred. Right-sided failure would produce backup in the periphery, the venous system.
III & IV, 2, Myocardial infarction

This is a simple factual knowledge question.

3.
③ Orthopnea refers to the need to assume an upright position to breathe.
III & IV, 2, Myocardial infarction

The PN needs to know the usual intended effects of a medication to answer this question.

4.
③ Inderal lowers the blood pressure and pulse rate, not raises it. It does sometimes cause depression in older patients.
III & IV, 2, Myocardial infarction/medication

The PN needs to know the common side effect of heparin, bleeding, and then what actions would help detect this problem.

5.
② Heparin can cause bleeding from mucous membranes if the level is too high. It is important to evaluate the urine for the presence of blood.
I & IV, 2, Myocardial infarction

To answer this question, the PN needs to know the correct way to administer heparin; this is simply a factual question.

6.
③ Subcutaneous heparin should be given in the fat of the abdomen. This area is less prone to trauma and bleeding. Do not massage the area because this increases bruising.
III, 2, Myocardial infarction/medication

The PN should remember that the client is often depressed after a close call with death, and exploring the client's fears and answering questions can help decrease depression.

7.
④ Depression is common after a myocardial infarction. It is important for clients to be able to express what is concerning them and have their questions answered fully.
III, 3, Myocardial infarction

This is a simple knowledge question.

8.
① According to the Food Guide Pyramid, 6 to 11 servings from the bread, cereal, rice, and pasta group are needed each day. In addition, 2 to 4 servings of fruit; 3 to 5 servings of vegetables; and 2 to 3 servings of milk, yogurt, and cheese are needed each day. Fats and sweets are to be used sparingly.
III, 4, Food Guide Pyramid

Again, this is a knowledge question, but breaking down the terms as described next will help you answer this question.

9.
③ The term "lacto" refers to milk, and "ovo" refers to egg. A lacto-ovo-vegetarian includes plant foods, dairy products, and eggs in the diet. All of the other choices contain meat and would not be included in the diet of a lacto-ovo-vegetarian.
III, 1, Vegetarian diet

This question asks for the most appropriate response. This means that more than one answer may be correct, but you are asked to make a judgment as to which is the most appropriate.

10.
② The body's most important source of energy is carbohydrates. Proteins are used in the formation of hemoglobin and as the essential component for tissue building. Fat promotes absorption of the fat-soluble vitamins.
III, 4, Nutrient functions.

Again, when the question asks for the best answer, more than one may be correct and you must choose the best answer. This also asks for a negative, which should be avoided. This tends to mean that some answers contain foods that would be recommended.

11. Foods high in cholesterol include foods of ani-
③ mal origin: meat, eggs, whole milk, and milk
products. Foods from plant sources are not
high in cholesterol.
III, 4, Sources of cholesterol

12. During an acute attack of diverticulosis, a clear
④ liquid diet is given. After the acute attack has
subsided, however, the client is maintained on
a high-fiber diet to increase the bulk of the
stool and propel the fecal matter through the
intestinal tract. The gluten-free diet, high-
protein diet, and low-fat diet are not helpful
in diverticulosis.
II, 1 & 2, Diverticulosis

**This is a simple knowledge question. You must know
what foods are high in fiber.**

13. Foods high in fiber include whole grain breads
② and cereals, peas, and lentils. Eggs, milk,
cheese, fish, and poultry are high in protein,
not fiber. Unsaturated vegetable oils contain
no fiber.
III, 4, Sources of fiber

**This question asks you to make a judgment. It is not
reasonable to tell a teenager not to eat any fast foods,
so you must go with the most reasonable answer.**

14. If selected wisely, "fast foods" can play a role
③ in meeting nutrient needs. Eating salads without high-fat dressings, omitting high-calorie
toppings, and modifying other meals to compensate are strategies that are helpful. "Junk
foods" are high in sugar and fat and contain
"empty" calories. Fast foods are not necessarily high in vitamins.
III, 4, Food selection

**You must know what problems might occur after
cataract surgery to know what is important in the
client's postoperative care plan.**

15. The client will probably be wearing a patch,
② and his vision will not be clear; assisting him
postoperatively in relation to his physical surroundings and other safety concerns is essential.
II, 1, Cataract

**This question and the next focus on the inappropriate
answer. This means that three of the answers will be
appropriate, and you are looking for the one that is
not correct for this client. This type of question is
often best treated as a true-false question, and you
want the one false answer.**

16. Complete bed rest is discouraged to avoid po-
④ tential development of thrombosis and pulmonary congestion. The rest of the items are all
routine areas of patient education related to
congestive heart failure.
III, 2, Congestive heart failure

17. Clients need a comprehensive understanding
④ of the disease and management to help allay
their anxiety.
II, 2, Respiratory

**Again, this question asks for the best response, mean-
ing that there may be more than one correct response.
It also asks you, as do the next two questions, to look
at the normal aging process as a basis for your answer.**

18. Basic intelligence is maintained but retrieval
① of information from long-term memory is
slowed.
III, 2, Age-related changes

19. There is a reduction in visual fields, the pupil is
③ less responsive to light, and depth perception
becomes distorted.
I, 1, Safety and falls

20. Depression in the elderly is often manifested
② by physical symptoms.
I, 3, Depression

**This is asking for basic information; however, you
must also remember the developmental level of the
young girl.**

21. At 8 weeks, all the basic body systems have
① formed and are ready for growth and maturation, the fetus is less than 2 inches long, and
the head is almost half the fetal length. A fetus
is approximately 12 inches long and covered
with lanugo by 24 weeks of gestation. External
sex identification is not usually possible until
11 to 12 weeks of gestation.
III, 4, Fetal development

**This question contains the key words "most likely."
This means that all may be correct, but one answer
is the best.**

22. A hands-and-knees position may help the fetus
② to rotate to a more favorable position and thus
hasten the delivery. Internal monitoring techniques facilitate monitoring fetal condition but
do not affect the timing of the delivery. Increasing the intravenous flow rate and giving oxygen are indicated in situations of fetal distress;
these actions do not hasten delivery. A cool

cloth and a back rub are comfort measures to help the patient cope with labor but do not directly assist the fetus to rotate to an anterior position.
II, 2, Labor and birth

The key word in this question is "next." You would do all these things, but one will be next in the sequence. Think to yourself what the priority of steps would be and then answer the question based on this.

23. Wiping the infant's face and suctioning help
② provide for a clear airway and should be done before the body is delivered and the baby takes his or her first breath. After clearing the airway, the nurse should check to see whether the cord is around the neck and then gently guide the infant's head downward to deliver the anterior shoulder, followed by a gentle upward maneuver to deliver the posterior shoulder. Although there is no need to rush once the head is delivered, the delivery should be accomplished shortly thereafter or the safety of the infant and mother will be compromised.
III, 1 & 2, Labor and birth (precipitous delivery)

You can treat this question as true-false. Three will be done, and one would be the least likely to be done. You are looking for the one false answer.

24. Performing eye prophylaxis interferes with
③ eye contact, which is important for bonding; this procedure can safely be delayed in the first hour after delivery. All other interventions listed are appropriate to facilitate parent-infant bonding.
III, 4, Parent-infant attachment

This is a priority-setting question. Again, think of what you would do and in what order. The key word here is "first."

25. One of the major side effects of epidural anes-
④ thesia and a supine position in the term pregnant woman is hypotension. Turning the woman to her side takes pressure off the major blood vessels, relieves supine hypotensive syndrome, and helps to restore a more normal blood pressure. Giving supplemental oxygen would be appropriate if the fetal monitor strip showed signs of distress but only after the pressure was relieved from the vena cava. The other actions are appropriate follow-ups to repositioning.
II (prioritizing) & III, 1 & 2, Labor and birth (pain management)

Be sure to read a question like this carefully, because all the answers may contain some correct information but one will be the most appropriate.

26. Application of cold appropriately suppresses
① the production of milk in the non–breast-feeding client and helps alleviate symptoms of engorgement. Applying warm compresses would be helpful to relieve engorgement for the client who is breast-feeding because it would stimulate the let-down reflex. Pumping and massaging the breasts tend to stimulate milk production, which is not desired in this situation.
II, 2, Postpartum care

In a question such as this, you must know several things. First, you need to know what each of the drugs listed does. Then you need to think which has an action that would decrease wound healing leading to an increased risk of dehiscence.

27. Corticosteroids decrease wound healing by in-
① hibition of fibroblast formation and collagen deposition. Heparin is an intravenous and subcutaneous anticoagulant that decreases platelet aggregation. Morphine is an analgesic that depresses the central nervous system. Aminophylline is a bronchodilator that opens up the airway and is a central nervous system stimulant.
I, 2, Steroid therapy

The next two questions focus on the side effects or toxic effects of medications. These are simple questions but require a knowledge of the effects of specific medications.

28. This is higher than the therapeutic range of
③ 0.5 to 2.0 ng/mL. The nurse should assess for symptoms of digoxin toxicity, which include arrhythmias, bradycardia, tachycardia, and irregular pulse. Other side effects include anorexia, nausea and vomiting, blurred vision, and yellow-green halos.
IV, 2, Digoxin therapeutic level

29. This level is in the toxic range. The nurse
④ should hold the drug because it may increase theophylline levels and then notify the physician. It is not in the scope of practice of the LPN or RN to change the amount of a drug ordered.
III, 2, Theophylline levels

This is a straight knowledge question, but two levels of knowledge are required. First, you must know the

action of aminophylline, then you must know the appropriate disease it is used to treat. Medication questions are often written this way.

30. Aminophylline is a bronchodilator and used
④ in the treatment of bronchospasm in restrictive types of diseases (chronic obstructive pulmonary disease, asthma, emphysema).
IV, 2, Aminophylline

This is another true-false question. Look for the incorrect answer.

31. Skin should be pulled to the side by tensing
② of the skin laterally. Bunching of the skin is used with subcutaneous administration. Placing 0.2 mL of air in the syringe after the correct amount of solution is drawn up prevents leaking and clears the needle of all the medication.
III, 2, Z tract

To answer this question, you must know the action of both medications even though the question asks you about only one of them. When studying medication questions, try to identify the classification of the medication, then think what you know about medications of that class. Chapter 4, Medication Administration, should help you with this.

32. Spironolactone (Aldactone) is a potassium-
② sparing diuretic and aids in replacing the potassium lost with furosemide (Lasix), a potassium-depleting diuretic. Potassium levels should still be determined periodically because potassium depletion is still possible. Dehydration is a side effect because the action of diuretics is to remove excess fluids. Clients are at lesser risk for thrombophlebitis in fluid excess because blood is more dilute. In fluid deficit or dehydration, there is an increased chance of blood clots or thrombophlebitis because of hypercoagulability of the blood.
IV, 2, Diuretics

You are again looking for the one incorrect answer. Try to find three symptoms of early shock and the remaining answer is the incorrect one. Remember, if you can eliminate one or two other answers, your chances of choosing the correct response increase.

33. Bradycardia is not a symptom of early shock.
② Tachypnea, restlessness, and cool, clammy skin are all signs of early shock and the body's compensation for the threat of shock.
I, 2, Emergency care

34. Peristalsis is decreased, leading to a buildup
② of gas and gastric secretions; this may result

in nausea and vomiting, which increases risk of aspiration. The gastrointestinal system would be hyperacidic with decreased peristalsis. Decreased peristalsis would lead to constipation, not diarrhea. Infection is not directly related to the gastrointestinal system.
II, 2, Burns

This is an assessment question. You are being asked to assess pain in a fresh postoperative client. You need to think about the client's condition at this time. Is the client alert enough to ask for pain medications? Always consider the best response in this given situation.

35. Because the client is still under the effects
③ of anesthesia, he or she will not be competent to ask for pain medication or to use self-administered medication. Not all clients require the same amount of pain relief; this would be an ineffective evaluation of adequate pain relief. Monitoring verbal and physical cues would provide the most effective evaluation of adequate pain management.
IV, 2, Postoperative care

This question requires you to know two things. First, what is the possible cause of the decreased respiratory rate? Next, what can a PN do about this problem? You need to know both parts to correctly answer the question.

36. This amount of decrease in respirations proba-
③ bly requires immediate intervention. As a PN, you are responsible for reporting this information to the RN. Currently, PNs do not receive phone orders from physicians or administer intravenous medications.
IV, 2, Respiratory

In this case, the client needs education to understand proper use of pain medications.

37. This client is showing lack of understanding
③ related to pain medications. Educating the client to the benefits of pain relief and helping him understand the minimal risk of addiction will most likely decrease his fears and increase his compliance level. This decreases the risk of postsurgical complications. Praising the client for wanting to be drug-free may lead him to believe that addiction is a high risk for him. Unless under legal commitment, clients have the right to refuse medications.
III, 2, Postoperative care

This asks for a noninvasive pain relief method. You must choose an answer that would be noninvasive.

38.
③
Altering the external stimuli is an external pain management intervention. Increasing fluids and administering oral pain medications are invasive techniques. Verbally belittling the client's pain will probably increase anxiety and increase the pain.
II, 2, Pain management

39.
②
Increasing fluids assists in decreasing the toxic effects of chemotherapeutic drugs on body organs. Clients with cancer are in a catabolic state and require an increased caloric intake. Because of low or ineffective white blood cell status, clients receiving chemotherapeutic drugs are at increased risk for infection and should avoid crowds.
II, 2, Cancer

This is a psychosocial question. You need to think about concepts associated with therapeutic communication when answering questions like this one. It is always a good idea to choose an answer that promotes communication and encourages the client to express feelings.

40.
②
This woman has had a procedure that has altered her body image. Refusal to look at the involved area suggests an altered self-concept. Allowing her to express her feelings about her body increases the potential for self-acceptance. Lack of looking at the incision suggests she is currently concerned about her body image more than cancer. Time alone may increase her sense of now being different. Informing her that she is going to change her own dressing is again not addressing her current needs.
III, 3, Mental health

This question asks you to understand the legal rights of clients and to answer the question based on that knowledge.

41.
②
Unless a client is physically or mentally incompetent, he or she has a right to decide how or where to live. The family's choice does not override the client's unless the client is incompetent. When incompetence exists, the client may not have a choice. Placing a client in a restrictive environment can lead to a decrease in functional status.
II, 1, Mental health

When answering this question and the next, think of what the environment is like in an intensive care unit or in isolation. This knowledge will help you focus your answer on what the client may be experiencing.

42.
①
A client in the intensive care unit experiences an increase in auditory, visual, and tactile stimulation. Because of the level of care required, the client also experiences altered sleep patterns. Clients in the intensive care unit are generally too ill to be bored. The monitors and frequent care contribute to sensory overload versus sensory deprivation. Clients are not usually addicted to narcotics in 3 days.
I, 3, Mental health

43.
③
A client who is confined to bed in a private room would be likely to experience a decrease in stimuli. This client is not ambulatory and would probably not be at risk for falls. The client's communication would remain unchanged.
III, 3, Mental health

44.
④
This client is suffering from sensory overload from the stimulation of the intensive care unit environment. The overstimulation has led to hallucinations. Clients in the intensive care unit are too ill for diversional activities. Although confusion is a symptom of a cerebrovascular accident, clients do not usually evidence symptoms of hallucinations.
I, 3, Mental health

Always read the information given to you about the client carefully. In this case, the important information is that the client has a regular alcohol intake. With this history, the PN should suspect alcohol withdrawal may be the problem.

45.
④
This client is experiencing withdrawal. It is the PN's responsibility to report changes in condition to the RN. It is the responsibility of the RN to call the physician. This client is not physically in control of calming down. This is a physical addiction. Asking the family to bring in beer would enable this client's condition; also, beer could interact with this client's other medical conditions, procedures, or medications.
III, 3, Mental health

These next few are simply factual questions.

46.
②
The first step in the CPR procedure, according to the American Heart Association, is to establish whether or not the client is responsive. Next, establish the *a*irway, restore *b*reathing, and then *c*irculation ("ABC").
III, 1, CPR

47. The tongue falls back into the throat when the
④ client loses consciousness. This can obstruct the airway and cause death.
I, 2, CPR

48. One rescuer should ventilate and compress at
① the rate of 2 breaths for every 15 compressions. If there are two rescuers, the ratio is 1 breath to every 5 compressions.
III, 1, CPR

49. CPR should be carried out until the person
② regains a satisfactory intrinsic pulse, the person is pronounced dead, or the rescuer is exhausted and unable to continue and no one else is available to perform CPR. Pupils may be dilated for other reasons.
III, 1, CPR

When a question asks for a goal, you should first think about what would be realistic and possible to accomplish. You should also consider which goal is the most important. In shock, increasing the oxygen level is the most important goal, through increasing the blood pressure and heart rate.

50. The primary goal in treating shock is to restore
② effective tissue perfusion. Oxygenation is the overall objective.
II, 2, Shock

This question asks for priorities; after giving you the first two, it asks what to do next.

51. The third priority in treating shock is establish-
① ing an intravenous line so that fluids, medications, and blood can be given immediately. Following this, blood gases are measured, an electrocardiograph monitor is attached, and a catheter is inserted.
III, 1, Shock

This question asks for the assessment findings most appropriate for hypovolemic shock.

52. When the client suffers from shock, vasocon-
④ striction is one of the first compensatory mechanisms associated with shock. The vasoconstriction causes the cold, clammy skin, and if the shock continues, hypotension occurs. Urine output is decreased to conserve fluids, and the heart rate increases.
I, 2, Shock

This question focuses on the assessment of anaphylactic shock. Compare it with the previous one to think about different findings with different kinds of shock.

53. Anaphylactic shock is the result of a severe
② antibody-antigen reaction. This reaction causes damage to the cells of the respiratory epithelium, resulting in edema.
I, 2, Shock

The next series of questions deals with an elderly client with a cataract extraction. Interventions and assessments are asked for. Read each answer carefully, and focus on whether it is an intervention or assessment.

54. Items in the environment should not be moved
③ after the client is oriented to her location to prevent her from tripping, falling, or walking into items. Thus, safety and client dignity are preserved.
III, 1, Cataract surgery

55. Sudden or severe pain in the eye can indicate
① increased intraocular pressure or hemorrhage.
I, 1 & 2, Cataract surgery

56. Any actions that increase intraocular pressure
② should be avoided, especially coughing or sneezing. The eye patch, if in place, is used to collect drainage and should not be applying pressure to the eye. Turning the client to the operative side might increase intraocular pressure, so it is an inappropriate nursing action. Complete bed rest is unnecessary.
II, 1 & 2, Cataract surgery

This question again asks for the most helpful answer, meaning that more than one answer may be correct but only one is helpful in planning a low-fat diet. With diet questions, first be sure you understand the prescription and then look for the foods that most meet that plan.

57. Linoleic acid, an essential fatty acid, cannot be
③ manufactured in the body and must be supplied in the diet. Fats contain 9 calories per gram. Fruits are not a source of dietary fat. Saturated fats come from animal sources.
II, 2 & 4, Diet planning

58. Foods high in potassium include citrus fruits,
① bananas, tomatoes, potatoes, meat, milk, legumes, and dark green leafy vegetables. Liver, organ meats, seafood, coffee, and nuts are not good sources of potassium.
III, 4, Sources of potassium

59. A saturated fat comes from an animal source
① and is solid at room temperature. An unsaturated fat is an oil and generally comes from a plant source. Omega-3 fatty acids are unsaturated forms of fat obtained from fish. The essential fatty acid is found in vegetable oils.
III, 4, Fats

60. Of the foods listed, pretzels have the highest
② sodium content. Broccoli, bananas, and fresh meat contain smaller amounts of sodium.
III, 4, Sources of sodium

61. Even though the Medicare program has under-
④ gone many changes and will continue to do so, its intent remains providing medical coverage to those older than age 65.
IV, 1, Health insurance

The next two questions deal with psychosocial issues. For these questions, remember that the best response is one that encourages the client to talk. Do not give advice or try to give the client the "answers."

62. It is generally noted that knowing oneself in
③ relation to mortality and death is necessary before being able to care successfully for the dying.
IV, 4, Death and dying

63. The nurse is showing understanding and ac-
① ceptance. She knows that the elderly experience many losses and that it is natural to have feelings of sadness.
III, 4, Grieving

This is a different kind of question, one that asks the least important point. To answer this question, try to list the important factors. It can also be seen as a true-false question in which the correct answer is the "wrong" one.

64. Nerve damage is indicated by pain, loss of
③ sensation, and no pulse.
IV, 2, Fractured hip

65. Sandbags at the thigh and lower leg assist in
① keeping the leg in proper position.
III, 2, Fractured hip

This is an evaluation question. You are asked to evaluate the client's knowledge by again looking for the incorrect response, the one showing that the client needs more teaching.

66. The use of tampons is not recommended dur-
① ing the postpartum period because of an in-

creased risk of infection and injury. All of the other statements made by the client demonstrate an understanding of postpartum self-care instructions.
IV, 4, Postpartum care

Again, consider this a true-false question looking for the inappropriate response.

67. The fundus may be gently palpated to deter-
② mine its location and tone after a cesarean section, but it should not be routinely massaged, as after a vaginal delivery. All other interventions would be appropriate for a client with either type of delivery.
II, 2, Postpartum care

This is a two-part question. You must first know the effects and adverse effects of magnesium sulfate and then what the priority nursing intervention would be if those adverse effects occur.

68. Absent reflexes and a respiratory rate below 12
② are symptoms of magnesium toxicity and indicate a need for the drug to be discontinued. Notification of the physician and close monitoring of the client are the next most appropriate interventions. Oxygen is administered, if ordered, usually by face mask. Magnesium sulfate is given to prevent seizures; toxicity causes central nervous system and respiratory depression; therefore, seizure activity is not expected.
II (prioritizing) and III, 1 & 2, Complications of childbearing (pregnancy-induced hypertension)

These questions require you to know the normal anatomy so that you can identify the abnormal findings.

69. A normal umbilical cord contains three vessels:
④ one vein and two arteries. A two-vessel cord is often associated with congenital anomalies and should be reported to the physician. All of the other findings are normal newborn characteristics.
I, 2, Newborn assessment

70. The so-called mongolian spot is found in ap-
② proximately 90% of infants of African, Indian, Asian, or Mediterranean descent and 10% of white babies. It is not associated with mistreatment or mental retardation, and it is not a bruise. The parents should be reassured that this is a normal finding and that mongolian spots usually fade in early childhood.
I, 2, Newborn assessment

This is again a two-part question. You must assess the cause of the tremors and then decide the priority nursing intervention to treat it.

71. ② Jittery behavior and tremors are symptoms of hypoglycemia, which has a tendency to develop in large infants (and infants born to diabetic mothers). The blood glucose should be checked and feedings of 5% or 10% glucose water given if the blood glucose is less than 40 mg/dL. The other interventions are not indicated at this time.
III, 1 & 2, Care of the newborn

To answer this question, you must know the side effects of heparin. You would then know that checking for bleeding is the correct response.

72. ② Heparin can cause bleeding from mucous membranes if the level is too high. It is important to evaluate the urine for the presence of blood.
I & IV, 2, Myocardial infarction

To answer this question, you would need to know what the risk factors are for heart disease and whether or not these risks can be modified.

73. ③ Lifestyle behavior that can be changed may reduce the risks of a heart attack but may not prevent it; therefore choices 1, 2, and 4 would not be correct. Because gender, age, and family history are major risk factors and they are not modifiable, the patient should be told that he can lower his risk through modifying behaviors but may not be able to prevent a heart attack.
I & II, 4, Cardiovascular disease.

74. ① The most likely problem after a catheterization is the formation of a hematoma. If a hematoma occurs, it may seriously impair circulation. The other choices are not likely to occur.
I & II, 1, Cardiac catheterization.

This again asks a true-false question: which of the following is unrelated to the presence of a urinary tract infection.

75. ① Signs of urinary tract infections include choices 2, 3, and 4. Nausea and vomiting would not occur as a result of a urinary tract infection, although these symptoms may be associated with pyelonephritis.
I, 2, Urinary tract infection

76. ③ "Dysuria" is the medical term for painful voiding. The usage of correct medical terminology is desirable for reporting information.
II, 1, Urinary tract infection

77. ② Cranberry juice is offered to clients with urinary tract infections because it increases the acidity of the urine. Acidic urine decreases the rate of bacterial multiplication. The other options are not known actions of cranberry juice.
II, 1, Urinary tract infection

As with most medication questions, this one requires you to know the side effects and intended effects and then decide what to teach the client.

78. ④ Gantrisin is a sulfa derivative that can cause crystal and stone formation in the urine. Clients taking Gantrisin should increase their fluid intake. It is not necessary to interrupt Mary's sleep.
III, 1, Urinary tract infection

A top priority in assessing a client is to ask questions about the condition and why the client thinks he or she has a problem.

79. ③ The first step should be to find out why the client believes that she has the disease. This information determines the second step. It is not within the role of the nurse to make judgments about the client's sexual activities. Choice 2 would not be done initially. Choice 4 is incorrect, in that most states provide for the treatment of sexually transmitted diseases without parental consent.
III, 4, Syphilis

This is a simple question that asks you to identify a problem based on a given set of symptoms.

80. ① Syphilis is a sexually transmitted disease that occurs in stages. In the primary stage, chancre, which is painless, appears, then disappears in 2 to 6 weeks. Primary syphilis can be cured with large doses of penicillin. Symptoms of primary herpes are dysuria, vaginal discharge, and a very painful lesion. Gonorrhea is characterized by vaginal discharge, pelvic pain, and dysuria. Symptoms of *Chlamydia* infection include burning on urination and vaginal discharge, although women are asymptomatic 70% of the time.
I, 4, Syphilis

This question asks for the most routine diagnostic test. Although several tests might be done, only one is the common test.

81.
② Although choices 1 and 3 can be correct in some cases, they are not routinely done. Cultures take 24 to 48 hours to grow and are impractical in many cases.
I, 4, Syphilis

Again, you must know the action of the medication to answer this question correctly.

82.
① Large doses of penicillin are administered for the treatment of syphilis. Penicillin is lost in the urine. Probenecid inhibits the excretion of penicillin. The PN should be able to explain the action of drugs that are administered.
II, 1, Syphilis/medication

You must know the normal assessment findings for a 4-month-old in order to answer this question. Three of the answers are normal findings, and one is an abnormal finding.

83.
② The other choices are all normal findings in a 4-month-old.
I, 2, Bronchiolitis

84.
③ The semi-Fowler's position allows for expansion of the lungs by lowering the contents of the abdominal cavity. A high Fowler's position is poorly tolerated by infants.
II, 2, Bronchiolitis

A question such as this may have more than one correct answer, but you need to identify the most appropriate action for a child in a mist tent.

85.
② Children in mist tents require a frequent change of clothing to keep dry. The child can be observed inside the tent, and parents may get into the tent for cuddling. Olivia should spend as much time as possible in the mist tent. She should not be disturbed for feeding every 3 hours.
III, 1, Bronchiolitis

Of the options given, rectal is the most appropriate. You might be thinking that the best way is with an ear thermometer, but that is not a choice. Remember, you can choose only from the options that are given.

86.
③ Olivia's temperature should be taken rectally. She is too young for oral temperatures. The cool mist tent would result in lower skin temperature.
II, 1, Basic skills

You need to know the correct specific gravity to answer this question. This way you can identify which data would show the best fluid balance.

87.
② Specific gravity measurement is ordered to determine the concentration of urine. Choice 1 indicates that the urine is dilute. Choices 3 and 4 indicate that the urine is highly concentrated.
IV, 2, Fluid balance

88.
③ This is the only option that is factually correct. It has been noted that children with a history of bronchiolitis frequently experience asthmatic allergic reactions. Choices 1, 2, and 4 are false statements.
III, 4, Bronchiolitis

You need to know the correct method for administering ear drops in a child for this question. Remember, it is different for an adult.

89.
② The correct method to administer ear drops to an infant is to pull the ear down and back. This action is necessary to straighten the eustachian tube.
III, 2, Medication administration

Again, you need to know the correct site for an injection in a child. The thigh is the most appropriate site because of the muscle development.

90.
④ Thigh muscles are the best site for intramuscular injections for infants. Other muscles are small and poorly developed.
III, 2, Medication administration

This is another true-false question with the correct answer being the false one.

91.
③ In response to pain, the pupils dilate. Pupil constriction may be observed following the administration of pain medication. Choices 1, 2, and 4 are other responses to pain.
I, 2 & 3, Bronchiolitis

This is a simple factual question that requires you to know the normal schedule for a DPT immunization.

92.
③ The normal schedule for DPT immunizations for an infant is 2, 4, and 6 months.
II, 1, Immunizations

This question asks you to understand the most appropriate way to administer pain medications for maximum pain relief.

93.
④ Administering pain medication on a routine schedule along with as-needed (p.r.n.) medication is the most effective pain relief. As-needed medication is not enough relief for the client who is in constant pain. Assessment of the pain is not an intervention.
III, 2, Pain management

This question requires that you know the appropriate role of the PN and what can be done by the PN.

94. As a PN, you are responsible for reporting this
④ finding to the RN. Currently, it is not within your practice to take orders over the phone from the physician. Applying pressure to the rectal area or educating the client not to strain does not facilitate finding the cause of the bleeding.
III, 2, Gastrointestinal care

95. Iron causes the stools to darken or turn green.
② Taking iron should lead to an increase in hemoglobin, which leads to an increased oxygen carrying capacity. Clients taking iron are more likely to suffer from constipation than diarrhea.
I, 2, Pharmacology

When a child has had a previous experience in a hospital, it is important to explore those experiences so you can understand what the child is actually feeling.

96. Jason's previous experience with hospitaliza-
④ tion will have resulted in certain preconceptions.
II, 3, Tonsillectomy

For this question, the PN needs to know the normal growth and development of children to understand the common fears of a child of this age.

97. Fear of body mutilation is a dominant fear of
① the preschool-aged child.
II, 3, Growth and development

It is always better to give any client, even a child, an honest answer. If you are not honest, the client will lose trust in you and any relationship will be difficult.

98. Choice 1 reflects honesty. Choices 2 and 3 indi-
① cate that the nurse is critical of Jason's fear. Choice 4 ignores the question.
III, 3, Perioperative care

The next two questions require you to calculate the correct dosages. You may not use a calculator on the examination but will be provided with scratch paper to figure your answer.

99. If one uses ratio and proportion, the correct
② response is choice 2. $50:1 = 35:X$.
III, 2, Medication administration

100. If one uses ratio and proportion, the only cor-
③ rect answer is choice 3. $100:2 = 12.5:X$.
III, 2, Medication administration

101. The compatibility chart is the correct source
④ of information. Choices 1 and 2 are incorrect practices. Choice 3 is a poor answer because the other nurse may not know the correct answer either.
III, 1, Medication administration

102. Jason must have the injection. In response 1,
② Jason's reaction is to the situation, not the nurse. Jason's parents should be allowed to stay because their presence may be a comfort.
III, 3, Medication administration

103. Of the listed choices, tepid water is the best
② option. Fluids that are too hot or too cold should be avoided. Orange juice is acidic and may cause burning. Milk causes coating of the membranes and thickened secretions.
III, 2, Tonsillectomy

104. This is the best response because after a
② tonsillectomy children are prone to experience hemorrhage as the membrane in the throat is sloughed. This occurs in about 5 days. There is nothing to indicate that Jason has choice 1 or 3. The ingestion of rough foods would more likely result in bleeding earlier.
III, 2 & 4, Tonsillectomy

105. The best time to schedule the procedure is
④ early morning. The parasites emerge at night and adhere to the sticky surface of the tape. A commercially prepared swab is also available.
III, 1, Pinworms

106. Good hand-washing technique helps prevent
① spread of the pinworm eggs from the hands to the mouth.
II, 1, Pinworms

107. Everyone caring for the child should be made
③ aware that the stools may be red. This information helps to avoid any misunderstanding of the finding.
III, 2, Pinworms

108. It is imperative that nurses avoid palpating the
① tumor because this could result in rupture of the tumor capsule. Choices 2 and 3 are not components of care for a child with Wilms' tumor. The child would most likely not be on complete bed rest.
II, 1, Wilms' tumor

109. Parents should be honest with their children.
② Choices 1 and 3 might cause the child to not want to go to sleep or to play. Choice 4 might result in a poor, nontrusting relationship between the child and the nurse.
III, 3, Growth and development

110. It is normal for the toddler to cry when she is
② left by her parents. Choices 1 and 4 would reflect a poor parent-child relationship. Hiding under the bed is not a behavior to anticipate in this situation.
I, 3, Growth and development

111. Choice 1 is incorrect, in that a large cuff results
② in a lower pressure reading. Choice 4 would result in a higher reading. The thigh would be the second choice.
I, 2, Basic skills

112. This is the first observable behavioral sign. All
① answers may be correct, but not observed first.
I, 2, Pain

113. Children with Legg-Calvé-Perthes disease fre-
① quently complain of hip and knee pain. The other symptoms are most likely due to other causes.
I, 4, Legg-Calvé-Perthes

114. The aim of conservative treatment is to prevent
④ pressure on the femoral head.
II, 1, Legg-Calvé-Perthes

115. Prolonged immobility is difficult for school-
④ aged children. There is usually no diet restriction. The disease does not cause fatigue. The child may return to school with braces.
IV, 3, Legg-Calvé-Perthes

116. Alcohol helps to toughen the skin. Choices 2
① and 3 should be performed daily. The child should be placed on bed rest until the braces are repaired.
III, 4, Legg-Calvé-Perthes

117. This is the only safe activity of those listed.
① The other activities could result in slippage of the head of the femur.
I, 2, Legg-Calvé-Perthes

118. The school-aged child is placed in the stage of
① industry versus inferiority. He should have

mastered trust and autonomy. He is too young to be mastering intimacy.
I, 3, Growth and development

119. Enlarged lymph nodes are a typical finding
④ of clients with infectious mononucleosis. The other symptoms might indicate a secondary diagnosis. Lesions of the gums are more common than lesions of the lip.
I, 2, Infectious mononucleosis

120. Infectious mononucleosis is slightly conta-
① gious. Good hand-washing technique is sufficient to prevent the spread of disease, and the various types of isolation are inappropriate in this situation.
III, 1, Infectious mononucleosis

121. Knowledge of diagnostic tests aids the PN in
③ client education. Choices 1, 2, and 4 would not confirm the diagnosis.
I, 4, Infectious mononucleosis

122. Orange juice, which is acidic, would not be
① given to Shannon because an extremely sore throat is a frequent complaint. Bland liquids and puddings are better tolerated. The remainder of the options are appropriate choices.
III, 2, Infectious mononucleosis

123. Hepatomegaly occurs in about 10% of the
④ cases. It usually resolves within 3 months. The other symptoms are not known complications of mononucleosis.
II, 4, Infectious mononucleosis

124. This reflects the best understanding of follow-
③ up convalescence. Shannon would not have to be on complete bed rest. She should slowly resume her normal activities with additional rest periods. Avoiding crowds would be appropriate only in the early stage of the disease.
IV, 4, Infectious mononucleosis

125. The major stress for hospitalized adolescents
④ is fear of loss of control in front of others. Although the other options may be true of a particular client, Choice 4 is considered the best of the options.
I, 3, Growth and development

126. Infectious mononucleosis is spread by contact
① with oral secretions. This knowledge aids the PN in preventing spread of the disease.
III, 1, Infectious mononucleosis

127. Rubella (German measles) can cause serious
② congenital malformations if contracted by a
pregnant woman, particularly during the first
trimester.
III, 1, Rubella

128. Koplik spots are bluish-white pinpoint spots
③ that appear in the mouth on about the second
or third day of the disease. They usually appear before the skin rash.
I, 2, Rubeola

129. The duration of the rubeola is about 7 days.
① Sometimes rubeola is referred to as the "7-day
measles."
II, 2, Rubeola

130. Nephrotic syndrome is characterized by proteinuria, hypoproteinemia, oliguria, and generalized edema. This excess extra fluid volume should be a nursing priority in care plan development.
I, 2, Nephrotic syndrome

131. The cause of nephrotic syndrome remains unknown. Parents frequently feel guilty and anxious when their child is ill, and every member of the health team should give consistent information.
I, 4, Nephrotic syndrome

132. The aim of steroid therapy is to prevent the
③ loss of protein in the urine by decreasing inflammation of the glomeruli. The benefits outweigh the numerous side effects in this situation.
II, 2, Nephrotic syndrome

133. The child will lose massive amounts of protein
② in the urine. Lowering the salt content may
aid in reducing edema.
III, 1, Nephrotic syndrome

134. Stored urine can result in false-positive results;
② thus, urine should either be stored in a refrigerator or transported immediately to the laboratory. Forcing fluids results in dilute urine. The specimen collected should be midstream. Betadine affects the results.
III, 1, Basic skills

135. Mononucleosis does not precede glomerulonephritis; glomerulonephritis is usually preceded by a group A beta-hemolytic streptococcal infection. The other three options may be caused by a streptococcal infection.
IV, 2, Glomerulonephritis

136. Urinalysis findings with glomerulonephritis include specific gravity less than 1.030, positive blood and protein, and white blood cells. Glucose and bacteria in the urine are not clinical findings with the disease.
I, 1, Glomerulonephritis

137. The PN should recognize that to complete the
④ assessment, he or she must first establish a rapport. Insurance information should be obtained by the financial department.
I, 3, Cast

138. Wet casts are easily indented. The other options are incorrect.
III, 1, Cast

139. Complaints 1 and 2 indicate decreased circulation. Increased respirations have many causes.
I, 2, Cast

140. This can be accomplished by using a fan. Nothing should ever be put inside the cast.
III, 1, Cast

141. Impetigo is a skin infection usually caused by
④ staphylococci or streptococci. It usually occurs on the face and hands. Impetigo is contagious, and steps should be taken to prevent the spread. The disease usually leaves no scars.
III, 2, Impetigo

142. Impetigo that is caused by streptococci can result in glomerulonephritis. Reye's syndrome is associated with viral infections and the use of aspirin.
I, 1, Impetigo

143. Normally, central facial injuries are unusual
④ because children protect this area. Children often cry during examinations. Bruises on the forehead and knees can be accidental. A broken arm in a child of 6 years of age is not as questionable as a broken arm in a child younger than 2 years of age.
I, 1, Child abuse

144. Documentation is extremely important. Care
③ should be taken to chart and report what you observe, but perceptions should never be charted. It is the law that suspected child abuse be reported.
III, 1, Child abuse

145. Aggressive behavior is not a cause of anxiety.
③ The other options refer to common causes of anxiety.
I, 3, Anxiety

146. One of the major side effects is the develop-
④ ment of extrapyramidal symptoms. The most common of these is tardive dyskinesia, which is a rumination-like effect characterized by facial grimaces and involuntary movements of the lips, tongue, and jaw. If this develops, the physician should be notified because non-phenothiazine tranquilizers could be substituted. The other options are common side effects that do not require physician interventions.
III, 3, Medications/anxiety

147. When the client is taking a drug such as Val-
③ ium, the use of any other central nervous system depressant is contraindicated. There is no need to take the drug with food or milk. The drug typically causes drowsiness, and the client should be warned of this; however, it does not require that the drug be stopped. Caffeine can inhibit the drug's effects.
III, 3, Medications/anxiety

148. Mask and gown are necessary only if there
① is a possibility of splash or droplet exposure. One should wear gloves when handling any material exposed to blood or other body fluids.
III, 4, Postpartum

149. The HIV-positive mother may need additional
② support in caring for her infant and in establishing bonding with the newborn. Rooming-in is not contraindicated for the mother or newborn.
III, 4, Postpartum

150. Hand washing is absolutely mandatory before
③ and after all procedures with *all* clients. It is the most basic and important action in infection control.
III, 4, Postpartum

151. HIV has been isolated in breast milk, and
① breast-feeding is discouraged. Approximately 40% of the infants born to HIV-positive mothers test seropositive themselves. If the newborn's status is negative, breast-feeding may pass the virus to it.
III, 4, Postpartum

152. The mother should care for the infant using
③ appropriate techniques. It is not necessary to wear gloves for contact with unsoiled articles or intact skin.
III, 4, Postpartum

153. Maturation (choice 1) refers to attaining maxi-
② mal development, and growth (choice 3) refers to an increase in size. Assessment of development should be a part of the admission process, which aids in all steps of the nursing process.
I, 4, Growth and development

154. The term "cephalocaudal" refers to a head-to-
③ tail or top-to-bottom direction. This knowledge should be used in assessment and in planning for client safety.
I, 2 & 4, Growth and development

155. Toddlers are not cooperative or competitive in
④ their play. Although they play alone for short periods, the type of play that is most characteristic of this age group is parallel.
I, 4, Growth and development

156. This information is important for the PN to
② know as a first step in nursing assessment of the infant.
I, 4, Growth and development

157. It is typical for preschoolers to view hospital-
② ization as punishment for real or imagined misdeeds. The response to such thinking is frequently a feeling of guilt.
IV, 4, Growth and development

158. Adolescents have the most difficulty in coping
④ with death, especially their own. Their concern is the present. They frequently feel alone.
I, 4, Growth and development

159. Because of an increased ability to compre-
③ hend, school-aged children experience fear in regard to death and dying. They frequently personify death as a devil, monster, or a bogeyman.
IV, 4, Growth and development

160. At 2 months, the infant develops a social smile
③ in response to various stimuli. Infants prefer people to objects.
I, 4, Growth and development

161. Erikson's first phase, from birth to 1 year, involves acquiring a basic sense of trust while overcoming a sense of mistrust. The crucial element of trust development is the consistent quality of care given to the infant by the mother. If this child-mother trust does not develop, mistrust is the outcome.
③ IV, 4, Growth and development

162. Stranger anxiety, in which the infant begins to fear strangers, appears between the age of 6 and 9 months. The friendly infant begins to cling to mother and become fretful when he cannot see his mother. The PN should assure parents that this is normal.
③ I, 4, Growth and development

163. Erikson's theory holds that the developmental crisis of adolescence leads to the formation of a sense of identity. The adolescent first identifies with a group and then develops a sense of personal identity.
④ I, 4, Growth and development

164. Adolescence is generally a time of turmoil. Adolescents demonstrate turbulent, rebellious, and unpredictable behavior. They experience frequent mood swings. They are idealistic and rather judgmental.
① I, 4, Growth and development

165. A history of genital herpes is a risk factor for cervical cancer. The other options are all risk factors for uterine cancer.
② III, 1, Uterine cancer

166. Uterine cancer can be diagnosed only through obtaining endometrial tissue. A fractional dilatation and curettage (D&C) provides this tissue. A Pap smear is positive only about 50% of the time in the presence of uterine cancer. A colposcopic examination is done to locate cervical lesions. Ultrasonography may be used in assessing for ovarian cancer.
③ III, 2, Uterine cancer

167. In the United States, heart disease is the leading cause of death in adults and cancer is the second leading cause of death in adults.
④ I, 4, Heart disease

168. Nitroglycerin dilates coronary arteries, causing increased blood flow to the coronary muscle.
③ I, 1, Coronary artery disease

169. Coronary vasodilators also dilate other arteries, causing side effects, such as headache, orthostatic hypotension, and fainting.
③ III, 2, Coronary artery disease

170. The coronary arteries provide blood to the myocardium. If these arteries are occluded, the client may suffer a heart attack.
④ I, 2, Coronary artery disease

171. Coronary artery disease includes any disease that affects the blood supply to the myocardium.
① I, 1, Coronary artery disease

172. When the muscle of the myocardium infarcts, isoenzymes are released. These can be measured, and they give an indication of how much damage has been done to the myocardium.
① III, 2, Coronary artery disease

173. The Holter monitor is a type of continuous electrocardiogram worn during normal activity so that any changes can be observed. The client is asked to keep an activity log during this time so that if any changes are noted on the electrocardiogram, the activity that caused them can be identified.
① III, 1, Coronary artery disease

174. Salt substitutes may be high in potassium and are not necessary on a restriction of 2 g. Substituting condiments such as lemon juice can provide the seasoning usually provided by salt.
④ III, 4, Coronary artery disease

175. It is important to assess for both bleeding and thrombus formation after an arteriogram. The pulses below the site should be taken before the arteriogram so that a baseline measurement can be established. Any changes should be reported to the physician immediately.
① III, 1, Coronary artery disease

176. It is important not only to protect the feet, but also to inspect them closely at regular intervals for injury. It is important to catch injuries early while treatment is more likely to be effective.
④ III, 1, Peripheral vascular disease

177. Intermittent claudication is defined as the pain caused by ischemia during exercise. When the pain occurs without activity, it is termed "rest pain."
③ IV, 1, Peripheral vascular disease

178.
① Stasis ulcers are venous ulcers and heal slowly because of the venous congestion associated with the vascular disease. The surgery that might be done to treat vascular ulcers is a skin graft to cover the ulcer once it is clean.
IV, 1, Peripheral vascular disease

179.
③ Thrombophlebitis is an inflammation of the vein associated with a blood clot within the vein. A thrombus is simply a clot, and phlebitis is inflammation of a vessel.
IV, 1, Peripheral vascular disease

180.
① Homans' sign is diagnostic of thrombophlebitis in the calf. When the calf muscle is contracted with a clot in the vessel, sharp pain is felt in the calf. The other symptoms may be associated with an arterial occlusion.
I, 1, Peripheral vascular disease

181.
① Elevating the leg with a clot is important to improve venous return. Peripheral pulses are checked with arterial disease, and the Berger-Allen exercises improve arterial flow. A pillow should never be used behind the knee in any patient with thrombophlebitis.
III, 1, Peripheral vascular disease

182.
② If a thrombus becomes dislodged, it becomes an embolus. Clots dislodged from the lower extremities travel to the lungs, becoming pulmonary emboli. This is a life-threatening complication of thrombophlebitis.
II & IV, 1, Peripheral vascular disease

183.
③ Walking and exercise are important to exercise the muscles and to help venous return, which is slowed from the incompetent veins. The other options are appropriate to treat varicose veins.
III, 1, Peripheral vascular disease

184.
② Excessive swelling postoperatively would be demonstrated by pain under the Ace wraps that are put on the legs after the stripping. Swelling may indicate bleeding postoperatively. The legs are elevated and never dangled.
III, 1, Peripheral vascular disease

185.
③ Tuberculosis is increasing in poor, elderly, and non-whites, especially Native Americans. The lower a person's resistance, the more malnutrition present, and the lower their immunity, the more likely is tuberculosis to develop.
IV, 1, Tuberculosis

186.
④ The tuberculin bacillus is an acid-fast bacillus. Obtaining a specimen of this bacillus for culture is diagnostic of tuberculosis. The skin test tells you only that the client has been exposed to tuberculosis and has formed antibodies. The chest radiograph cannot differentiate between active or encapsulated tuberculosis.
IV, 1, Tuberculosis

187.
③ The tuberculin bacillus is difficult to control. Treatment can never cure or eradicate the bacillus. The bacteria become encapsulated only after 1 to 2 years of treatment with the antibiotics.
III & IV, 1, Tuberculosis

188.
② A tuberculin skin test is simply an antigen-antibody response. It takes about 72 hours for the full reaction to be seen.
III & IV, 1, Tuberculosis

189.
④ A positive skin test result indicates only that the person has antibodies against tuberculosis. It does not mean that the person has active or inactive tuberculosis.
IV, 2, Tuberculosis

190.
③ Prophylactic treatment for a person who has been exposed to tuberculosis but has not developed it lasts at least 1 year.
III & IV, 1, Tuberculosis

191.
② Tuberculosis is an acid-fast bacillus. It can affect almost any organ, such as the kidneys.
I, 2, Tuberculosis

192.
① Unfortunately, the only early symptom of lung cancer is a persistent cough. Many smokers, the largest group of people to have lung cancer, have a chronic cough anyway. Many people do not notice the cough until they begin to cough up blood.
I, 2, Lung cancer

193.
③ A magnetic resonance imaging scan does not require any preparation. The MRI scan is not a radiographic examination but instead uses magnetically stimulated images.
III, 2, Lung cancer

194.
② When a client has a bronchoscopy, local anesthesia is used in the back of the throat to deaden the gag reflex. Nothing can be taken by mouth until the gag reflex returns so that the client does not choke. It usually takes several hours for this reflex to return.
III, 1, Bronchoscopy/lung cancer

195. Specimens can be obtained without the surgery. Chest tubes are required if a wedge resection is done. This procedure would be performed if a small tumor had already been diagnosed and needed to be resected.
④
IV, 2, Lung cancer

196. The highest risk factor for lung cancer is cigarette smoking. Smoking is also the most modifiable cause of disease.
③
I, 2, Lung cancer

197. It is important for the client and family to be well informed of tests and procedures to be done. Fear of the unknown is one of the most anxiety-producing problems for the ill client. Visitors can provide much support to the client. The client should not be bombarded with a lot of information at this time.
①
III, 3, Lung cancer

198. After a thoracotomy, it is important for the client to be positioned so that the affected lung can best reexpand. Lying on the affected side could slow or interfere with this reexpansion.
③
III, 1, Lung cancer

199. Chest tubes are inserted to reexpand the lung. A pneumonectomy means that the entire lung is removed so there is nothing to be reexpanded. The other procedures require chest tubes for reexpansion.
①
IV, 2, Lung cancer

200. The chest tube drains fluid and removes air from the pleural space after the integrity of
②
this space has been violated. A chest tube can be used for access of chemotherapy, but this is a minor use.
IV, 2, Lung cancer

201. Continuous bubbling during ventilation indicates that air is leaking into the drainage system or pleural cavity. The other observations are normal with the three-bottle system.
④
III, 1, Lung cancer

202. The tube is clamped if it becomes dislodged because if it is left open to the air, the lung will collapse. The tube should be clamped close to the chest wall so that no further leakage can occur. The tubing should then be repaired and reattached properly to water-seal drainage so that it can be unclamped as soon as possible.
④
III, 1, Lung cancer

203. The elderly are often dehydrated preoperatively and have difficulty maintaining homeostasis. None of the other clients are at particular risk.
④
I, 1, Surgical intervention

204. Demerol 50 mg/1 mL = 100 mg/$\times$ mL, $50\times = 100$, $\times = 2$. Atropine 0.4 mg/1 mL = 0.3 mg/$\times$ mL, $0.4\times = 0.3$, $\times = 0.75$.
④
III, 2, Medication administration

205. Atropine acts to reduce tracheobronchial secretions and dries the mucous membranes. It increases the pulse, is not a muscle relaxant, and does not affect Demerol.
③
IV, 2, Medications

The Nursing Process and Basic Skills

3

I. THE NURSING PROCESS

A. Assessment

1. Collection of subjective and objective data about clients to aid in the planning, implementing, and evaluating of client care
2. Methods
   a. observe client and environment
   b. perform physical assessment, including procedures such as vital signs, height, weight, and other objective data
   c. communicate with client to obtain an accurate and complete history
   d. collect all laboratory specimens ordered

B. Planning

1. The act of setting reasonable, prioritized goals designed to meet client needs either independently or, in some states, working under the RN
2. Must be based on the client's assessed needs
3. Becomes basis of nursing interventions
4. Goals must be clearly stated to aid in evaluation of goal achievement
5. Goals should be *mutually* set between the PN and client (with RN oversight in some states)

C. Implementation

1. Provision of nursing care designed to meet established goals
2. Includes both physical and psychosocial care of clients and their environment
3. Recording, reporting, and documentation of all pertinent data is an important part of nursing care

D. Evaluation

1. Participate in identifying whether established goals set for each client were accomplished and whether nursing care was effective in meeting goals
2. Evaluation should lead to revision of the plan of care if needs are unmet while effective interventions are continued

II. BASIC SKILLS

A. Skills Associated with Sexuality

1. Privacy
   a. always drape client who is potentially exposed for examination
   b. draw curtain and close door when client might be exposed
2. Perineal care
   a. always wipe or wash from front to back
   b. daily cleanse area with soap and water in both men and women
   c. type of solutions used for cleansing varies and may require a physician's order
   d. change and remove soiled perineal pads front to back
3. Vaginal douche
   a. done to cleanse vagina
   b. client should void first
   c. client is placed on bedpan in dorsal recumbent position with knees flexed
   d. solution varies from soap solution to vinegar in warm water
   e. irrigation administered under low pressure to avoid trauma; hold container just above client's hips
   f. nozzle is inserted with solution running and is pointed down and back into vagina
   g. rotate nozzle gently to clean all vaginal folds
4. Pap smear
   a. test to detect changes in cervix that are either premalignant or malignant
   b. performed on women beginning at age 18 years or earlier if they are sexually active

c. frequency of examination yearly in high-risk women and then according to physician's decision in others; guidelines vary

d. must refrain from douching 24 hours before test

e. patient in lithotomy position; drape carefully

f. when physician scrapes tissue from cervix, apply to glass slide and spray with fixative agent

5. Breast self-examination

a. systematic observation and palpation of breasts to detect cysts or tumors

b. should be done by women over age 20 years, monthly about 1 week following menstrual period

c. encourage correct technique

6. Testicular self-examination

a. systematic observation and palpation of testicles to detect tumors

b. should be done monthly by men between age 20 and 40 years

c. encourage correct technique

B. Skills Associated with Oxygenation

1. Ace bandages/TED hose/compression stockings

a. used to encourage venous return from extremities and prevent thrombi formation

b. pressure should not be great enough to interfere with circulation

c. should be applied before client gets out of bed and worn while client is in bed

d. remove every 8 hours to check for undue pressure on skin

2. Heat and cold application

a. heat application

(1) produces muscle relaxation

(2) promotes suppuration

(3) helps localize infections

(4) increases metabolic rate

(5) increases local blood flow to relieve circulatory congestion

b. apply heat and cold only with physician's order

c. K-pads have exact temperature settings

d. monitor closely for redness, pain, and swelling; prevent burning

e. cold application

(1) constricts blood vessels and reduces blood flow

(2) aids in control of hemorrhage

(3) reduces inflammatory process

(4) prevents suppuration

f. fill ice packs about 2/3 full of ice; remove all air

g. cover pack before application

h. refill about every 2 hours; remove periodically to maintain circulation

i. monitor skin closely for excess cold: white, mottled skin, numbness

j. monitor body temperature

3. Coughing and deep breathing

a. done to effectively remove secretions from the respiratory tract

b. improves oxygenation by preventing atelectasis

c. method of effective coughing and deep breathing

(1) sit patient up in high Fowler's position

(2) splint abdomen or chest with pillows or hands, if necessary, to prevent incisional pain

(3) request deep inspiration through mouth several times

(4) bend client forward and instruct to contract thorax and abdomen to expel air forcibly

d. medicate for pain before coughing to improve effort

e. encourage in preoperative and postoperative clients and those with decreased mobility

4. Vaporizer/nebulizer

a. provision of air with a high humidity to

(1) soothe irritated mucous membranes

(2) provide extra moisture to respiratory tract

(3) liquefy thick secretions

(4) loosen crusts on mucous membranes

(5) administer medications directly to respiratory tract

b. administered by a wide variety of equipment

c. possibility of bacterial growth in warm water reservoir

d. monitor for bronchospasms and overhydration

5. Blow bottles/Triflow

a. used to encourage deep breathing and coughing

b. client exhales against pressure of water or balls in Triflow

c. should be done hourly while awake

6. Inspiratory/incentive spirometer

a. helps client to inspire deeply, thereby expanding lung capacity

b. with lips sealed over mouthpiece, client takes a deep breath, holds 3 seconds, then exhales slowly

c. encourage client to use hourly while awake

7. Intermittent positive-pressure breathing (IPPB) treatments

a. administration of higher-than-ambient pressures and higher-than-client's normal tidal volume to force oxygen into respiratory tract

b. IPPB used to
  (1) promote deep breathing in clients with decreasing levels of consciousness
  (2) mobilize secretions through stimulation of coughing
  (3) increase O_2 intake and CO_2 removal
  (4) produce mechanical bronchodilation
  (5) administer aerosol medications
  (6) prevent atelectasis by hyperinflation of alveoli
  (7) decrease work of breathing temporarily
  c. should be administered only by trained personnel
8. Postural drainage
  a. technique of positioning client so that gravity assists with the drainage of secretions from the lobes of the lungs
  b. improves removal of secretions when combined with clapping and vibration over affected areas of lungs
  c. position client so that gravity helps to drain affected areas of lung
9. Suctioning
  a. mechanical aspiration of secretions from the tracheobronchial tree, when client is unable to remove
  b. tracheal suctioning is a sterile procedure; oral or nasal suctioning is a clean procedure
  c. administer O_2 in high levels before and after suctioning
  d. apply suction after inserting the catheter
  e. do not suction for more than 10 seconds continuously
  f. withdraw catheter slowly with rotating motion
  g. give a breath with ambu bag or pause to give client a chance to breathe between suctioning attempts
10. Sputum specimen
  a. performed to inspect sputum for infective agents or malignancy
  b. best obtained in morning before breakfast
  c. use proper container, sterile for culture, and with preservative for cytology
  d. have client breathe deeply to induce cough
  e. avoid contamination of inside of container
11. Tracheostomy care
  a. monitor client closely for signs of obstruction of tube
  b. suctioning and cleaning of tracheostomy: sterile procedure
  c. monitor and maintain skin around stoma
  d. always provide humidified air

12. Oxygen administration
  a. used to treat hypoxemia (low blood oxygen); determined by blood gas analysis or pulse oximeter
  b. can be given in many concentrations and through many devices
    (1) ordered in L/minute
    (2) various devices provide higher or lower concentrations; mask higher, nasal cannula lower (Fig. 3–1)
  c. post signs against smoking because oxygen supports combustion
  d. avoid high levels of oxygen in clients with chronic obstructive pulmonary disease (COPD) or over long times for any client
13. CPR (see Chapter 7)
14. Intake and output
  a. must be measured accurately to determine client's fluid balance
  b. learn volumes of containers commonly used for fluids
  c. measure urine, liquid feces, and other bodily drainage for accurate output

C. Skills Associated with Sensory/Perception

1. Eye and ear irrigations
  a. use of a large volume of therapeutic agent to wash or flush the eye or ear
  b. to flush eye
    (1) use sterile technique when irrigating eye; treat each eye separately
    (2) position client to drain fluids and any foreign bodies from eye
    (3) expose conjunctival sac and direct irrigation from inner canthus toward outer angle
    (4) use little force when irrigating
  c. to flush ear
    (1) draw auricle down and back for children and up and back for adults to straighten ear canal
    (2) tilt client's head so ear to be treated is uppermost
    (3) direct stream toward wall of ear canal, not eardrum
2. Level of consciousness (LOC)
  a. describe what client is doing or is able to do; avoid labels
  b. assess orientation to person, place, and time
  c. test protective reflexes (gag and corneal)
  d. test neuromuscular function to determine purposeful activities by asking client to move extremities and push against resistance

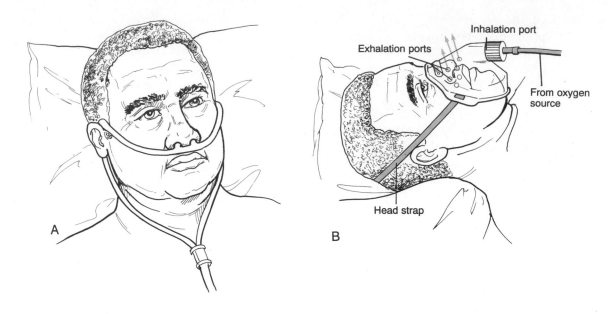

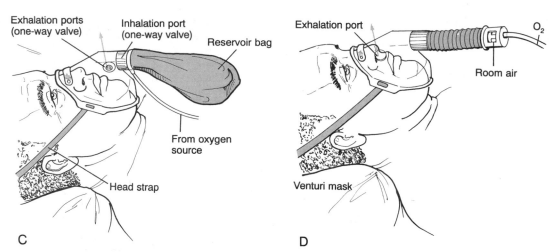

FIGURE 3-1 Oxygen delivery systems. *A,* Nasal cannula; *B,* standard oxygen mask; *C,* partial rebreathing oxygen mask; *D,* Venturi oxygen mask. (From Linton, A.D., Matteson, M.A., & Maebius, N.K. (1995). *Introductory nursing care of adults.* Philadelphia; W.B. Saunders Co.)

3. Neurologic assessment
    a. pupil reactions
        (1) normal pupils are equal, round, react to light with accommodation (PERRLA)
        (2) size and shape
        (3) speed of reaction to light
        (4) equality of pupil size and reaction
    b. eye movements, ability to follow finger vs. erratic and uncontrolled movement
    c. movement of extremities
        (1) voluntary and purposeful
        (2) equality of strength and movement
    d. reflexes: normal responses and equal on both sides of the body
    e. vital signs
    f. level of consciousness
4. Protective devices/restraints
    a. protectors used to prevent clients from harming either themselves or others
    b. require physician's order
    c. select the least restrictive device of proper type and size
    d. investigate all alternatives to eliminate the precipitating problem before resorting to restraints
    e. use restraints as a last resort and only on a short-term basis
    f. involve the client (if possible) and the family in the decision making

g. document need for restraints clearly on chart

h. assess the client frequently for
    (1) damage to tissue under restraint
    (2) damage to other body parts, such as shoulder dislocation
    (3) problems related to immobility
    (4) damage to joints
    (5) safety; client may be unable to call for help, reach water, or relieve pressure on areas; anticipate needs

i. check every hour, release for 15 minutes, and reapply at least every 2 hours

j. avoid client isolation, encourage interaction

k. maintain restraint record per institutional policy

l. reevaluate need for restraints frequently

5. Pain control
  a. assessment of pain
    (1) history of pain development and occurrence
    (2) location of pain
    (3) nature of pain: onset, intensity, depth, radiation, duration, quality
    (4) physical signs: grimacing, crying, change in vital signs, restlessness, insomnia
    (5) what relieves pain
    (6) associated symptoms: nausea, restlessness, constipation
  b. methods of controlling pain
    (1) medication
      (a) narcotic analgesics: oral, parenteral, rectal, transdermal, intrathecal
      (b) non-narcotic analgesics: oral most common
    (2) noninvasive methods
      (a) relaxation exercises
      (b) repositioning
      (c) therapeutic interaction with client
      (d) rhythmic breathing
      (e) heat and cold applications, as ordered
      (f) cutaneous stimulation, back rubs
      (g) diversional activities

D. Skills Associated with Protective Functions

1. Culture and sensitivity specimens
  a. culture identifies infective organisms from multiple body sites and fluids
  b. sensitivity identifies drugs that should effectively combat the identified microorganism
  c. requires sterile container and sterile collection techniques

d. collect specimen before beginning antibiotics

e. antibiotic treatments based on results

2. Hygiene needs
  a. bed bath
    (1) avoid chilling or exposure
    (2) water should be between 105° F and 115° F
    (3) change bath water frequently, as needed
    (4) use soap sparingly to avoid drying skin; rinse well
    (5) assess skin during bath
    (6) soak hands and feet in warm water
  b. skin care
    (1) use oils and lotions to restore natural oils to skin
    (2) massage skin gently
    (3) turn and reposition client frequently
    (4) assess for reddened or broken areas
    (5) keep bed linen clean, dry, and wrinkle-free
    (6) use special beds or mattresses to avoid skin breakdown in high-risk clients
    (7) wash and clean client thoroughly after using bedpan
  c. nail care
    (1) daily cleaning
    (2) physician's order needed to cut nails
      (a) especially true in diabetic clients
      (b) cut evenly across ends of fingers and toes
  d. oral care
    (1) brush teeth before meals, if necessary, and after
    (2) use mouthwashes unless mouth ulcers or dry mucous membranes are present (mouthwashes contain alcohol)
    (3) provide mouth care to unconscious clients every 2 hours
    (4) remove dentures for thorough cleaning and examine gums underneath for sores
    (5) keep unused dentures in container labeled with client's name
  e. hair care
    (1) needs daily brushing and periodic shampooing if possible
    (2) apply alcohol or vinegar to hair to help remove matting or tangles
    (3) braid long hair to prevent tangling
    (4) never cut a client's hair without permission

3. Bed making
  a. types of beds
    (1) unoccupied: top covers fan-folded to bottom of bed and ready for client

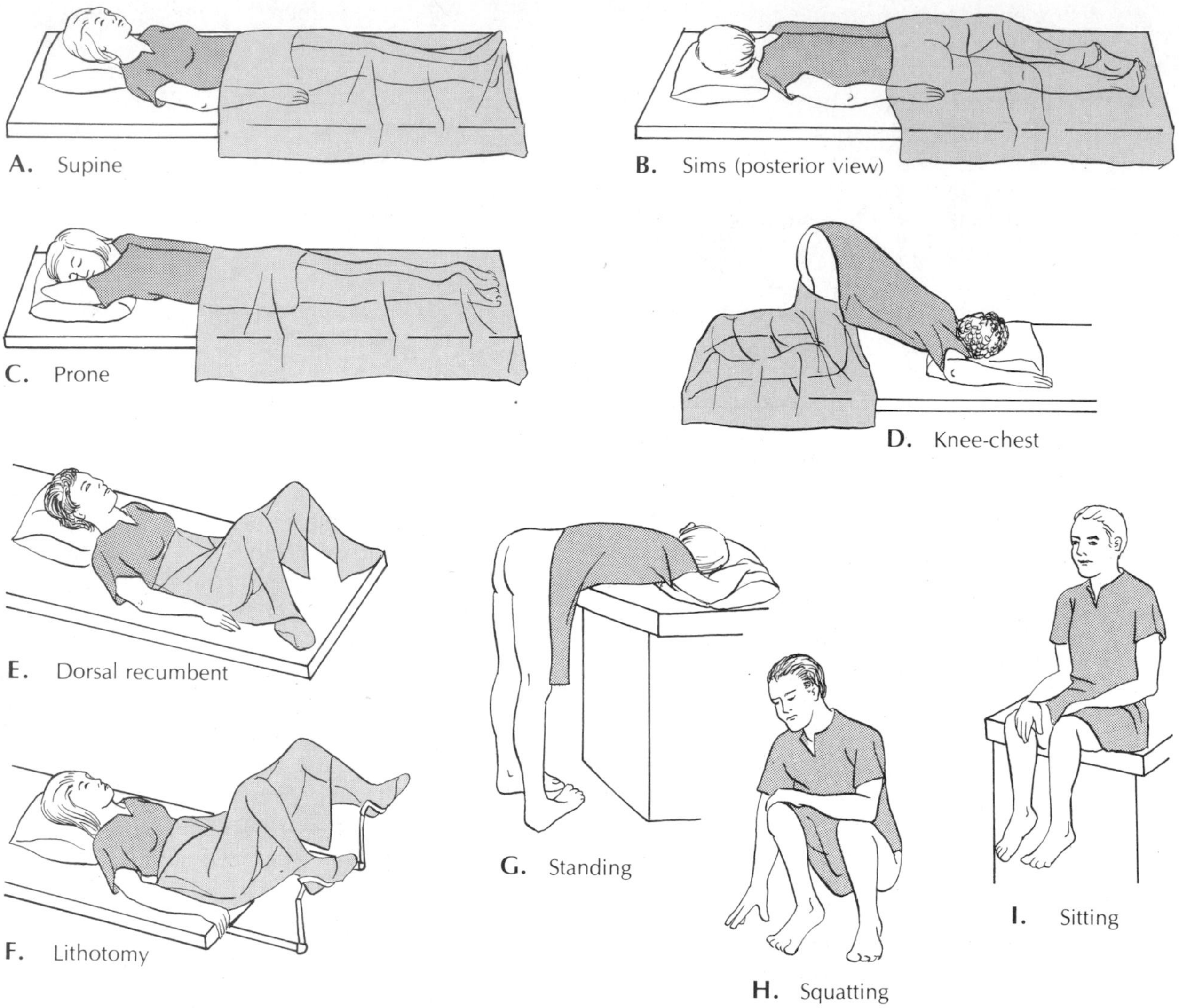

A. Supine

B. Sims (posterior view)

C. Prone

D. Knee-chest

E. Dorsal recumbent

F. Lithotomy

G. Standing

H. Squatting

I. Sitting

FIGURE 3-2 *A–I,* Common examination positions. (From Lammon, C.B., Foote, A.W., Leli, P.G., Ingle, J., & Adams, M.H. (1995). *Clinical nursing skills.* Philadelphia: W.B. Saunders Co.)

      (2) occupied: made with the client in the bed; turn client from side to side or can be made top-to-bottom, especially for orthopedic clients who cannot turn

      (3) surgical: prepared for a client returning from surgery; top covers not tucked in but fan-folded to side or bottom

   b. linen must be tightly pulled to avoid wrinkling

   c. do not shake out linens, to avoid spreading of dust and microorganisms

   d. avoid holding linens close to nurse's clothing

   e. complete one side of the bed at a time

   f. use good body mechanics to avoid injury or straining

 4. Positioning and body alignment

   a. client positioning (Fig. 3–2)

      (1) prone: lying flat in bed on abdomen (Fig. 3–2C)

      (2) semi-Fowler's: head of bed raised 45 degrees

      (3) supine: lying flat on back (Fig. 3–2A)

      (4) high Fowler's: head of bed elevated to a 90-degree position with client's knees slightly flexed

      (5) knee-chest: client on knees with shoulders flat on bed (Fig. 3–2D)

      (6) Lateral position: on left or right side with opposite hip and knee acutely flexed, client slightly forward

      (7) lithotomy: client on back with legs widely separated, thighs acutely flexed to abdomen, and feet in stirrups; modified lithotomy with less flexion common for geriatric clients (Fig. 3–2F)

      (8) orthopneic: client fully upright leaning over padded overbed table, resting head on arms

      (9) Trendelenburg: head lower than feet and legs

          (10) reverse Trendelenburg: head elevated, feet and legs lower

    b. alignment

        (1) always prevent pressure on bony prominences

        (2) use pillows and blanket rolls to position client for comfort

        (3) rule is no skin on skin

5. Wound care

    a. sterile dressing: used to protect wound from contaminants

        (1) wash hands

        (2) assemble sterile equipment and field

        (3) remove old dressing wearing clean gloves

        (4) carefully note drainage for later charting

        (5) place old dressing in watertight container and dispose of properly

        (6) carefully assess wound

        (7) put on sterile gloves

        (8) cleanse wound per institutional policy or physician's order from clean area to dirty

        (9) apply sterile dressing

        (10) anchor securely with tape or binder

    b. wet-to-dry dressings

        (1) similar to sterile

        (2) done to cleanse wound and remove debris

        (3) sterile saline usually used to moisten dressing

        (4) avoid saturating dressing to avoid leakage

        (5) cover with dry sterile sponges to increase wicking action

        (6) secure dressing

6. Bandages and binders

    a. types of and uses for bandages

        (1) circular: holds dressings in place

        (2) spiral: immobilizes part of extremity or decreases swelling

        (3) figure-of-eight: applies pressure, supports or immobilizes joint, shapes stump

        (4) triangular: sling to hold forearm immobile

        (5) recurrent: shapes stumps, head dressings

    b. Montgomery straps

        (1) consists of two large pieces of tape with cloth straps that tie over dressing to immobilize it

        (2) used for frequently changed dressings to prevent constant retaping

    c. abdominal or chest binders

        (1) apply tightly enough to support chest or abdomen

        (2) avoid an overtight binder that prevents adequate chest expansion

    d. scultetus or "many-tailed" binder

        (1) made of rectangular cloth with many long tails attached

        (2) used either for support or to hold dressings in place

        (3) apply while client is supine

        (4) starting at bottom of binder, bring each tail across abdomen, pulling taut

        (5) overlap tails at slight upward angle

        (6) anchor each tail with next one

        (7) pin final tail in place

    e. T-binder: used to secure rectal or perineal dressings

7. Isolation precautions

    a. universal or body fluid precautions: used with all clients

        (1) gloves worn for any contact with body fluids

        (2) gown and mask with goggles worn if potential contamination from body fluids, such as hemorrhaging client in emergency department

        (3) separate disposal of sharps without breaking; do not recap needles

    b. strict isolation: used for airborne and contact spread of highly contagious pathogens

        (1) private room

        (2) gown, gloves, and mask when entering room

        (3) double bag linens; disposable eating utensils, dishes, and cups; trash; and other contaminated articles

        (4) flush urine and feces down toilet in room

        (5) keep a stethoscope and a glass thermometer in the room

        (6) hand washing after client contact

    c. respiratory isolation: used with airborne pathogens

        (1) private room

        (2) wear mask when entering room

        (3) hand washing after client contact

        (4) double bag contaminated articles

    d. drainage secretion precautions

        (1) private room preferable, if excessive drainage

        (2) wear gown and gloves for direct contact, mask if excessive secretions

        (3) double bag linens and dressings and other contaminated articles

        (4) hand washing after client contact

    e. enteric precautions: used for infections spread through fecal contact

(1) private room for children or uncooperative adults

(2) wear gown for direct contact

(3) wear gloves for contact with fecal material; ie, bedpans or cleaning up client

(4) double bag linens and dressings; use disposable dishes

(5) flush feces down toilet immediately

  f. blood precautions: used for blood-borne infections

(1) dispose of all blood-contaminated equipment separately; double-bag

(2) dispose of sharps in container without breaking; do not recap needles

(3) flush urine and feces down toilet immediately

  g. reverse isolation: used for immunosuppressed clients

(1) private room

(2) no one allowed in with any respiratory or other infection

(3) neutropenic diet with no fresh fruits or vegetables, meat well cooked

(4) no fresh flowers, stuffed animals, or any other objects in room that may harbor bacteria

8. Care of the dying

  a. psychosocial issues

(1) client's need to know of impending death

(2) PN's attitude toward death influences care of dying

(3) cultural or ethnic responses to dying

(4) client and family ability to cope with dying varies

(5) client's reactions to dying, described by Kubler-Ross (1975)

    (a) denial

    (b) anger: difficult for PN and family to handle

    (c) bargaining

    (d) depression: difficult for PN and family to handle

    (e) acceptance

(6) all actions should be directed at opening communication with client

  b. spiritual needs

(1) provide clergy for client as appropriate

(2) allow client to participate in appropriate religious practices

(3) provide for family comfort and time with client

  c. physical changes of approaching death

(1) facial muscles relax, cheeks flaccid, dentures do not fit, mumbling speech

(2) pale, ashen skin that is cool and clammy

(3) sight gradually fails

(4) hearing believed to be sense retained longest

(5) muscles become flaccid

(6) respirations become irregular, rapid and shallow or very slow, Cheyne-Stokes—periods of hyperpnea regularly alternate with periods of apnea; may be very restless

(7) pulse becomes weak, irregular, and thready

(8) mental status varies from clarity to coma

(9) reflexes decreased or absent

(10) bowel and bladder retention or incontinence

  d. nursing care

(1) all care directed at client comfort and safety

(2) provide for relief of unpleasant symptoms

(3) maintain good hygiene and oral care

(4) turn client frequently and position for maximum comfort

(5) keep linens fresh and dry

(6) allow family sufficient time with client

(7) support client and family as needed

(8) continue pain medications and treatments as appropriate

  e. postmortem care

(1) performed after the physician pronounces the client dead

(2) position client flat in bed in a natural position with one pillow under head

(3) close eyes

(4) return dentures to mouth as soon as possible and close mouth

(5) clean body and remove all tubes per institutional policy

(6) allow family time with body after it is prepared

(7) wrap in shroud and label body per policy

(8) remove body to morgue or funeral home per policy

(9) pack all belongings, give to family, and document in chart

(10) complete institutional death record

9. Discharging clients

  a. done only after written physician's order

  b. nursing care

(1) help client gather all belongings

(2) review discharge instructions, prescriptions, and follow-up appointments

(3) help client obtain transportation from family or contact social service if assistance needed

(4)   accompany client to exit per institution policy

(5)   chart information per policy

E.   Skills Associated with Mobility

1.   Rest and sleep
   a.   position client in individualized comfort position
   b.   maintain quiet and darkness to help with sleep
   c.   provide comfortable environment, blankets or cooling as needed
   d.   promote relaxation
      (1)   warm bath
      (2)   back rub
   e.   avoid overuse of prescribed sleep agents
2.   Body mechanics
   a.   lifting or moving
      (1)   feet apart to width of shoulder
      (2)   move object to be lifted close to body before lifting
      (3)   keep back only slightly flexed
      (4)   contract abdominal and lumbar muscles during lifting
      (5)   use shoulder and arm muscles to pull
      (6)   flex knees slightly and then straighten as object lifted
   b.   transferring client from bed to stretcher
      (1)   use at least two or three people
      (2)   use drawsheet to move client
      (3)   move client toward edge of bed
      (4)   adjust stretcher next to bed at level of bed
      (5)   lock both bed and stretcher
      (6)   reach across stretcher and, using drawsheet, pull client toward you, first to edge, then to center of stretcher
   c.   assisting client from bed to chair
      (1)   lower bed to lowest position
      (2)   move chair close to bed and firmly anchor or lock wheelchair
      (3)   help client to sitting position, then to side of bed with legs dangling
      (4)   face client, maintain wide base of support, hands around client's lower chest
      (5)   keep client's knees between your legs to prevent falls
      (6)   have client lean forward and place hands on your shoulders, not neck
      (7)   pull client to standing position
      (8)   pivot client and lower into chair or wheelchair
   d.   positioning client up in bed
      (1)   adjust bed height to below your waist
      (2)   position the client flat in bed

(3)   stand at side of bed with feet pointed in direction you are to move client

(4)   reach under client's shoulders and back to slide client without lifting

(5)   have client bend knees and use feet to push self up if possible

(6)   use draw sheet, if possible, to avoid shearing force on client's back

   e.   turning client
      (1)   client should be turned every 2 hours while in bed
      (2)   adjust bed to mid or upper thigh level
      (3)   lower bed rail on the side where you are standing
      (4)   cross client's arms on chest and cross legs
      (5)   reach across client, placing your hands on the client's far shoulder and hip, or use a draw sheet
      (6)   turn client toward you using your whole body
      (7)   put pillow(s) behind client's back and between legs; raise side rail
3.   Range-of-motion (ROM) exercises
   a.   definitions
      (1)   passive: movement of client's joints through complete range of mobility when client is unable to perform this activity independently
      (2)   active: client moves joints through complete range of mobility independently
   b.   always exercise only to limit of mobility or pain
   c.   support limb by cupping or cradling extremity to avoid stress on joints
   d.   often done easily during bath

F.   Skills Associated with Metabolism/Elimination

1.   Feeding clients
   a.   wash client's hands and provide oral care
   b.   place tray so client can see food being served
   c.   if possible, raise head of bed to ease swallowing
   d.   prepare foods, but allow client as much independence as possible
   e.   tell client what foods are on the tray
   f.   use straws for fluids and allow client to eat finger foods independently
   g.   offer food in small amounts
   h.   vary foods being offered or ask clients what they want next
   i.   alternate liquids with solid foods
   j.   blind clients: describe what foods offered and position of foods on plate

    k. always strive to make mealtimes pleasant to promote a good appetite

    l. do not rush client

    m. wash client's hands and provide oral care after meals

2. Nasogastric (NG) tubes
   a. used either to drain gastric contents or to administer tube feedings
   b. NG tubes (Levin, Salem Sump, Miller-Abbott, Cantor) may be connected to continuous or intermittent suction
   c. check proper tube placement before irrigating
      (1) aspirate stomach contents with a syringe
      (2) inject 10 mL of air into tube while listening with stethoscope for whooshing sound over stomach
   d. irrigate with normal saline at intervals to prevent clogging
   e. note and chart amount, color, and consistency of drainage at end of shift, being sure to subtract irrigating solution
   f. provide mouth care every 2 hours

3. Tube feedings
   a. done through nasogastric or gastrostomy tube for clients unable to swallow or take in sufficient nutrients
   b. feedings either continuous at slow drip rates or intermittently throughout the day and night
   c. many prepared solutions available; also may be made by dietary department
   d. always serve feedings at room temperature to prevent cramping
   e. flush feeding tube with water before and after each feeding as well as before and after any medication given per tube
   f. give feedings by gravity infusion; never force the feeding under pressure
   g. raise head of bed during feedings and maintain elevated position for 45 minutes following feeding
   h. administer feedings slowly to prevent nausea and overdistention of stomach
   i. follow feedings with prescribed amount of water
   j. aspirate stomach contents 1 hour after feeding, as ordered, to check for residual feedings left in stomach
   k. provide client with emotional support because inability to eat independently is often distressing
   l. administer mouth care every 2 hours

4. Assisting with normal bowel function
   a. assess each client's normal bowel pattern and attempt to maintain it
   b. encourage adequate intake of fluids unless contraindicated and fiber to prevent constipation, often associated with decreased mobility
   c. if possible, have client sit on toilet, commode, or bedpan for natural position for defecation
   d. tell client not to ignore urge to defecate
   e. provide privacy
   f. help cleanse client after defecation
   g. monitor amount, color, and consistency of stool

5. Rectal tubes
   a. insert to relieve distention due to flatus
   b. lubricate tube before inserting 2–4 inches into rectum
   c. position client in left lateral Sims' position
   d. tape in place and leave no longer than 30 minutes
   e. report and record results

6. Enemas
   a. requires physician's orders for most, especially for cardiac clients
   b. cleansing
      (1) can be tap water, mixture of soap and water, or saline
      (2) temperature of solution should be no more than 105° F
      (3) administer 500–1000 mL of fluid
      (4) position client in left lateral Sims' position
      (5) hold fluid container about 18 inches above anus
      (6) lubricate tube and insert 3–4 inches
      (7) if cramping occurs, stop and have client take deep breaths until cramping passes
      (8) observe results and record amount of feces
      (9) if ordered "until clear," return should eventually be free of feces; no more than three enemas unless specified by physician
   c. oil retention
      (1) given to soften feces to ease defecation
      (2) oil heated to 100° F
      (3) use only about 100 mL; encourage client to try to retain it for 30 minutes
      (4) may require cleansing enema afterward
      (5) commercially prepared prefilled enemas available

7. Manual extraction of impaction
   a. requires physician's order for cardiac clients
   b. apply gloves and adequately lubricate index finger
   c. position client in left lateral Sims'

d. gently insert finger into hardened stool and break off small pieces and remove
e. assess client's condition throughout; stop if client's vital signs change or if discomfort experienced
f. place client on bedpan following procedure to allow evacuation of remaining stool

8. Stool specimens
   a. to determine presence of blood, ova, and parasites or microorganisms
   b. all specimens except for blood require sterile container, and collection must be sent to laboratory warm and fresh

9. Colostomy irrigation
   a. done to empty bowel and regulate the passage of feces and flatus
   b. presently not considered a necessary procedure in colostomy management
   c. not all clients require irrigation to regulate defecation
   d. irrigation takes about 45 minutes and is best done at client's established routine time
   e. irrigation done daily or every other day
   f. equipment and procedure same as for enema administration
   g. irrigation done with warm normal saline or tap water
   h. special ostomy pouch worn for irrigation to collect fecal drainage
   i. record results of irrigation

10. Assisting with urinary elimination
    a. altered patterns of urinary elimination
       (1) incontinence: inability to control voiding
       (2) retention: inability to void
       (3) dysuria: painful urination
       (4) polyuria: excessive urination
       (5) oliguria: output less than 400 mL/day
       (6) anuria: no urine output
    b. offer bedpan or urinal at regular intervals or leave within client's reach
    c. provide client privacy
    d. encourage client to sit or stand, if able, to promote ease of voiding
    e. if client has difficulty voiding
       (1) run water in his or her hearing
       (2) place client's hand in basin of warm water
       (3) pour warm water over perineum
    f. help client wash hands after voiding

11. Catheters
    a. purposes
       (1) to obtain sterile urine specimens
       (2) to relieve retention
       (3) to keep bladder decompressed
       (4) to measure residual urine following voiding
       (5) to irrigate bladder or instill medication
    b. "straight" catheters inserted for single bladder decompression and then removed
    c. Foley catheter inserted and left in for length of time ordered
    d. general principles of catheterization
       (1) use sterile procedure
       (2) use smallest size possible to avoid trauma
       (3) explain procedure to client before beginning
       (4) provide privacy; position client
       (5) put on sterile gloves and set up sterile field
       (6) cleanse the urinary meatus front to back for women and in a circular motion for men
       (7) lubricate catheter well before inserting
       (8) insert catheter about 3–4 inches in women and 6–8 inches in men
       (9) if using indwelling catheter, fill balloon with 5–10 mL of sterile water and anchor with tape to thigh, straight for women and at right angle in men, and connect to drainage tubing and bag
    e. removal of indwelling catheter
       (1) position client and provide privacy
       (2) withdraw water from balloon port with syringe
       (3) release tape, have client take deep breath, and remove catheter with steady, gentle pull
       (4) monitor client for voiding within 8 hours after removal
       (5) encourage fluid intake to improve output
       (6) warn client that some burning may occur with first voiding

12. Urine specimens
    a. sterile specimen collected by straight catheterization
    b. voided specimen
       (1) wash perineal area well first
       (2) collect midstream specimen by having client start voiding, stop voiding, and restart voiding into sterile container
    c. clean specimen collected for urinalysis
    d. single specimen or up to 24-hour specimens may be collected
    e. container and preservative dependent on type of specimen collected
    f. 24-hour specimens: discard first void and record time; collect all urine for next 24 hours

g. double-voided specimen: client empties bladder; collect next voided specimen. Done when testing for glucose and acetone

13. Bladder irrigation

   a. must be done using aseptic technique

   b. can be done as manual irrigation using syringe or constant bladder irrigation (CBI), using an intravenous-type setup

   c. done to clear catheter of obstructions, remove clots from urine, wash the bladder with medication, or decrease bleeding from bladder or prostate, usually after surgery

   d. can be done without disconnecting catheter if three-way Foley used

   e. amount and type of solution determined by physician's orders

   f. account for amount of solution on output record

14. Tests for glucose and acetone

   a. done before meals and at bedtime or sometimes every 6 hours if client receiving intravenous fluids

   b. done either on urine or fingerstick with glucose monitor

   c. use double-voided specimen to insure fresh urine

   d. use glucose monitor per product instructions

BIBLIOGRAPHY

Bolander, V.R. (1994). *Sorensen and Luckmann's basic nursing: A psychophysiologic approach*, 3rd ed. Philadelphia: W.B. Saunders Co.

Betz, C.L., Hunsberger, M., & Wright, S. (1994). *Family-centered nursing care of children*, 2nd ed. Philadelphia: W.B. Saunders Co.

Kubler-Ross, E. (1975). Death: *The final stage of growth.* Englewood Cliffs, NJ: Prentice-Hall.

Linton, A.D., Matteson, M.A., & Maebius, N.K. (1995). *Introductory nursing care of adults.* Philadelphia: W.B. Saunders Co.

Monohan, F.D., Drake, T., & Neighbors, M. (1994). *Nursing care of adults.* Philadelphia: W.B. Saunders Co.

Perry, A.G., & Potter, P.A. (1994). *Clinical nursing skills and techniques*, 3rd ed. St. Louis: Mosby–Year Book.

Potter, P.A, & Perry, A. G. (1993). *Fundamentals of nursing: Concepts, process, and practice*, 3rd ed. St. Louis: Mosby–Year Book.

Thompson, J. M., et al. (1993). *Mosby's manual of clinical nursing*, 3rd ed. St. Louis: Mosby–Year Book.

❓QUESTIONS

1. The nursing process is composed of which of the following steps in the correct order?

   ① Planning; assessment; implementation; evaluation
   ② Assessment; planning; implementation; evaluation
   ③ Assessment; nursing diagnosis; intervention; evaluation
   ④ Nursing diagnosis; planning; implementation; evaluation

2. Although terminology differs, the steps in the nursing process and in the problem-solving approach to nursing care are quite similar. Stating the client's problem correlates with which step in the nursing process?

   ① Planning
   ② Assessment
   ③ Implementation
   ④ Evaluation

3. When a soapsuds enema is given, the soapsuds have the effect of:

   ① Soothing the mucosal lining of the colon
   ② Cleansing the intestinal tract of bacteria
   ③ Allowing easier passage of feces
   ④ Irritating the mucosal lining of the colon

4. An oil retention enema, such as a Fleet enema, is given primarily to:

   ① Stimulate peristalsis
   ② Soften fecal material
   ③ Cleanse the bowel before a diagnostic test
   ④ Relieve distention from flatus

5. When heating the oil for an oil retention enema, the nurse must remember that:

   ① Oil should not be heated to more than 100° F because it retains heat longer than water
   ② Oil must be heated to over 100° F for it to flow freely through the rectal tube
   ③ Oil will mix with water only after it has been heated
   ④ Oil does not conduct heat as well as water, so it must be heated to more than 100° F.

6. Before administering an enema, the nurse should tell the client to:

   ① Try to go to the bathroom before the enema is given
   ② Expel the enema as soon as possible after it is given
   ③ Hold it until the urge to defecate is strong
   ④ Hold it for at least an hour

7. The amount given for a tap water enema is usually no greater than:

   ① 1000 mL
   ② 500 mL
   ③ 300 mL
   ④ 100 mL

8. To decrease the client's urge to defecate, the nurse should insert a rectal suppository:

   ① Very quickly
   ② Well beyond the sphincter
   ③ At least 2 inches into the rectum
   ④ Only at body temperature

9. When applying a dressing to the rectal area, the nurse should use a:

   ① Velcro binder
   ② Scultetus binder
   ③ T-binder
   ④ Straight binder

10. The client who requires frequent dressing changes experiences fewer skin problems if the nurse applies:

    ① Wide strips of adhesive tape
    ② A tight abdominal binder
    ③ A T-binder
    ③ Montgomery straps

11. A *disadvantage* associated with a circular Ace bandage is that:

    ① Movement is permitted
    ② Circulation increased
    ③ It can cause a tourniquet effect
    ④ Temperature increases

12. The advantage of using a figure-of-eight bandage is:

    ① Decreasing temperature
    ② Decreasing circulation
    ③ Preventing a tourniquet effect
    ④ Restricting movement

13. When wrapping the ankle or wrist in an Ace bandage, the foot and hand should be included in the Ace wrap to:

  ① Prevent edema
  ② Permit movement
  ③ Cause blanching
  ④ Decrease pain

14. When wrapping the wrist or ankle in an Ace bandage, the toes and fingers should *not* be included in Ace wraps to:

  ① Improve circulation
  ② Permit circulation check
  ③ Allow movement
  ④ Decrease pain

15. The term "implementation" refers to the:

  ① Measurement of the effectiveness of the nursing care plan in meeting client needs
  ② Management and performance of the nursing care plan
  ③ Systematic approach to data collection and analysis
  ④ Link between the identification of client needs and the actual performance of health care activities

16. Performance of nursing care requires that the nurse:

  ① Delegate responsibility for some nursing actions to others
  ② Is responsible for all the nursing care of every assigned client
  ③ Limit interaction with the client
  ④ Plan at the beginning of the nursing process

17. Documentation for nursing care needs to be:

  ① Written objectively
  ② Read by the client
  ③ Reported verbally to the physician
  ④ Written after each nurse–client interaction

18. Documentation is an important source for:

  ① Proving what procedures the nurse can perform
  ② Recording the nurse's verbal responses to the client
  ③ Recording the client's response to treatment
  ④ Specifying the responsible person for each procedure

19. The purpose of recording information throughout a client's stay is to:

  ① Establish the same format in all hospitals
  ② Eliminate interpersonal relationships among the health care personnel
  ③ Aid the nurse in coordinating and directing continuous care for each client
  ④ Protect the client from being sued

20. A sterile urine specimen should be obtained by:

  ① Having the client void in a sterile bedpan
  ② Straight catheterizing the client
  ③ Cleansing the external genitalia before the client voids
  ④ Obtaining a midstream voided urine

21. For a clean urine specimen, the nurse should:

  ① Give the client a clean urine cup to void into
  ② Straight catheterize the client
  ③ Cleanse the external genitalia before the client voids
  ④ Have the client drink a full glass of water first

22. To collect a 24-hour urine specimen correctly, the nurse should:

  ① Discard the first void and save all urine for 24 hours
  ② Save the first and last void in a 24-hour period
  ③ Randomly collect a single specimen during a 24-hour period
  ④ Collect all urine from the first void at 7 A.M. for 24 hours

23. To ensure an accurate result when testing the urine of a diabetic client for glucose and acetone, the nurse should:

  ① Keep the client NPO for 4 hours
  ② Withhold all fluids for at least 1 hour before the test
  ③ Cleanse the external genitalia before the client voids
  ④ Have the client void, drink water, and then void again in 30 minutes

24. The optimum time to collect a sputum specimen is:

  ① At bedtime
  ② Early morning
  ③ After lunch
  ④ In the midmorning

25. A sputum specimen must contain material from the:

    ① Lungs and bronchi
    ② Nasal secretions
    ③ Lining of the trachea
    ④ Salivary glands

26. When collecting a stool specimen for ova and parasites, it is important to remember that the specimen must be:

    ① Refrigerated until examined
    ② In a sterile container
    ③ In an airtight container
    ④ Warm until examined

27. When collecting a specimen for culture and sensitivity, the nurse must remember that the specimen will be:

    ① Potentially contaminated with pathogenic bacteria
    ② A urine or stool specimen
    ③ A large amount, usually 500 mL
    ④ Collected only by an RN

28. The container for a specimen collected for a culture must be:

    ① Covered with a sterile gauze
    ② Plugged with cotton
    ③ Filled completely
    ④ Checked for cracks before it is used

29. After the specimen for culture is obtained, the container must be:

    ① Kept warm until sent to the laboratory
    ② Taken to the laboratory promptly
    ③ Kept in an upright position until it can be sent to the laboratory
    ④ Wrapped in a sterile wrapper

30. Which of the following would *not* be the responsibility of the LPN/LVN in obtaining a culture specimen?

    ① Instruct the client what is to be done
    ② Accurately label the specimen container
    ③ Determine the type of test to be done
    ④ Avoid contaminating the specimen

ANSWERS AND RATIONALES

Guide to item identification (see pp. 4–5 for further details about each category)

I, II, III, or IV for the phase of the nursing process
1, 2, 3, or 4 for the category of client needs
A, B, C, D, E, F, or G for the category of human functioning

Specific content category by name; i.e., cholecystectomy

1. The nursing process consists of four basic steps
② performed in a specific order for the purpose of obtaining maximum benefit to the client.
I, 1, G, Nursing process

2. Both assessment and stating the client's problem
② require collection and organization of data from a variety of sources to plan care based on client needs.
III, 1, G, Nursing process

3. Soapsuds irritate the lining of the intestine, lead-
④ ing to increased peristalsis and bowel evacuation.
I, 1, F, Enema

4. The oil retention enema is given to soften the
② feces with the oil and to lubricate the lining of the bowel.
IV, 1, F, Enema

5. Oil retains heat longer than water, and there is
① a greater risk of injury if it is heated too much.
III, 1, F, Enema

6. It is important for the client to hold the enema
③ for at least a short time for the maximum effect.
III, 1, F, Enema

7. A tap water enema usually does not need more
② than 500 mL to achieve the maximum effect. A greater volume can lead to fluid and electrolyte problems, and a lesser volume may not be effective.
III, 1, F, Enema

8. Unless the suppository is inserted well past the
② sphincter, the client will feel the urge to defecate too quickly before the suppository liquefies.
III, 5, F, Suppository

9. A T-binder is used to hold a rectal dressing in
③ place.
III, 1, D, Dressings

10. Montgomery straps allow the dressing to be
④ changed without constantly removing tape.
III, 1, D, Dressings

11. A circular bandage applied too tightly creates a
③ tourniquet effect, which would prevent adequate circulation and probably cause necrosis.
IV, 1, F, Bandages

12. Circulation needs to be maintained while sup-
③ porting the muscles to prevent edema. A figure-of-eight bandage accomplishes all of these.
IV, 1, F, Bandages

13. If the foot and hand were not included in an Ace
① wrap, a tourniquet effect could possibly form, which would decrease the blood supply, decrease venous return, and promote edema formation.
IV, 1, F, Bandages

14. Visibility is necessary to insure that proper circu-
② lation is maintained.
III, 1, F, Bandages

15. Implementation is assigning the workload to ap-
② propriately trained personnel and the performance of skills according to procedure.
III, 1, G, Nursing process

16. No one nurse can do everything for all clients;
① it is a team coordinated effort.
III, 1, G, Nursing process

17. Documentation proves what observation was
① made, when it was made and by whom.
IV, 1, G, Documentation

18. Documentation is an ongoing written communi-
③ cation concerning a client's response to treatment.
IV, 1, G, Documentation

19. Client care is based on the continual assessment
③ of changes noted in documentation.
IV, 1, G, Nursing process

20. The only way to obtain a sterile specimen is
② with a catheter; a voided specimen is always contaminated to some degree.
III, 2, F, Urine specimen

21. A clean specimen requires that the nurse clean
③ the client's external genitalia with an antiseptic solution before voiding.
III, 2, F, Urine specimen

22.
①
A 24-hour specimen is collected by discarding the specimen that has been sitting in the bladder, the first void, and then collecting all urine voided in a 24-hour period, including having the client void the last specimen exactly 24 hours later.
III, 2, F, Urine specimen

23.
④
The first void contains urine that has been in the bladder for an indeterminate time. Having the client void and then drink and revoid gives a picture of the client's current status.
III, 2, F. Urine specimen

24.
②
The most sputum is available first thing in the morning. Also, these specimens are most likely to contain cells and bacteria.
III, 2, B, Specimens/basic skills

25.
①
To test the specimen, there must be actual material from the lungs and bronchi.
III, 2, B, Sputum specimens

26.
④
For ova and parasites to survive until testing, the stool must be kept warm.
III, 2, F, Stool specimens

27.
①
A culture and sensitivity is done when infection is suspected, so there is a good chance the specimen will contain a large number of potentially pathogenic organisms.
III, 2, D, Culture and sensitivity

28.
④
A culture and sensitivity specimen must be collected in an intact sterile container.
III, 2, D, Culture and sensitivity

29.
③
To prevent contamination of the specimen, it must be kept upright.
III, 2, D, Specimens/basic skills

30.
③
The LPN is responsible for all actions except determining the actual test to be done. This action is solely the responsibility of the physician.
III, 2, D, Diagnostic tests/basic skills

Medication Administration

I. OVERVIEW OF PHARMACOLOGY

A. Names of Drugs

1. Chemical name: description of drug using nomenclature of chemistry
2. Generic name
   a. name assigned by government to drug
   b. also known as nonproprietary name
   c. universal drug name
3. Trade name
   a. created by drug companies to sell a product
   b. also known as proprietary or brand name
   c. generic drug may have many trade names

B. Drug Information Sources

1. Nursing drug books
   a. many different books available
   b. both pharmacology texts and drug handbooks
   c. focus on nursing implications of drugs
2. *Physician's Desk Reference*
   a. published yearly
   b. similar to drug inserts supplied by manufacturers
   c. easy to find drug by brand name
3. *Drug Facts and Comparisons*
4. United States Pharmacopeia (USP) and National Formulary (NF)
   a. revised every 5 years, with supplements in between
   b. establishes legal standards for drugs
5. Package inserts
   a. supplied by manufacturer
   b. regulated by Food and Drug Administration (FDA)

C. Drug Legislation and Regulation

1. FDA maintains strict control of all drugs for use in humans

2. Food, Drug, and Cosmetic Act
   a. first legislation to regulate drug safety
   b. ensures that drugs are safe and effective
   c. requires physician's prescription for dispensing of drugs
3. Harrison Narcotic Act
   a. passed in 1914
   b. first federal law to help prevent drug addiction
   c. established word "narcotic" as legal term
4. Comprehensive Drug Abuse Prevention and Control Act of 1970, also known as the Controlled Substances Act
   a. sets rules for manufacture and distribution of drugs that have potential for abuse
   b. sets categories into which various controlled substances are divided
      (1) *Schedule I:* drugs with a high potential of abuse and not approved for medical use
      (2) *Schedule II*
         (a) drugs with a high potential for abuse but that have been approved for medical use
         (b) no refills without new prescription
         (c) no telephone refills
         (d) prescription good for only 3 days
         (e) in some states, require triplicate prescriptions
      (3) *Schedule III*
         (a) drugs with a lower potential for abuse but that have high risk of psychologic dependence and low-to-moderate potential of dependence
         (b) may refill up to five times; new prescription must be written every 6 months
         (c) telephone refills permitted
      (4) *Schedule IV*
         (a) drugs with some potential for abuse
         (b) prescription must be rewritten after 6 months and five refills
         (c) telephone refills permitted

(5) *Schedule V*
    (a) drugs with little potential for abuse, often in combination with small amounts of controlled substances
    (b) some may be dispensed without prescription
5. Orphan Drug Act provides funding for drugs used to treat rare diseases as incentive for companies to research and produce them

D. Sources of Drugs

1. Chemicals
2. Plants
3. Animal products
4. Food substances
5. Microorganisms
6. Biotechnology
7. Minerals

E. Forms of Drugs

1. Liquid
   a. solution: drug dissolved in a liquid, usually water
   b. suspension: drug in finely divided, undissolved state dispersed in a liquid substance
   c. elixir: solutions containing alcohol, sugar, and water
   d. emulsion: suspension of fat globules and water
   e. tincture: drugs dissolved in alcohol alone or plus water
   f. lotion: liquid suspension or dispersion of drug for topical use
   g. liniment: drug in oily, soapy, or alcohol mixture applied to skin as counterirritant
2. Transdermal
   a. fat-soluble form of medication
   b. applied directly to skin on covered patch
   c. longer absorption and action
3. Solid or semisolid drug forms
   a. capsule
      (1) liquid or solid drug inside gelatinous capsule that dissolves after swallowing
      (2) sustained-release form: drug in small particles coated with substances to vary solubility, contained inside capsule; released slowly, should not be crushed
   b. tablet: solid form of drug pressed into various sizes and shapes
      (1) buccal: solid form that dissolves when held between cheek and gum and directly absorbed by oral mucosa
      (2) sublingual: solid form that dissolves when held under tongue and directly absorbed by oral mucosa
      (3) enteric coated: drug coated with substance that delays release of drug until it reaches intestine, should not be crushed
   c. suppository: drug mixed in soft material that melts at body temperature when inserted into body orifice
   d. ointment: semisolid preparation, usually fatty substance, for external application
   e. troche or lozenge: drug incorporated into mass made of sugar and mucilage or fruit base made to dissolve in mouth

F. Pharmacokinetics: Study of Drug Movement Throughout Body

1. Pharmacodynamics
   a. Absorption
      (1) movement of drug from site of administration into blood stream
      (2) drugs must first be dissolved
      (3) affected by
          (a) rate at which drug dissolves
          (b) surface area exposed to dissolved drug
          (c) blood flow to site of drug absorption
          (d) how fat soluble drug is (more fat soluble, faster absorption)
          (e) route of administration
          (f) condition of client
   b. Distribution
      (1) movement of drug throughout body
      (2) affected by
          (a) blood flow through tissues, to move drug
          (b) ability of drug to leave vascular system
          (c) ability of drug to enter cells
          (d) chemical properties as with carriers
   c. Metabolism
      (1) enzymatic alteration of drug structure; also known as biotransformation
      (2) usually occurs in liver
      (3) prepares the drug either for action or excretion
      (4) affected by
          (a) age of client; under 1 year old, liver not fully functional
          (b) liver function
          (c) nutritional status

(d) competition of two drugs for same enzymes

(e) time administered

d. Excretion
(1) removal of drugs from body
(2) usually occurs through kidneys and urine
(3) affected by renal function
(4) some excretion through nonrenal sources
(a) breast milk
(b) bile and feces
(c) lungs
(d) skin
(e) tears
(f) saliva

e. mechanisms of action
(1) drug action
(2) drug effect

f. drug receptor interaction

g. dose-response curve

h. drug potency and efficacy

i. therapeutic index

2. Pharmacotherapeutics
a. types of therapy
(1) acute
(2) empiric
(3) supportive
(4) palliative
(5) maintenance
(6) supplemental
(7) replacement

b. clinical response

c. route

d. onset and duration of action

e. drug interactions

G. Factors Affecting Drug Action

1. Dose of drug and route of administration

2. Patient age
a. newborns and infants with immature systems for metabolism and excretion
b. elderly may have deterioration of systems affecting pharmacokinetics

3. Diet: some foods may alter action of drugs

4. Other drugs
a. additive effects: two drugs taken together lead to increased effect
b. potentiation: effect of two drugs greater than sum of effects if drugs taken separately
c. antagonism: one drug acts on another to decrease its effectiveness

5. Body size: both height and weight affect dose of drug needed

6. Pregnancy

7. Disease processes

H. Reactions to Medication

1. Intended effect: that effect for which drug was designed

2. Side effect: drug effect other than that intended

3. Local effect: action of drug limited to area of application

4. Systemic effect: potential effect on any body system resulting from absorption of drug into blood

5. Adverse effects
a. idiosyncratic reaction: unusual or unexpected reaction to a drug
b. allergic reaction: stimulation of antibodies in reaction to foreign antigen; categories of drug allergies I–IV
c. untoward reaction: one harmful to one or more body systems
d. teratogenic effect: drug that causes fetal abnormalities when given to pregnant client
e. dependency: physical or psychologic need for further doses of drug

6. Tolerance: drug given over a period of time no longer producing same effect, requires larger doses to achieve same effect

I. Nursing Process Applied to Drug Therapy

1. Assessment
a. medication history
b. food or drug allergies
c. past medical history
d. identifying actual or potential problems
e. knowledge deficits/teaching needs

2. Planning
a. purpose and goal of therapy
b. proper dosage
c. equipment

3. Implementation
a. use of five rights
b. adaptations for individual clients

4. Evaluation
a. assess response
b. report any untoward effects

II. COMMON CATEGORIES OF DRUGS
(See each section for more details on specific drugs)

A. Drugs Affecting Sexuality

1. Uterine smooth muscle stimulants
a. *description:* drugs that stimulate uterine smooth muscle, especially gravid uterus; sensitivity of uterus increases during gestation and increases sharply before parturition

b. *uses:* for initiation and improvement of uterine contractions for term or preterm delivery in maternal or fetal distress situations; postpartum to control postpartum bleeding or hemorrhage; nasal oxytocin indicated for initial let-down of milk

c. *side effects:* fetal bradycardia, anaphylaxis, hemorrhage, nausea, vomiting, uterine hypertonicity, rupture of uterus, water intoxication

d. *nursing implications:* obtain good obstetric history; do not administer intravenously (IV) without physician available; have MgSO$_4$ on hand to treat tetany; use infusion pump with IV infusion; monitor mother and fetus continually during administration; monitor for postpartum bleeding; monitor uterine contractions

e. *example:* oxytocin (Pitocin)

2. Beta-receptor antagonist
   a. *description:* drugs that have an antagonistic effect on beta$_2$-adrenergic receptors, such as those in uterine smooth muscle
   b. *uses:* management of preterm labor in suitable clients; safe and effective under 20 weeks' gestation
   c. *side effects:* dose-related alterations in maternal and fetal heart rates and maternal blood pressure; palpitations; tremors; nausea; vomiting; headache; erythema; malaise
   d. *nursing implications:* check maternal vital signs and monitor fetus; monitor uterine contractions; run as IV piggyback; use IV infusion pump; teach client use of oral form; keep in left lateral position during IV administration
   e. *example:* ritodrine hydrochloride (Yutopar)

3. Hormones
   a. androgens
      (1) *description:* drugs that produce anabolic and androgenic effects
      (2) *uses:* replacement therapy for men; to treat dysmenorrhea and menopause in women; treatment of inoperable breast cancer in certain women
      (3) *side effects:* **males**—impotence, gynecomastia, epididymitis, bladder irritation; **females**—hirsutism, amenorrhea, masculinization; **both**—nausea, vomiting, diarrhea, fluid retention
      (4) *nursing implications:* warn client about possible changes in sexual characteristics; use with caution in clients on oral anticoagulants; monitor input and output (I&O); check for edema; monitor calcium levels
      (5) *example:* testosterone propionate
   b. estrogens
      (1) *description:* drugs that act by inhibiting pituitary activity; increase tone of breasts and genitourinary structures and insure proper menstrual flow in premenopausal women
      (2) *uses:* postmenopausal syndrome, amenorrhea caused by ovarian failure, suppression of lactation; prostatic cancer in men
      (3) *side effects:* nausea, vomiting, anorexia, abdominal distention and bloating, spotting, menstrual changes, fluid retention, depression, hypercalcemia, migraines, breast tenderness and enlargement, reduced glucose tolerance, possible uterine cancer, hypersensitivity; men have similar side effects but also development of female secondary sexual characteristics
      (4) *nursing implications:* contraindicated in pregnancy, some breast cancers, thrombophlebitis, thyroid and liver disease; use cautiously in clients with hypertension, migraines, diabetes mellitus, and asthma; monitor for edema and congestive heart failure; watch for depression
      (5) *example:* diethlystilbestrol (DES)
   c. oral contraceptive agents
      (1) *description:* drugs that work in a variety of ways either to prevent ovulation or to provide barrier at the cervix to prevent sperm from penetrating
      (2) *uses:* to prevent pregnancy
      (3) *side effects:* nausea and vomiting; fluid retention; migraines; cerebrovascular accident; bloating; weight gain; breast tenderness; breakthrough bleeding, spotting; thrombophlebitis, especially in women who smoke
      (4) *nursing implications:* monitor blood pressure, weight, pregnancy status, liver function studies; use with caution in women over 35 or who have smoked more than 15 years; follow package information for missed doses; notify physician about breakthrough bleeding
      (5) *example:* norgestrel (Ovrette)

B. Drugs Affecting Oxygenation

1. Antihypertensives and fluid volume regulators
   a. *description:* drugs that act to reduce blood pressure through a wide variety of mechanisms and drugs that produce diuresis

b. *uses:* control of moderate-to-severe hypertension
c. thiazide diuretics
  (1) *side effects:* hypokalemia, hyponatremia, hyperuricemia, hyperglycemia, orthostatic hypotension
  (2) *nursing implications:* maintain K^+ level; teach high K^+, low Na^+ diet; monitor I& O, blood pressure
  (3) *example:* hydrochlorothiazide (Hydro-DIURIL)
d. loop diuretics
  (1) *side effects:* orthostatic hypertension, hypokalemia, hyponatremia, constipation, urinary frequency
  (2) *nursing implications:* maintain K^+ level; give in early morning to prevent nocturia; weigh client to monitor fluid loss; give with food to reduce gastrointestinal distress; encourage high K^+ diet
  (3) *example:* furosemide (Lasix)
e. potassium-sparing diuretic
  (1) *side effects:* hyponatremia, hyperkalemia, gastrointestinal disturbances, allergic reactions
  (2) *nursing implications:* monitor K^+ intake to insure excess not ingested; monitor I& O, blood pressure
  (3) *example:* spironolactone (Aldactone)
f. sympathetic-inhibiting agents, sympatholytic
  (1) *side effects:* orthostatic hypotension, depression, drowsiness, gastrointestinal disturbances, impotence (Aldomet), bradycardia, Na^+ and water retention
  (2) *nursing implications:* caution client to change position slowly; monitor for side effects altering compliance; maintain low Na^+ diet; restrict alcohol use (may increase hypotension)
  (3) *example:* methyldopa (Aldomet)
2. Cardiac glycosides
  a. *description:* drugs that act directly on myocardium to increase force of contraction; cardiac output increased while heart rate slowed
  b. *uses:* congestive heart failure, dysrhythmias (especially those with increased rate), cardiogenic shock with pulmonary edema
  c. *side effects:* dysrhythmias, heart block, bradycardia, gastrointestinal upset, muscle weakness, diplopia
  d. *nursing implications:* take apical pulse for 1 full minute before administration; if above 120 or below 60, hold medication and notify physician; monitor for toxicity and hypokalemia if client is also taking diuretics; teach client to check pulse rate at home and eat high K^+ diet if taking diuretics
  e. *example:* digoxin (Lanoxin)

3. Vasodilators
  a. *description:* drugs that act on blood vessels to cause increase in diameter, thereby improving blood flow; most effective in dilating coronary arteries and less effective in dilating peripheral vessels
  b. *uses:* antianginal, some action on cerebral and peripheral circulation
  c. *side effects:* generalized vasodilation (headache, flushing, orthostatic hypotension, tachycardia)
  d. *nursing implications:* know correct form and schedule of administration; e.g., p. r. n. (as needed) vs. regular, oral, sublingual, chewable, or transdermal
  e. *types and examples:* nitrites/nitrates, nitroglycerin (Nitro-Bid); calcium channel blockers, verapamil (Calan); cerebral vasodilators, dipyridamole (Persantine); peripheral vasodilators, isoxsuprine hydrochloride (Vasodilan)
4. Anticoagulants
  a. *description:* drugs that act to prevent blood clotting; parenteral forms act by inhibiting formation of prothrombin activator, which then diminishes conversion of prothrombin to thrombin; also form plasma antithrombin and block activation of fibrin-stabilizing factor; oral forms block synthesis of vitamin K–dependent clotting factors in liver; neither form has any effect on existing clots
  b. *uses:* prevention and treatment of thromboses; parenteral drugs can also be used to prevent clotting of blood outside body
  c. *side effects:* hemorrhage
  d. *nursing implications:* avoid use of any other product that increases anticoagulation or causes bleeding (e.g., aspirin); teach client safety precautions to avoid bleeding (e.g., soft toothbrush, electric razor); monitor laboratory tests: parenteral—partial thromboplastin time (PTT); oral—prothrombin time (PT)
  e. *types and examples:* parenteral, heparin; oral, warfarin (Coumadin)
5. Anticoagulant antagonists
  a. *description:* drugs that act as antagonists to block action of anticoagulants
  b. *uses:* overdose of anticoagulants; bleeding; hypoprothrombinemia
  c. *side effects:* flushing, gastrointestinal upset, allergic reactions
  d. *nursing implications:* monitor client during administration, assess effectiveness by noting decrease in bleeding
  e. *examples:* parenteral, protamine sulfate; oral, vitamin K (AquaMEPHYTON)

6. Antihyperlipidemics
   a. *description:* drugs that lower blood cholesterol or triglycerides through a variety of actions; bile acid sequestrants inhibit reabsorption of bile acids leading to increased excretion
      (1) HMC-CoA reductase inhibitors inhibit cholesterol biosynthesis
      (2) fibric acid drugs decrease serum triglycerides
   b. *uses:* to lower serum cholesterol, triglycerides, or both
   c. *side effects:* constipation or diarrhea; nausea and vomiting; abdominal pain; headache; cholelithiasis; dyspepsia
   d. *nursing implications:* monitor cholesterol levels; take with or shortly before meals; monitor presence of side effects; may need to supplement fat-soluble vitamins with bile acid sequestrants
   e. *examples:*
      (1) bile acid sequestrants—cholestyramine (Questran)
      (2) HMC-CoA reductase inhibitors— pravastatin (Pravachol)
      (3) fibric acid drugs—gemfibrozil (Lopid)
7. Bronchodilators—xanthine derivatives
   a. *description:* drugs that relax bronchial smooth muscle and inhibit release of histamine and slow-release substance A (SRS-A) from mast cells; mild diuretics and cardiac stimulants
   b. *uses:* symptomatic relief of asthma and bronchial spasms
   c. *side effects:* gastrointestinal upset, nausea, nervousness, frequency, diarrhea, insomnia, tachycardia, palpitations, esophageal reflux
   d. *nursing implications:* use with caution in clients with hypertension, tachycardia, hypoxemia, glaucoma, hyperthyroidism, benign prostatic hypertrophy, diabetes; monitor for central nervous system (CNS) symptoms; give with food or antacids; client should avoid smoking and maintain upright position after meals
   e. *example:* theophylline (Theo-Dur)
8. Cough preparations
   a. expectorants
      (1) *description:* drugs that facilitate removal of thick mucus from lungs and act as soothing demulcent by stimulating secretion of lubricant
      (2) *uses:* facilitate productive cough
      (3) *side effects:* nausea, vomiting, gastrointestinal irritation, drowsiness
      (4) *nursing implications:* instruct client not to use for more than 1 week without seeing physician; use high fluid intake and humidity to loosen secretions; do not follow with water except potassium iodide
      (5) *example:* guaifenesin (Robitussin)

   b. antitussives
      (1) *description:* drugs that suppress cough reflex
      (2) *uses:* to treat nonproductive coughs
      (3) *side effects:* dizziness, sedation, sweating, nausea, dry mouth, urinary retention, constipation
      (4) *nursing implications:* never use in clients with productive coughs; administer with caution in clients with asthma, COPD, cardiac disease, convulsions, renal or hepatic disease; if cough continues more than 1 week, client should see physician
      (5) *example:* codeine
9. Antibiotics
   a. *description:* group of drugs that are either bacteriostatic (inhibiting or arresting growth of microorganisms) or bactericidal (killing of microorganisms); terms ''antibacterial,'' ''antimicrobial,'' ''antiinfective,'' and ''antiseptic'' are often used synonymously with antibiotic
   b. penicillins
      (1) *uses:* treatment of common infections caused by penicillin-sensitive microorganisms
      (2) *side effects:* allergic reactions including anaphylaxis; diarrhea; development of resistant organisms; superinfection; gastrointestinal distress
      (3) *nursing implications:* watch closely for rash or early signs of allergic reactions; check all clients for allergy before giving; obtain appropriate culture and sensitivity before starting drug; teach client to take full course of drugs as ordered
      (4) *example:* ampicillin (Polycillin)
   c. aminoglycosides
      (1) *uses:* treatment of gram-negative infections (often nosocomial or iatrogenic); effective in treating serious, systemic, gram-negative infections
      (2) *side effects:* ototoxicity, nephrotoxicity, superinfections; allergic potential small
      (3) *nursing implications:* monitor closely for hearing changes; monitor renal function; watch for development of superinfection
      (4) *example:* gentamicin (Garamycin)
   d. cephalosporins
      (1) *uses:* treatment of septicemia and most systemic infections; effective against some penicillin-resistant organisms
      (2) *side effects:* allergic reactions (two thirds of penicillin-sensitive clients are also cephalosporin sensitive), superinfection, nephrotoxicity with higher doses, phlebitis at IV site, diarrhea

(3) *nursing implications:* monitor known penicillin-sensitive clients closely for allergies; give IV preparations over 30 minutes to reduce phlebitis; give oral preparations 1 hour before or 2 hours after meals for maximum effectiveness; monitor for superinfection, especially oral or vaginal fungal infections

(4) *example:* cephalothin (Keflin)

e. tetracyclines

(1) *uses:* effective against wide variety of pathogens, including many of those causing diarrhea and pneumonia; used to control acne

(2) *side effects:* diarrhea, nausea, vestibular disturbances (minocycline), hypersensitivity reactions, gastrointestinal upset, permanent discoloration of teeth (especially in children), impairment of bone growth, superinfection

(3) *nursing implications:* check for symptoms of hypersensitivity; do not give to pregnant women or children under age 8 years; do not administer with milk or antacids; give with sufficient water; watch for superinfection

(4) *example:* tetracycline (Achromycin)

f. monobactams

(1) *uses:* to treat aerobic gram-negative rod infections

(2) *side effects:* anaphylaxis, diarrhea, nausea and vomiting, rash, neutropenia

(3) *nursing implications:* make sure client knows to take full course of medication; intramuscular (IM) injections painful; watch for phlebitis at IV site; monitor for reduction of symptoms; report abnormalities in white blood count (WBC) to physician

(4) *example:* aztreonam (Azactam)

g. carbapenems

(1) *uses:* to treat aerobic and anaerobic gram-positive and gram-negative infections

(2) *side effects:* nausea and vomiting, diarrhea, rash, fever, hypotension, cross allergy for penicillin-sensitive clients

(3) *nursing implications:* monitor for the development of pain and phlebitis at IV site; watch blood pressure; not given IM; use cautiously with elderly or clients with history of renal disease

(4) *example:* imipenem/cilastatin (Primaxin)

h. macrolides

(1) *uses:* treatment of gram-positive infections in penicillin-sensitive clients, used for legionnaire's disease and *Mycoplasma* pneumonia

(2) *side effects:* nausea and vomiting, hearing loss, dyspepsia, abdominal pain, hepatitis

(3) *nursing implications:* avoid IM injections if possible because they are very painful; do not take medication with food; report adverse reactions to physician; monitor for history of allergies; use cautiously in clients with liver disease; safety in pregnancy not established

(4) *example:* erythromycin ethylsuccinate (E.E.S)

i. antiretrovirals

(1) *uses:* treatment of human immunodeficiency virus (HIV) seroconverted clients with a T-cell (CD4) level less than $500/mm^3$

(2) *side effects:* headache, insomnia, hypersensitivity, nausea, anemia, leukopenia, infection, myalgia

(3) *nursing implications:* contraindicated in clients with known hypersensitivity; use cautiously in clients with bone marrow suppression, renal impairment, or hepatic dysfunction or in children under 3; administer around the clock if possible; protect medication from light; treat pain carefully because of interaction of most pain medications with antiretroviral

(4) *example:* zidovudine (Retrovir)

10. Antitubercular agents

a. *description:* drugs that act specifically on tubercular bacillus to inhibit growth of organism and cause it to become walled off; made up of first-line drugs (most effective with fewest side effects) and second-line drugs (more side effects and less effective)

b. *uses:* to treat tuberculosis (TB) and for TB prophylaxis

c. *side effects:* isoniazid (INH)—peripheral neuropathy, gastrointestinal distress, hepatic toxicity, agranulocytosis, hemolytic anemia; rifampin (Rifadin)—red-orange urine and secretions, gastrointestinal distress, liver dysfunction, hematologic reaction; ethambutol hydrochloride (Myambutol)—loss of visual acuity, disturbance of color discrimination, dermatitis, gastrointestinal symptoms, elevated liver function tests, precipitation of gout

d. *nursing implications:* emphasize importance of finishing medication; instruct client about side effects; monitor drug dosage and liver and renal function; administer pyridoxine to prevent peripheral neuropathy from INH; administer INH on empty stomach or 1 hour before intake of antacids to increase absorption; monitor visual acuity and color discrimination

e. *examples:* first-line drugs—isoniazid (INH) and pyridoxine (vitamin B$_6$), rifampin (Rifadin), ethambutol (Myambutol); second-line drugs—para-aminosalicylic acid (PAS), streptomycin

11. Iron preparations
   a. *description:* acts to build hemoglobin in iron-deficient clients
   b. *uses:* iron deficiency anemia; prophylactically in pregnancy, childhood, menopause, and heavy menses
   c. *side effects:* nausea, vomiting, gastrointestinal distress, constipation, headache, lethargy; do not use in clients with cirrhosis, peptic ulcers, or ulcerative colitis
   d. *nursing implications:* do not give tetracycline or antacids; use straw with solutions to avoid staining teeth; warn client that stools will turn black; give with meals to prevent gastrointestinal distress; increase iron in diet; give IM Z-track
   e. *examples:* ferrous sulfate (Feosol), iron dextran (Imferon)

C. Drugs Affecting Perception

1. Analgesics
   a. nonnarcotic
      (1) *description:* drugs that act to decrease pain, often through antiinflammatory actions without side effects of narcotics; major drugs either salicylate (aspirin) or paraaminophenols (acetaminophen)
      (2) *uses:* for relief of mild-to-moderate pain
      (3) *side effects: salicylate*—salicylism (headache, nausea, vomiting, palpitations, hyperventilation), hypersensitivity, gastrointestinal distress and bleeding, anticoagulant effect, liver damage; *acetaminophen*—hypersensitivity, CNS stimulation, liver and renal damage, palpitations
      (4) *nursing implications:* avoid use of salicylate in clients with gastrointestinal disorders, antiinflammatory or anticoagulant therapy, or history of aspirin sensitivity; avoid overuse; keep supply away from children; monitor liver and renal function; warn client to avoid over-the-counter medicines that contain "hidden" aspirin
      (5) *examples: salicylate*—acetylsalicylic acid (aspirin); *paraaminophenols*—acetaminophen (Tylenol)
   b. narcotics
      (1) *description:* drugs that act to decrease pain by inhibiting transmission of pain impulses, reducing cortical responses to pain stimuli, or altering activity in pain-perception center of brain
      (2) *uses:* treatment of moderate or severe pain
      (3) *side effects:* drowsiness, dizziness or light-headedness, euphoria, respiratory depression, constipation, urinary retention, hypersensitivity, hypotension
      (4) *nursing implications:* monitor effectiveness of analgesia; watch for hypotension and respiratory depression; monitor I& O, bowel movements; watch for possible tolerance and dependence
      (5) *examples:* morphine sulfate, meperidine (Demerol)

2. Miotic-cholinergics
   a. *description:* drugs that mimic effects of cholinergic nerve stimulation and produce response similar to acetylcholine
   b. *uses:* glaucoma (miotic), urinary retention, postoperative abdominal distention, myasthenia gravis, antidote for curare
   c. *side effects:* headache, conjunctival hyperemia (otic), urinary urgency, severe hypotension, bronchospasms, respiratory paralysis, cholinergic crisis
   d. *nursing implications:* administer miotic preparations on time; note CNS irritability; monitor vital signs; have atropine available as antidote; avoid IM or IV use, may cause vascular collapse
   e. *examples:* **direct-acting cholinomimetic**—bethanechol (Urecholine), pilocarpine (Isopto Carpine); **indirect-acting cholinomimetic**—physostigmine sulfate (Eserine Sulfate)

3. Carbonic anhydrase inhibitors
   a. *description:* drugs that increase urine output by blocking carbonic anhydrase in kidneys; also decrease production of aqueous humor
   b. *uses:* to treat glaucoma, edema not responding well to single-drug therapy, adjuvant to anticonvulsant therapy for epilepsy
   c. *side effects:* paresthesia, lethargy, anorexia, tinnitus, headache, hypokalemia, hyponatremia, ureteral colic, metabolic acidosis
   d. *nursing implications:* use cautiously in clients with respiratory acidosis, diabetes, and gout; monitor Na$^+$ and K$^+$ levels; watch for hypersensitivity; monitor visual improvement
   e. *example:* acetazolamide (Diamox)

4. Barbiturates
   a. *description:* drugs that act by reversibly depressing activity of all excitable tissues; CNS is particularly sensitive; sleep induced has decreased rapid eye movement (REM) time

b. *uses:* sedation, sleeplessness, anticonvulsant (phenobarbital), general anesthesia adjunct

c. *side effects:* drowsiness, lethargy, headache, depression, hangover, hypersensitivity, blood dyscrasias

d. *nursing implications:* warn client about potential drug interactions, especially other CNS depressants; use other means to promote sleep; avoid overuse or dependence; monitor for overdose

e. *example:* secobarbital (Seconal)

5. Nonbarbiturates

a. *description:* drugs that act by increasing non-rapid eye movement (NREM) sleep while decreasing REM sleep by depressing subcortical levels in CNS

b. *uses:* sleeplessness, preoperative sedation

c. *side effects:* nausea, vomiting, constipation, hangover, headache, rash, urinary frequency

d. *nursing implications:* use with care in elderly, COPD, depressed clients; avoid other CNS depressants; use natural methods to induce sleep; monitor for overuse or abuse

e. *example:* flurazepam (Dalmane)

6. Antianxiety agents (benzodiazepines)

a. *description:* drugs that act selectively as presynaptic inhibitors of neural pathways throughout CNS; have similar activities to CNS depressants but act more selectively

b. *uses:* to treat anxiety, preoperative sedation, status epilepticus, acute alcohol withdrawal syndrome, mild muscle relaxant

c. *side effects:* confusion, headache, agitation, oversedation, drowsiness, constipation, decreased libido, urinary retention, hypersensitivity; may be habit forming

d. *nursing implications:* avoid use with alcohol or CNS depressants; food and antacids decrease absorption; avoid overuse and abuse; withdraw drugs slowly, assess mood and affect

e. *example:* diazepam (Valium)

7. Antipsychotic agents

a. *description:* drugs that produce strong antipsychotic effects, possibly by blockade of postsynaptic dopamine receptors in brain; act on hypothalamus and reticular formation to produce strong sedation; strong alpha-adrenergic effect and weak anticholinergic effect

b. *uses:* to control manic phase of manic-depressive illness; to treat severe nausea/vomiting; severe anxiety and agitation; intractable hiccoughs

c. *side effects:* laryngospasms, dyspnea, extrapyramidal syndrome, agranulocytosis, jaundice, photosensitivity, orthostatic hypotension, tachycardia, sedation, constipation, dry mouth, tardive dyskinesia (abnormal facial grimaces and movements of the lips, tongue, and jaw)

d. *nursing implications:* avoid other CNS depressants; monitor for development of extrapyramidal syndrome, liver function changes, signs of blood dyscrasias; check blood pressure; watch for constipation; do not give with antacids; teach about orthostatic changes

e. *example:* chlorpromazine (Thorazine)

D. Drugs Affecting Protective Functions

1. Antineoplastics

a. *description:* a wide variety of drugs that act to destroy rapidly dividing cells; classified as "cell-cycle specific" (those that attack cells at a specific point in process of cell division) or "cell-cycle nonspecific" (those that act at any time during cell division)

b. alkylating agents
   (1) *uses:* leukemias, lymphomas, multiple myelomas
   (2) *side effects:* bone marrow depression, nausea/vomiting, vesicant action if extravasated, alopecia, hemorrhagic cystitis
   (3) *nursing implications:* monitor blood counts closely; teach client safety precautions concerning low counts; avoid any contact with skin; prevent nausea
   (4) *example:* cyclophosphamide (Cytoxan)

c. antimetabolites
   (1) *uses:* leukemias, testicular cancer, ovarian cancer, colon tumors
   (2) *side effects:* gastrointestinal ulceration, stomatitis, bone marrow depression, nephrotoxicity, ototoxicity, anaphylaxis
   (3) *nursing implications:* give leucovorin as ordered to prevent toxicity from methotrexate; hydrate well; monitor blood counts closely; watch for gastrointestinal bleeding
   (4) *example:* methotrexate (Mexate)

d. antitumor antibiotics
   (1) *uses:* to treat breast, ovarian, testicular, and lung cancer; leukemia; and lymphoma
   (2) *side effects:* bone marrow depression, severe tissue necrosis with extravasation, nausea/vomiting, cardiotoxicity, alopecia, stomatitis, red discoloration of urine
   (3) *nursing implications:* avoid extravasation; maintain adequate food and fluid intake; monitor cardiac function and blood counts
   (4) *example:* doxorubicin (Adriamycin)

e. vinca alkaloids
   (1) *uses:* to treat testicular, lung, ovary, and breast cancers; leukemia; and lymphoma
   (2) *side effects:* neurotoxicity, constipation, depression, mild bone marrow depression, alopecia, inflammation with extravasation
   (3) *nursing implications:* monitor for sensory or motor changes; administer stool softeners; administer IV slowly
   (4) *example:* vincristine (Oncovin)
f. hormones
   (1) *uses:* to treat hormone-dependent tumors such as breast and prostate cancers
   (2) *side effects:* minimal bone marrow depression, mild hypoglycemia, nausea, hypercalcemia in women with bone metastasis
   (3) *nursing implications:* monitor menstrual function; monitor blood calcium levels
   (4) *example:* tamoxifen (Nolvadex)

E. Drugs Affecting Mobility

1. Antiinflammatory drugs
   a. nonsteroidal
      (1) *description:* large group of drugs with antiinflammatory and often analgesic properties; act to reduce symptoms of inflammation such as redness, swelling, fever, and pain
      (2) *uses:* to treat mild-to-moderate pain caused by inflammatory conditions; symptomatic relief of arthritic conditions
      (3) *side effects:* gastrointestinal irritation, ulcers, bleeding, dyspepsia, bone marrow depression, headache, dizziness, bowel changes, allergy
      (4) *nursing implications:* take with food or antacid to decrease gastrointestinal distress; monitor blood counts; watch for gastrointestinal bleeding; monitor for aspirin allergy; do not administer aspirin or other antiinflammatories
      (5) *example:* ibuprofen (Motrin)
   b. steroids
      (1) *description:* drugs that block inflammatory, allergic, and immune responses by a variety of processes, including both naturally occurring and synthetic glucocorticoids
      (2) *uses:* replacement for primary or secondary adrenocortical insufficiency; to treat wide variety of inflammatory, allergic/autoimmune disorders including rheumatoid disease, collagen disease, allergic reactions, dermatologic responses, oph-

thalmic problems, ulcerative colitis, Crohn's disease, neoplasms
   (3) *side effects:* salt and water retention, gastrointestinal ulceration from increased hydrochloride secretion, hypertension, congestive heart failure, hirsutism, striae, impaired wound healing, fat redistribution, decreased growth in children, protein catabolism, osteoporosis, emotional lability, leukopenia, increased susceptibility to infection, sterility, cataracts, diabetes, hypokalemia
   (4) *nursing implications:* warn client about need to avoid infections and increased need for steroids during times of physical and emotional stress; monitor decreased response to stress and side effects; help client learn to minimize side effects as much as possible (eg, low Na^+, high K^+, low carbohydrate diet); give with antacid or histamine receptor antagonist; give on diurnal schedule (high in A.M.); stress need for client to adhere strictly to medication regimen; offer support to clients experiencing changes in body image; suggest Medic Alert
   (5) *examples:* dexamethasone (Decadron), cortisone acetate (prednisone)
2. Skeletal muscle relaxants
   a. *description:* drugs that act by interfering with nerve impulses in muscle tissues; CNS depressants with sedative properties; act on spinal and supraspinal sites to decrease frequency and amplitude of muscle spasms
   b. *uses:* acute painful muscle spasms, muscle tension and pains associated with anxiety; to treat spastic disorders such as multiple sclerosis
   c. *side effects:* headache, lethargy, dizziness, nausea/vomiting, hypotension, blurred vision, hypersensitivity, hypotonia
   d. *nursing implications:* give with meals; avoid orthostatic changes; warn about drowsiness; warn client urine may change color; avoid alcohol or other CNS depressants; use cautiously with elderly and clients with seizure disorders; withdraw drugs slowly
   e. *examples:* methocarbamol (Robaxin), baclofen (Lioresal)
3. Anticonvulsants
   a. *description:* a wide variety of drugs that act to decrease nerve cell excitability in various ways
   b. *uses:* treatment of epilepsy and other seizure disorders
   c. *side effects:* gastrointestinal irritation, dizziness, apathy, nervousness, ataxia, gum hyperplasia, blurred vision
   d. *nursing implications:* teach client to comply

with consistent medication regimen; avoid use of alcohol; warn client about drowsiness or decreased alertness; give with meals to decrease gastrointestinal distress

e. *types and examples:* **barbiturates**—phenobarbital; **hydantoins**—phenytoin (Dilantin)

4. Antiparkinsonian agents
   a. *description:* drugs that increase level of dopamine in CNS; often given in conjunction with anticholinergics because cholinergic activity is increased when deficit of dopamine exists
   b. *uses:* control of symptoms of Parkinson's disease
   c. *side effects:* nausea/vomiting, anorexia, orthostatic hypotension, dry mouth, dysphagia, ataxia, headache, insomnia, anxiety, hypertension, urinary retention
   d. *nursing implications:* use cautiously in clients with cardiovascular, respiratory, endocrine, or hepatic disease; peptic ulcers; wide-angle glaucoma; diabetes; and psychoses; watch blood pressure
   e. *example:* levodopa and carbidopa (Sinemet)

F. Drugs Affecting Metabolism/Elimination/Nutrition

1. Antiemetics
   a. *description:* drugs that act to treat and prevent nausea and vomiting; most act by inhibiting chemoreceptor trigger zone or by depressing vestibular apparatus in inner ear
   b. *uses:* prevention and treatment of nausea and vomiting; motion sickness
   c. *side effects:* drowsiness, dry mouth, flushing, hypotension, restlessness, fatigue, extrapyramidal effects (parkinsonism, akathisia, tardive dyskinesia, dystonia)
   d. *nursing implications:* monitor I&O, blood pressure; when client on long-term phenothiazine therapy, monitor for liver disease and extrapyramidal symptoms; warn client about drowsiness; monitor effectiveness; use preventively
   e. *types and examples:* **phenothiazines**—prochlorperazine (Compazine); **nonphenothiazines**—trimethobenzamide (Tigan)

2. Antidiarrheals
   a. *description:* drugs that act to reduce liquidity of feces; local agents act within bowel to soothe intestinal tract and increase absorption of water, electrolytes, and nutrients; systemic agents act systemically to inhibit peristaltic reflex and reduce gastrointestinal motility
   b. *uses:* treatment of acute and chronic diarrhea
   c. *side effects:* nausea/vomiting, acute glaucoma (Lomotil), headache, drowsiness, hypersensitivity, nystagmus
   d. *nursing implications:* identify cause of diarrhea and eliminate cause; do not use Lomotil in clients with glaucoma or benign prostatic hypertrophy; avoid overuse; prevent constipation; protect drugs from light and moisture
   e. *types and examples: local*—kaolin and pectin (Kapectolin); *systemic*—diphenoxylate hydrochloride with atropine (Lomotil)

3. Laxatives
   a. *description:* drugs that facilitate evacuation of bowel by wide variety of mechanisms
   b. *uses:* treatment of constipation; preparation for certain diagnostic tests
   c. *nursing implications:* suggest alternate methods to promote bowel movements: diet, fluids, exercise; time administration according to action; do not use if obstruction suspected; give adequate fluids.
   d. *types and examples:* **irritants**—bisacodyl (Dulcolax); **bulk formers**—psyllium (Metamucil); **saline/osmotic**—MgOH (milk of magnesia); **emollients**—docusate sodium (Colace); **lubricants**—mineral oil

4. Hypoglycemics
   a. *description:* drugs that either stimulate islet cells in the pancreas to secrete more insulin (oral) or act as insulin replacement when pancreatic function ceases (parenteral)
   b. *uses:* treatment of diabetes mellitus
   c. *side effects:* hypoglycemic reactions, gastrointestinal distress, neurologic symptoms, alcohol intolerance (oral), allergic reactions
   d. *nursing implications:* know onset and duration of action for each agent and teach to client; monitor for and teach client to monitor for hypoglycemic reactions; stress compliance with total diabetic regimen; check for pork or beef allergy; teach client insulin self-administration, site rotation, care of equipment, proper storage, and glucose and urine self-testing
   e. *examples:* **oral agents**—acetohexamide (Dymelor); **insulins**—rapid-acting, regular insulin; intermediate-acting, insulin suspension (NPH); long-acting, protamine zinc insulin (PZI)

5. Sulfonamides
   a. *description:* drugs that are bacteriostatic against both gram-positive and gram-negative organisms; drugs excreted unchanged and undissolved and dissolve well in urine; therefore excellent for treating urinary tract infections
   b. *uses:* urinary tract infections, acute otitis media, ulcerative colitis, chronic bronchitis

c. *side effects:* gastrointestinal distress, allergic reactions, headache, peripheral neuritis, hearing loss, crystalluria, hypoglycemia

d. *nursing implications:* administer with large amounts of fluid; monitor serum glucose levels (may produce false-positive urine glucose); monitor for allergies; check I&O; maintain alkaline pH because drugs more soluble in alkaline urine; teach client to take full course of drugs

e. *examples:* trimethoprim (Bactrim, Septra), sulfisoxazole (Gantrisin)

6. Quinolones

a. *description:* drugs that exhibit a bactericidal effect by interfering with bacterial DNA gyrase to prevent bacterial DNA synthesis

b. *uses:* for treating gram-negative and gram-positive infections

c. *side effects:* dizziness, insomnia, nausea, vomiting, diarrhea, rash, joint or back pain

d. *nursing implications:* antacids impair absorption; use with caution in clients with a history of CNS disease; avoid alkalinization of urine; safe use during pregnancy or lactation has not been established; maintain good hydration; teach client to take complete course of medication even if symptoms disappear

e. *examples:* ciprofloxacin (Cipro), norfloxacin (Noroxin)

7. Anticholinergics

a. *description:* drugs that act as competitive antagonists at cholinergic-receptor sites, thereby blocking action of acetylcholine

b. *uses:* to produce mydriasis; preoperative to decrease salivation and prevent laryngospasms and bradycardia; decrease gastrointestinal motility; antiparkinsonian; decrease nasopharyngeal and bronchial secretions

c. *side effects:* blurred vision, photophobia, urinary hesitancy, increased intraocular pressure, palpitations, flushing, tachycardia, dry mouth, allergic reactions, restlessness

d. *nursing implications:* contraindicated in clients with glaucoma, gastrointestinal obstruction, benign prostatic hypertrophy, renal or hepatic disease; caution client against driving; warn about usual side effects; monitor vital signs; give 30 minutes before meals

e. *examples:* atropine; propantheline bromide (Pro-Banthīne)

8. Antacids

a. *description:* drugs that act to neutralize hydrochloride and provide protective coating on lining of stomach

b. *uses:* to treat duodenal ulcers; reduce gastric acid concentration and prevent stress ulcers;

prevent ulcer recurrence; relieve flatus (simethicone)

c. *side effects:* **aluminum**—constipation; **magnesium**—diarrhea

d. *nursing implications:* check bowel movements; watch for rebound acidity and ulcer recurrence when drug discontinued

e. *types and examples:* **aluminum**—Amphojel; **magnesium**—milk of magnesia; *aluminum and magnesium*—Maalox, Gelusil

9. Histamine H_2 receptor antagonist

a. *description:* drugs that decrease gastric acid secretion, total acidity, and pepsin activity

b. *uses:* to prevent and treat duodenal ulcers; reduce gastric acid secretion and concentration; prevent stress ulcers; prevent ulcer recurrence

c. *side effects:* diarrhea, dizziness, rash, gynecomastia, alopecia, neutropenia, impotence, bradycardia, headache

d. *nursing implications:* do not give within 1 hour of antacids; monitor for relief of symptoms; does not cause rebound acidity when discontinued

e. *examples:* cimetidine (Tagamet), ranitidine (Zantac)

10. Antithyroid drugs

a. *description:* drugs that interfere with uptake of iodine and block synthesis of thyroxine (T_4) and triiodothyronine (T_3); does not interfere with release and use of stored thyroid; takes days or weeks for effect to be seen; hormone reduction leads to increased thyroid-stimulating hormone (TSH), which leads to hyperplasia and increased vascularity of gland; euthyroidism occurs in 6–12 weeks

b. *uses:* to establish euthyroidism preoperatively; palliative care of toxic goiter

c. *side effects:* nausea, vomiting, diarrhea, loss of taste, skin changes, headache, dizziness, drowsiness, lymphadenopathy, hypersensitivity, agranulocytosis, hypothyroidism

d. *nursing implications:* monitor blood counts; should not be used in last trimester of pregnancy or during lactation; report any symptoms of infection; urge continued compliance because of slow response

e. *example:* propylthiouracil (PTU)

11. Thyroid drugs

a. *description:* synthetic thyroid preparation of controlled potency; contains T_4, which is converted to T_3; acts as replacement for thyroid hormone

b. *uses:* to treat hypothyroidism

c. *side effects:* rare; hyperthyroidism, tremors, hunger, weight loss

d. *nursing implications:* use with caution in clients with acute myocardial infarctions, hypertension, renal insufficiency, diabetes, and elderly or pregnant clients; give a single dose in A.M.; watch for adverse effects early in treatment; monitor for improvement of symptoms

e. *example:* levothyroxine sodium (Synthroid)

III. PRINCIPLES OF MEDICATION ADMINISTRATION

A. Five Rights of Medication Administration and Safety

1. Right drug
2. Right dose
3. Right route
4. Right time
5. Right client
6. Some sources say six rights and add "right documentation"

B. Methods to Ensure Five Rights Followed

1. Do not administer any drug you are not familiar with; look it up first
   a. know intended action and uses for drug; does it fit this client's diagnosis?
   b. know side and toxic effects
   c. know safe dosage range for clients of this age, weight, and health status
   d. be familiar with allergies and possible idiosyncracies
   e. know possible interactions with other drugs or foods
   f. be aware of any special precautions associated with drug
2. Be sure that drug ordered is what is given
   a. compare drug card to physician's order
   b. check label three times
      (1) when container taken from shelf or medication cart
      (2) before drug is poured
      (3) when container is replaced in cabinet or empty container discarded
3. Always keep medication card, sheet, or other form of medication order with drug and check it against client's arm band to insure that the right client is receiving the right drug
4. Never take medication from an unmarked container or one with an illegible label (return to pharmacy for identification and correct relabeling)
5. Check to be sure that medication is being given by right route

6. Watch client take medication; do not leave it at bedside or in client's room
7. If the medication cannot be given for any reason, chart why it was not given and notify physician
8. Never leave medication tray unattended
9. Administer medications at correct time; no more than 30 minutes before or 30 minutes after appointed time

C. Routes of Administration

1. Oral: p.o.—by mouth
2. Injection
   a. subcutaneous: SC—under the skin; also called hypodermic
   b. intradermal: in between the layers of skin
   c. intramuscular: IM—into muscle tissues
   d. intravenous: IV—into a vein
3. Transdermal: through the skin
4. Topical: onto the skin
5. Rectal: per rectum
6. Vaginal: per vagina
7. Inhalation: inhaled into respiratory tract
8. Sublingual: SL—placed under tongue until dissolved
9. Buccal: held against cheek until dissolved

D. Correct Methods of Medication Administration for Adults

1. Oral
   a liquids
      (1) measured in ounces (oz), drams, minims, milliliters (mL), or cubic centimeters (cc)
      (2) hold container so that you are pouring away from label
      (3) position medicine cup at eye level; pour so that bottom of meniscus is at level of ordered dosage
      (4) never open a new bottle until the old one is empty
      (5) wipe lip of bottle before replacing cap
      (6) if medicine ordered in drops, use eye dropper provided with medication
   b. solid medications
      (1) only scored tablets may be broken; capsules and unscored tablets may never be broken
      (2) dissolve powders as ordered
      (3) crush pills only after checking safety of doing so; i.e., never crush enteric-coated tablets or time release capsules
2. Injections
   a. special points

(1) maintain sterility of syringe and all its parts

(2) carefully choose correct site for injection; measure site properly

(3) always cleanse site of injection with disinfectant before injection

(4) after needle is inserted, draw back plunger except for intradermal injections and subcutaneous heparin injections; if blood returns, withdraw needle, discard medication contaminated with blood, and start over

(5) pediatric considerations

    (a) site, thigh for premobile children

    (b) use smaller needle size

    (c) be aware of age considerations

(6) dispose of needle attached to syringe in safe, puncture-proof container

(7) wear gloves with injection administration

b. subcutaneous injections

(1) given into any subcutaneous tissues, especially upper arm, thigh, and abdomen

(2) use small-gauge, #25, short needle, 3/4 inch

(3) amount usually under 2 mL

(4) administer at 90- or 45-degree angle

    (a) at 90-degree angle, pinch skin and insert needle, release skin and inject medication

    (b) insert at 45-degree angle if ample subcutaneous tissues

(5) check carefully to ensure that it is safe to administer drug by this route

c. intradermal injections

(1) usually given in inner part of forearm

(2) use 3/8- to 1/2-inch #25-gauge needle

(3) dosage usually under 1 mL

(4) insert needle at 10- to 15-degree angle to skin

(5) most often used for vaccines or skin tests

d. intramuscular injections

(1) choose site and needle carefully

    (a) deltoid small muscle, little mass for injection

    (b) choose needle long enough to insert into muscle

(2) position client for best access to muscle chosen; ensure complete exposure so site can be properly palpated

(3) volume administered dependent on site chosen, 2 to 2.5 mL

e. IV therapy

(1) assessment must be made of the injection site at least each shift, to insure that IV infusion is flowing properly and vein not inflamed

(2) if vein inflamed or IV infiltrated

    (a) remove IV line from vein

    (b) apply warm packs to area

    (c) notify physician

(3) redress site of infusion per hospital policy

(4) monitor type of fluids running and rate of infusion carefully and frequently

(5) calculate IV rate: rate in drops/minute = amount of IV fluid (in mL) × drip factor/time (in minutes)

3. Ocular medications

a. terminology: OD—right eye; OS—left eye; OU—both eyes

b. have client look up and instill drops into inner canthus

c. do not touch the dropper to the eye

d. have client gently close eye, do not squeeze shut

e. gently wipe excess away with clean tissue

4. Otic medications

a. ear drops usually warmed to body temperature

b. straighten adult ear canal by gently pulling lobe upward and backward, and child ear canal by gently pulling lobe downward and backward

c. have client tilt head away from affected side

d. after drops instilled, leave head tilted for a few minutes

e. use a cotton ball to gently plug ear, if ordered

5. Transdermal medications

a. medication that can be absorbed through intact skin

b. check skin for irritation before application; do not apply over irritated skin

c. apply measured dose or premeasured pad without rubbing medication into skin

d. leave medication on skin, covered, for specified time

e. apply to upper back, upper chest, or upper arms

f. nurse should wear gloves during application

g. wash hands before and after application

6. Suppositories

a. rectal

(1) position client in left lateral Sims' position

(2) wear gloves for procedure

(3) lubricate suppository and gloved index finger with water-soluble lubricant

(4) insert suppository past rectal sphincter; if client is tense, encourage deep breaths

(5) have client hold suppository for required length of time (20–60 minutes)

b. vaginal
    (1) wear gloves during procedure
    (2) have client lie down with knees bent and slightly separated
    (3) insert foam or suppository into vagina
    (4) have client lie down for required length of time

E. Pediatric Modifications for Correct Methods of Medication Administration

1. General principles
  a. correct drug therapy based on child's age, weight, and growth and development
  b. always approach child with assumption that child will take medication
  c. be honest with children and tell them about medication as appropriate for their developmental level
  d. administer distasteful medications with Jello or other tasteful food
  e. never call medication "candy," and never use medication as a threat
  f. calculate drug doses using one of following rules
    (1) body surface area: child's dose = body surface area (in square meters)/1.73 m^2 × adult dose
    (2) Clark's rule: child's dose = weight (in pounds) ÷ 150 pounds × adult dose
    (3) Fried's rule: child's dose = age (in months) ÷ 150 × adult dose
2. Oral medication
  a. infants
    (1) give liquids through syringe without needle
    (2) insert syringe into infant's mouth and gently expel medication
    (3) medication can be mixed with baby food unless contraindicated
  b. toddlers: allow them to drink from cup if possible

3. Topical medications
  a. area may need to be covered to prevent child from rubbing medication off or spreading it
  b. child may have to be restrained until medication dries
4. Injections
  a. infants and young children have to be adequately restrained
  b. use gluteal or vastus lateralis sites for injections if child is walking and has developed gluteal muscle, otherwise use vastus lateralis
  c. always talk to child and try to calm him or her without restraints if possible, but always restrain for safety

F. Modifications for Elderly Patients

1. Carefully check for special precautions or warnings
2. Modify adult doses for elderly who weigh less than 150 pounds
3. Check closely for drug interactions because elderly often take multiple medications
4. Monitor closely for overmedication
5. In long-term care facilities, clients may be identified by pictures rather than arm bands

BIBLIOGRAPHY

Brown, M., and Mullholland, J.L. (1988). *Drug calculations,* 3rd ed. St. Louis: C.V. Mosby Co.

Clark, J.F., Queener, S.F., and Karb, V.B. (1990). *Pharmacological basis of nursing practice,* 3rd ed. St. Louis: C.V. Mosby Co.

Clayton, B.D. (1993). *Mosby's handbook of pharmacology in nursing,* 5th ed. St. Louis: Mosby–Year Book.

Govoni, L., and Hayes, J. (1992). *Drugs and nursing implications,* 7th ed. Norwalk, CT: Appleton & Lange.

Hodgson, B.B., Kizior, R.J., & Kingdon, R.T. (1995). *Nurse's drug handbook, 1995.* Philadelphia: W.B. Saunders Co.

Lehne, R.A., Moore, L., Crosby, L., & Hamilton, D. (1994). *Pharmacology for nursing care,* 2nd ed. Philadelphia: W.B. Saunders Co.

Mathewson-Kuhn, M. (1994). *Pharmacotherapeutics: A nursing process approach,* 3rd ed. Philadelphia: F.A. Davis.

Roth, L.S. (1995). *1995 Mosby's nursing drug reference.* St. Louis: Mosby–Year Book.

Wilson, B.A., Shannon, M.T., & Strang, C.L. (1995). *Nurse's drug guide, 1995.* Norwalk, CT: Appleton & Lange.

? QUESTIONS

1. Which of the following medications may be administered to reduce target symptoms seen in psychotic episodes?

   ① Valium
   ② Thorazine
   ③ Tofranil
   ④ Lithium

2. Which medication would best control extrapyramidal side effects caused by many antipsychotic medications?

   ① Cogentin
   ② Ativan
   ③ Mellaril
   ④ L-Dopa

3. Mrs. Davis is receiving Thorazine. What objective finding would indicate an early sign of tardive dyskinesia?

   ① Cogwheel rigidity at the elbow
   ② Drying of the mucous membranes
   ③ Akathisia of the lower extremities
   ④ Vermiform movements of the tongue

4. Medications administered in suppository form:

   ① Are always administered rectally
   ② Produce bowel evacuation
   ③ Are soothing to mucous membranes
   ④ Have a base that melts at body temperature

5. A medication consisting of a suspension of fat globules and water is classified as a(an):

   ① Emulsion
   ② Ointment
   ③ Tincture
   ④ Elixir

6. Tablets that are enteric coated are:

   ① Absorbed through the skin
   ② Dissolved by intestinal juices
   ③ Dissolved by gastric acid
   ④ Held in the mouth until dissolved

7. When administering a troche or lozenge, the nurse should instruct the client to:

   ① Always dissolve it in water to protect the teeth

   ② Follow the medication with a full glass of water
   ③ Hold it in the mouth until dissolved
   ④ Take it on an empty stomach

8. Sustained-release tablets are forms of drugs given to clients:

   ① To increase the duration of action of the drug
   ② To increase the rapid absorption of the drug
   ③ For prevention of gastrointestinal irritation
   ④ Who need a delayed reaction because of hypersensitivity

9. When administering an antibiotic or a vaccine, the nurse must be alert for the possibility of:

   ① Overdosage and CNS depression
   ② Hypersensitivity and possible anaphylaxis
   ③ Signs of increasing infection
   ④ Orthostatic hypotension

10. Drugs that are administered to relieve pain are classified as:

    ① Analgesics
    ② Anxiolytics
    ③ Hypnotics
    ④ Tranquilizers

11. Drugs that are administered to induce and maintain sleep are classified as:

    ① Analgesics
    ② Antipyretics
    ③ Hypnotics
    ④ Tranquilizers

12. A drug commonly used for the treatment of arthritis is:

    ① Phenobarbital
    ② Aspirin
    ③ Morphine sulfate
    ④ Codeine sulfate

13. Digoxin is an example of a cardiac glycoside that:

    ① Increases and strengthens the contractions of the heart
    ② Raises the blood pressure
    ③ Slows the contraction of the heart
    ④ Slows and strengthens the contractions of the heart

14. Because of the potential for severe side effects, before administering digoxin, the nurse must always:

  ① Check the client's blood pressure
  ② Determine the client's prothrombin time
  ③ Count the client's apical pulse for 1 minute
  ④ Monitor the client's radial pulse for 30 seconds

15. The most common route used for administering nitroglycerin to treat acute angina is:

  ① Subcutaneous
  ② Intramuscular
  ③ Oral
  ④ Sublingual

16. Which of the following medications should *not* be followed by water?

  ① Cough syrups
  ② Antacids
  ③ Laxatives
  ④ Iron preparations

17. Before administering an antibiotic to a client with a severe wound infection, the nurse must:

  ① Obtain an ordered culture of the wound
  ② Verify the order with the physician
  ③ Check the client's temperature
  ④ Wait until the client has had something to eat

18. Mr. Wilson, a client with COPD, is receiving theophylline, which will act to:

  ① Relax the diaphragm and intercostals to increase chest expansion
  ② Decrease contraction of the smooth muscles of the bronchi
  ③ Increase the contraction of the bronchi and alveoli
  ④ Decrease the amount of mucus secretion from the bronchi

19. A nursing intervention used to decrease reflux esophagitis, a side effect of theophylline, is:

  ① Administering the drug at bedtime
  ② Having the client sit up after meals
  ③ Encouraging the client to eat three large meals a day
  ④ Administering the medication with large quantities of water

20. While you are administering a rectal suppository, your client asks, "Will I have a bowel movement after this suppository?" To answer this, the nurse must know that rectal suppositories are given to:

  ① Relieve constipation
  ② Treat hemorrhoids
  ③ Clients who cannot tolerate enemas
  ④ Clients for a variety of reasons, depending on the medication in the suppository

21. To decrease the gastrointestinal side effects, iron preparations should be administered:

  ① At bedtime
  ② Before breakfast
  ③ With meals
  ④ Between meals

22. Pilocarpine, a miotic, causes:

  ① Dilation of the pupil
  ② Inhibition of bacteria in the eye
  ③ Local anesthesia to the pupil
  ④ Constriction of the pupil

23. Because of its action, the nurse knows that pilocarpine will be used to:

  ① Treat glaucoma
  ② Treat cataracts
  ③ Examine the retina
  ④ Prevent night blindness

24. Atropine, a mydriatic, causes:

  ① Dilation of the pupil
  ② Inhibition of bacteria in the eye
  ③ Local anesthesia to the pupil
  ④ Constriction of the pupil

25. Because of its action, the nurse knows that atropine is contraindicated in clients with:

  ① Glaucoma
  ② Cataracts
  ③ Nearsightedness
  ④ Night blindness

26. The classification of drugs used to treat the symptoms of an allergic reaction is:

  ① Antibiotic
  ② Antihistamine
  ③ Cholinergic
  ④ Sulfonamide

27. You notice that the label on the cough syrup bottle is difficult to read. Your most appropriate action is to:

① Return the drug to the pharmacy for relabeling

② Hold the medication and chart that it was not given

③ Make out a new label and apply it over the old one

④ Pour the medication because you know what it is

28. You notice that the medication you are about to administer has changed color since yesterday; you know that this means that:

① This is not uncommon and has no significance

② The drug can be given if you check first with the charge nurse

③ The drug should be held and charted as not given

④ The drug is not given, and a fresh supply is obtained and given

29. When you enter Mr. Smith's room to administer his 9 A.M. medications, you find that he and his wife are engaged in an argument about the cost of this hospitalization and the impact on their finances. When you offer him his medication, he refuses, stating, "Those pills make me sick to my stomach." When charting the event, the nurse should write that the client:

① Refused medication because it makes him sick

② Refused medication because upset by fight with wife

③ Refused medication, stating the pills made him sick to his stomach

④ Worried about the cost of hospitalization so refused to take medication

30. It is important to chart a client's refusal of the medication to:

① Document the client's response

② Cover yourself in case there is trouble later

③ Notify the physician of the client's refusal to take the drug

④ Warn the other nurses that the client is uncooperative

31. When you are charting later that day, you make an error. The proper way to correct an error is to:

① Cross it out with multiple lines and initial it as an error

② Use correction fluid and erase it

③ Ask the charge nurse to co-sign it as an error

④ Draw a single line through it and write the word "error" above it and initial it

32. It is important that the nurse is able to convert from pounds to kilograms because medication dosages are based on kilograms of body weight. A 106-lb woman weighs approximately:

① 52 kg

② 48 kg

③ 42 kg

④ 36 kg

ANSWERS AND RATIONALES

Guide to item identification (see p. 4–5 for further details about each category)
I, II, III, or IV for the phase of the nursing process
1, 2, 3, or 4 for the category of client needs
A, B, C, D, E, F, or G for the category of human functioning

Specific content category by name; ie, cholecystectomy

1. Chlorpromazine (Thorazine) reduces psychotic
② symptoms. Essentially the client's behavior becomes more socially acceptable.
III, 2 & 3, G, Psychiatric medications

2. Pseudoparkinsonism is drug induced; therefore,
① antiparkinsonian agents, such as Cogentin, Artane, and Benadryl, relieve these symptoms.
III, 2 & 3, G, Psychiatric medications

3. Check the client's tongue regularly for vermi-
④ form (wormlike) movements, which are often the first sign of tardive dyskinesia.
I, 2 & 3, G, Psychiatric medications

4. Suppositories may be given vaginally, orally, or
③ rectally. They contain medication in a base that melts at body temperature.
III, 2, D, Medication administration

5. An emulsion is a suspension of fat in water that
① must be shaken before administration to mix the two.
I, 2, D, Medication administration

6. Enteric-coated tablets resist dissolution by gas-
② tric acids but are made to dissolve in the basic intestinal secretions.
I, 2, D, Medication administration

7. These medications are designed to act on the
③ oral mucous membranes or upper throat, so they must be allowed to dissolve completely in the mouth. They should never be diluted with water, which would decrease their action.
III, 2, D, Medication administration

8. The action of these tablets is prolonged and
① gradual over time, allowing for less frequent administration.
I, 2, D, Medication administration

9. These agents are often allergens in sensitive indi-
② viduals, and anaphylaxis is always a risk.
III & IV, 2, D, Medication administration

10. Analgesics, both narcotic and nonnarcotic, are
① the drugs given for pain relief.
I, 2, D, Medications/analgesics

11. Hypnotics is the class of drugs to which most
③ sleeping pills belong. The other common class is sedatives.
I & IV, 2, C, Medications/hypnotics

12. Nonsteroidal antiinflammatories are the drugs
③ of choice to treat arthritis, an inflammatory condition.
IV, 2, D, Medications/antiinflammatories

13. Digoxin acts by strengthening the contraction of
④ the heart to improve cardiac output. It also slows the rate, making each beat more efficient and effective.
IV, 2, B, Medications/cardiac

14. Digoxin slows the heart rate as part of its action;
③ however, an early symptom of overdose or toxicity is abnormal slowing of the heart. Digoxin should not be given without checking with the physician if the apical pulse is <60 or >120 over 1 full minute.
III, 2, B, Medications/cardiac

15. Nitroglycerin for acute angina is needed imme-
④ diately. The most rapid absorption is through the mucous membranes under the tongue.
III, 2, B, Medications/cardiac

16. Cough syrups are intended to coat the throat
① with a soothing medication and therefore should never be followed with water.
III, 2, B, Medications/expectorants

17. If antibiotics are started before the ordered
① wound culture is obtained, an accurate culture is impossible. Whenever possible, the culture should be obtained before the drugs are started.
III, 2, D, Medications/antibiotics

18. The action of theophylline, a bronchodilator, is
② to relax the bronchial smooth muscles.
IV, 2, B, Medications/bronchodilators

19. Sitting up after meals helps the food remain in
② the stomach and not reflux into the esophagus.
IV, 2, B, Medications/bronchodilators

20. Any form of medication that can be absorbed
④ through mucous membranes can technically be administered rectally. The nurse must find out why a medication is being given in order to give the client an accurate explanation.
III, 1, F, Medication administration

21. Iron is irritating to the gastrointestinal tract, and
③ administering it with food decreases this.
II, 1, F, Medications/iron

22. Miotics constrict the pupil.
④ I, 2, C, Medications/optic

23. To increase the outflow of the humor in the eye,
① the canal of Schlemm must be open. Constricting
the pupil increases the angle and therefore the
outflow.
IV, 2, C, Medications/optic

24. Mydriatics dilate the pupil.
① I, 2, C, Medications/optic

25. Atropine causes the pupil to dilate. A client with
① glaucoma should never have the pupil dilated
because this interferes with the outflow of aqueous humor, possibly leading to acute glaucoma.
I, 2, C, Medications/optic

26. Antihistamines counter the histamine produced
② by an allergic reaction.
IV, 2, D, Medications/antihistamines

27. The only person legally licensed to label medica-
① tion is the pharmacist.
III, 2, D, Medication administration

28. That drug should not be given because a color
④ change may indicate an alteration in the chemical composition of a drug as a result of age,
light, or moisture. A new supply should be obtained and administered as ordered.
III, 2, D, Medication administration

29. This is the most objective statement of the inci-
③ dent. When charting, the nurse should avoid
subjective statements.
III, 1 & 2, G, Medication administration

30. Charting is an important way to document accu-
① rately and objectively the client's responses to
therapy.
IV, 2, G, Medication administration

31. The correct way to alter the legal chart record
④ is to cross out the error with a single line, write
"error," and initial it.
III, 1, G, Medication administration

32. The conversion is 2.2 lb per kilogram.
② III, 2, D, Medication administration

Diet Therapy

5

I. PRINCIPLES OF NORMAL NUTRITION

A. Requirements
Vary according to age, sex, activity level, state of health, and climate

B. Optimal Nutrition

1. Intake matches energy expenditure
2. Proper amounts of each essential nutrient
3. Need for balanced diet to provide good nutrition (accomplished by following food guide pyramid)

C. Essential for

1. Normal growth, development, organ function
2. Maintenance of bodily function
3. Optimal activity status
4. Resistance to infection
5. Repair of injuries to cells and tissues

D. Nutritional Deficiencies of Either Calories or Specific Nutrients

1. Primary deficiencies: inadequate intake
2. Secondary deficiencies
   a. interference with ingestion, digestion, absorption, or usage of proper nutrients
   b. increased requirements as a result of stress or illness

E. Six Classes of Essential Nutrients

1. Fats
2. Proteins
3. Carbohydrates
4. Minerals
5. Vitamins
6. Water

F. USDA Food Guide Pyramid (Fig. 5–1)

1. Bread, cereal, rice, and pasta group
   a. 6–11 servings per day
   b. composed of
      (1) 1 slice bread
      (2) 1 ounce cereal
      (3) 1/2 cup cooked cereal, rice, or pasta
   c. contain starch and incomplete proteins
   d. whole grain cereals contain fiber
   e. grains often enriched to become good sources of iron, thiamine, riboflavin, and niacin
2. Vegetable group
   a. 3–5 servings per day
   b. composed of
      (1) 1 cup raw leafy vegetables
      (2) 1/2 cup of cooked or raw other vegetable
      (3) 3/4 cup of vegetable juice
   c. dark green and deep yellow vegetables are good sources of vitamin A
   d. leafy green vegetables are a good source of iron
   e. potatoes are high in iron, thiamine, and vitamin C
3. Fruit group
   a. 2–4 servings per day
   b. composed of
      (1) 1 medium apple, banana, or orange
      (2) 1/2 cup chopped, cooked, or canned fruit
      (3) 3/4 cup fruit juice
   c. contain sugar, starch, cellulose, and varying amounts of vitamins and minerals
   d. primary source of vitamin C
4. Milk, yogurt, and cheese group
   a. 2–3 servings per day
   b. composed of
      (1) 1 cup milk or yogurt
      (2) 1 1/2 cup milk or yogurt
      (3) 2 ounces processed cheese

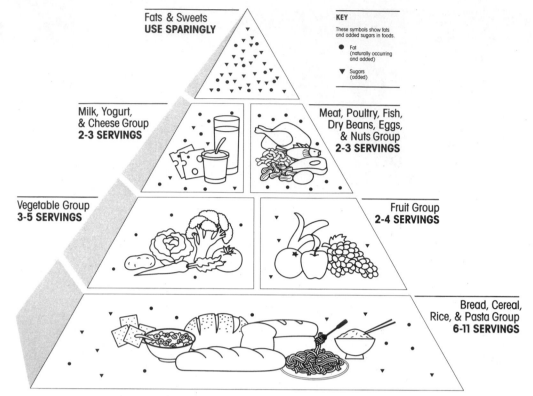

FIGURE 5-1 U.S.D.A. Food Pyramid/U.S. Department of Health and Human Services. A guide to daily food choices. (From Peckenpaugh, N.J., & Poleman, C.M. (1995). *Nutrition: essentials and diet therapy,* 7th ed. Philadelphia: W.B. Saunders).

c. provides adequate amounts of calcium and riboflavin

d. also contains protein, carbohydrates, phosphorus, thiamine, vitamin D, and possibly vitamin A

e. whole milk has higher amounts of fat than low-fat milk or skim milk with no fat

5. Meat, poultry, fish, dry beans, eggs, and nuts group

a. 2–3 servings per day

b. composed of

    (1) 2–3 ounces cooked lean meat, poultry, or fish

    (2) 1/2 cup cooked dry beans, 1 egg, or 2 tablespoons peanut butter count as 1 ounce lean meat

c. source of protein, iron, thiamine, niacin, fat, phosphorus, and riboflavin

d. liver is an excellent source of iron and vitamin A

e. saltwater seafood contains iodine

f. eggs are high in protein, iron, thiamine, phosphorus, and riboflavin, with yolk high in vitamin A and fat (cholesterol)

g. legumes contain incomplete protein which leads to some problems in vegetarian diet

h. nuts high in protein, iron, thiamine, riboflavin, niacin, and fat

6. Fats, oils, and sweets

a. use sparingly

b. all may be added or naturally occurring

c. decrease use of saturated fats

G. Vitamins

1. Fat-soluble vitamins

a. can reach toxic amounts

b. not easily lost in cooking

c. vitamin A

    (1) requirements: men—5000 IU; women—4000 IU; pregnancy— +1000 IU; lactation— +2000 IU

    (2) functions: purple vision development, which allows vision in dim light; normal growth and development of bones and teeth; formation and maintenance of skin and mucous membranes

    (3) sources: liver, egg yolks, fortified dairy products, dark green and yellow vegetables

d. vitamin D

    (1) requirements: age 19–22 years— 300 IU; after 22 years—200 IU; pregnancy or lactation— +200 IU

(2) functions: helps maintain optimal level of calcium and phosphorus for normal bone mineralization

(3) sources: fortified milk and breakfast cereals, egg yolks, sardines, liver, salmon, and tuna fish (fish oils)

e. vitamin E

(1) requirements: men—10 mg; women—8 mg; pregnancy— +2 mg; lactation—+3 mg

(2) functions: antioxidant that protects vitamin A and polyunsaturated fatty acid (PUFA); protects cell membrane

(3) sources: vegetable oils, wheat germ, leafy vegetables, corn, nuts, and soybeans

f. vitamin K

(1) requirements: 70—140 μg

(2) function: essential for formation of clotting factor prothrombin; salicylates interfere with vitamin K production

(3) sources: green leafy vegetables, egg yolks, and liver

2. Water-soluble vitamins

a. easily lost in cooking or by sitting

b. not usually toxic even in large amounts because excess lost in urine

c. vitamin C

(1) requirements: men and women—60 mg; pregnancy— +20 mg; lactation—+40 mg

(2) function: antioxidant; essential in formation of collagen; strengthens mucous membranes; enhances absorption of iron in gut; converts folic acid to active form; involved in metabolism of selected amino acids

(3) sources: green vegetables, citrus fruits, potatoes, tomatoes, and cabbage

(4) relatively unstable vitamin

d. thiamine (vitamin B_1)

(1) requirements: men and women—5 mg/1000 calories; pregnancy—+0.4 mg/1000 calories; lactation—+0.5 mg/1000 calories

(2) function: carbohydrate metabolism; normal function of central nervous system

(3) sources: pork, liver, organ meats, whole and enriched grains, legumes, potatoes, eggs, and milk

e. riboflavin (vitamin B_2)

(1) requirements: men and women—0.6 mg/1000 calories; pregnancy—+0.3 mg/1000 calories; lactation—+0.5 mg/1000 calories

(2) functions: fat, carbohydrate, and protein metabolism

(3) sources: dairy products, organ meats, eggs, enriched grains, and green leafy vegetables

f. niacin (vitamin B_3)

(1) requirements: men and women—6.6 mg/1000 calories; pregnancy—+2 mg/1000 calories; lactation—+3 mg/1000 calories

(2) function: fat, carbohydrate, and protein metabolism

(3) sources: organ meat, poultry, lean meats, peanut butter, whole and enriched grains, dried beans and peas, and nuts

g. pyridoxine (vitamin B_6)

(1) requirements: men—2.2 mg; women—2 mg; pregnancy—+0.6 mg; lactation—+0.5 mg

(2) functions: metabolism of amino acids; blood formation; maintenance of nervous system; conversion of tryptophan to niacin

(3) sources: wheat germ, yeast, organ meats, pork, egg yolks, whole grain cereals, corn, potatoes, and bananas

h. folic acid (folacin)

(1) requirements: men and women—400 μg; pregnancy—+400 μg; lactation—+100 μg

(2) functions: amino acid metabolism; proliferation of cells; blood formation

(3) sources: green leafy vegetables, organ meats, eggs, milk, yeast, wheat germ, and kidney beans

i. cobalamin (vitamin B_{12})

(1) requirements: men and women—3 μg; pregnancy—+1 μg; lactation—+1 μg

(2) functions: RNA and DNA synthesis; blood formation; maintenance of nervous tissue; folic acid metabolism; fat, protein, and carbohydrate metabolism

(3) sources: liver, kidney, fresh shrimp and oysters, milk, eggs, and cheese

(4) the nutrient most commonly missing on a total vegetarian diet

j. pantothenic acid

(1) requirements: men and women—4–7 mg

(2) function: fat, protein, and carbohydrate metabolism

(3) sources: organ meats, egg yolks, salmon, fresh vegetables, yeast, and whole grains

k. biotin

(1) requirements: men and women—100–200 μg

(2) function: fat, protein, and carbohydrate metabolism

(3) sources: organ meats, peanuts, mushrooms, milk, egg yolks, and yeast

H. Daily Balanced Diet (Table 5–1)

1. Calculation of calories for ideal body weight
   a. consult weight table for ideal body weight
   b. basal caloric need = 10–11 × ideal weight; add ideal weight × 3 for sedentary people; add ideal weight × 5 for moderately active people; add ideal weight × 10 for people with strenuous activity
   c. 1 pound body fat = 3500 calories; add or subtract for each pound to lose per week
2. Milk
   a. children under age 9 years: 2–3 servings
   b. children ages 9–12 years: 3 or more servings
   c. teenagers: 4 or more servings
   d. adults: 2–3 servings
   e. pregnant women: 3 or more
   f. nursing mothers: 4 or more
3. Meats
   a. 2–3 servings per day
   b. meats lower in fat should be used
   c. number of eggs per week should be limited because of high cholesterol content
4. Breads and cereals
   a. 6–11 servings per day
   b. enriched products preferable

I. Special Nutritional Needs by Age

1. Infants
   a. higher protein and calorie requirements because of high rates of growth and activity
   b. breast milk provides all essential nutrients
   c. solid food introduced at 5–6 months
   d. add new foods one at a time to assess for digestive tolerance and allergies
   e. formulas able to meet nutritional needs
2. Preschoolers
   a. growth rate erratic
   b. dietary needs fluctuate throughout period
   c. child learns lifetime eating habits, so offer wide variety of foods
   d. finger food best
   e. give foods in small amounts
   f. avoid refined sweets
   g. risk of iron deficiency anemia if intake of milk too great with toddlers and preschoolers
3. School age
   a. growth rate increases gradually, requiring increased nutrients
   b. between-meal snacks are often a problem because of poor nutritional content, so offer nutritional snacks
   c. reinforce nutritional education
   d. concerns for developing good eating habits for a lifetime
      (1) introduction of wide variety of foods at early age
      (2) avoid obesity and other eating disorders in childhood
      (3) importance of exercise and low fats important to learn at early age
4. Adolescents
   a. tremendous growth spurt; usually increased activity
   b. girls
      (1) usually 10–13 years old
      (2) usually gain fat tissue and lean muscle
   c. boys
      (1) usually 13–16 years old
      (2) usually gain lean muscle tissue
5. Pregnancy
   a. increase
      (1) protein intake by 50%
      (2) calories
      (3) calcium, phosphorus, and vitamin D
   b. no need to limit salt excessively
   c. weight gain within medical recommendations, but not severely limited
6. Nursing mothers
   a. high protein with increased calories
   b. all nutrients need to be increased
   c. increased fluid intake important
7. Young and middle adulthood
   a. too busy to eat
   b. overuse of fast foods
   c. development of deficiencies for later in life, such as low calcium levels in osteoporosis

TABLE 5-1 Daily Balanced Diet

Meal Pattern	Sample Menu
Breakfast	
Fruit	1/2 cup orange juice
Cereal or breadstuff	1 cup oatmeal
Hot food	1 soft boiled egg
Beverage	Coffee or tea, 1 cup milk
Lunch	
Sandwich	Sandwich with 2 slices whole wheat bread, 2 oz chicken, mustard, lettuce, and tomato
Salad	1 cup fruit salad
Dessert	1 cup yogurt
Beverage	Coffee or tea
Dinner	
Soup	1/2 cup tomato soup with crackers
Meat	2 oz broiled ground beef
Salad	Lettuce salad with low-fat dressing
Vegetable	1/2 cup broccoli
Dessert	1 banana
Beverage	1 cup milk

8. Elderly
   a. lower metabolic rate and decreased activity mean fewer calories needed
   b. decreased food intake
      (1) senses of smell and taste decrease resulting in decreased appetite
      (2) loss of teeth, poor-fitting dentures, and social isolation all impair eating
      (3) decreased bowel motility leads to constipation, which lowers appetite
      (4) diets low in protein, vitamin C, and calcium
      (5) shopping and cooking may be impaired because of other disabilities
      (6) financial difficulties may contribute to poor intake, especially of fresh fruits and vegetables
      (7) depression may lead to decreased or increased intake
   c. great safety risk due to decreased sense of smell may cause inability to detect spoiled foods
   d. diet planning with older adults should take all these areas into consideration
   e. significance of Senior Centers and food services for shut-ins such as Meals on Wheels

II. THERAPEUTIC DIET MODIFICATIONS

A. Postsurgical Diets

1. Clear liquid
   a. tea or coffee without cream or milk, fat-free broth, and gelatin
   b. carbonated beverages allowed, although carbonation may increase intestinal gas in post-surgical clients
   c. nutritionally inadequate diet
   d. reduces colonic residue
   e. allows evaluation of tolerance of oral intake
2. Full liquids
   a. any food that is liquid at body temperature
   b. foods allowed include milk, cream, ice cream, juices without pulp, gelatin, strained soups, broth, tea, coffee, and carbonated beverages
   c. lacks some necessary nutrients
   d. provides some calories and liquids
   e. still low residue
3. Soft diet
   a. composed of easily chewed and digested foods
   b. can be nutritionally adequate and high in calories
   c. includes most foods except fried, high-fiber, and strongly flavored foods

B. Low-Sodium Diets (Table 5–2)

1. Mild restriction
   a. used for mild edema or hypertension
   b. 2–3 g (2000–3000 mg) of sodium daily
   c. minimal restrictions; no brine foods or those prepared with monosodium glutamate (MSG)
   d. no added table salt to food
   e. usually palatable and easily followed
2. Moderate restriction
   a. used for hypertension, more severe edema
   b. 1 g (1000 mg) sodium daily
   c. meat, milk, and bakery goods restricted
   d. no table salt added during or after cooking
   e. some vegetables omitted

TABLE 5-2 Low-Sodium Diets: Sodium Content of Common Food Groups

Dairy products	
Naturally high	None
High in added sodium	Buttermilk; cheese and cottage cheese; milk products such as ice cream, malts, milk shakes, and sherbet
Low sodium	Skim, 2% evaporated, and low-sodium milk and low-sodium cheeses
Fruits and vegetables	
Naturally high	Spinach, celery, carrots, white turnips, greens, beets, and artichokes
High in added sodium	Glazed fruits, maraschino cherries, fruits with sodium preservatives, canned vegetables and juices, frozen vegetables with added salt
Low sodium	Fresh fruits and vegetables, frozen or canned vegetables and fruit without added sodium
Breads and cereals	
Naturally high	None
High in added sodium	Mixes, bread and rolls made from premixed dough, crackers, instant cereals, most dry cereals, self-rising flour, baking soda and powder, and egg whites
Low sodium	Low-sodium breads, crackers, and cereals; puffed rice; puffed wheat; cornmeal; shredded wheat; barley; unsalted matzo; and rice
Meats	
Naturally high	Seafoods, shellfish, brain, and kidney
High in added sodium	Bacon, lunch meat, corned beef, chipped beef, hot dogs, sausage, salt pork, codfish, smoked meats and fish, kosher meats and chicken, egg substitutes, and peanut butter
Low sodium	Low-sodium products, fresh fish such as bass, catfish, flounder, sole, trout, and tuna; and low-sodium tuna and salmon

TABLE 5-3 High-Potassium Foods

Dairy products	Raisins
Whole milk	Watermelon
Evaporated and canned milk	
Condensed sweetened milk	*Breads and cereals*
	Barley
Fruits and vegetables	Raisin bread
Baked potato with skin	Pumpernickel bread
Asparagus	Whole wheat bread
Lima beans	Bran flakes
Green beans	Buckwheat flour
Beets	Angel food cake
Broccoli	Coffeecake
Brussels sprouts	Gingerbread
Lettuce	Chocolate cake
Spinach	Fruitcake
Tomato	
Apricot	*Meats*
Avocado	Lean meats
Banana	Flounder
Oranges	Raw shrimp
Dates	Legumes
Grapefruit juice	Sunflower seeds
Peaches	

3. Strict sodium restriction
   a. for severe hypertension, renal and liver disease, severe edema
   b. 0.5 g (500 mg) sodium daily
   c. used only for severe disease states, such as severe congestive heart failure
   d. many foods not allowed; severe meat and egg restriction
   e. not well accepted by clients

C. High- or Low-Potassium Diet (Table 5–3)

1. Typical adult intake 2000–4000 mg/day
2. Restrictions required for clients with renal disease
3. Increased amounts needed for clients on potassium-wasting diuretics; better handled through dietary means rather than supplements

D. Low-Cholesterol Diet (Table 5–4)

1. Moderate restriction: 300–500 mg/day
   a. increase polyunsaturated fats and decrease saturated fats
   b. up to 3 egg yolks/week can be substituted for 3 oz of lean meat
   c. use lean meats, fish, and poultry
   d. use skim milk and low-fat products
2. Strict restriction of 100–300 mg/day
   a. increase polyunsaturated fats and decrease saturated fats to a 2:1 ratio
   b. limit meat intake; use mostly fish, chicken, turkey, and veal
   c. eliminate egg yolks
   d. use only skim or low-fat milk

TABLE 5-4 High-Cholesterol Foods in Descending Order (Highest to Lowest)

Organ meats—beef, pork, and lamb	Halibut
Egg yolks	Tuna
Shrimp	Oysters
Lamb	Salmon
Veal	Butter
Crab	Whole milk
Beef	Cheddar cheese
Pork	Ice cream
Lobster	Half-and-half
Chicken and turkey, dark meat with skin	Creamed cottage cheese
Chicken and turkey, white meat with skin	Light cream
	Lard
	Plain cottage cheese
Clams	Skim milk

3. Either diet may be associated with decreased caloric intake
4. Remind client that lowering cholesterol intake does not automatically lead to immediate drop in serum cholesterol

E. Low-Fat Diet (Table 5–5)

1. Reduction of all fats in diet, eating only foods that are 1/3 or less fat
2. Foods should not be fried or prepared with added fat; baking, broiling, or boiling are appropriate cooking methods
3. Trim all visible fat from meats and remove skin from poultry
4. Lean meat and up to 3 egg yolks/week
5. No more than 6 servings of fat/day, unsaturated to saturated fat 2:1

TABLE 5-5 Fat Content of Foods

Low-fat foods	Shortening
Lean meats	Cold cuts
Fish	Oil
Skinless poultry	Mayonnaise
Egg whites	Avocados
Egg substitutes	Bacon
Skim milk	Heavy cream
Low-fat cheese	Salad dressings
Low-fat yogurt	Nuts
All fresh fruits and	Olives
vegetables except	Fatty meats
avocados	Whole milk
Plain cereals	Oil-packed fish
Pasta	Peanut butter
Rice	Cheese
Enriched or whole	Yogurt
grain breads	Ice cream
Sherbet	Bread products prepared
Fruit ices	with added fats: waffles,
Gelatin	muffins, pancakes,
Angel food cake	biscuits, sweet rolls,
Skim or low-fat milk	danishes
	Gravy
High-fat foods	Desserts
Butter	Chocolate
Margarine	

TABLE 5-6 High-Calcium Foods

Highest amounts	
Milk	Cabbage
Milk products	Molasses
Green leafy vegetables	
Shellfish	*Lesser amounts*
Cheese	Egg
Mustard and turnip greens	Carrot
Clams	Celery
Oysters	Orange
Broccoli	Grapefruit
Cauliflower	Figs
	Breads made with milk

TABLE 5-7 Low-Calorie, Reducing Diet (1200 cal)

Breakfast	lettuce
1/2 cup orange juice	1 medium apple
1/2 cup bran flakes with raisins	Coffee/tea
	Dinner
1 cup skim milk	3 oz roast beef
1 slice whole wheat toast	1 medium baked potato
Coffee/tea	2 T low-fat sour cream
Lunch	1/2 cup broccoli
Sandwich	1 cup skim milk
2 slices enriched bread	Snack
2 oz ham	1 small cucumber, sliced
1 oz cheese slice	3–4 carrot sticks, 3 inches long
1/2 medium tomato	

F. High-Calcium Diet (Table 5–6)

1. Recommend daily amount is about 800 mg/day for men and up to 1500 mg/day for women
2. Increased need with various endocrine disorders, osteoporosis, and pregnancy and lactation
3. Milk and milk products are the best source, although other sources good in client with lactose intolerance
4. Canned fish with bones is also good
5. Vitamin D is necessary for normal calcium absorption

TABLE 5-8 Meal Planning for Insulin-Dependent Diabetic Using a Combination of Regular and Intermediate-Acting Insulin*

Diet Prescription: 2000 kcal (275 g carbohydrate, 70 g protein, 65 g fat)

Mealtime Division:
20% Breakfast
30% Lunch
10% Midafternoon snack
30% Dinner
10% Bedtime snack

Total Daily Division of Food into Exchanges:

EXCHANGE LIST	NO. OF EXCHANGES
Starch/bread	8
Meat, lean	4
Vegetables	3
Fruit	8
Milk, nonfat	2
Fats	9

% Energy Nutrient Distribution:

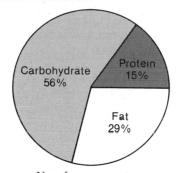

Sample Meal Plan	No. of Exchanges	Sample Menu
Breakfast		
Fruit	1	1/2 banana
Starch/bread	2	3/4 cup bran flakes
		1 slice whole wheat toast
Fat	2	2 tsp safflower margarine
Milk	1	1 cup skim milk
Free		2 tsp sugar-free jam
Lunch		
Meat, lean	2	2 oz lean broiled pork chop
Starch/bread	2	1/2 cup scalloped potatoes
		1 whole wheat roll
Vegetable	1	1/2 cup cooked carrots
Free		1/2 cup cabbage slaw
Fats	3	1 tbsp reduced-kilocalorie mayonnaise (in slaw)
		2 tsp safflower margerine (in scalloped potatoes and for roll)
Fruit	3	1/3 cup pineapple chunks (in slaw)
		1 baked apple

Sample Meal Plan	No. of Exchanges	Sample Menu
Snack		
Fruit	1	2 pear halves canned in juice
Starch/bread	1	6 crackers
Dinner		
Meat, lean	2	2 oz beef cubes
Starch/bread	3	1/2 cup noodles
		2 slices whole wheat bread
Vegetable	2	1/2 cup broccoli
		1/2 cup steamed summer squash
Free		Relishes: cherry tomato, celery sticks, radishes, cucumber slices
Fat	2	2 tsp safflower margarine
Fruit	2	1 1/2 cup fresh blueberries
Bedtime snack		
Milk, nonfat	1	1 cup plain yogurt
Fruit	1	2 tbsp raisins (in yogurt)
Fat	2	2 tbsp chopped nuts (in yogurt)

From Davis, J., and Sherer, K. (1994). *Applied nutrition and diet therapy for nurses,* 2nd ed. Philadelphia: W.B. Saunders Co.
* Coffee, tea, and artificially sweetened beverages are allowed as desired.

G. Low-Calorie, Reducing Diet (Table 5–7)

1. First, identify amount of calories to maintain weight
   a. restrict calories to promote 1- to 2-pound weight loss/week
   b. subtract 500 calories/day for each pound to be lost
2. Important that balanced diet be maintained
3. Use supportive techniques to help client maintain diet

H. Diabetic Diet (Tables 5–8, 5–9, and 5–10)

1. American Diabetes Association recommendations
   a. carbohydrates should provide 50%–60% of total calories
      (1) complex carbohydrates best choice, such as grains and vegetables
      (2) limit simple carbohydrates, such as sugar
   b. protein should provide 12%–20% of total calories
      (1) sources should be low in saturated fat and cholesterol
      (2) high biologic value proteins should be used
   c. fats should provide 30%–38% of calories
      (1) limit saturated fats and cholesterol
      (2) slight increase in polyunsaturated fats
2. Number of calories allowed on diet may vary greatly
   a. may need calorie reduction if client is obese
   b. calories may be to maintain weight and minimize insulin requirements
3. Foods allowed should be similar to a normal balanced diet for the specific client
   a. major limitations in high refined sugars
   b. ethnic foods included in exchange lists

TABLE 5-9 Meal Planning for a Noninsulin-Dependent Diabetic Client*.†

Diet Prescription: 1200 kcal (125 g carbohydrate, 70 g protein, 45 g fat)

Mealtime Division:
Equally divided into 3 meals

Total Daily Division of Food into Exchanges:

EXCHANGE LIST	NO. OF EXCHANGES
Starch/bread	5
Meat, lean	4
Vegetables	2
Fruit	4
Milk, nonfat	1
Fats	4

% Energy Nutrient Distribution:

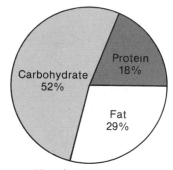

Sample Meal Plan	No. of Exchanges	Sample Menu
Breakfast		
Fruit	1	1/2 banana
Starch/bread	2	3/4 cup bran flakes
		1 slice whole wheat toast
Fat	1	1 tsp safflower margarine
Milk, nonfat	1/2	1/2 cup skim milk
Free		2 tsp sugar-free jam
Lunch		
Meat, lean	2	2 oz lean broiled pork chop
Starch/bread	1	1/2 cup scalloped potatoes
Vegetable	1	1/2 cup cooked carrots
Free		1/2 cup cabbage slaw
Fats	2	1 tbsp reduced-kilocalorie mayonnaise (in slaw)
		1 tsp safflower margarine (in scalloped potatoes and for roll)
Fruit	2	1 baked apple

Sample Meal Plan	No. of Exchanges	Sample Menu
Dinner		
Meat, lean	2	2 oz beef cubes
		1/2 cup noodles
Starch/bread	2	1 slice whole wheat bread
Vegetable	2	1/2 cup broccoli
		Relishes: cherry tomato, celery sticks, radishes,
Free		cucumber slices
Fat	1	1 tsp safflower margarine
Milk, nonfat	1/2	1/2 cup skim milk
Fruit	1	1 3/4 cup fresh blueberries

From Davis, J., and Sherer, K. (1994). *Applied nutrition and diet therapy for nurses,* 2nd ed. Philadelphia: W.B. Saunders Co.
* Coffee, tea, and artificially sweetened beverages are allowed as desired.
† Supplement with multivitamin supplement and calcium.

TABLE 5-10 Diabetic Diet Exchange Lists

Milk exchanges
   1 exchange = 12 g CHO, 8 g protein, and 80 cal (1 cup serving)
   Skim or nonfat milk
   Yogurt made from skim milk
   Whole milk, contains 2 fat exchanges
   Buttermilk, contains 2 fat exchanges

Vegetable exchanges
   1 exchange = 5 g CHO, 2 g protein, and 25 cal (1/2 cup serving)
   Asparagus
   Bean sprouts
   Beets
   Brussels sprouts
   Cabbage
   Cauliflower
   Celery
   Eggplant
   Green pepper
   Greens
   Mushrooms
   Okra
   Onions
   String beans
   Summer squash
   Tomato
   Turnips
   Zucchini

Free vegetables (used as desired)
   Cucumbers
   Endive
   Escarole
   Lettuce
   Parsley
   Dill pickles
   Radishes
   Watercress

Fruit exchanges
   1 exchange = 10 g CHO and 40 cal
   Apple—1 small
   Apple juice—1/3 cup
   Unsweetened applesauce—1/2 cup
   Apricots—2 medium
   Banana—1/2 small
   Blackberries—1/2 cup
   Blueberries—1/2 cup
   Raspberries—1/2 cup
   Strawberries—3/4 cup
   Cherries—10 large
   Cider—1/3 cup
   Dates—2
   Fresh figs—1
   Grapefruit—1/2
   Grapefruit juice—1/2 cup
   Grapes—12
   Grape juice—1/4 cup
   Mango—1/2 small
   Cantaloupe—1/4 small
   Honeydew—1/8 medium
   Watermelon—1 cup
   Nectarine—1 small
   Orange—1 small
   Orange juice—1/2 cup
   Papaya—3/4 cup
   Peach—1 medium
   Pear—1 small
   Persimmons, native—1 medium

   Pineapple—1/2 cup
   Pineapple juice—1/3 cup
   Plums—2 medium
   Prunes—2 medium
   Prune juice—1/4 cup
   Raisins—2 tbsp
   Tangerine—1 medium

Bread exchanges
   1 exchange = 15 g CHO, 2 g protein, and 70 cal
   White, French, and Italian bread—1 slice
   Whole wheat bread—1 slice
   Rye or pumpernickel—1 slice
   Bagel, small—1/2
   English muffin, small—1/2
   Plain bread roll—1
   Hamburger bun—1/2
   Frankfurter roll—1/2
   Dried bread crumbs—3 T
   Tortilla, 6-inch—1

Low-fat items
   Bran flakes—1/2 cup
   Unsweetened cereal—3/4 cup
   Puffed cereal—1 cup
   Cooked cereal—1/2 cup
   Cooked grits—1/2 cup
   Cooked rice or barley—1/2 cup
   Pasta, cooked—1/2 cup
   Popcorn popped without butter—3 cups
   Dry cornmeal—2 T
   Flour—2 1/2 T
   Wheat germ—1/4 cup
   Graham crackers—3
   Matzo, 4 inches × 6 inches—1/2
   Oyster crackers—20
   Pretzels, 3 1/8 inches long × 1/8 inches diameter—25
   Rye wafers 2 inches × 3 1/2 inches—3
   Saltines—6
   Soda crackers, 2 1/2 inches sq—4
   Beans, peas, lentils (dried and cooked)—1/2 cup
   Baked beans, no pork (canned)—1/4 cup
   Corn—1/3 cup
   Corn on cob—1 small
   Lima beans—1/2 cup
   Parsnips—2/3 cup
   Green peas—1/2 cup
   White potato—1 small
   Mashed potato—1/2 cup
   Pumpkin—3/4 cup
   Winter, acorn, or butternut squash—1/2 cup
   Sweet potato—1/4 cup

Prepared foods with added fat
   Biscuit, 2-inch diameter—1, contains 1 fat exchange
   Corn bread, 2 inches × 2 inches × 1 inch—1 contains 1 fat exchange
   Corn muffin 2-inch dia.—1, contains 1 fat exchange
   Crackers, round butter type—5, contains 1 fat exchange
   Muffin, plain small—1, contains 1 fat exchange

   Potatoes, french fried, 2 inches to 3 1/2 inches—8, contains 1 fat exchange
   Potatoes or corn chips—15, contains 2 fat exchanges
   Pancake, 5 inches × 1/2 inches—1, contains 1 fat exchange
   Waffles, 5 inches × 1/2 inches—1, contains 1 fat exchange

Meat exchanges
   1 exchange lean meat × 7 g protein, 3 g fat, and 55 cal (1 oz serving)
   Beef: Baby beef, chipped beef, chuck, flank steak, tenderloin, plate ribs, skirt steak, round (top and bottom), all cuts rump, spare ribs, and tripe
   Lamb: Leg, rib, sirloin, loin (roast and chops), shank, and shoulder
   Pork: Leg (whole rump, center shank), ham, smoked (center slices)
   Veal: Leg, loin, rib, shank, shoulder, cutlets
   Poultry: Meat, without skin, of chicken, turkey, Cornish hen, guinea hen, pheasant
   Fish: Any fresh or frozen, clams, oysters, scallops, shrimp
   Canned salmon, tuna, mackerel, crab, and lobster—1/4 cup
   Drained sardines—3
   Cheese containing less than 5% butterfat—1 oz
   Cottage cheese, dry and 2% butterfat—1/4 cup
   Dried beans and peas—1/2 cup; contains 1 bread exchange
   1 exchange medium-fat meat = 7 g protein, 5 g fat, and 75 cal, and 1/2 extra fat exchange (1 oz serving)
   Beef: Ground (15% fat), corned beef (canned), rib eye, and round (ground commercial)
   Pork: Loin (all cuts tenderloin), shoulder arm, shoulder blade, boston butt, canadian bacon, and boiled ham
   Liver, heart, kidney, and sweetbreads (high cholesterol)
   Cheese: Mozzarella, ricotta, farmer's, neufchatel
   Creamed cottage cheese—1/4 cup
   Parmesan cheese—3 T
   Egg—1 (high cholesterol)
   Peanut butter—2 T, contains 2 extra fat exchanges
   1 exchange high-fat meat = 7 g protein, 8 g fat, and 100 cal and 1 extra fat exchange (1 oz serving)
   Beef: Brisket, corned beef brisket, ground beef (more than 20% fat), hamburger (commercial), chuck (ground commercial), rib roasts, and club and rib steaks
   Lamb: Breast
   Pork: Spare ribs, loin (back ribs), pork (ground), country-style ham, deviled ham
   Veal: Breast
   Poultry: Capon, duck (domestic), and goose
   Cheese: Cheddar
   Cold cuts, 4 1/2 inches × 1/8—1 slice
   Frankfurter—1 small

Fat exchanges
   1 exchange = 5 g fat and 45 cal

Polyunsaturated fats
   Margarine, soft, tub, or stick—1 tsp
   Avocado, 4-inch diameter—1/8
   Corn, cottonseed, safflower, soy, sunflower oil—1 tsp
   Olive oil—1 tsp
   Peanut oil—1 tsp
   Olives—5 small
   Almonds—10 whole
   Pecans—2 large whole
   Spanish peanuts—20 whole
   Virginia peanuts—10 whole
   Walnuts—6 small
   Other nuts—6 small

Saturated fats
   Margarine, regular stick—1 tsp

Table continued on following page

TABLE 5-10 Diabetic Diet Exchange Lists *Continued*

Butter—1 tsp	Mayonnaise—1 tsp	Restrict simple CHO
Bacon fat—1 tsp	Salad dressing, mayonnaise	Protein should provide 30%–38% of calories; use sources low in fat and cholesterol; increase polyunsaturated fats
Bacon, crisp—1 strip	type—2 tsp	
Light cream—2 T	Salt pork—3/4-inch cube	Include at least minimum servings of four basic food groups
Sour cream—2 T	*Principles of diabetic diet*	
Heavy cream—1 T	Diet set by physician's order	Increase fiber by using high-fiber foods or highly refined carbohydrates low in fiber
Cream cheese—1 T	Diet based on patient's age, weight, type of diabetes, and type of hypoglycemic agent used	
French dressing—1 T		Calculate grams of each nutrient, then convert to exchanges
Italian dressing—1 T	Carbohydrates should provide 50%–60% of total calories	
Lard—1 tsp	Emphasize complex CHO	

CHO, carbohydrate.

I. Low-Protein Diet (Table 5–11)

1. Lowered protein in renal or liver disease
2. Goal to maintain nitrogen balance while keeping blood urea nitrogen and serum ammonia levels as low as possible
3. 40 g protein usually lowest level; may range from 40 to 90 g
4. Limited amounts of protein of highest biologic value used
   a. protein containing essential amino acids
   b. high biologic proteins include foods such as eggs, milk, yogurt, meat, fish, poultry, and tuna
   c. include breads, cereal, fruits, and vegetables

TABLE 5-11 Low-Protein Diet

Grams of protein per exchange
Milk—8 g
Vegetable—2 g
Bread—2 g
Meat—7 g
40-g protein diet
Lacks calcium, iron, riboflavin, and niacin. Omit peas, lima beans, and dried legumes.
Sample pattern for 40-g protein diet

BREAKFAST	LUNCH	DINNER
Fruit	Cheese, 1 oz	Meat, 2 oz
Cereal	Vegetable	Potato, butter
Bread, 1 slice	Bread, 1 slice	Salad, dressing
Butter	Salad, dressing	Bread, 1 slice
Milk, 1 cup	Butter	Butter
Beverage	Fruit	Vegetable
Sugar	Beverage	Fruit
	Sugar	Beverage
		Sugar

100-g protein diet
Nutritionally adequate diet. Still based on food exchanges. Sugar, fats, and fruits may be used as desired. Increase fluid intake as protein intake increases

BIBLIOGRAPHY

American Medical Association and American Diabetic Association. (1991). *Targets for adolescent health: Adolescent nutrition and physical fitness.* Chicago: Authors.

Davis, J., & Sherer, K. (1994). *Applied nutrition and diet therapy for nurses,* 2nd ed. Philadelphia: W.B. Saunders Co.

Pipes, P.L. (1993). *Nutrition in infancy and childhood,* 5th ed. St. Louis: Mosby–Year Book.

U.S. Department of Agriculture, US Department of Health and Human Services. (1990). *Nutrition and health: Dietary guidelines for Americans,* 3rd ed. Home and Garden Bulletin, No. 232. Washington, DC: Government Printing Office.

Williams, S. R. (1992). *Basic nutrition and diet therapy,* 9th ed. St. Louis: Mosby–Year Book.

? QUESTIONS

1. A therapeutic diet is based on:

   ① Cultural preferences
   ② A well-balanced diet
   ③ Previous dietary habits
   ④ Financial income

2. A full liquid diet is one that contains:

   ① Clear liquids at body temperature
   ② Any liquid at body temperature
   ③ Only liquids that have residue
   ④ Only liquids that have no residue

3. To increase protein and not fat to the diet, one could add:

   ① Bread
   ② Egg
   ③ Nonfat milk
   ④ Vegetables

4. The best foods with which to increase dietary iron content are:

   ① Pork, apples, Karo syrup, corn
   ② Liver, raisins, molasses, soybeans
   ③ Chicken, cranberry juice, honey, tomatoes
   ④ Fish, oranges, brown sugar, red beets

5. The minimum fat diet is often used for:

   ① Colitis
   ② Kidney stones
   ③ Gallbladder and cardiac conditions
   ④ Gout

6. Which of the following foods would be *limited* on a low-cholesterol diet?

   ① Skim milk
   ② Eggs
   ③ Oranges
   ④ Peas

7. A low-cholesterol diet includes foods that are primarily low in:

   ① Animal proteins and carbohydrates
   ② Sodium
   ③ Saturated fats
   ④ Vitamins and minerals

8. The prescribed diet for a client with kidney disease would limit:

   ① Glucose
   ② Vitamins
   ③ Fats
   ④ Proteins

9. Clients who need to improve wound healing need an increase in:

   ① Protein
   ② Fiber
   ③ Fat
   ④ Fried food

10. For infants, cow's milk can be supplemented to be equivalent to human milk *except* in:

    ① Sugar content
    ② Vitamin level
    ③ Water amounts
    ④ Natural immunity

11. Low-purine diets are indicated for:

    ① Atonic constipation
    ② Peptic ulcer
    ③ Celiac disease
    ④ Gouty arthritis

12. Obesity is defined as the following percent above the ideal weight:

    ① 5%
    ② 10%
    ③ 20%
    ④ 25%

13. Which of the following foods should be *excluded* from a low-residue diet?

    ① Cooked vegetables
    ② Whole grain products
    ③ Broiled foods
    ④ White rice

14. Fats used in a diabetic diet should be mainly:

    ① Polyunsaturated
    ② Monounsaturated
    ③ Saturated
    ④ Hydrogenated

15. An example of a complex carbohydrate is:

    ① A monosaccharide
    ② Flour
    ③ Corn syrup
    ④ A disaccharide

16. For a diabetic diet, bacon is included in the exchange group of:

    ① Bread
    ② Milk
    ③ Fat
    ④ Meat

17. When a diabetic client dislikes a carbohydrate food served, the nurse should:

  ① Call the physician
  ② Tell the client to eat it anyway
  ③ Give the client an orange to eat
  ④ Substitute another equal carbohydrate

18. Nutritional anemia may develop if the pre-school child's or infant's diet consists chiefly of:

  ① Milk
  ② Vegetables
  ③ Meat
  ④ Fresh fruits

19. Vitamins are defined as:

  ① Inorganic compounds supplied in large amounts to serve as catalysts
  ② Elements that prohibit bacterial production
  ③ Organic substances needed in small amounts for growth and maintenance of life
  ④ Enzymes that prohibit the acid-base balance

20. If fats were completely excluded from the diet, the result would be a deficiency in:

  ① Vitamins A, D, E, and K
  ② All vitamins
  ③ Water-soluble vitamins only
  ④ Vitamins B and C

21. A deficiency of vitamin K results in:

  ① Poor bone formation
  ② Extreme irritability of the nerves
  ③ Muscle spasms
  ④ Delay in the clotting of blood

22. Night blindness may occur as a result of a deficiency of vitamin:

  ① A
  ② C
  ③ D
  ④ E

23. Whole grain cereals are considered nutritional breakfast food because they:

  ① Contain large quantities of protein
  ② Supply great amounts of glucose
  ③ Contain vitamin B complex
  ④ Are easily digested

24. When the strength of the walls of the capillaries is reduced, resulting in small hemorrhages, as is the case in bleeding gums, the diet contains too little:

  ① Vitamin E
  ② Vitamin A
  ③ Vitamin C
  ④ Vitamin B_6

25. The highest quantity of vitamin C is found in:

  ① Potatoes
  ② Cereals
  ③ Citrus fruits
  ④ Milk

26. Fish liver oils are an important source of:

  ① Riboflavin
  ② Vitamin D
  ③ Vitamin C
  ④ Thiamine

27. Scurvy is a deficiency disease resulting from an extreme lack of:

  ① Phosphorus
  ② Vitamin D
  ③ Vitamin C
  ④ Calcium

28. Hypervitaminosis is caused by the vitamins:

  ① C and E
  ② A and D
  ③ B complex
  ④ C and D

29. The most *unstable* of all vitamins in cooking or storage is:

  ① A
  ② C
  ③ Thiamine
  ④ Riboflavin

30. The following oil is *not* to be used in food preparation:

  ① Mineral
  ② Safflower
  ③ Sunflower
  ④ Soybean

31. Which of the following medications interferes with vitamin K production?

  ① Diuretics
  ② Vitamin C
  ③ AquaMEPHYTON
  ④ Salicylates

32. Vitamin B_{12} is found naturally in:

    ① Meat
    ② Breads
    ③ Fruits
    ④ Sugars

33. Daily selection of foods as recommended in the food pyramid will:

    ① Make it easier to plan a reducing diet
    ② Always prevent malnutrition
    ③ Inform people about the basis of good nutrition
    ④ Help plan diets that satisfy minimum nutritional needs of most people

34. Nutrients are substances needed by the body for maintaining life and growth. Essential nutrient groups include:

    ① Meats; breads and cereals; milk; citrus fruits
    ② Fats; carbohydrates; meats; calcium; sodium and water
    ③ Proteins; minerals; starches; vitamins; fats
    ④ Proteins; fats; carbohydrates; vitamins; minerals; water

35. The kilocalorie refers to a unit of measurement indicating the amount of fuel value provided for the body in a given quantity of food. Which nutrients can be converted into kilocalories?

    ① Fats, starches, and vitamins
    ② Sugars, starches, and minerals
    ③ Proteins, carbohydrates, and fats
    ④ Vitamin and mineral supplements, fats, and starches

ANSWERS AND RATIONALES

Guide to item identification (see pp. 4–5 for further details about each category):

I, II, III, or IV for the phase of the nursing process
1, 2, 3, or 4 for the category of client needs
A, B, C, D, E, F, or G for the category of human functioning
Specific content category by name; ie, cholecystectomy

1. A therapeutic diet is simply an adaptation of a
② well-balanced diet that provides the nutritional needs for a client.
III, 3, F, Nutrition

2. A full liquid diet includes a clear liquid diet and
② all liquids with residue at body temperature.
I, 2, F, Nutrition

3. Nonfat milk increases protein without increas-
③ ing other significant nutrients, specifically fat.
III, 2, F, Nutrition

4. These foods have more iron content than the
② other choices.
III, 2, F, Nutrition

5. The gallbladder would need to produce addi-
③ tional bile to emulsify the fat. Fat increases the cholesterol level of the blood, which may cause atherosclerosis of the coronary vessels.
II & III, 2, F, Nutrition

6. Egg yolks contain a high percentage of choles-
② terol.
III, 2, F, Nutrition

7. Foods low in saturated fats may contain polyun-
③ saturated fats, which reduce the level of satu-rated fats. These indirectly reduce the choles-terol level.
III, 2, F, Nutrition

8. Kidney dysfunctions retain the toxic by-prod-
④ ucts of protein metabolism. A limited daily amount of protein, 40 g (normal, 70 g), is recom-mended.
II & III, 2, F, Nutrition

9. Clients who need to heal need increased
① amounts of protein, sometimes up to 70 g a day.
II & III, 2, F, Nutrition

10. Natural immunity is transferred through the co-
④ lostrum of breast milk. IV, 2, F, Nutrition

11. Pyruvic acids are absorbed in the joints, espe-
④ cially the big toe. Diets low in purine (pyruvic acid) may diminish the occurrence of gouty arthritis.
I, 2, F, Nutrition

12. Ten percent is considered overweight. Twenty
③ percent is termed obesity.
I, 2, F, Nutrition

13. Whole grain products contain more fiber than
② other foods.
III, 2, F, Nutrition

14. Polyunsaturated fats reduce the level of satu-
① rated fats, monounsaturated fats, and choles-terol, which may reduce weight and increase the efficiency of insulin.
III, 2, F, Nutrition

15. Flour is a complex carbohydrate made from
② combined grains.
III, 2, F, Nutrition

16. Bacon is predominantly fat with a small amount
③ of protein.
III, 2, F, Nutrition

17. Carbohydrate foods are interchangeable within
④ the amount of grams, as long as the food is not out of limits for protein and fats.
III, 2, F, Nutrition

18. Milk contains only a slight amount of iron. More
① than the normal volume of milk would have to be consumed to obtain the necessary amounts of iron.
I & IV, 2 & 4, F, Nutrition

19. Minerals are inorganic compounds, and vita-
③ mins are organic compounds needed in small amounts for growth and maintenance of life. Both are catalysts.
I & IV, 2 & 4, F, Nutrition

20. A, D, E, and K are fat-soluble vitamins, and
① small amounts of fats are necessary for their absorption and metabolism.
I & IV, 2 & 4, F, Nutrition

21. Vitamin K is a necessary component of the clot-
④ ting factor. I & IV, 2 & 4, F, Nutrition

22. Vitamin A is a component of rhodopsin (visual
① purple) affecting the rods and cones of the ret-ina, permitting sight at night.
I & IV, 2 & 4, F, Nutrition

23. Vitamin B complex is necessary for a sound
③ nervous system and carbohydrate metabolism.
Most cereals do not contain protein and large
amounts of carbohydrates are not useful. Cereals are not more easily digested than other
foods.
I & IV, 2 & 4, F, Nutrition

24. Ascorbic acid (vitamin C) strengthens the mu-
③ cous membranes.
I & II, 4, F, Nutrition

25. Citrus fruits contain more ascorbic acid (vitamin
③ C) than the other foods.
I, 4, F, Nutrition

26. Vitamin D is a fat-soluble vitamin found in fish
② liver. Other vitamins are water soluble.
I & II, 4, F, Nutrition

27. Vitamin C (ascorbic acid) promotes mucous
③ membrane and tissue development. Scurvy is
characterized by thinning of the mucous membranes and tissues. I, 4, F, Nutrition

28. A and D are fat-soluble vitamins that are re-
② tained by the body, especially in the liver and
skin.
I, 4, F, Nutrition

29. Vitamin C is the most unstable of all vitamins
② with cooking or storage. This is one of the reasons for covering citrus juices after opening,
when refrigerating.
I, 4, F, Nutrition

30. Mineral oil blocks the absorption of the fat-
① soluble vitamins.
I, 4, D, Nutrition

31. Salicylates interfere with vitamin K production,
④ which is a component of the clotting factor.
I & III, 4, F, Nutrition

32. Meat contains vitamin B_{12}; whereas the other
① foods do not contain it naturally. Some fortified
breads may contain it.
I, 4, F, Nutrition

33. The four food groups show how minimum daily
③ requirements can be met.
II, 1, F, Nutrition

34. Essential nutrients are divided into six catego-
④ ries. They are proteins, fats, carbohydrates, vitamins, minerals, and water.
I, 1, F, Nutrition

35. The body can use three nutrients for fuel: carbo-
③ hydrates, fats, and proteins. Minerals and vitamins simply assist in the body's regulatory functions.
I, 1, F, Nutrition.

Special Needs of Older Adults

6

I. PHYSIOLOGIC ALTERATIONS RELATED TO AGING

A. Generalized Physiologic Changes

1. Decreased physical reserve
   a. diminishes recuperative powers
   b. homeostatic changes occur much more slowly
   c. cells and tissues less able to repair themselves, especially neurons, muscle, and kidney cells
   d. stress poses special problems with diminished reserves
2. Body systems begin to function less efficiently
   a. cardiovascular system
   b. nervous system
   c. endocrine system

B. Generalized Changes in Sensory System

1. Decreased efficiency
2. General decline of awareness of environmental stimuli
3. After age 75 years, three of five elderly have some sensory deficits

C. Generalized Changes in Nervous System

1. Nervous transmission slows
2. Loss of recent memory without loss of distant memory
3. Slower reaction time
4. Fine motor movement affected
5. Less able to react to painful stimuli
6. Impaired temperature regulation, more prone to hypothermia and hyperthermia

D. Changes in Proprioception—Position Sense

1. Impaired
2. Balance and coordination affected: decreased
3. Increased risk of injury

E. Visual Changes

1. Loss of visual acuity—presbyopia
   a. decreases progressively greater in women than men
   b. leads to problems with close work
2. Arcus senilis, rings around corneal periphery, not pathologic
3. Cataracts
4. Altered color vision
   a. color transmission from green to violet decreases
   b. sensitivity to blue and possibly red decreases
5. Loss of accommodation
   a. rate diminishes
   b. after age 60 years, no further loss
   c. decreased adaptation to dark occurs
   d. vision strongly affected by glare
6. Reduced pupil size and reactivity
7. Depth perception less accurate
8. Glaucoma more common
9. Decreased tear production leading to drying of the eyes

F. Hearing Changes

1. Auditory threshold decreases
2. Unilateral or bilateral loss common over age 65 years
3. Greater loss of high-frequency sounds
4. Lack of ability to discriminate volume or pitch; hard to understand speech
5. Long exposure to noise pollution of modern world increases hearing loss
6. Can lead to psychologic difficulties
7. May be mistaken for confusion or other mental status changes
8. Monitor for cerumen impactions

9. Safety implications related to driving, crossing streets, alarms

G. Changes in Taste, Smell, and Touch

1. Taste appears to change with aging
   a. often "picky" about foods
   b. increased preference for tart tastes
   c. decreased sensitivity leading to use of more salt and sugar
2. Smell seems to decrease with aging, can't tell if food spoiled, and can't smell smoke—thus safety an issue
3. Sense of touch decreased, which affects adaptation to environment

H. Metabolic and Gastrointestinal Changes

1. Decreased enzyme secretion
2. Decreased nutrient and drug absorption
3. Decreased peristalsis
4. Often poor nutritional status
5. Changes in dentition
6. Decreased metabolic rate
7. Less ability to withstand stress and to maintain homeostasis
8. Constipation common
9. Endocrine changes
   a. decreased response to stress
   b. most hormones normally decrease with aging

I. Cardiovascular Changes

1. Arteriosclerosis
2. Arterial blood pressure: rate of systolic increase greater than rate of diastolic increase
3. Baroreceptor sensitivity decreases
4. Increased circulation time
5. Decreased thirst mechanism may lead to dehydration, hemoconcentration, and decreased volume
6. Heart
   a. without disease, its pump function is relatively normal, but cardiac output decreases 40% between ages 25 and 65
   b. loss of physiologic reserve
   c. decreased coronary artery blood flow
   d. difficulty maintaining homeostasis when stressed
   e. contractility
      (1) decreased
      (2) time prolonged, leading to increasing oxygen requirement

f. stroke volume decreased
   g. cardiac output decreased
   h. electrocardiogram: usually shows no sign of change from aging alone
   i. atrial gallop common, even in absence of disease
7. Organ perfusion decreases
8. Peripheral vascular resistance increases
9. Postural hypotension
   a. happens fairly frequently
   b. increased with febrile diseases
   c. a side effect of many medications
10. Pulse pressure generally widens with age
11. Few changes in hematopoietic system
    a. anemia often associated with poor nutrition, not simply aging
    b. with decreased immunity, white blood cells may decrease

J. Respiratory Changes

1. Decreased ventilatory volumes
2. Decreased capacity for gas exchange
3. Increased risk of disease
4. Decreased cough effectiveness
5. Fragile mucous membranes
6. Decreased ciliary action
7. Decreased alveoli
8. Decreased Po_2: about 15%

K. Changes in Genitourinary Function

1. Benign prostatic hyperplasia with resultant urinary changes
2. Decreased blood flow to kidneys
3. Ureters, bladder, and urethra lose muscle elasticity, leading to decreased urinary sphincter control; incontinence may occur
4. Nephrons are lost
5. More alkaline vaginal environment in women
6. Decreased bladder capacity
7. Decreased tubular function

L. Changes in Musculoskeletal System

1. Osteoporosis
2. Increase in fibrous connective tissue with stiffening
3. Arthritic changes; joint cartilage erodes
4. Muscle atrophy
   a. muscle cells reduced in size and number
   b. protein building in muscle diminished
5. Intervertebral discs dehydrate
   a. may fracture more easily
   b. shorten height up to 2 inches

6. Slight kyphosis
7. Slight knee flexion
8. Slight hip flexion
9. Slight wrist flexion
10. Mobility may be decreased due to changes

M. Skin Changes

1. Decreased activity of oil and sweat glands
   a. increase in dry skin and itching
   b. decrease in perspiration leading to decrease in cooling effect
2. Increased skin fragility and susceptibility to trauma
3. Delayed wound healing
4. Decreased tone and elasticity causing wrinkles
5. Decrease in subcutaneous tissue
6. Decreased hair and nail growth
7. Hair thinning and loss of color
8. Pigmentation changes

II. PSYCHOLOGIC ALTERATIONS RELATED TO AGING

A. Retirement

1. May be difficult to live on fixed income
2. May alter self-concept because of lifestyle changes
3. New concerns about leisure time and what to do
4. Physical limitations may prevent enjoyment of these years
5. May be welcomed as new experience with growth potentials, especially if prepared for retirement in earlier years
6. May be difficult to adjust to decreased social contact

B. Role Changes

1. May vary from independent one to dependent one
2. May be difficult without role of worker
3. May be that of widow or widower
4. Take on role of grandparent

C. Erikson's Stage of Ego Integrity versus Despair

1. Successful adaptation shown through satisfaction with life and acceptance of eventual death
2. Unsuccessful adaptation shown by sense of failure and futility, desire to redo life, sense of worthlessness

D. Body Image Changes May Lead to Depression

1. Diminished strength
2. Actual physical changes of aging may alter appearance
3. May not see themselves as "old," but others identify them that way

E. Confusion As a Problem, Not a Disease

1. May result from any change in living conditions
2. May be due to medications
3. May be result of a disease

F. Confidence in Cognitive Function Decreases

1. Slower response time
2. Slowed nerve impulse transmission
3. General intelligence not affected
4. Capacity to learn intact, but learning may take longer and may require more repetition and different methods

G. Environment

1. Possible need to change living arrangements
2. Limitations imposed by illness or infirmity increase
3. Likelihood that residence will change increases
4. Need for assistance with transportation increases
5. Need for safety features increases

H. Financial Changes

1. Income usually decreased, often drastically
2. Usually on fixed income; financial planning may have been neglected
3. Inflation adjustments restricted

I. Problems Associated with Aging and Loss

1. Less desire for new experiences
2. Planning impaired by decreased energy levels
3. Difficulty sustaining anticipation
4. Sense of decreased worth to others
5. Loss of friends or spouse to death

J. Sexuality

1. Sexual function still present
2. Slowed or decreased capacity for orgasm

3. Slower to achieve erection and decreased pressure of ejaculation
4. Water-soluble lubricant or hormone therapy sometimes needed for vaginal dryness
5. Often decreased opportunities for intimacy if institutionalized or loss of significant other
6. More women alive than men
7. Sexual expression in elderly often viewed negatively by society

K. Society's View of the Elderly

1. Discrimination
2. Negative image in media
3. Ageism

III. LEGAL CONCERNS OF OLDER ADULTS

A. Legal Rights

1. Unchanged unless shown in courts to be incompetent
2. Right to refuse medical treatments, advanced directives
3. Entrance into nursing home does not mean automatic loss of rights
4. Encourage client to obtain legal help as needed for financial matters, wills, and generalized legal counseling about his or her rights
5. Encourage client to consider appropriate person to grant power of attorney, for health care decisions or for monetary purposes
6. Guardianship may be necessary to protect the older adult

B. Elder Abuse

1. Occurs much more frequently than previously imagined
2. May occur when living with children or in nursing home
3. Assess injuries in older adults for signs of abuse
4. Abuse can be physical, verbal, or sexual
5. If abuse is suspected, it must be reported to proper authorities
6. Exploitation is also a form of neglect

IV. COMMON HEALTH PROBLEMS OF OLDER ADULTS

See Chapter 7, The Adult Patient.

A. Cataracts

B. Glaucoma

C. Herpes Zoster

D. Parkinson's Disease

E. Alzheimer's Disease

F. Heart Disease

1. Angina
2. Arrhythmias
3. Hypertension
4. Congestive heart failure

G. Peripheral Vascular Disease

1. Stasis ulcers
2. Arterial occlusions
3. Varicose veins

H. Chronic Obstructive Pulmonary Disease

I. Anemia

J. Chronic Lymphocytic Leukemia

K. Malignant Lymphomas

L. Benign Prostatic Hyperplasia

M. Osteoarthritis

1. Osteoporosis
2. Hip fractures

N. Cancer

O. Cerebrovascular Accident

P. Diabetes

V. MEDICATIONS AND OLDER ADULTS

A. General Principles of Drug Therapy for Older Adults

1. Alterations in pharmacokinetics
   a. absorption often slower
      (1) decreased intestinal blood flow
      (2) delayed gastric emptying

    (3) increased gastric pH

    (4) multiple drugs ingested simultaneously may alter absorption of all or interact unfavorably

  b. distribution may be altered

    (1) lower fluid intake leads to increased plasma concentration of drugs

    (2) lean muscle mass decreased with increased body fat

    (3) fat-soluble drugs more dangerous because more accumulation in body fat

    (4) decreased serum proteins lead to problems with protein-bound drugs

  c. altered metabolism of drugs

    (1) liver function vital and decreased with age

    (2) blood flow to liver decreased

    (3) liver microsomal action decreased

  d. changes in elimination

    (1) renal function vital to drug elimination

    (2) approximately 50% loss of nephrons

    (3) decreased glomerular and tubular filtration

    (4) low fluid intake and decreased output

    (5) renal blood flow decreased

    (6) constipation may affect drugs eliminated through feces

  e. drug sensitivity

    (1) sudden development of new allergies

    (2) decreased T cells

    (3) increased permeability of blood-brain barrier

    (4) drug dosages often must be lowered to prevent problems

2. Drug interactions

  a. older adults often have multiple chronic problems and take multiple prescription and nonprescription drugs

  b. alcohol interacts with many medications, causing excessive effects, such as alcohol and sedatives

  c. drugs may interact with food

    (1) drugs may cause nutrients to be poorly absorbed

    (2) nutrients may interfere with drug actions

B. Other Problems

1. Older adults with limited resources may have problems affording drugs

2. Self-medication practices may be dangerous

  a. overuse of over-the-counter drugs

  b. Difficulty in remembering to take drugs

  c. Multiple physicians and multiple medications often present

  d. may not understand dangers of increasing or decreasing dosages

  e. may not understand dangers of taking drugs ordered for their friends with similar problems

VI. NURSING PROCESS APPLIED TO THE SPECIAL NEEDS OF OLDER ADULTS

A. Assessment

1. Assess older adult's level of development

2. Identify physiologic changes that have occurred and their effect on the client

3. Identify psychologic changes that have occurred and their effect on the client

4. Be aware of impaired communication potential, such as client being hard of hearing or forgetful

5. Assess client's level of functioning and independence

6. Find out what the client's expectations are for this hospitalization

7. Take detailed medication and nutritional history

8. Identify role within the family—support system

9. Common nursing problems

  a. altered communication

  b. chemical and physical restraints

B. Planning

1. Identify reasonable goals with client and RN if appropriate

2. Discuss possible outcomes with client

3. Establish priorities

C. Implementation

1. Care related to general physiologic changes

  a. decrease stress as much as possible

  b. monitor for changes in health status

  c. prevent injury through good safety precautions because recuperative powers are less

    (1) provide adequate lighting

    (2) avoid hazards such as throw rugs and objects on floor

    (3) teach client to rise from sitting or lying slowly

    (4) use side rails and safety bars

    (5) teach client to allow time for eyes to adjust to darkness

2. Care related to sensory/perceptual changes

  a. allow longer for responses because reaction time slower

   b. maintain body temperature; avoid extremes of heat or cold
   c. provide adequate pain medication
   d. monitor for development of cataracts or glaucoma; refer to physician if either develops
   e. monitor for hearing loss; refer to physician if this develops
   f. assess signs of confusion carefully; may be related to external causes
   g. orient to changes in environment
   h. monitor food intake
      (1) provide high-nutrition, appealing foods
      (2) find out client likes and dislikes
      (3) provide socialization at mealtimes
      (4) frequent small feedings may be better tolerated
3. Care related to metabolic changes
   a. provide increased fluid and fiber to decrease constipation
   b. stool softeners may be necessary if stools are hard
   c. encourage activity and exercise
   d. provide consistent toileting
   e. monitor serum proteins for signs of malnutrition
   f. check for presence and condition of teeth and gums
      (1) poor-fitting dentures
      (2) long-time established food habits
   g. assess ability to swallow
   h. monitor for hormonal deficiencies
      (1) increased antidiuretic hormone: observe for diluted urine and increased urine
      (2) decreased glucose tolerance: observe for frequent and excessive urination, excessive thirst, excessive eating, fatigue, visual blurring
      (3) hypothyroidism: observe for constipation, lethargy, dry skin, mental deterioration, weight changes
4. Care related to cardiovascular changes
   a. remember increased systolic blood pressure is normal in aging adult·
   b. monitor fluid intake carefully
   c. offer liquids frequently; make sure liquids are within reach; encourage intake
   d. monitor for signs of decreased organ perfusion, such as decreased urine output and edema
   e. monitor for presence of anemia
   f. avoid abrupt position changes
   g. have client avoid people with infections
5. Care related to respiratory changes
   a. turn, cough, and deep breathe if client on bed rest and following surgery
   b. provide rest periods during exercise or increased activity

   c. assess for abnormal breathing patterns
   d. limit contact with people with respiratory infections
   e. frequent mouth care to keep mucous membranes moist to help prevent infections
6. Care related to genitourinary changes
   a. monitor male clients for signs of benign prostatic hyperplasia
   b. treat incontinence, if possible
      (1) encourage use of bedpan, urinal, or toilet, every 2 hours
      (2) respond promptly to client's need to void
   c. monitor output; urine often much more diluted
   d. observe for signs of urinary tract infection, such as confusion, urinary frequency, color and odor of urine
   e. if incontinent, clean skin and monitor condition of skin frequently
7. Care related to musculoskeletal changes
   a. prevent falls and monitor for fractures
   b. encourage joint-sparing movements
   c. treat arthritic changes as ordered
   d. prevent pressure on bony prominences
   e. encourage exercise, as tolerated
   f. do not rush the client
   g. moist heat provides comfort, e.g., showers
   h. teach proper body mechanics
8. Care related to skin changes
   a. daily baths not necessary
   b. temperature of bath water no more than 105° F
   c. use superfatted soap or bath oil
      (1) avoid using soap, unless necessary
      (2) safety precautions if oil in bathtub or shower to prevent falls
   d. apply emollient lotions to skin; avoid using alcohol or dusting powders
   e. discourage scratching, and keep nails short
   f. Using proper technique, turn client on bed rest every 2 hours establish turning schedule
   g. use pillows for proper positioning
   h. avoid friction when positioning client
   i. provide for client's safety to prevent skin trauma
9. Care related to psychosocial alterations
   a. assess developmental status and intervene if inappropriate
   b. watch for development of depression
   c. allow more time for learning activities
   d. encourage client to remain as independent as possible
   e. be aware of financial difficulties and recommend social service involvement
   f. allow for appropriate sexual expression

(1) provide privacy

(2) allow couples to room together in extended-care facilities, if possible

(3) provide sexual counseling as needed

(4) teach clients about expected changes in sexual functioning

10. Care related to legal concerns

a. allow competent adults rights of decision making

b. monitor for signs of elder abuse

11. Care related to common health problems (see Chapter 7, The Adult Patient)

12. Care related to medications

a. read precautions of all drugs before administering

b. use drugs with care in clients with impaired liver function

c. monitor serum protein levels and administer drugs appropriately

d. monitor renal function and report changes to physician

e. encourage adequate intake to ensure drug excretion

f. monitor closely for idiosyncratic reactions to drugs

g. check for potential interactions between drugs when the client is taking multiple medications

h. check for possible food-drug interactions

i. teach client principles of self-medication

(1) provide client with written reminders of teaching

(2) teach client importance of following medication prescription orders exactly

(3) assess client's ability to be dependable in self-medication

(4) include family member or person who can help in home setting in teaching

D. Evaluation

1. Decide whether identified goals are met based on criteria

2. Identify changes required to meet unmet goals

3. Modify nursing care as necessary to meet established goals

BIBLIOGRAPHY

Betz, C.L., Hunsberger, M., & Wright, S. (1994). *Family-centered nursing care of children*, 2nd ed. Philadelphia: W.B. Saunders Co.

Bolander, V.R. (1994). *Sorensen and Luckmann's basic nursing: A psychophysiologic approach*, 3rd ed. Philadelphia: W.B. Saunders Co.

Davis, J., & Sherer, K. (1994). *Applied nutrition and diet therapy for nurses*, 2nd ed. Philadelphia: W. B. Saunders Co.

Ebersole, P., and Hess, P. (1994). *Toward healthy aging*, 4th ed. St. Louis: Mosby–Year Book.

Hogstel, M. O. (1990). *Geropsychiatric nursing*. St. Louis: Mosby–Year Book.

Lehne, R.A., Moore, L., Crosby, L., and Hamilton, D. (1994). *Pharmacology for nursing care*, 2nd ed. Philadelphia: W.B. Saunders Co.

Linton, A.D., Matteson, M.A., & Maebius, N.K. (1995). *Introductory nursing care of adults*. Philadelphia: W.B. Saunders Co.

Maas, M., et al. (1991). *Nursing diagnoses and interventions for the elderly*. Redwood City, CA: Addison-Wesley.

Matteson, M.A., & McConnell, E.W. (1988). *Gerontological nursing: Concepts and practice*. Philadelphia: W.B. Saunders Co.

Monohan, F.D., Drake, T., & Neighbors, M. (1994). *Nursing care of adults*. Philadelphia: W.B. Saunders Co.

Potter, P.A., & Perry, A.G. (1993). *Fundamentals of nursing: Concepts, process, and practice*, 3rd ed. St. Louis: Mosby–Year Book.

1. Mary Nelson, age 80 years, is admitted after falling at home and fracturing her femur. At the time of admission, she is confused and disoriented. Based on your knowledge of aging and her history, you may conclude that Mrs. Nelson is:

   ① Probably suffering from the trauma of the fall and will need time to adjust to the situation
   ② Behaving normally for her age and cannot be expected to show any improvement
   ③ In need of special attention and a lot of "babying" during her stay
   ④ Unable to control herself and will be totally dependent on the staff during her stay

2. Mrs. Nelson, age 80, who fell at home, seems to confuse you with her daughter Anne during the first postoperative day and frequently calls you by her name. Your best response would be:

   ① Reassure her by telling her that Anne will visit soon even if you are not sure that she is coming in today
   ② Tell her that Anne went home for a rest and will return and that in the meantime you will take good care of her
   ③ Pretend that you are Anne and answer her questions so she will not be frightened
   ④ Tell her your name and explain that you are her nurse and will do anything you can to help her

3. Two days later, Mrs. Nelson, age 80, who fell at home, apologizes for being so much trouble for the nurses and says, "I don't know what is wrong; I always take care of myself. If I just hadn't broken my hip, I could take care of myself." The LPN realizes that she is probably:

   ① Expressing a desire to become more dependent
   ② Regressing into senility and childishness
   ③ Anxious that she is losing self-control and independence
   ④ Expressing guilt about her carelessness

4. It is important that Mrs. Nelson, age 80, suffering from a fractured hip, receive skin care daily, but a daily bath is unnecessary for older adults because their:

   ① Activity level is decreased
   ② Sweat and oil glands are less active
   ③ Interest in hygiene is decreased
   ④ Body odor is diminished

5. Mrs. Nelson, an 80-year-old who is in for repair of a fractured hip, needs a diet in the hospital that must include:

   ① Fewer calories because she is less active
   ② More protein and calcium for adequate healing
   ③ More calories because she is less active
   ④ Higher fat and carbohydrates for energy

6. You suggest to Mrs. Nelson, age 80, who fell at home and has had a fractured hip repaired, that she wear a nice robe and apply some makeup before going to physical therapy. Your intervention is:

   ① Appropriate because she needs to be clean to prevent infection
   ② Inappropriate because she is unaware of her surroundings
   ③ Appropriate because it will increase her self-esteem
   ④ Inappropriate because makeup can be harmful to her skin

7. Because of decreased muscle tone in the digestive tract of elderly individuals, their diet should emphasize sufficient intake of:

   ① Fiber and calcium
   ② Whole grain cereals, fresh fruits, vegetables, and plenty of fluids
   ③ Increased amounts of meat and cheese
   ④ A bulk laxative daily with plenty of fluids

8. The term that applies to research and study of the aging process is:

   ① Gerontology
   ② Senility
   ③ Geriatrics
   ④ Bariatrics

9. Which of the following statements regarding aging is correct?

   ① Old age begins at 65 years
   ② People age in different ways and at different rates
   ③ The majority of old people live in retirement homes or in convalescent facilities
   ④ Elderly people generally lack the financial resources necessary for independent living

10. Characteristics that best describe the process of aging include:

① Increased flexibility in most situations and loss of rigidity of body parts
② Mental and physical deterioration
③ Inability to cope with the stress of everyday living
④ Decreased flexibility in some situations and increased rigidity of certain body parts

11. According to Erikson's stages of development, healthy aging for an elderly person would be characterized by:

① An acceptance of eventual death
② Reliving of past events
③ Refusal to retire well beyond normal retirement age
④ Reassessment of relationship with spouse after children leave home

12. Constipation is a common health problem in the elderly usually caused by:

① Decreased activity and poor eating habits
② Failure to use bulk laxatives daily
③ Too much residue in their diet
④ Decreased appetite

13. What kind of personality change is common in clients with dementia?

① Docile, compliant personality
② Exaggeration of basic personality
③ Aggressive, uncooperative personality
④ Opposite of usual personality

14. What kind of group work can the PN initiate for clients with dementia?

① Groups that focus on "here and now" issues
② Groups that focus on reasons for feelings
③ Groups that focus on reasons for behavior
④ Groups that focus on personality issues

15. Which of the following is an example of using reminiscing to help bring a client with dementia to the present?

① "It sounds as if you are lonely since your husband died 5 years ago. Tell me about him."
② "Your husband has been dead for 5 years. You're at The Happy Trails Mental Health Center now."

③ "Don't you remember? I told you yesterday that you were widowed 5 years ago."
④ "You need to accept that your husband is dead. He died of a heart attack 5 years ago."

16. Which of the following is appropriate recreational therapy for the client with dementia?

① Individual physically active games
② Mind-stimulating games
③ Concrete, repetitious crafts
④ Noncompetitive team sports

17. Which of the following would be a physical change associated with the older adult between ages 75 and 80 years?

① Decreased response to physical stress
② Inability to carry out normal activities of daily living
③ Rapid progression of aging changes
④ Normal response time to stimuli

18. Older adults have a decrease in total body fluids, which can cause:

① Increased thirst
② Decreased risk of dehydration
③ Increase in urine output
④ Increased incidence of side effects from water-soluble drugs

19. Older adults are more susceptible to overdoses from fat-soluble drugs because they have a(an):

① Decreased percentage of body fat
② Increased percentage of body fat
③ Decrease in renal function
④ Increase in bowel transit time

20. Respiratory changes in older adults include:

① Decrease in dead space
② Increased vital capacity
③ Decreased cough effectiveness
④ Increased respiratory rate

21. Which of the following is *not* a typical problem associated with skin changes in older adults?

① Increased ability for wound healing
② Dry cracking skin from decreased turgor
③ Decreased sweating because decreased sweat glands
④ Increased risk of hypothermia

22. A normal visual change associated with aging is:

① Development of tunnel vision
② Decreased accommodation to light or dark

③ Loss of central vision
④ Decreased vision from clouding of the lens

23. The average number of calories a 65-year-old woman should eat daily to maintain an ideal body weight is about:

① 1000
② 1500
③ 2000
④ 2500

24. Which of the following is *not* a likely cause of nutritional problems in older adults?

① Difficulty chewing because of lost teeth
② Difficulty shopping for food
③ Decreased caloric needs
④ Social isolation during meals

25. Older adults are more prone to drug overdoses from a variety of drugs because:

① They have a lower fat content
② Their water content is proportionally high
③ They often forget to take their medication
④ Their serum albumin levels are lower

26. Your older client is exhibiting severe confusion. The family says that the client had been perfectly clear at home and never confused before. The most likely cause of the confusion is:

① Relocation trauma
② Alzheimer's disease
③ Organic brain syndrome
④ Related to medication

27. A common developmental task of the older adult is:

① Preparation for retirement
② Continued parenting of adult children
③ Preparation for death
④ Reassessment of roles within the family

28. Because older adults are more prone to accidents and fractures, the nurse should protect them by:

① Encouraging their families to put them in nursing homes
② Providing a safe environment for them
③ Keeping them confined to a chair; up only with help
④ Maintaining them on bed rest

ANSWERS AND RATIONALES

Guide to item identification (see pp. 4–5 for further details about each category):
  I, II, III, or IV for the phase of the nursing process
  1, 2, 3, or 4 for the category of client needs
  A, B, C, D, E, F, or G for the category of human functioning
  Specific content category by name; ie, cholecystectomy

1. Confusion often occurs in the elderly with
① trauma and a sudden, unexpected alteration in the environment.
I, 3, A & G, Older adult/fractured hip

2. Never reinforce confusion by lying to a client.
④ Reorient the client to reality when confusion occurs.
III, A & G, Older adult/fractured hip

3. The client was suffering from temporary confu-
③ sion, but loss of independence is one of the greatest fears of older adults.
IV, 3, A & G, Older adult/fractured hip

4. The older adult does not need bathing daily
② owing to the decrease in function of the sweat and oil glands, but for the same reasons, they must have frequent skin care.
III, 2, A & D, Older adult/fractured hip

5. The older adult is often protein malnourished.
② Anyone suffering an injury requires more protein for healing. Calcium is needed for bone repair.
I & III, 2, F, Older adult/fractured hip

6. Wearing clothes of their own and good groom-
③ ing help older adults maintain self-esteem.
III, 2, A & G, Older adult/fractured hip

7. In the elderly, constipation is a common prob-
② lem attributable to decreased gastrointestinal muscle tone, which causes inability to move waste effectively through the system. Fresh fruits, vegetables, and water provide bulk, which stimulates peristalsis.
II, 2 & 4, F, Older adult

8. Gerontology refers to research and study of the
① aging process.
I, 4, A, Older adult

9. The aging process is different for each person
② and is more related to feelings and behavior than to chronologic age alone.
IV, 4, A, Older adult

10. Aging involves the loss of ability to withstand
④ change and increased rigidity of joints, muscles, lung tissue, and so forth.
IV, 4, E, Older adult

11. It is healthy for an elderly person to begin to
① accept the inevitability of death.
I, 4, A & G, Older adult

12. Older adults experience a slowing of peristalsis
① because of their decreased activity. Fiber and bulk are often deficient in their diets.
IV, 4, F, Older adult

13. Clients with dementia tend to maintain their
② basic personality only with more exaggerated behavior.
IV, 3, C & G, Organic mental disorder/older adult

14. Groups focusing on "here and now" issues offer
① a concrete basis for dealing with specific items the clients can grasp. Such groups are led by a wide spectrum of health providers who do not need special training in group dynamics.
II, 3, C & G, Organic mental disorder/older adult

15. Using the client's past memories may bring the
① client into the present. For example, say "You are in a nursing home now. But tell me about the time that you had a farm." This helps to orient the client to the present while encouraging the client to share experiences from the past with you.
IV, 3, C & G, Organic mental disorder/older adult

16. Using concrete, repetitious tasks helps create fa-
③ miliarity and comfort in a demented client.
III, 3, C & G, Organic mental disorder/older adult

17. The major physical change experienced by the
① "middle" old is a decreased ability to respond to stress. They are still able to carry out normal activities of daily living but do have a slightly slower response time. Aging is usually gradual.
I, 4, A & D, Older adult

18.
④ Because older adults have a decrease in body water, water-soluble drugs can become increasingly concentrated leading to an increase in side effects. Thirst is normally decreased, with an increased risk of dehydration. Urine output is usually decreased and concentrated.
I, 4, F, Older adult

19.
② Older adults have an increase in the percentage of fat in the body resulting in an increase in the amount of fat-soluble drugs that can be absorbed, leading to possible overdose. Renal function should not affect these drugs, and an increase in bowel transit time would decrease their absorption, leading to underdosing.
I, 4, F, Older adult

20.
③ Older adults have an increase in dead space, a decrease in vital capacity, and little change in rate. A decrease in the effectiveness of the cough is the most common and potentially serious change.
I, 4, B, Older adult

21.
① There is a decreased ability to form granulation tissue in older adults, which impairs healing and normal scar formation.
I, 4, D, Older adult

22.
② Tunnel vision may be a sign of glaucoma, loss of central vision, a retinal detachment, and cloudy vision characteristic of cataracts. Decreased accommodation is the only normal visual change associated with aging.
I, 4, C, Older adult

23.
② The rule is that the caloric intake should decrease about 7.5% per decade after age 25 years.

The normal caloric intake would be about 1500 calories from age 65 years on.
III, 4, F, Older adult

24.
③ Older adults often need more calories than they receive and more nutritious foods.
I, 4, F, Older adult

25.
④ Many drugs that older adults take, such as cardiac glycosides, are protein-bound drugs. The low serum albumin common in many older people means that higher levels of the drugs are in circulation, leading to overdose. Older adults have a higher percentage of fat and a low level of body water and forgetting their drugs would lead to underdosing, not overdoses.
I, 4, F, Older adult

26.
① The most common cause of sudden acute confusion in this client is probably relocation trauma associated with the change in the environment. Alzheimer's disease and organic brain syndrome occur gradually, and the family would have noticed some changes. There is no mention of medication administration and it *cannot* be assumed.
I, 4, G, Older adult

27.
③ One of the common developmental tasks of older adults is acceptance of and preparation for death. The other options are tasks of the middle-aged person.
II, 4, A, Older adult

28.
② If a safe environment is maintained, an older adult can remain independent and still be accident-free.
III, 4, D & E, Older adult

The Adult Client

GROWTH AND DEVELOPMENT

Life Stages

I. MIDDLE-AGED ADULT

A. Physiologic Alterations

1. Hormonal changes
   a. menopause (see p. 87)
      (1) cessation of reproductive ability
      (2) women are usually between age 40 and 50 years
      (3) men are usually between age 50 and 60 years, but symptoms may not be as pronounced
   b. benign prostatic hyperplasia in men begins usually by age 50 years
   c. decreasing hormonal production by both sexes may alter sexual function to some degree
2. Skeletal changes
   a. osteoporosis from decalcification of bones
      (1) women often lose up to 2 inches of height from shrinking of intervertebral discs
      (2) "dowager's hump" in cervical thoracic spine
   b. women are much more susceptible to hip and other bone fractures at age 55 years than men are
3. Skin changes
   a. cell atrophy and decreased repair
   b. shrinkage of body
   c. loss of subcutaneous tissue
4. Nerve conduction slows and muscle function decreases
   a. leads to increased muscle atrophy
   b. impaired heat and cold sensation
5. Vision
   a. presbyopia, decreasing accommodation
   b. glasses, often bifocals, needed

6. Hearing
   a. decreased sensitivity to high-pitched sounds
   b. decreased sound discrimination
7. Cardiovascular changes
   a. decreased elasticity of vessels, especially coronary arteries
   b. rise in serum cholesterol in women after menopause, with increase in coronary heart disease
   c. cardiac output decreased
   d. glomerular filtration rate decreased
8. Metabolic changes
   a. altered nutritional needs
      (1) decreased basal metabolic rate
      (2) reduce calories by 7.5% per decade after age 25 years
      (3) maintain high fluid intake
   b. rest and activity
      (1) activity level often relatively unchanged
      (2) development of a new sense of energy in some people
      (3) no reason to decrease activity or increase rest unless a disease state is present

B. Psychosocial Alterations

1. Cognitive changes
   a. reaction time usually unchanged
   b. ability to learn unchanged
   c. time for learning increased
   d. memory not impaired, but less ability to memorize or remember new material
   e. problem-solving abilities unchanged
2. Emotional development
   a. climacteric
   b. transitional period
      (1) prime of work life
      (2) role changes: children, spouse, own parents
      (3) time when goals are reached or never achieved

    c. Erikson's stage of generativity versus self-absorption and stagnation
      (1) success means sense of parenthood or other generative activity and creativity, guiding new generation, establishing continuity
      (2) not necessarily biologic in nature
      (3) negative development seen as lack of acceptance of self and accomplishments, regression to earlier stages, and self-absorption

3. Midlife crisis
    a. "empty nest" syndrome when children leave home
    b. change in roles from mother or father to spouse again
    c. upheaval, which may be internal or external
    d. time for reexamination of self, role, and life
    e. sandwich generation, especially women caring for teenaged children and older parents
    f. reproductive ability lost in women

C. Common Health Problems

1. Fractures and dislocations are the leading types of injury
2. Sinusitis and upper respiratory infections are common
3. Hiatal hernia and esophagitis may be mistaken for myocardial infarction
4. Peptic ulcers, especially with increased stress
5. Angina pectoris
6. Essential hypertension
7. Hyperuricemia and gout
8. Type II diabetes mellitus (non–insulin-dependent diabetes mellitus)
9. Prostatitis, acute and chronic
10. Benign prostatic hyperplasia
11. Lumbosacral strain
12. Sexual dysfunction, of both physical and psychological causes
13. Dental problems, gum disease, loss of teeth
14. Decreasing eyesight and hearing

II. THE OLDER ADULT (see also Chapter 6)

A. Physiologic Alterations

1. Nervous system changes
    a. nervous transmission slows
    b. recent memory loss
    c. slower reaction time
    d. sense of balance sometimes decreased
    e. fine motor movement affected
    f. less ability to react to painful stimuli

    g. impaired temperature regulation; higher susceptibility to hypothermia and hyperthermia
    h. decreased tactile sensation

2. Visual changes
    a. normal
      (1) loss of visual acuity, presbyopia
      (2) arcus senilis (rings around corneal periphery), not pathologic
      (3) altered color vision
      (4) loss of accommodation
    b. pathologic
      (1) cataracts
      (2) glaucoma more common
      (3) macular degeneration possibly increased, leading to severely impaired vision

3. Hearing changes
    a. unilateral or bilateral hearing loss common over age 65 years
    b. lack of ability to discriminate volume or pitch

4. Metabolic changes
    a. decreased enzyme secretion
    b. decreased nutrient and drug absorption
    c. decreased peristalsis
    d. loss of sense of taste and smell
    e. changes in dentition
    f. decreased metabolic rate
    g. less ability to withstand stress and to maintain homeostasis
    h. constipation common

5. Cardiovascular changes
    a. arteriosclerosis
    b. decreased coronary artery blood flow
    c. hypertension common
    d. few changes in hematopoietic system

6. Respiratory changes
    a. decreased ventilatory volumes
    b. decreased capacity for gas exchange
    c. increased risk of disease

7. Genitourinary function changes
    a. benign prostatic hyperplasia with resultant urinary changes
    b. decreased blood flow to kidneys
    c. incontinence, especially in women who had children with resultant perineal muscle weakness

8. Musculoskeletal changes
    a. osteoporosis
    b. increase in fibrous connective tissue with stiffening
    c. arthritic changes
    d. muscle atrophy

B. Psychosocial Alterations

1. Retirement
2. Role changes

3. Erikson's stage of ego integrity versus despair
   a. successful adaptation shown through satisfaction with life and acceptance of eventual death
   b. unsuccessful adaptation shown by sense of failure and futility, desire to redo life, and a sense of worthlessness
4. Body image changes can lead to depression
5. Cognitive changes
   a. slower
   b. slowed nerve impulse transmission
   c. general intelligence not affected
   d. capacity to learn intact, but learning time longer and more repetition sometimes necessary

C. Common Health Problems (see Chapter 6)

Reproductive System in Women

I. NORMAL FUNCTION

A. To provide nourishment and protection for the developing fetus

B. To assist in the birth of the child through muscular contractions

C. To assist in the production of required hormones during pregnancy

D. To nourish the newborn child

Reproductive Changes and Disorders in Women

I. BREAST

A. Benign Tumors, Cysts

1. Assessment
   a. definition: painless or tender lumps in breast tissue
   b. incidence: most often occurring in women between ages 30 and 50 years
   c. predisposing factors
      (1) possible genetic link
      (2) diet high in caffeine
   d. signs and symptoms
      (1) enlargement of area in breast
      (2) pain when area pressed
   e. diagnostic tests
      (1) mammography: radiographic picture of breast tissue; no special preparation necessary except explanation to client
      (2) biopsy: removal of section of tissue to be examined under microscope; procedure

performed on outclient basis; explanation necessary
      (3) aspiration: fluid removed from the cyst using a needle and syringe; performed by the physician; explanation of procedure necessary
   f. usual treatment: excision or aspiration

B. Breast Carcinoma

1. Assessment
   a. definition: cancerous growth in breast tissue
   b. incidence
      (1) higher in women with family history
      (2) higher in women over age 40 years
   c. predisposing/precipitating factors
      (1) genetic predisposition; mother, sister, or grandmother with breast cancer
      (2) age over 40 years
      (3) childless or first child after age 30 years
      (4) presence of other cancers (ovarian, endometrial)
   d. signs and symptoms
      (1) painless lump in breast
      (2) "dimpling" of skin
      (3) retraction of nipple
      (4) discharge from nipple
      (5) asymmetry of breasts
   e. diagnostic tests
      (1) biopsy
      (2) mammography
         (a) all women: baseline at age 35 years, every other year after age 40 years, and yearly after age 50 years
         (b) high-risk women: baseline at age 35 years and yearly after age 40 years
   f. usual treatments
      (1) chemotherapy: see explanation in discussion on cancer under "Immune Disorders."
      (2) radiation therapy
      (3) surgical procedure: mastectomy; lumpectomy; simple or modified radical mastectomy
2. Planning, goals, expected outcomes
   a. client performs monthly breast self-examination correctly
   b. client complies with breast self-examination
   c. assist client to alleviate emotional distress associated with breast disease
   d. assist in reducing complications of surgery and reducing recurrence of cancer
3. Implementation
   a. teach monthly breast self-examination techniques taught to client; importance of early detection should be stressed

b. palpation examination by physician should be performed on yearly basis

c. mammography examination should be performed as ordered

d. assist client to verbalize fears related to breast disease and the diagnosis of cancer

e. explain procedures and side effects as they relate to treatment

f. implement routine postoperative care and specific arm exercises to reduce postoperative complications

g. advise client to modify diet to decrease caffeine intake

4. Evaluation

a. client performs monthly breast self-examinations

b. client maintains regular check-up appointments

c. client fully recovers from any surgical procedures without complications

d. client performs postoperative exercises as instructed

e. client verbalizes feelings related to body image

f. referrals to self-help agencies made as needed, including American Cancer Society, Reach for Recovery, and other social service agencies

g. client verbalizes diet changes and modifies diet, such as decreased caffeine intake

II. UTERINE TUMORS: BENIGN

A. Assessment

1. Definition: abnormal growth within uterus; usually benign uterine myomas; also known as fibroids

2. Incidence: common between ages 24 and 40 years

3. Signs and symptoms

a. bleeding most common

b. as size increases, pressure may be felt

4. Diagnostic tests

a. physical pelvic examination; emotional support of client necessary

b. nurse assists with preparing and labeling specimens

c. proper draping of client to preserve modesty

5. Usual treatments

a. surgical excision, determined by age of client

b. conservative treatment if bleeding not excessive or if children still desired

III. CERVICAL CANCER

A. Assessment

1. Definition: abnormal growth in cervical area of uterus

2. Incidence: women over age 40 years

3. Predisposing factors

a. first pregnancy at an early age

b. frequent sexual relations with numerous partners

c. multiparity

d. history of venereal disease

e. presence of human papillomavirus

4. Signs and symptoms

a. postmenopausal bleeding

b. bleeding with intercourse

5. Diagnostic tests

a. Pap smear (see Chapter 3)

b. cervical biopsy

c. colposcopy

d. Schiller test

e. cone biopsy

6. Complications: metastasis (spread) to other areas in the body

a. local spread to bladder or bowel

b. possibly lymphatic spread

c. metastasis to liver

7. Usual treatments

a. surgical excision

b. radiation therapy—either internal implants or external

c. chemotherapy

B. Planning, Goals, Expected Outcomes

1. Reduce emotional stress associated with diagnosis of cancer

2. Assist client to recover fully from surgical procedure

3. Client complies with prescribed treatment plan

C. Implementation

1. Client receives preoperative and postoperative teaching as covered under "Perioperative Care" (see p. 195)

2. Offer support by allowing client to verbalize fears and worries

3. Explain all procedures and activities to be performed

D. Evaluation

1. Client recovers completely from surgical procedure

2. Client verbalizes feelings and demonstrates an understanding of continued treatments

3. Family members aware of need for their assistance and social service agencies notified if needed

IV. ENDOMETRIOSIS

A. Assessment

1. Definition: endometrial tissue found outside uterus
2. Incidence: common disorder in women of child-bearing age
3. Predisposing factors
   a. unknown
   b. possibly related to family history
4. Signs and symptoms
   a. pain
   b. excessive menstrual flow
   c. bleeding between periods
   d. painful intercourse
5. Complications: infertility
6. Usual treatments
   a. conservative: administration of birth control pills
   b. surgical: excision of abnormal tissue outside uterus, possible hysterectomy

B. Planning, Goals, Expected Outcomes

1. Client experiences a reduction of discomfort
2. Client completely recovers from surgical procedure

C. Implementation

1. Administer medications and explain their schedule properly
2. Encourage client to verbalize feelings concerning diagnosis
3. Provide appropriate preoperative and postoperative care

D. Evaluation

1. Client is pain-free
2. Client takes medications correctly
3. Client recovers completely from surgical procedure

V. MENOPAUSE

A. Assessment

1. Definition: end of woman's reproductive period; total cessation of menstruation
2. Incidence
   a. between age 45 and 50 years; may occur between 35 and 58 years
   b. statistics
      (1) 25% by age 47 years
      (2) 50% by age 50 years
      (3) 75% by age 52 years
      (4) 95% by age 55 years
   c. artificial menopause occurs with surgical removal of ovaries
3. Signs and symptoms
   a. menstrual irregularity
   b. flushing of skin: "hot flashes"
   c. excessive perspiration
   d. fatigue
   e. emotional instability
   f. depression
4. Usual treatment: medical therapy (estrogen replacement via oral medications) is controversial

B. Planning, Goals, Expected Outcomes

1. Client adjusts to menopause
2. Client maintains normal lifestyle and function
3. Client experiences decrease in symptoms of menopause
4. Client verbalizes understanding of possible problems related to menopause

C. Implementation

1. Encourage good nutrition to maintain normal weight
   a. reduce amount of fat in diet
   b. reduce amount of carbohydrates eaten
   c. reduce amount of red meat eaten
   d. encourage consumption of fish and poultry, fresh fruits, and vegetables
   e. encourage client to exercise daily
2. Encourage client to verbalize feelings related to this time in her life
3. Teach client to report any unusual bleeding or spotting to physician
4. Lubricant may be necessary with intercourse because of dry vaginal walls
5. Encourage use of nonhormonal remedies to treat symptoms
6. Encourage woman to discuss use of estrogen with health care provider

D. Evaluation

1. Client adjusts to menopause and maintains normal activities

2. Symptoms of menopause reduced and made more tolerable
3. Client verbalizes understanding of what is happening to her body
4. Client verbalizes understanding of potential problems, such as bleeding after menses has stopped

Reproductive Disorders in Men

I. BENIGN PROSTATIC HYPERPLASIA

A. Assessment

1. Definition/pathophysiology: enlargement of prostate not caused by inflammation or neoplasm; enlarged prostate pushes on urethra, causing difficulties in urination
2. Incidence: common in men over 45 to 50 years of age
3. Predisposing or precipitating factors
   a. aging process
   b. chronic urinary tract infections
4. Signs and symptoms
   a. decreased force of urine flow
   b. hesitancy in starting to void
   c. inability to empty bladder totally
   d. urgency and frequency
   e. nocturia
   f. dysuria
   g. overflow urinary incontinence
   h. hematuria
   i. enlarged prostate palpable on rectal examination
5. Diagnostic tests
   a. history and physical examination with rectal examination
   b. urine for culture and sensitivity, urinalysis
   c. cystoscopy
   d. intravenous pyelogram
   e. complete blood count (CBC)
   f. blood urea nitrogen (BUN), serum acid phosphatase, alkaline phosphatase
6. Complications
   a. total blockage of urine output
   b. hydronephrosis
   c. pyelonephritis
   d. renal failure
7. Usual treatment
   a. urinary catheterization to drain bladder
   b. pharmacology
      (1) antibiotics
      (2) urinary tract antiseptics
      (3) antispasmodics
   c. suprapubic catheter possible for long-term drainage of bladder
   d. surgery
      (1) transurethral prostatectomy
         (a) performed with resectoscope inserted into penis, follows urethra to point of hyperplasia
         (b) electrocautery loop inserted and excess tissue removed
         (c) only enlarged tissue removed, leaving normal tissue and prostatic capsule intact
         (d) may be combined with laser treatment
         (e) treatment of choice for clients with simple hyperplasia, elderly clients, or poor-risk clients
         (f) continuous bladder irrigation set up with three-way Foley catheter afterward
         (g) remaining tissue continues to hyperplasia
      (2) suprapubic prostatectomy
         (a) incision made into bladder through abdominal wall and prostatic tissue removed
         (b) continuous bladder irrigation set up through cystotomy catheter from abdominal puncture site and Foley catheter inserted for drainage
         (c) large, draining abdominal wound; may heal with fistula
         (d) cause of sterility
      (3) retropubic prostatectomy
         (a) performed through low abdominal incision between pubic arch and prostatic capsule
         (b) prostatic capsule incised and prostatic tissue removed
         (c) benefit—bladder not entered
         (d) causes sterility
      (4) perineal prostatectomy
         (a) approach through incision between scrotum and anus
         (b) prostatic capsule opened and prostatic tissue removed
         (c) used only for prostatic cancer
         (d) cause of impotence
         (e) slow healing with risk of infection
   e. bilateral vasectomy sometimes performed at time of prostatectomy to reduce risk of epididymitis

B. Planning, Goals, Expected Outcomes

1. Client understands need for medical and surgical regimen
2. Client is relieved of acute or chronic urinary retention
3. Client is free of pain

4. Client does not have complications of surgical procedure
5. Client has safe hospital stay

C. Implementation

1. Assist client to understand surgical procedure
2. Provide emotional support for client and significant others during diagnostic workup and postoperative period
3. Explain to client and significant others the possibility of continuous bladder irrigation and hematuria; hematuria for 3–5 days
4. Monitor urinary drainage for blockage in drainage tubes, presence of clots, hematuria, oliguria, pyuria; report abnormal findings to team leader
5. Postoperative period
   a. monitor vital functions
      (1) particularly blood pressure if client has had spinal anesthesia: danger of hypotension
      (2) intake and output: record each drainage tube separately
      (3) continuous bladder irrigation at rate as ordered by physician
   b. institute early ambulation as ordered; cough and deep breathe
   c. perform catheter care using sterile technique
   d. observe sterile technique for dressing changes
   e. avoid rectal tubes or suppositories
   f. use stool softeners to avoid straining at bowel movement
6. Administer pain medications per physician's order; watch for adverse effects in elderly population
7. Assist RN in assessment of geriatric client in preoperative and postoperative periods for functions in sight, hearing, musculoskeletal function, steadiness on feet, vital signs, orientation
8. Provide safe environment, such as having bed in lowest position, call light easily available, side rails up at night; assist with activities of daily living and ambulation
9. Notify team leader immediately of any potential or actual problems in safety, such as confusion

D. Evaluation

1. Client's voiding returned to normal
2. Client complied with treatments
3. Client's pain controlled
4. Client recovered from surgery without complications
5. Client resumed normal sexual activity as appropriate

II. CANCER OF THE PROSTATE

A. Assessment

1. Definition/pathophysiology: malignant tumor of prostate gland
2. Incidence: men over 60 years of age
3. Predisposing/precipitating factors
   a. cause unknown
   b. chronic urinary tract irritation
   c. cancer metastasized from other part of genitourinary tract
4. Signs and symptoms
   a. early stage, asymptomatic
   b. later stage, may be similar to prostatic hyperplasia
   c. symptoms of metastasis, such as back pain
5. Diagnostic tests
   a. similar to those for benign prostatic hyperplasia
   b. digital rectal examination, hard nodule felt in posterior lobe
   c. transrectal ultrasound
   d. cystoscopy with biopsy
   e. prostate-specific antigen (PSA), serum acid and alkaline phosphatase; acid phosphatase level rises as cancer spreads outside prostatic capsule
6. Complications
   a. complete obstruction of urinary flow
   b. metastasis to other parts of genitourinary system
   c. metastasis to other parts of body
   d. perforation of bladder after surgery
7. Usual treatment
   a. early stages, probably transurethral approach (see under "Benign Prostatic Hyperplasia")
   b. later stages, radical retropubic or perineal prostatectomy, in which prostate, capsule, seminal glands, and bladder neck removed
   c. radiation therapy
   d. chemotherapy
   e. supportive measures, such as hydration and pain control

B. Planning, Goals, Expected Outcomes

1–5. Similar to planning under "Benign Prostatic Hyperplasia"
6. Client understands need, function, and side effects of radiation therapy
7. Client understands need, function, and side effects of chemotherapy
8. Client feels supported by nursing staff
9. Client's spiritual needs are met

C. Implementation

1–5. Similar to implementation under ''Benign Prostatic Hyperplasia''
6. Assist client to understand need, function, and adverse effects of radiation therapy (see under ''Cancer'')
7. Assist client to understand need, function, and adverse effects of chemotherapy (see under ''Cancer'')
8. Provide environment so client feels comfortable enough to express feelings and fears; use verbal and nonverbal supportive nursing care
9. If appropriate, assist client to contact clergy of choice or meet needs on individual basis

D. Evaluation

1. Client complied with radiation therapy
2. Client complied with chemotherapy
3. Client remained in stable emotional state
4. Client received spiritual support

❓QUESTIONS

1. Margaret Simmons, age 62 years, calls her physician, by whom you are employed, to report that for the past 3 weeks she has been having episodes of vaginal bleeding. Your most appropriate response would be to:

    ① Suggest she wait a few more weeks to see if the bleeding stops
    ② Tell her it probably doesn't mean anything, but you will arrange an appointment with the physician
    ③ Suggest, jokingly, that she may need to resume taking birth control measures
    ④ Arrange an appointment with the physician as soon as possible

2. Mrs. Simmons, a 62-year-old with vaginal bleeding, makes an appointment to see the physician for a pelvic examination and a Pap smear. The nurse explains to Mrs. Simmons that:

    ① A vaginal douche is not to be taken before the examination
    ② A vaginal douche should be taken immediately before the appointment to ensure clear visualization of the area
    ③ It is most important to be on time for the appointment so the physician can spend sufficient time with her
    ④ If the bleeding stops, she is to cancel her appointment

3. Cancer of the cervix is one of the most treatable cancers if it is detected early. Women at the greatest risk for this cancer include women who had:

    ① Early onset of menstruation and malnutrition
    ② Children before the age of 20 or after 35 years
    ③ Frequent early sexual relations and multiple partners
    ④ Abstained from sexual intercourse and are obese

4. Breast self-examination is important for all women but is especially important for those who:

    ① Are over age 50 years and had children before the age of 20
    ② Have very large breasts and breast-fed their children

    ③ Have a history of fibrocystic disease and are under age 40 years
    ④ Never had children and have a grandmother and aunt with breast cancer

5. Which of the following explains the importance of assessing the client's present functioning (growth and development) level?

    ① Assists staff in excusing current behaviors
    ② Assists staff in developing realistic goals for care
    ③ Assists clients in understanding own behavior
    ④ Assists staff in determining admission status

6. Mrs. Simon is admitted for a modified radical mastectomy for a malignant breast tumor. Preoperative teaching for Mrs. Simon should include:

    ① Preparation for a skin graft
    ② Beginning arm exercises
    ③ Use of an arm sling
    ④ Fitting of a prosthesis

7. Mrs. Simon returns from a modified radical mastectomy for breast cancer with a Hemovac in place. Nursing interventions for a client with a Hemovac include:

    ① Irrigating the tube as needed
    ② Not emptying the Hemovac
    ③ Avoiding kinks in the tubing
    ④ Pinning the Hemovac to the back of the client's gown

8. Following a modified radical mastectomy with axillary lymph node dissection, to decrease the postoperative lymphedema of the affected arm, the client should:

    ① Elevate her arm on pillows above the heart
    ② Keep the arm fixed at her side
    ③ Apply a warm pad over the affected arm
    ④ Use only the unaffected arm for all activities

9. On the first postoperative day following a modified radical mastectomy for breast cancer, the nurse recommends that Mrs. Simon begin arm exercises. The best exercise at this time is:

    ① Abducting the arm and flexing the elbow
    ② "Wall walking" every 4 hours
    ③ Using a rope pulley to extend her shoulder
    ④ Combing her hair with her affected arm

10. Mrs. Simon, who had a radical mastectomy for breast cancer yesterday, seems depressed about her loss at times and happy about the positive outcome of her surgery at other times. The nurse realizes that:

① Mrs. Simon is neurotic and should see the social worker

② Clients often have a difficult time adjusting to this type of surgery

③ Mrs. Simon is simply vain and needs time to adjust

④ Clients often need some time alone after a loss like this

11. Mrs. Simon, who had a radical mastectomy for breast cancer, asks if she still has to do a monthly breast self-examination. Your best response would be:

① Yes, the cancer is likely to spread to the other breast

② No, there is no further risk of breast cancer

③ No, the physician will do it every 3 months

④ Yes, there is an increased risk of a new cancer in the other breast

12. Mrs. Sands has been diagnosed with cervical cancer and is to have an internal radium implant for the next 48 hours. In caring for Mrs. Sands, you know that a problem during the time the implant is in place is often:

① Fear and isolation

② Nausea and vomiting

③ Vaginal bleeding

④ Pain from the implant

13. When caring for Mrs. Sands after the insertion of a radium implant for cervical cancer, the nurse must protect herself from undue exposure to the radiation. To do this the nurse should:

① Care for the client no more than 10 minutes per day

② Wear a lead apron and stand anywhere when giving direct care

③ Stand at the head of the bed whenever possible while giving care

④ Ask a family member to be present and to assist with client care

14. Your client has an internal radium implant to treat cervical cancer. To ensure that no more radiation than the prescribed dose is received by the client's internal organs, the nurse should:

① Encourage the client to turn side to side every 2 hours

② Elevate the head of the bed for meals

③ Administer laxatives as ordered to prevent constipation

④ Carefully maintain the patency of the urinary catheter

15. When it is time for an internal radium implant inserted to treat cervical cancer to be removed, the nurse has the responsibility of:

① Calling the radiology department to remind them

② Assisting the surgeon with the removal

③ Removing the implant and placing it in a lead container

④ Waiting until the radiology department has time to remove it

16. After removal of an internal radium implant used to treat cervical cancer, it is important to teach the client to:

① Avoid all pregnant women

② Limit her exposure to children to 30 minutes a day

③ Not sleep in the same bed as her husband for 1 month

④ Avoid sexual intercourse and douches for 6 weeks

17. Which of the following problems would *not* be expected following removal of an internal radium implant for cervical cancer and would require that the client call the physician?

① She experiences moderate constipation

② She notes brown, foul-smelling vaginal drainage

③ She develops urinary incontinence spontaneously

④ Her urine is slightly blood-tinged

18. Mike Dawson, 70 years old, has been experiencing symptoms of frequency, urgency, and nocturia, which have been increasing over the last 2 months. The physician performed a rectal examination on Mr. Dawson. The purpose of this examination is to:

① Diagnose an enlarged prostate

② Check for the presence of blood

③ Definitively diagnose prostatic cancer

④ Diagnose the presence of an infection

19. A client with benign prostatic hyperplasia is scheduled for a suprapubic prostatectomy. In doing preoperative teaching, the nurse should be sure to include:

① Information about his inevitable impotence

② The need for frequent postoperative dressing changes

③ That the client will not have an external incision

④ That there is a chance cancer will be found

20. Following a suprapubic prostatectomy for benign prostatic hyperplasia, your client is complaining of pain in the bladder and bladder spasms. The best medication to administer at this time would be:

① Demerol (meperidine)
② Morphine
③ Pro-Banthīne (propantheline bromide)
④ Aspirin

21. On the first day following a suprapubic prostatectomy for benign prostatic hyperplasia, large amounts of urine are draining through the dressing and little is draining through the catheter. Your appropriate nursing intervention is to:

① Irrigate the catheter as ordered
② Change the dressing and record the approximate output
③ Call the physician
④ Reinforce the dressing and irrigate the catheter

22. When the catheter is removed following a suprapubic prostatectomy for benign prostatic hyperplasia, the client is experiencing some dribbling and urinary incontinence. Which of the following should the nurse include in client teaching?

① Recommending the use of an external catheter
② Advising the client's partner to purchase protective adult underpads
③ Instructing him to limit his intake
④ Instructing him to do perineal exercises to strengthen his urinary muscles

23. It is important for the client who has just had a suprapubic prostatectomy for benign prostatic hyperplasia to avoid straining for a bowel movement because this can increase the risk of bleeding. The medication or treatment most likely to be administered to aid with a bowel movement would be:

① Fleet enema
② Milk of magnesia
③ Colace (docusate sodium)
④ Dulcolax suppository (bisacodyl)

24. Middle-aged persons should:

① Exercise less each decade after age 50 years
② Increase their sleep after age 50 years
③ Decrease their calories by 7.5% for each decade after age 25 years
④ Increase their diversional activities to prepare for retirement

25. The major cause of death in middle-aged men is:

① Heart disease
② Lung cancer
③ Cirrhosis
④ Stroke

26. Major physiologic changes that occur in middle age include:

① Increased peristalsis
② Increased metabolic rate
③ Increased rigidity of lung tissue
④ Increased visual accommodation

27. Martha Hayes is a 44-year-old mother of two who has been experiencing excessive vaginal bleeding for the past 2 months. She is in the gynecologist's office for her yearly Pap smear. Before the pelvic examination, the nurse should:

① Have the client void
② Administer an enema
③ Catheterize the client
④ Scrub the perineal area with antiseptic soap

28. Women should be encouraged to void before a pelvic examination to:

① Prevent incontinence during the pelvic examination
② Obtain a sterile urine specimen
③ Decrease discomfort during the pelvic examination
④ Prevent the bladder from interfering with the Pap smear

29. The physician performed a Pap smear on your client, which returned as a class III smear. This means that the cells are:

① Normal
② Inflammatory
③ Malignant
④ Dysplastic

30. Your client is scheduled for a total abdominal hysterectomy. The night before surgery she receives a povidone-iodine (Betadine) douche. The purpose of this is to:

① Minimize vaginal bleeding
② Cleanse the vaginal canal
③ Sterilize the vaginal canal
④ Decrease the number of malignant cells present

31. Following an abdominal hysterectomy, your client is encouraged to ambulate frequently after surgery. The nurse knows that for this type of surgery, it is important to prevent:

① Abdominal distention
② Wound infection
③ Diarrhea
④ Urinary retention

32. Your client who had a total abdominal hysterectomy asks if she will continue to have periods postoperatively. You would explain that because of the surgery she will:

① Experience surgical menopause
② Not have the uncontrolled bleeding she had preoperatively
③ Experience some changes associated with menses, but not have a period
④ Continue to have normal periods

ANSWERS AND RATIONALES

Guide to item identification (see pp. 4–5 for further details about each category):

I, II, III, or IV for the phase of the nursing process
1, 2, 3, or 4 for the category of client needs
A, B, C, D, E, F, or G for the category of human functioning
Specific content category by name, i.e., cholecystectomy

1. Bleeding at times other than normal menstrual periods may be abnormal. In this case, the bleeding is postmenopausal and has lasted longer than 2 weeks, which makes it a possible warning sign of cancer.
④ III, 4, A, Uterine cancer

2. Douching can wash away material that can assist the physician in diagnosing the cause of any possibly abnormal bleeding or discharge.
① III, 1 & 2, A, Pap smear

3. One risk for cervical cancer is anything that causes chronic cervical irritation.
③ I, 2, A & F, Cervical cancer

4. Family history is one of the greatest risk factors for breast cancer. Never having children is also a risk factor.
④ I & III, 2 & 4, A & F, Breast cancer

5. Understanding the client's developmental level can help the staff anticipate certain needs. This understanding should help in realistic goal setting.
② I & IV, 4, A, Adult growth and development

6. It is important that the client be taught arm exercises preoperatively so that she can begin basic ones immediately after surgery.
② III, 1, A & E, Breast cancer

7. The tubing must remain patent for the Hemovac to function properly.
③ III, 2, D, Breast cancer

8. Elevating the arm will help decrease the possibility of postoperative lymphedema.
① III, 2, B & D, Breast cancer

9. Combing the hair provides some movement without initiating vigorous exercises too early.
④ III, 2, A & D, Breast cancer

10. It is common for the client to experience this ambivalence over the loss of the breast com-
② bined with the positive removal of the cancer.
I, 2 & 4, A, F, & G, Breast cancer

11. There is an increased risk of a second primary cancer in the opposite breast after a woman has cancer in one breast.
④ III, 1, A & D, Breast cancer

12. While the implant is in place, she will be in a private room with staff and visitors allowed in for only limited periods. Also, the presence of an implant is usually frightening for the client.
① I, 2, D, F, & G, Cervical cancer

13. The important factors to remember when caring for a client with an implant are time, distance, and shielding. The nurse is most shielded, by the client's body, when standing at the head of the bed.
③ III, 2, D, Cervical cancer

14. Bladder distention would move the bladder closer to the source of radiation.
④ III & IV, 2, D & F, Cervical cancer

15. It is the nurse's responsibility to note the time for the removal and to notify the radiologist if it is not done on time.
① III, 2, D, Cervical cancer

16. Because of the trauma to the vaginal and cervical mucosa caused by the radiation, all forms of irritation should be avoided for at least 6 weeks.
④ III, 4, A & D, Cervical cancer

17. The sudden development of urinary incontinence could indicate the presence of a vesico-vaginal fistula, which often occurs spontaneously after radiation therapy because of tissue breakdown between the bladder and vagina.
③ IV, 2, A & F, Cervical cancer

18. The prostate is easily palpated rectally, and enlargement is easily detected.
① IV, 2, A & F, Benign prostatic hyperplasia

19. A suprapubic prostatectomy involves an incision into the bladder, which drains large amounts of urine postoperatively.
② III, 2 & 4, A & F, Benign prostatic hyperplasia/prostatectomy

20. Pro-Banthīne is an antispasmodic and best treats the bladder spasms.
③ I & III, 2, B, Benign prostatic hyperplasia/prostatectomy

21. It is normal for the majority of the drainage
② to come out through the dressing in the early
postoperative period until the edema around
the urethra decreases.
III, 2, F, Prostatectomy

22. Perineal exercises help the client regain urinary
④ control gradually.
III, 2, D & F, Prostatectomy

23. Colace is a stool softener that decreases the
③ amount of straining the client will have to do.
Any direct stimulation of the rectum should be
avoided because it could lead to increased bleeding from the prostatic bed.
I & III, 2, F, Prostatectomy

24. The middle-aged adult has a natural decrease
③ in metabolism, requiring a 7.5% decrease in calories to maintain the same body weight.
III, 4, A & F, Adult growth and development

25. Heart disease is the leading cause of death in
③ middle-aged men; therefore, the major health
need in this group is centered on prevention of
cardiovascular disease.
I, 4, A & B, Adult growth and development

26. The flexibility of lung tissue decreases during
③ the middle-aged years.
IV, 4, A & B, Adult growth and development

27. A full bladder can interfere with the pelvic ex-
① amination because the client is experiencing severe discomfort.
III, 1, A & F, Female reproductive disorders

28. A full bladder can cause discomfort during the
③ pelvic examination.
II, 1, A & C, Female reproductive disorders

29. A class III smear means that the cells are
④ dysplastic. It may also indicate carcinoma in
situ.
IV, 2, A & F, Female reproductive disorders

30. Because the cervix will be removed, it is impor-
② tant to cleanse the vaginal canal before surgery.
II, 2, D & F, Cervical cancer

31. Abdominal distention is one of the most com-
① mon problems after a hysterectomy.
II, 2, D & F, Cervical cancer

32. A total abdominal hysterectomy does not in-
③ volve the removal of the ovaries, so the client
will still have some of the symptoms associated
with menses but no actual menstruation.
III, 2, A & D, Cervical cancer

OXYGENATION AND CARDIOPULMONARY DISORDERS

The need of every cell for oxygen requires balance
in supply and demand; oxygenators are heart and
lungs, and disorders associated with these organs are
the greatest threat to life in the United States.

Cardiovascular Disorders

I. ARTERIOSCLEROSIS/ATHEROSCLEROSIS

A. Assessment

1. Definitions/pathophysiology
   a. arteriosclerosis: condition in which arteries
      harden and narrow, causing them to lose
      their elasticity
   b. atherosclerosis: condition in which fatty de-
      posits (plaques) form on inner lining of
      blood vessels
2. Incidence
   a. most common condition in United States
   b. increasing risk with age
   c. more common in men; women's rate rises
      after menopause
3. Predisposing/precipitating factors
   a. high-fat diet
   b. smoking
   c. familial tendency
   d. obesity
   e. sedentary lifestyle
4. Signs and symptoms (*vary depending on degree and
   location of involved blood vessels*)
   a. coronary involvement
      (1) chest pain
      (2) dyspnea
      (3) palpitations
      (4) fainting
      (5) fatigue
   b. cerebral involvement
      (1) transient ischemic attacks
      (2) loss of memory
      (3) headaches
      (4) deterioration of personality
   c. extremities
      (1) leg cramps
      (2) cool skin

TABLE 7-1 Antianginals (Vasodilators)

Class	Example	Action	Use	Common Side Effects	Nursing Implications
Vasodilators	Nitroglycerin, dipyridamole (Persantine), isoxsuprine hydrochloride (Vasodilan), isosorbide dinitrate (Isordil)	Act on blood vessels to increase diameter, effective on coronary arteries	To treat angina, cerebral vasoconstriction, and peripheral vascular disease	Excessive vasodilation, headache, orthostatic hypotension, tachycardia	Monitor blood pressure closely, teach how to take correctly, check for relief
Calcium channel blockers	Verapamil (Calan, Verelan)	Reduce oxygen demand, dilate coronary arteries	To treat vasospastic or stable angina	Hypotension, dizziness, congestive heart failure, peripheral edema, gastrointestinal upset	Monitor for signs of congestive heart failure, may also treat hypertension

    (3) color changes
    (4) numbness and tingling
    (5) reduced or absent peripheral pulses
    (6) skin ulcerations and gangrene
5. Diagnostic tests
    a. history and physical examination
    b. arteriograms
6. Usual treatment
    a. reduce cholesterol in blood with diet and drugs
    b. coronary, cerebral, and peripheral vasodilators (Table 7–1)
    c. reduce risk factors, such as smoking, obesity, lifestyle, stress
    d. surgery to remove plaque or bypass obstructions

B. Planning, Goals, Expected Outcomes

1. Client attains lower cholesterol level
2. Client avoids trauma to extremities
3. Pain of ischemia is relieved
4. Client understands and complies with therapeutic restrictions

C. Implementation

1. Teach low-fat, low-calorie, low-cholesterol diet and counseling (Table 7–2; see also Tables 5–5, 5–6, and 5–8)

TABLE 7-2 Foods Low in Cholesterol

Skim milk	Sherbet	Fish
Buttermilk	Egg whites	Low-fat cottage cheese
Coffee	Vegetable oils	Potatoes
Tea	Low-fat margarine	Rice
Carbonated beverages	Oil and vinegar dressings	Spaghetti (nonegg noodles)
Whole grain breads	Lean meat	Noncream soups
	Chicken with skin removed	Sugar
Most cereals	Turkey with skin removed	All vegetables
Fresh fruits		

2. Teach client to protect extremities from trauma
3. Encourage meticulous skin care
4. Teach client to observe for and report any change in skin color, temperature, pain or numbness, pulse volume, or breaks in skin
5. Teach client to avoid tight clothing
6. Use protective devices such as bed cradles
7. Teach client methods to relieve or reduce pain
8. Teach client need for taking appropriate prescribed vasodilators (see Table 7–1)
    a. teach client to use warmth for vasodilation with care, such as warm baths or hot water bottle to lower abdomen
    b. teach client to use sufficient activity to increase blood flow without causing ischemia
    c. educate client and family regarding diet, medication, activity, and risk factors

D. Evaluation

1. Client's serum cholesterol lowered
2. Client had no trauma to extremities
3. Client's ischemic pain controlled or lessened
4. Client understood and complied with therapeutic restrictions

II. HYPERTENSION

A. Assessment

1. Definition/pathophysiology: persistently high blood pressure greater than 140 systolic or greater than 90 diastolic; must be consistently above this level to be classified as hypertension
    a. primary or essential (idiopathic)
        (1) most common type
        (2) cause unknown
        (3) known risk factors

b. secondary
   (1) follows other conditions such as renal disease, pregnancy, heart defects, or endocrine disorders
   (2) treated by treating primary condition
2. Incidence and predisposing factors
   a. age 30–70 years
   b. African-Americans are affected 2:1
   c. obesity
   d. smoking
   e. stress
   f. birth control pills and estrogen
   g. genetic factors, heredity
   h. males
3. Signs and symptoms (*may be vague and usually late*)
   a. headache
   b. fatigue
   c. irritability
   d. tachycardia
   e. blurred vision
   f. tinnitus
   g. nose bleeds
4. Diagnostic tests
   a. history of high blood pressure, hypertension treatments, family history
   b. postural blood pressure measurement (lying, sitting, standing)
   c. comparison of present with previous blood pressure readings (must be high on at least three separate occasions to be hypertension)
   d. chest radiograph
   e. funduscopic eye examination
   f. laboratory examinations: BUN, hematocrit, urinalysis
5. Complications
   a. cardiac hypertrophy
   b. congestive heart failure
   c. transient ischemic attacks
   d. accelerated atherosclerosis, nephrosclerosis
   e. aneurysms and hemorrhages
   f. papilledema
6. Usual treatment
   a. reduce risk factors, such as smoking, obesity, lifestyle, stress
   b. reduce cholesterol in blood with diet and drugs
   c. antihypertensives (Table 7–3)

B. Planning, Goals, Expected Outcomes

1. Client's blood pressure is lowered through use of antihypertensives
2. Client follows low-sodium, low-cholesterol diet and loses weight (Table 7–4; see also Tables 5–3 and 7–2)
3. Client's blood pressure is maintained through stress management
4. Client understands and complies with therapeutic regimen

C. Implementation

1. Teach client to take prescribed antihypertensives (see Table 7–3)
2. Assess and document symptoms and response to treatment
3. Teach concepts of prescribed diet
4. Teach client to weigh daily
5. Teach client to have blood pressure monitored regularly in both arms
6. Assist in planning of exercise regimen
7. Educate client and family about importance of blood pressure control

D. Evaluation

1. Client's blood pressure returned to and maintained at normal levels
2. Client followed low-sodium and low-cholesterol diet and attained normal weight
3. Client followed stress reduction and exercise regimen
4. Client understood and complied with therapeutic regimen

III. CORONARY ARTERY DISEASE

A. Assessment

1. Definition/pathophysiology: coronary arteries provide the only blood supply to the myocardium, and any significant interference with flow through these vessels impairs the entire function of circulatory system; the heart has the vital function of pumping blood by its rhythmic contractions; dangerous disorder of heart, in which heart muscle can be so damaged by diminished oxygen supply or so weakened it can no longer function effectively as pump
2. Incidence
   a. leading cause of death in United States (myocardial infarction)
   b. mortality rate declining due to improved prevention methods and improved treatments
3. Predisposing/precipitating factors
   a. obesity
   b. hypertension
   c. smoking
   d. sedentary lifestyle

TABLE 7-3 Antihypertensives

Class	Example	Action	Use	Common Side Effects	Nursing Implications
Thiazide diuretics	Hydrochlorothiazide (HydroDiuril)	Diuretic, K⁺ wasting	To treat hypertension	Hypokalemia, hyponatremia, orthostatic hypotension, hyperglycemia	Teach high-K⁺, low-Na⁺ diet, check I & O, BP
Potassium-sparing diuretics	Spironolactone (Aldactone)	Diuretic, increase Na⁺ and water excretion	To treat hypertension	Hyponatremia, hyperkalemia, gastrointestinal upset, allergies	Monitor Na⁺ and K⁺, I & O, BP
Loop diuretics	Furosemide (Lasix)	Inhibit reabsorption of Na⁺ and water	To treat hypertension	Orthostatic hypotension, hypovolemia, hyponatremia, hypokalemia	Watch for dehydration, monitor electrolytes, check BP, give high-K⁺ diet, store in light-resistant bottle
Sympathetic inhibitors	Methyldopa (Aldomet)	Lower BP by blocking of sympathetic impulses	To treat hypertension	Orthostatic hypotension, depression, impotence, bradycardia, Na⁺ and water retention	Have client change position slowly, use low-Na⁺ diet, avoid alcohol
Vasodilators	Hydralazine (Apresoline)	Lower BP by causing vasodilation	To treat hypertension	Excessive vasodilation, headache, tachycardia, Na⁺ and water retention	Monitor I & O, BP, maintain low-Na⁺ diet
Angiotensin-converting enzyme inhibitors	Enalapril maleate (Vasotec)	Suppresses renin-angiotensin-aldosterone system, preventing conversion of angiotensin I to angiotensin II, a potent vasoconstrictor	To treat hypertension	Headache, dizziness, fatigue, rash, diarrhea, nausea, loss of taste perception	Obtain baseline BP, then monitor regularly watching for fluctuations and effectiveness of medications, monitor K⁺, warn client about possible orthostatic changes, teach client to change position slowly

BP, blood pressure; I & O, intake and output; K, potassium.

TABLE 7-4 High- and Low-Sodium Foods

Low-Sodium Foods	High-Sodium Foods
Chicken	Milk
Fish	Cheese
Lean meat	Tomato juice
Most fresh vegetables	Canned vegetables, soups
Most fresh fruits	Lunch meats
Bread	Salted foods, such as chips or nuts
No salt-added foods	Condiments
Salt substitutes	Relish, pickles
Cereal	Peanut butter
Cooked rice	Processed foods
Fresh cooked beans	Butter
	Soft drinks
	Celery

    e. age

    f. stress

    g. hereditary

    h. elevated lipids and blood pressure

4. Signs and symptoms

    a. chest pain

    b. fatigue

    c. palpitations

    d. dyspnea on exertion

    e. syncope

    f. edema

5. Diagnostic tests

    a. Electrocardiogram (ECG): graph of electrical activity of heart

TABLE 7-5 Cardiac Glycosides

Example	Action	Use	Common Side Effects	Nursing Implications
Digoxin (Lanoxin)	Acts on myocardium to increase force of contraction and cardiac output while slowing rate	To treat congestive heart failure, tachycardia	Arrhythmias, heart block, bradycardia, gastrointestinal upset, muscle weakness, diplopia	Take apical pulse before giving, hold if >120 or <60, check K^+ if on diuretics, watch for toxicity

b. exercise stress test: shows ECG during physical exercise, usually treadmill or stationary bike

c. echocardiogram: uses ultrasonic beams to demonstrate shape, location, and size of heart

d. angiography: uses contrast media to demonstrate blood flow through coronary arteries and aorta

e. chest radiograph: to demonstrate size, shape, and location of heart

f. continuous cardiac monitoring

g. Holter monitor: portable monitor that records heart activity during 24-hour period—client keeps log of activity during this time; gives picture of ECG changes as client goes through usual activities

h. laboratory studies

  (1) CBC: to determine whether anemia or infection is present

  (2) erythrocyte sedimentation rate: to check for inflammation

  (3) serum enzymes and isoenzymes: serum glutamic-oxaloacetic transaminase (SGOT), lactate dehydrogenase (LDH), creatine phosphokinase (CPK) taken soon after admission

  (4) lipids: elevation indicates risk of heart disease

  (5) BUN and creatinine: elevated with renal or liver damage

6. Usual treatment

a. medications

  (1) cardiac glycosides slow and strengthen heart (Table 7–5)

  (2) antiarrhythmics restore and maintain rhythm of heart (Table 7–6)

  (3) vasodilators improve blood supply to myocardium (see Table 7–1)

  (4) antianginals decrease pain in myocardium (see Table 7–1)

  (5) anticoagulants treat abnormal clotting patterns or decrease risk of clot formation (Table 7–7)

  (6) diuretics reduce blood volume to correct hypertension and edema (see Table 7–3)

  (7) analgesics control pain and relieve anxiety (Table 7–8)

  (8) calcium channel blockers relax muscles in coronary arteries (see Table 7–1)

b. diet (see Chapter 5)

  (1) low sodium (see Tables 5–3 and 7–4)

  (2) low fat and cholesterol (see Table 7–7)

  (3) often high potassium if client is taking thiazide diuretic (Table 7–9; see also Table 5–4)

  (4) low calorie if weight reduction needed

c. exercise

  (1) rest required in acute phase

  (2) exercise regimen to improve oxygenation, ordered by physician

  (3) oxygen therapy, as needed, based on blood gas values

d. surgery: coronary artery bypass, valve replacements

TABLE 7-6 Antiarrhythmics

Example	Action	Use	Common Side Effects	Nursing Implications
Procainamide hydrochloride (Procan)	Decreases cardiac irritability	To treat PVCs, tachycardia	Severe hypotension, bradycardia, GI upset, rash	Monitor BP, watch for side effects, use carefully in clients with CHF
Quinidine gluconate (Quinaglute)	Slows conduction through AV node	To treat atrial flutter or fibrillation	Vertigo, headache, PVCs, hypotension, tinnitus, CHF, GI upset	May increase digoxin toxicity, check apical rate, give with meals
Propranolol hydrochloride (Inderal)	Decreases impulses through AV node and increases refractory period	To treat supraventricular, ventricular, and atrial arrhythmias	Fatigue, hypotension, CHF, bradycardia, GI upset, depression, bronchial constriction	Do not use with asthmatics, withdraw drug slowly, check pulse, monitor BP, watch for peripheral edema

AV, atrioventricular; BP, blood pressure; CHF, congestive heart failure; GI, gastrointestinal; PVCs, premature ventricular contractions.

TABLE 7-7 Anticoagulants

Example	Action	Use	Common Side Effects	Nursing Implications
Heparin sodium	Acts to inhibit formation of prothrombin activator	To treat and prevent blood clots	Hemorrhage	Avoid use of other anticoagulants at same time, teach client to avoid bleeding, monitor partial thromboplastin time, protamine sulfate antidote
Warfarin (Coumadin)	Acts to inhibit formation of prothrombin in liver	To treat and prevent blood clots	Hemorrhage	Avoid use of other anticoagulants at same time; vitamin K antidote

7. Complications
   a. angina pectoris
   b. myocardial infarction

B. Planning, Goals, Expected Outcomes

1. Client has coronary artery disease controlled without surgery
2. Client complies with medical therapy
3. Client is prepared for surgery as needed

C. Implementation

1. Teach client to take medications as ordered
2. Teach client diet modifications
3. Teach client to monitor for any increase or change in pain
4. Provide preoperative teaching as needed with RN
5. Monitor postoperatively as directed
6. Teach lifestyles for a healthy heart

D. Evaluation

1. Client complied with prescribed therapy
2. Client had disease controlled without surgery

3. Client recovered from surgery without complications

IV. ANGINA PECTORIS

A. Assessment

1. Definition/pathophysiology: chest pain caused by reduced blood flow from coronary arteries to myocardium
2. Predisposing/precipitating factors
   a. long-term result of atherosclerosis, hypertension, or diabetes mellitus
   b. immediate precipitating factors
      (1) emotional upset
      (2) exposure to cold
      (3) exertion
      (4) overeating
3. Signs and symptoms
   a. sudden severe chest pain, substernal, radiating to left arm, shoulder, and neck
   b. pallor
   c. cold clammy skin
   d. dyspnea
   e. anxiety

TABLE 7-8 Analgesics

Class	Example	Action	Use	Common Side Effects	Nursing Implications
Non-narcotics	Acetylsalicylic acid (aspirin), acetaminophen (Tylenol), ibuprofen	Act to decrease pain as anti-inflammatory	To treat less severe pain	Salicylism, allergic reactions, gastrointestinal distress, ulcerogenic, anticoagulant, liver damage	Avoid use in clients with ulcers, on anticoagulants, do not overuse, keep away from children, monitor liver function
Narcotics	Morphine, meperidine (Demerol), codeine (Tylenol #3)	Act by inhibiting transmission of pain impulses, reduce cortical response, alter pain perception areas of brain	To treat and prevent pain	Drowsiness, dizziness, euphoria, respiratory depression, constipation, urinary retention, allergy, hypotension	Monitor effectiveness, watch for hypotension and respiratory depression, monitor I & O, bowel movements, tolerance

I & O, intake and output.

TABLE 7–9 Foods High in Potassium

Whole milk	Cantaloupes	Mustard greens
Coffee in quantity	Oranges	Baked potatoes
Bread	Peas	Salt substitutes
Bran cereals	Spinach	Peanuts
Dried apricots	Lima beans	Molasses
Dried prunes	Soybeans	Broiled beef
Bananas	White beans	
Watermelons	Squash	

4. Diagnostic tests
   a. history and physical examination
   b. ECG and Holter monitoring
   c. exercise stress test
5. Usual treatment
   a. nitroglycerin, sublingually, to relieve acute pain (see Table 7–1)
   b. vasodilators, such as nitroglycerin and isosorbide, may prevent anginal attacks (see Table 7–1)
   c. diet to reduce fat and cholesterol and maintain normal weight
   d. coronary bypass surgery

B. Planning, Goals, Expected Outcomes

1. Client's pain is relieved without progressing to myocardial infarction
2. Client learns to reduce or cope with physical and emotional stress
3. Client learns to avoid risk factors
4. Client reduces fat in diet and alters calories as needed to manage weight

C. Implementation

1. Assess and document symptoms of stress and pain
2. Ask client to report chest pain promptly
3. Administer vasodilators and teach client their actions
   a. can be used as a preventive measure, taken before pain occurs if activity usually causes pain, such as climbing stairs
   b. teach proper administration
      (1) sublingual forms, rapid onset
      (2) transdermal application every 24 hours
      (3) some chewable and others slow release
4. Teach client to stop activity when pain appears
5. Provide emotional support and assurance
6. Reinforce dietary instructions
7. Teach client and family importance of drug therapy, dietary restrictions, management of stress, and exercise

D. Evaluation

1. Client's pain kept to minimum
2. Client exercised according to ability and physician's order
3. Client avoided exposure to cold, emotional stress, heavy meals, and overexertion
4. Client maintained normal weight and followed ordered dietary modifications

V. MYOCARDIAL INFARCTION

A. Assessment

1. Definition/pathophysiology: obstruction of branch of coronary artery leading to areas of necrosis resulting from ischemia; heart's ability to recover depends on size and location of infarction
2. Incidence: same as for coronary artery disease
3. Predisposing/precipitating factors
   a. emotional stress
   b. obesity
   c. smoking
   d. high-fat diet
   e. familial tendency
   f. diabetes mellitus
   g. history of angina
   h. atherosclerosis
4. Signs and symptoms
   a. sudden, severe crushing chest pain, radiating down left arm or to jaw; may be mistaken for indigestion
   b. dyspnea
   c. symptoms of shock (anxiety, pallor, diaphoresis)
   d. leukocytosis
   e. elevated cardiac enzymes (CPK, LDH, SGOT)
   f. arrhythmias
5. Diagnostic tests
   a. history and physical examination
   b. ECG
   c. laboratory tests, serum cardiac enzymes, white blood count
6. Complications
   a. cardiogenic shock
   b. congestive heart failure
   c. pulmonary edema
   d. dysrhythmias
   e. death
7. Usual treatment
   a. intravenous morphine for chest pain (see Table 7–8)
   b. thrombolytic therapy to dissolve clots
   c. oxygen for respiratory distress
   d. cardiac monitoring

e. drugs as required for arrhythmias (see Table 7–6)
f. bed rest
g. cardiopulmonary resuscitation as needed

B. Planning, Goals, Expected Outcomes

1. Client does not experience life-threatening arrhythmias
2. Client's pain is relieved promptly
3. Client does not experience oxygen deprivation
4. Client understands importance of and complies with exercise and dietary restrictions
5. Client's anxiety is reduced

C. Implementation: assist RN to

1. Record vital signs every hour during acute phase
2. Monitor pulse during activity
3. Provide prompt pain relief
4. Monitor oxygenation
5. Provide activity as permitted
6. Provide prescribed diet, sodium and caffeine restricted, and teach client restrictions
7. Provide counseling as needed to reduce anxiety
8. Educate client on need to stop smoking

D. Evaluation

1. Client had no arrhythmias
2. Client's pain relieved
3. Client's oxygen levels maintained within normal range
4. Client understood and followed exercise and dietary restrictions
5. Client's anxiety reduced

VI. CONGESTIVE HEART FAILURE

A. Assessment

1. Definition/pathophysiology: congestive heart failure occurs when heart fails to pump as it should, causing congestion when blood is not adequately circulated
    a. right-sided heart failure: symptoms of congestion in periphery with edema
    b. left-sided heart failure: symptoms of congestion in lungs, pulmonary edema
    c. cor pulmonale or complete failure: symptoms of both right-sided and left-sided heart failure
2. Incidence
    a. may follow myocardial infarction
    b. increases with age

3. Predisposing/precipitating factors
    a. complication of other cardiovascular disorders
        (1) myocardial infarction
        (2) hypertension
        (3) arteriosclerosis
        (4) congenital and acquired heart defects
    b. hypervolemia
4. Signs and symptoms: vary according to degree of failure
    a. heart failure may be either right-sided or left-sided; however, either leads to complete heart failure
    b. left-sided heart failure
        (1) dyspnea
        (2) orthopnea
        (3) productive cough with frothy, blood-tinged sputum
        (4) rales
        (5) fatigue
        (6) anxiety
    c. right-sided heart failure
        (1) dependent edema
        (2) distended neck veins
        (3) abdominal distention
        (4) liver enlargement
        (5) nausea and vomiting
        (6) anorexia
        (7) oliguria
        (8) weight gain
        (9) increased venous pressure
5. Diagnostic tests
    a. history and physical examination
    b. ECG
    c. arterial blood gases
    d. chest radiograph
6. Usual treatment
    a. limited activity or bed rest
    b. drug therapy
        (1) digitalis (see Table 7–5)
        (2) diuretics (see Table 7–3)
    c. oxygen therapy
    d. restricted sodium intake

B. Planning, Goals, Expected Outcomes

1. Client's cardiac workload is reduced
2. Prescribed medications to reduce pulse rates, to reduce fluid volume, and to strengthen heart muscle are taken
3. Oxygenation of tissues is maintained
4. Client and family understand and comply with diet therapy, medication therapy, and activity

C. Implementation (Varies According to Severity of Failure)

1. Monitor vital signs including apical pulse for 1 full minute before giving digitalizing drugs; teach client and family to do so
2. Record intake and output
3. Restrict fluids as ordered
4. Weigh daily
5. Monitor peripheral edema; elevate feet when sitting
6. Assess exercise tolerance
7. Provide and teach client low-sodium diet (see Table 7–4)
8. Explain expected outcomes of therapy
9. Listen to client concerns
10. Teach client and family importance of diet and exercise regimen

D. Evaluation

1. Client's cardiac workload reduced
2. Prescribed medications taken as ordered
3. Oxygen concentration level maintained to all tissues
4. Client understood and complied with diet therapy, medication therapy, and activity

VII. PERIPHERAL VASCULAR DISORDERS

Peripheral vascular disorders are chronic problems in blood vessels outside the heart that cause cellular changes in these peripheral tissues, especially lower extremities.

A. Arterial Vascular Disease (Atherosclerosis Obliterans)

1. Assessment
   a. definition and pathophysiology: arterial insufficiency of lower extremities caused by atherosclerosis and usually affecting one extremity more than the other, although both are impaired
   b. incidence: same as for arteriosclerosis
   c. predisposing or precipitating factors
      (1) atherosclerosis and all its risk factors
      (2) smoking
      (3) cold
      (4) anything causing arterial constriction
   d. signs and symptoms: all apparent below level of obstruction and dependent on extent, location, degree of occlusion, and amount of collateral circulation
      (1) pain
         (a) intermittent claudication: cramping pain brought on by exercise and relieved by rest
         (b) rest pain: burning, tingling, and numbness, noticeable at night and not associated with activity
      (2) cyanosis or pale color
      (3) skin temperature cool to cold below level of obstruction, with potential areas of blue-black necrosis
      (4) trophic changes, such as smooth, shiny, thin skin; little or no hair; and thick nails
      (5) impaired or absent peripheral pulses
   e. diagnostic tests
      (1) history and physical examination
      (2) arteriogram
      (3) Doppler studies
      (4) digital subtraction angiography
      (5) exercise tests
   f. usual treatment
      (1) disease not curable; treatment done only to relieve ischemic pain and improve blood flow
      (2) peripheral vasodilators, such as isoxsuprine (Vasodilan) (see Table 7–1)
      (3) progressive structured exercise to increase collateral circulation
      (4) surgery
         (a) endarterectomy
         (b) femoral-popliteal bypass graft
         (c) sympathectomy
      (5) clot-dissolving medication
   g. complications
      (1) infection
      (2) amputation of affected part
2. Planning, goals, expected outcomes
   a. client has arterial blood flow maintained to lower extremities
   b. client does not develop further injury to extremities
   c. client understands and complies with exercises to improve collateral circulation
3. Implementation
   a. teach client proper vascular care (Chart 7–1)
   b. teach client to avoid vasoconstrictors
      (1) avoid caffeine
      (2) stop smoking
      (3) avoid cold
      (4) avoid constricting clothing
   c. teach client Buerger-Allen exercises
      (1) client lies with legs elevated to 45- to 90-degree angle until skin turns dead white
      (2) client lowers legs below level of rest of body without pressure behind knees
      (3) when legs become red, client lies flat for 3 to 5 minutes

Chart 7–1
Information for Patients with Peripheral Vascular Disease

ARTERIAL

1. Keep warm without overheating.

2. Do not use tobacco in any form.

3. Take great care to be sure that foot is not injured. Do not go barefoot.

4. Wear wide-toed shoes that cause no pressure and have adequate support for the arches. Wear cotton socks.

5. Do not wear circular garters. Support hose may be contraindicated.

6. Do not sit with the knees crossed.

7. If the weight of the bedclothes is uncomfortable, use a pillow or bed cradle to hold the bedclothes off the feet.

8. Soak the feet in a basin of warm water for 5 minutes every day. Dry thoroughly, especially between the toes, by dabbing not rubbing.

9. Do not apply any medications to the feet without physician's directions.

10. If the feet are dry and scaly, apply lanolin and blot off excess.

11. If feet are moist, use talcum powder.

12. Before filing nails, soak feet in warm (not hot) water for 5 minutes to soften nails. File straight across. Do not use a razor blade, knife, or scissors. If arterial disease is severe, see a podiatrist.

13. Proper first aid treatment is important. Consult your physician immediately for any redness, blistering, pain, or swelling.

14. Do not attempt to treat corns or calluses. Ask your physician what should be done.

VENOUS

1. Do not sit for long periods without exercising legs.

2. Do not cross legs when sitting.

3. Wear good-fitting support stockings or hose.

4. Elevate legs at intervals throughout the day and in the evening.

5. Avoid hot baths or other vasodilators.

d. teach client to take vasodilators and analgesics as ordered

e. teach client to promote vasodilation safely

4. Evaluation

a. client's arterial blood flow to lower extremities maintained

b. no further tissue damage occurred

c. client understood and followed instructions to improve and maintain collateral circulation

B. Venous Disorders

1. Thrombophlebitis and embolism

a. assessment

(1) definition/pathophysiology:

(a) thrombus: clump of platelet and fibrin, which form clot; usually occurs as result of injury or sluggish venous blood flow or an increase in number of platelets or red blood cells

(b) embolus: clot that becomes dislodged and travels through circulation until it obstructs an artery

(2) predisposing/precipitating factors

(a) venous stasis

(b) irritation or inflammation of vein wall

(c) long periods of standing or sitting

(d) increased platelets or red blood cells

(e) general surgery

(f) obesity

(g) bed rest

(h) oral contraceptives

(3) signs and symptoms of thrombophlebitis (*embolus signs and symptoms depend on location*)

(a) positive Homans' sign if clot in calf

(b) redness and heat over area

(c) swelling and hardness over area

(d) distention of surrounding veins

(e) possible cyanosis

(4) diagnostic tests

(a) history and physical examination

(b) arteriogram or venogram

(c) nuclear scans

(d) Doppler studies

(5) usual treatment

(a) complete bed rest

(b) warm, moist packs to affected area

(c) anticoagulants

(i) intravenous heparin immediately for prevention of clot extension or further clot formation

(ii) oral coumarin for long-term anticoagulant therapy to prevent recurrence (see Table 7–7)

(iii) antiplatelet aggregants

(d) surgery

(i) vein ligation to trap thrombus and prevent embolus

(ii) plication of vena cava to filter out clots

(iii) embolectomy to remove clot

(6) complications

(a) pulmonary embolus

(b) stroke

(c) death

b. planning, goals, expected outcomes

(1) client does not develop thrombophlebitis or embolus

(2) client who develops thrombophlebitis does not develop an embolus

(3) client understands and complies with therapeutic regimen

c. implementation

(1) preventive measures

(a) avoid activities that promote venous stasis

(b) use support stockings or antiembolic hose

(c) exercise legs frequently during standing or sitting for long periods; do not cross legs

(d) avoid constricting clothing

(e) elevate legs when sitting

(f) teach and promote all preventive measures

(2) treatment

(a) administer anticoagulants as ordered

(i) monitor anticoagulant laboratory values

(ii) know drugs to reverse effects of heparin or coumarin

(b) apply warm, moist packs to affected area

(c) maintain bed rest

(d) apply antiembolus stocking to unaffected leg

(3) educate client about anticoagulant therapy and prevention of recurrence

d. evaluation

(1) client did not develop thrombophlebitis or embolus as a result of preventive measures

(2) client with thrombophlebitis did not develop embolus

(3) client followed therapeutic regimen to treat and prevent thrombophlebitis and emboli

2. Varicose veins
    a. assessment
        (1) definition/pathophysiology: enlarged, tortuous veins distended with pooled blood caused by stasis and incompetent valves
        (2) incidence: people with jobs requiring prolonged sitting or standing; more common in women
        (3) predisposing/precipitating factors
            (a) obesity
            (b) prolonged sitting or standing
            (c) incompetent venous valves
            (d) multiple pregnancies
        (4) signs and symptoms
            (a) enlarged tortuous veins
            (b) fatigue and heaviness in legs after prolonged sitting or standing
            (c) dull or sharp leg pains
            (d) itching along course of vein
        (5) diagnostic tests
            (a) history and physical examination
            (b) plethysmography
            (c) phlebography
            (d) Doppler flowmeter
            (e) Brodie-Trendelenburg test
        (6) usual treatment
            (a) external support with elastic bandages or support stockings
            (b) weight reduction
            (c) surgical therapy: vein ligation and stripping, sclerotherapy
    b. planning, goals, expected outcomes
        (1) client does not develop varicose veins
        (2) client recovers from surgery without complications
    c. implementation
        (1) teach client to avoid standing and sitting for prolonged periods of time
        (2) avoid garters, girdles, and crossing legs at knee
        (3) provide diet counseling for weight reduction
        (4) encourage use of support hose
        (5) encourage activities such as walking, stair climbing, and swimming
        (6) postoperative care
            (a) monitor Ace wraps, thigh high
            (b) encourage walking without standing or sitting for long periods
            (c) monitor peripheral pulses in affected extremity

    d. evaluation
        (1) client did not develop varicose veins
        (2) client recovered from surgery without complications

3. Venous stasis ulcers
    a. assessment
        (1) definition/pathophysiology: ulcers, usually around ankles; result from venous stasis; heal slowly and often become chronic
        (2) incidence: result of chronic venous stasis
        (3) predisposing/precipitating factors
            (a) chronic venous stasis
            (b) prolonged sitting or standing
            (c) injury or trauma
        (4) signs and symptoms
            (a) ruddy red-brown coloration around ankles
            (b) edema
            (c) pink to reddish ulcer
        (5) usual treatment
            (a) warm, moist dressings
            (b) debridement
            (c) skin grafts to cover ulcer
    b. planning, goals, expected outcomes
        (1) client's ulcer heals without problems
        (2) client does not develop further ulceration
    c. implementation
        (1) teach client to prevent leg ulcer by wearing support hose, avoiding prolonged sitting or standing, and avoiding trauma
        (2) apply dressings and teach client correct application technique
        (3) prevent infection
        (4) encourage regular exercises, calf pumping exercises
    d. evaluation
        (1) client's ulcer healed without complications
        (2) client's ulcer did not recur

C. Amputations

1. Assessment
    a. definitions/pathophysiology: traumatic or planned removal of upper or lower extremity
    b. predisposing/precipitating factors
        (1) peripheral vascular disease
        (2) crush injuries
        (3) malignancy
        (4) severe lacerations that disrupt circulation
        (5) any severe circulatory impairment

c. signs and symptoms—if caused by peripheral vascular disease
   (1) cold, cyanotic limb
   (2) gangrene present or absent
   (3) pulses decreased or absent
   (4) ischemic pain
d. diagnostic tests
   (1) arteriogram
   (2) radiographs

2. Planning, goals, expected outcomes
   a. client is psychologically prepared for amputation
   b. client recovers from surgery without complications
   c. client copes with amputation and participates in rehabilitation
   d. client can care for own stump and prosthesis

3. Implementation
   a. help client prepare psychologically for amputation
   b. elevate stump for 24 hours postoperatively to decrease bleeding and swelling; do not flex hip if possible (raise foot of bed)
   c. position stump to prevent flexion contractures after 24 hours
      (1) do not continue to elevate leg to prevent flexion contracture of hip and knee
      (2) position client prone 1 hour out of 4
   d. monitor for hemorrhage
      (1) check dressing for bleeding
      (2) do not suction drainage
      (3) check vital signs
   e. begin rewrapping stump daily to prevent edema and to shrink, shape, and prepare it for prosthetic fitting
   f. explain phantom limb pain to client
   g. offer client emotional support
   h. begin range-of-motion exercises
   i. exercise upper extremities to increase strength
   j. support physical therapy exercises
   k. encourage client to participate actively in rehabilitation

4. Evaluation
   a. client adequately prepared for amputation
   b. client recovered from surgery without complications
   c. client coped with amputation and begins rehabilitation
   d. client safely cares for stump and prosthesis

Diseases of the Blood

I. LEUKEMIA

A. Assessment

1. Definition/pathophysiology: malignant disorders of the blood affecting white blood cells; abnormal reproduction usually leading to immature stem cells; classified by maturity of cells and origin of normal cells
   a. acute
      (1) preponderance of primitive cells called blasts
      (2) sudden onset with rapid progression
      (3) if remission is not achieved rapidly, death occurs
   b. chronic
      (1) predominant cells more mature
      (2) gradual onset and slow progression
      (3) more common in adults
      (4) longer survival time
   c. myeloid leukemias: arise from bone marrow
   d. lymphoid leukemias: arise from lymphatic system

2. Incidence
   a. acute lymphocytic leukemia more common in children
   b. acute lymphocytic leukemia most common cancer in children
   c. acute nonlymphocytic leukemia most common in adults
   d. chronic myelogenous leukemia and chronic lymphocytic leukemia more common in older adults

3. Predisposing/precipitating factors
   a. exposure to radiation in large doses
   b. exposure to certain chemicals, such as benzene
   c. possibly viruses

4. Signs and symptoms
   a. anemia
   b. white blood count may be above 50,000 with abnormal cells with certain types of leukemia
   c. severe neutropenia
   d. severe infections
   e. enlarged lymphatic tissue: liver, spleen, lymph nodes
   f. weakness and weight loss
   g. headache, confusion, central nervous system (CNS) symptoms as cells invade CNS
   h. bruising and bleeding due to low platelet counts

5. diagnostic tests
   a. CBC with differential
   b. bone marrow aspiration and biopsy
      (1) keep client calm
      (2) apply pressure dressing to site
      (3) watch for excessive bruising or bleeding
   c. history and physical examination
   d. lymph node biopsy

6. Usual treatment
   a. chemotherapy to slow growth and produce remission of symptoms (see Table 7–22)

b. blood and platelet transfusions to maintain blood levels
c. antibiotics to combat potential infections (Table 7–10)
d. bone marrow transplant
7. Complications
a. infection
b. hemorrhage
c. death

B. Planning, Goals, Expected Outcomes

1. Client does not suffer from life-threatening infections
2. Client does not hemorrhage
3. Client has side effects of chemotherapy controlled
4. Client maintains ideal body weight
5. Client and family cope with diagnosis and possible terminal prognosis

C. Implementation

1. Protect from infection
a. reverse isolation if necessary
b. avoid crowds
c. avoid people with infections
2. Bleeding precautions; prevent trauma
a. use soft toothbrush
b. do not use aspirin or nonsteroidal drugs
c. do not use safety razor
d. avoid injections
3. Encourage well-balanced diet and teach client about nutritious foods (see Chapter 5)
4. Monitor urinary function and maintain adequate hydration
a. force fluids
b. administer allopurinol (Zyloprim) to prevent increased uric acid and possible urinary stones
5. Provide emotional support
6. Prepare client for self-care in home setting
7. Teach client about long-term medication regimen to treat chronic leukemia

D. Evaluation

1. Client did not develop infection
2. Client did not hemorrhage
3. Side effects of chemotherapy controlled
4. Client's ideal body weight maintained
5. Client and family coped with diagnosis

II. LYMPHOMA

A. Assessment

1. Definition/pathophysiology: cancers of cells of lymphoid system, lymphocytes, and histiocytes; referred to as Hodgkin's disease or non-Hodgkin's lymphoma; tumors usually start in lymph nodes
2. Incidence
a. more common in males
b. peaks in early 20s and after age 50 years
3. Predisposing or precipitating factors
a. unknown cause
b. may be associated with virus
c. alkylating chemical agents
4. Signs and symptoms
a. painless enlargement of lymph nodes, either in neck or groin, usually beginning unilaterally and progressing bilaterally
b. generalized pruritus
c. symptoms of pressure on organs as internal lymph nodes enlarge
d. enlarged spleen and liver
e. low-grade fever
f. night sweats
g. anemia
h. increased white blood cells
i. weight loss
5. Diagnostic tests
a. CBC
b. lymph node biopsy
c. bone marrow biopsy
d. liver/spleen scan
e. computed tomography (CT) of thorax or abdomen
f. magnetic resonance imaging (MRI)
g. lymphangiogram
(1) invasive test done by injection of radiopaque dye into lymph channels in feet and using x-rays to visualize lymph nodes throughout abdomen
(2) takes 3 or more hours to complete
(3) top of feet remain blue from dye for up to 1 year
(4) encourage coughing and deep breathing because dye is excreted from body through lungs
h. staging laparotomy to determine extent of disease
6. Usual treatment
a. exploratory laparotomy with splenectomy and lymph node biopsy
b. radiation therapy
c. chemotherapy (see Table 7–22)

B. Planning, Goals, Expected Outcomes

1. Client has lymphoma diagnosed and treated early
2. Client understands diagnostic tests
3. Client recovers from surgery without complications
4. Client has side effects of chemotherapy controlled
5. Client has side effects of radiation therapy controlled
6. Client maintains ideal body weight
7. Client and family cope with diagnosis

TABLE 7-10 Antibiotics

Class	Example	Action	Use	Common Side Effects	Nursing Implications
Penicillin	Ampicillin (Polycillin), amoxicillin	Bactericidal against sensitive organisms	To treat penicillin-sensitive organisms	Allergic reactions, gastrointestinal upset, development of resistant organisms, anaphylaxis	Monitor for rash, check for allergy before administration, obtain C & S before starting
Aminoglycosides	Gentamicin (Garamycin), kanamycin (Kantrex)	Bactericidal	To treat gram-negative infections	Ototoxicity, nephrotoxicity, superinfections, small allergic potential	Monitor for hearing or renal changes, watch for superinfections
Cephalosporins	Cephalothin (Keflin), cephalexin (Keflex)	Bactericidal	To treat septicemia, penicillin-resistant organisms	Allergic reactions in many penicillin-sensitive clients, superinfections, nephrotoxicity, phlebitis (IV), diarrhea	Monitor for allergies, do not give with food, watch for superinfections
Tetracycline	Tetracycline (Achromycin)	Bactericidal	To treat pneumonia and bacterial diarrhea	Diarrhea, nausea, permanent discoloration of teeth and bones in children, superinfections, impaired bone growth	Monitor for allergies, do not give to children under 12 years of age or pregnant women, do not give with milk or antacids, give with enough water
Monobactams	Aztreonam (Azactam)	Bactericidal	To treat aerobic gram-negative rod infections	Anaphylaxis, diarrhea, nausea and vomiting, rash, neutropenia	Make sure client knows to take full course of medication; IM injections painful; watch for phlebitis at IV site; monitor for reduction of symptoms; report abnormalities in white blood cells to physician
Carbapenems	Imipenem/cilastatin (Primax)	Bactericidal	To treat aerobic and anaerobic gram-positive and gram-negative infections	Nausea and vomiting, diarrhea, rash, fever, hypotension, cross allergy for penicillin-sensitive clients	Monitor for the development of pain and phlebitis at IV site; watch blood pressure; not given IM; use cautiously with elderly or clients with history of renal disease
Macrolides	Erythromycin ethylsuccinate (EES)	Bactericidal	Treatment of gram-positive infections in penicillin-sensitive clients, used for legionnaires' disease and *Mycoplasma* pneumonia	Nausea and vomiting, hearing loss, dyspepsia, abdominal pain, hepatitis	Avoid IM injections if possible because they are painful; do not take medication with food; report adverse reactions to physician; monitor for history of allergies; use cautiously in clients with liver disease; safety in pregnancy not established
Antiretrovirals	Zidovudine (Retrovir)	Inhibits DNA replication	Treatment of HIV-seroconverted clients with a CD4 level less than 500/mm^3	Headache, insomnia, hypersensitivity, nausea, anemia, leukopenia, infection, myalgia	Contraindicated in clients with known hypersensitivity; use cautiously in bone marrow suppression, renal impairment, hepatic dysfunction, or children under age 3; administer around the clock if possible; protect medication from light; treat pain carefully because of interaction of most pain medications with antiretroviral

C & S, culture and sensitivity; IV, intravenous; IM, intramuscular; HIV, human immunodeficiency virus; DNA, deoxyribonucleic acid.

C. Implementation

1. Teach client about diagnostic tests
2. Provide standard postoperative care
3. Encourage well-balanced diet and teach client nutritious foods (see Chapter 5)
4. Provide emotional support
5. Prepare client for radiation therapy as outpatient
6. Prepare client for chemotherapy

D. Evaluation

1. Client had lymphoma diagnosed and treated early
2. Client understood diagnostic tests
3. Client recovered from surgery without complications
4. Client had side effects of chemotherapy controlled
5. Client had side effects of radiation therapy controlled
6. Client maintained ideal body weight
7. Client and family coped with diagnosis

III. SICKLE CELL DISEASE

A. Assessment

1. Definition/pathophysiology
   a. hereditary disease, occurring predominantly in African-Americans
   b. hemoglobin takes on characteristic crescent shape
   c. unable to carry adequate amounts of oxygen
   d. cells more fragile and rupture easily in small capillaries
   e. chronically low red blood count leads to cardiomegaly and tachycardia to compensate for low oxygen
   f. during periods of crisis, cells clump together leading to obstructed blood flow and pain
2. Predisposing/precipitating factors
   a. race and heredity: mainly in African-Americans; nearly 10% of African-Americans are carriers of trait
   b. trait sometimes found in those of Mediterranean ancestry
3. Signs and symptoms
   a. crisis can be triggered by variety of stressors
      (1) dehydration
      (2) infection
      (3) overexertion
      (4) cold weather changes
      (5) alcohol intake
      (6) smoking
   b. anemia
   c. enlarged liver and spleen
   d. painful swollen fingers and toes (dactylitis)
   e. chronic leg ulcers
   f. cerebral infarcts, strokes
   g. aplastic anemia from overstress on bone marrow
   h. aseptic necrosis of bones
   i. vaso-occlusion
   j. renal infarcts, renal failure
   k. cholelithiasis
   l. pulmonary infarct and stasis
   m. cardiomegaly, congestive heart failure
   n. infections
   o. jaundice
4. Diagnostic tests
   a. CBC
   b. sickle cell preparation
   c. genetic studies and history
5. Usual treatment
   a. treatment symptomatic and preventive
   b. drug therapy to combat sickling of red blood cells

B. Planning, Goals, Expected Outcomes

1. Client remains in remission as long as possible
2. Client suffers from minimal complications
3. Client does not develop life-threatening infections
4. Client's pain is controlled

C. Implementation

1. Educate client and family about disease and avoidance of precipitators of crisis
2. Provide emotional support
3. Teach client about adequate nutrition and hydration
4. Provide for genetic counseling
5. Teach clients about prevention of infections
6. Provide adequate pain medication as ordered

D. Evaluation

1. Client remained in remission as long as possible
2. Client had minimal complications
3. No life-threatening infections occurred
4. Client's pain was controlled

IV. SHOCK

A. Assessment

1. Definitions/pathophysiology: variety of causes—hemorrhagic, neurogenic, septic, vasogenic, anaphylactic, and cardiogenic—leading to cellular hypoxia and tissue necrosis
2. Predisposing/precipitating factors

a. inadequate blood volume
b. decreased cardiac output
c. shift in body fluids from one compartment to another
d. vascular collapse
e. nervous system overstimulation
f. exposure to allergens
3. Signs and symptoms
a. hypotension
b. tachycardia
c. cold clammy skin
d. pallor or cyanosis
e. thirst
f. restlessness
g. oliguria
h. decreasing level of consciousness
4. Diagnosis
a. blood gas values
b. vital signs
c. other tests specific to cause of shock
5. Usual treatment
a. identify and reverse cause
b. emergency situation that requires quick action to stop hemorrhage
c. vasopressors (Table 7–11)
d. replacement of lost volume and blood components

B. Planning, Goals, Expected Outcomes

1. Shock does not develop
2. Client ensures that shock is diagnosed and treated rapidly
3. Client recovers from shock without long-term complications

C. Implementation

1. Assess client frequently; monitor vital signs
2. Keep client calm
3. Keep client warm without overheating
4. Administer intravenous fluids, as ordered
5. Position client with feet up to increase venous return, if possible (modified Trendelenburg); contra-

indicated if increased intracranial pressure suspected
6. Give oxygen as ordered

D. Evaluation

1. Client did not develop shock
2. Client was treated for shock immediately
3. Client recovered from shock without complication

Pulmonary Disorders

I. PNEUMONIA

A. Assessment

1. Definition/pathophysiology: extensive inflammation of lung with consolidation of tissue as it fills with exudate
2. Predisposing/precipitating factors
a. children or elderly
b. weak, debilitated, chronically ill clients
c. immobilized clients
d. after surgery
e. vomiting and aspiration
f. inhalation of toxins
g. trauma
h. immunosuppressed clients
i. smoking
3. Signs and symptoms
a. high fever, chills except in older clients
b. productive cough often with rusty or blood-tinged sputum
c. pleural pain
d. general malaise and general weakness
e. abnormal breath sounds
4. Diagnostic tests
a. chest radiograph indicating areas of consolidation
b. physical assessment of chest
c. sputum culture and sensitivity
5. Usual treatment
a. anti-infective agents, such as penicillin or erythromycin (see Table 7–10)
b. treatment specific to cause

TABLE 7-11 Vasopressors

Class	Example	Action	Use	Common Side Effects	Nursing Implications
Adrenergics	Dopamine	Cause vasoconstriction of peripheral vascular system while increasing blood flow to vital organs and kidneys	To treat shock	Hypertension, tachycardia, dizziness, headache, palpitations	Use with care in clients with hypertension, benign prostatic hypertrophy, chronic obstructive pulmonary disease, check I & O, BP

BP, blood pressure; I & O, intake and output.

B. Planning, Goals, Expected Outcomes

1. High-risk client does not develop pneumonia
2. Client recovers without complications

C. Implementation

1. Control high temperatures with antipyretics
2. Maintain fluid and electrolyte balance; monitor input and output
3. Maintain good nutrition
4. Cough and deep breathe client hourly
5. Monitor vital signs and respiratory status
6. Provide good oral hygiene
7. Preventive measures for high-risk clients, such as mobilization and respiratory therapy
8. Suction as needed
9. Administer antimicrobials as ordered

D. Evaluation

1. High-risk client did not develop pneumonia
2. Client recovered without complications

II. TUBERCULOSIS

A. Assessment

1. Definition/pathophysiology
   a. infectious lung disease caused by *Mycobacterium tuberculosis*
   b. characterized by encapsulated lesions containing bacilli
   c. lesions degenerate and become necrotic or heal with fibrosis and calcification
   d. disease never cured, just in remission
   e. can infect extrapulmonary sites, such as intestine, kidneys, and CNS
2. Incidence
   a. African-Americans, Native Americans
   b. increasing in recent years
   c. high in human immunodeficiency virus (HIV) and immunosuppressed clients
3. Predisposing/precipitating factors
   a. not highly contagious
   b. poor living conditions, overcrowding with poor sanitation
   c. malnutrition
   d. highest rates among elderly, men, non-whites, and immigrants
   e. immunocompromised and HIV clients
4. Signs and symptoms
   a. onset gradual
   b. cough
   c. low-grade fever in afternoon
   d. night sweats
   e. weight loss
   f. fatigue
   g. occasional hemoptysis
5. Diagnostic tests
   a. skin testing: positive test (induration, swelling at injection site after 72 hours) means only that person has been exposed to tubercle bacillus and has formed antibodies against it, not that the person has active tuberculosis; further evaluation needed
   b. chest radiographs and tomograms
   c. positive sputum culture: only accurate method of diagnosis
6. Usual treatment
   a. antitubercular agents effective almost always with combination therapy; must treat for 2 years (Table 7–12)
   b. prophylactic treatment for 1 year for those exposed and most susceptible
   c. hospitalization only for diagnosis and early treatment, then outpatient treatment
   d. bacille Calmette-Guérin (BCG) vaccine for high-risk, noninfected groups

B. Planning, Goals, Expected Outcomes

1. Client has diagnosis of tuberculosis made early
2. Client complies with drug therapy
3. Tuberculosis is in remission

C. Implementation

1. Control spread of infection through respiratory isolation until chemotherapy begun

TABLE 7-12 Antitubercular Agents

Example	Common Side Effects	Nursing Implications
Isoniazid	Peripheral neuritis, hepatitis, hypersensitivity	Give pyridoxine (vitamin B_6) to prevent neuropathy, check liver enzymes, teach client to take all medication for 2 years
Ethambutol	Optic neuritis, rash	Monitor color vision, monitor renal function
Rifampin	Hepatitis, febrile reaction	Turns urine red-orange, potentiates actions of other antibiotics
Streptomycin	Eighth cranial nerve damage, nephrotoxicity	Monitor hearing, use with caution in elderly, monitor renal function

a. use masks to prevent spread
b. laminar-flow air systems for resistant organisms
2. Teach client good hygiene with respiratory wastes, mucus, saliva, and urine and feces
3. Administer medications as ordered
4. Immunize high-risk groups
5. Ensure client compliance for full course of drugs, usually 1 year for prophylaxis and 2 years for treatment
    a. teach client that not taking full course of drugs can lead to the development of resistant organisms
    b. vitally important that those living in close contact receive prophylactic treatment
6. Educate family of client and other high-risk groups
7. Stress importance of testing family and those in close contact
8. Notify Public Health Department, reportable disease

D. Evaluation

1. Diagnosis of tuberculosis was made early
2. Client complied with drug therapy
3. Client experienced a remission

III. CHRONIC OBSTRUCTIVE PULMONARY DISEASE OR CHRONIC OBSTRUCTIVE LUNG DISEASE

A. Assessment

1. Definition/pathophysiology
    a. term used to describe three diseases: asthma, bronchitis, and emphysema; may occur singly or mixed types
    b. general pathology obstruction of small bronchioles and alveoli
    c. emphysema characterized by permanent distention of bronchioles and destruction of alveolar walls; air trapped after inhalation
2. Incidence
    a. among top 10 leading causes of death in United States
    b. increasing morbidity and mortality rates directly attributable to cigarette smoking and air pollution
3. Predisposing/precipitating factors
    a. smoking
    b. air pollution
    c. genetic predisposition
    d. respiratory allergies
    e. chronic bronchitis

4. Signs and symptoms
    a. barrel chest
    b. pink skin color due to hypercapnia (high P_{CO_2})
    c. hypoxia (low O_2 concentration level)
    d. cough with thick, tenacious sputum or none
    e. shortness of breath and dyspnea on exertion
    f. severe activity intolerance
    g. abnormal breath sounds
5. Diagnostic tests
    a. pulmonary function tests show air trapping
    b. blood gas analysis shows CO_2 retention
    c. abnormal breath sounds and percussion of trapped air
6. Usual treatment
    a. antibiotics to prevent infections (see Table 7–10)
    b. bronchodilators (Table 7–13)
    c. mucolytics and expectorants to aid in liquefying secretions
    d. oxygen in low levels for severe dyspnea; never more than 2 L/min of 20% to 24% oxygen
7. Complications
    a. congestive heart failure
    b. cor pulmonale
    c. pneumonia

B. Planning, Goals, Expected Outcomes

1. Client maintains P_{O_2} of at least 60 mm Hg
2. Client maintains maximal activity level
3. Client remains free from infection
4. Client complies with therapy, especially avoiding respiratory irritants
5. Client stops smoking cigarettes

C. Implementation

1. Teach client:
    a. to avoid respiratory irritants, especially cigarette smoking
    b. pursed lip and diaphragmatic breathing
    c. to drink plenty of fluids unless contraindicated
    d. to eat multiple small meals a day rather than three large ones
    e. to avoid people with infections
    f. to avoid over-the-counter drugs, especially antihistamines and inhalers
2. Help client to maintain optimal health status
3. Include family in educational programs
4. Achieve balance of rest and activity

TABLE 7-13 Bronchodilators

Example	Action	Use	Common Side Effects	Nursing Implications
Theophylline (Theo-Dur)	Relaxes bronchial smooth muscle and inhibits release of histamine, mild diuretics and cardiac stimulants	To treat asthma and bronchial spasms	GI upset, nervousness, frequency, diarrhea, insomnia, tachycardia, palpitations	Use with care in clients with hypertension, glaucoma, BPH and diabetes, monitor for CNS symptoms, give with food to decrease GI upset, avoid smoking

BPH, benign prostatic hyperplasia; CNS, central nervous system; GI, gastrointestinal.

D. Evaluation

1. Client's P_{O_2} remained above 60 mm Hg
2. Client remained active within limits of disease
3. Client remained infection-free
4. Client complied with therapy and stopped cigarette smoking

IV. LUNG CANCER

A. Assessment

1. Definition/pathophysiology
   a. no early signs and symptoms
   b. leading cause of cancer deaths in both men and women
   c. often widely metastatic at diagnosis
2. Incidence
   a. more common in men than women, although number of women is increasing dramatically
   b. most common cancer
3. Predisposing/precipitating factors
   a. smoking
   b. air pollution
   c. environmental pollutants
   d. asbestos
   e. usually over age 40 years
4. Signs and symptoms
   a. no early signs or symptoms
   b. cough, especially early morning
   c. late symptoms
      (1) chest pain
      (2) exertional dyspnea
      (3) hemoptysis
      (4) compression on surrounding areas
5. Diagnostic tests
   a. sputum cytology
   b. chest radiograph
   c. bronchoscopy: nursing responsibilities
      (1) client takes nothing by mouth (NPO) for 8 to 10 hours pretest
      (2) after test, client is on NPO status until gag reflex returns
      (3) check for gag reflex with tongue blade at back of throat before allowing food or fluids

      (4) monitor for bleeding or respiratory distress
   d. mediastinoscopy
   e. thoracentesis: nursing responsibilities
      (1) client must be cooperative and able to hold still and hold breath
      (2) monitor vital signs before and after procedure
      (3) watch for development of respiratory distress
      (4) make sure no air leak at insertion site
   f. needle biopsy
   g. open biopsy
   h. lung scan
6. Usual treatment
   a. surgical resection
      (1) wedge resection
      (2) lobectomy
      (3) pneumonectomy
   b. chemotherapy
   c. radiation therapy
   d. immunotherapy

B. Planning, Goals, Expected Outcomes

1. Client and family cope with diagnosis and potentially terminal nature of disease
2. Client understands diagnostic tests
3. Client recovers from surgery without complications
4. Side effects of chemotherapy are controlled
5. Side effects of radiation therapy are controlled

C. Implementation

1. Assist client through diagnostic workup in clinic
2. Provide emotional support
3. Request clergy or other counselors as needed
4. Monitor for postoperative complications (see under "Chest Surgery")
5. Teach client to avoid infections
6. Help client cope with radiation or chemotherapy

D. Evaluation

1. Client accepted diagnosis and coped with potentially terminal nature of disease
2. Client recovered from surgery without complication
3. Side effects of chemotherapy were controlled
4. Side effects of radiation therapy were controlled
5. Client and family coped with diagnosis

V. CHEST SURGERY

A. Preoperative Preparation

1. Often done in clinic or outpatient setting and admitted to hospital day of surgery
2. On admission day of surgery, check to be sure that all tests done
   a. Assess respiratory status and function
   b. Ensure that client understands postoperative exercises, especially breathing exercises
   c. Be sure that client understands special exercises to strengthen shoulder muscles and improve breathing efficiency

B. Postoperative Care

1. Position for maximum ventilation, drainage, and comfort
   a. do not allow client to lie on unaffected side after pneumonectomy
   b. position client on unaffected side after all other chest surgery
   c. prevent tension pneumothorax and mediastinal shift by maintaining patency of chest tubes
   d. prevent rupture of bronchial stump
2. Assist RN in monitoring function of chest tubes using either bottles or the Pleur-Evac (Fig. 7–1)
   a. do not allow tubing to become kinked
   b. do not empty bottle if it becomes full of drainage; notify physician
   c. never raise drainage bottle above level of client's chest
   d. do not clamp tube unless specifically ordered for short periods of time; can cause tension pneumothorax—have clamps available per hospital policy
   e. do not dislodge tubes
   f. watch for fluctuation of water level with respiration or bubbling in water seal bottle until negative pressure is restored
   g. monitor rate of fluid drainage; no more than 100 to 150 mL/hour is normal first few days
   h. monitor for occurrence of subcutaneous emphysema
   i. tape junctions of tubing to prevent leakage
   j. milk or strip only if specifically ordered
3. Apply occlusive dressing as tubes are removed
4. Monitor respiratory status, especially return of breath sounds as lung reexpands
5. Check vital signs frequently

VI. LARYNGEAL CANCER

A. Assessment

1. Definition/pathophysiology: common malignancy of head and neck; may affect glottis, supraglottis, or true cords
2. Incidence
   a. more common in men than women
   b. highest among smokers and those with heavy alcohol intake
   c. increased after age 50 years
3. Predisposing/precipitating factors
   a. cigarette smoking and alcohol ingestion
   b. voice abuse
   c. may be associated with bronchiogenic cancer
4. Signs and symptoms
   a. hoarseness only early symptom
   b. late
      (1) pain
      (2) dysphagia
      (3) lymphadenopathy in throat
      (4) feeling of lump in throat
5. Diagnostic tests
   a. direct examination with laryngoscopy
   b. CT scan of neck
   c. laryngogram
   d. biopsy
6. Usual treatment
   a. depends on stage of disease and spread
   b. radiation therapy: preoperatively, postoperatively, or instead of surgery in high-risk or elderly clients
   c. surgery
      (1) partial laryngectomy
      (2) hemilaryngectomy
      (3) total laryngectomy and tracheostomy with or without radical neck dissection
      (4) laryngoplasty after resection

B. Planning, Goals, Expected Outcomes

1. Client understands diagnostic tests
2. Client is physically and psychologically prepared for surgery

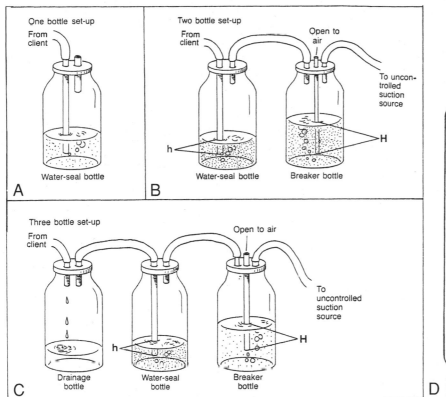
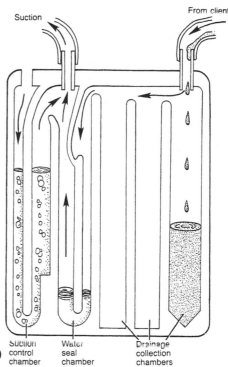

FIGURE 7-1 One-, two-, and three-bottle methods for providing a closed drainage system. *A,* In the one-bottle system, the drainage from the chest tube enters the bottle through the glass tube that has one end submerged under water to form a seal. This provides a one-way valve that prevents a backflow of air into the pleural cavity, which could collapse the lung. As fluid and air from the pleural cavity enter the drainage bottle, the air that is displaced in the bottle is vented through the short tube above water level. *B,* The second bottle in the two-bottle system acts as a trap to control and decrease the amount of suction within the chest tube. Otherwise, the suction might be too forceful and damage the pleural membrane. No drainage enters this bottle. Its only purpose is to control the force of suction applied. *C,* The third bottle in the three-bottle system also is used to regulate the amount of suction. This can be done by adjusting the length of the glass tube that is under water. *D,* Pleur-Evac-type drain. (From Matassarin-Jacobs, E. (1994). *Saunders review for NCLEX-RN,* 2nd ed. Philadelphia: W.B. Saunders Co., pp. 133, 134.)

3. Client recovers from surgery without complications
4. Client learns acceptable, alternate form of communication
5. Client understands and tolerates radiation therapy without complications
6. Client copes with altered body image
7. Client maintains adequate nutritional status
8. Client is free from pain
9. Client and significant others learn self-care activities
10. Client and significant others cope with terminal prognosis

C. Implementation

1. Preoperative—beginning of discharge planning
   a. allow verbalization of fears
   b. establish alternate form of communication

   c. provide meticulous mouth care
   d. provide adequate nutritional intake
     (1) liquids
     (2) enteral nutrition
     (3) hyperalimentation
   e. prepare client for preoperative radiation therapy
     (1) provide skin care as needed
     (2) provide artificial saliva for decreased salivation

2. Postoperative—at beginning of period, PN assists RN with care
   a. suction as needed through mouth and tracheostomy
   b. monitor for hemorrhage
      (1) monitor drain output closely
      (2) assess dressings frequently
   c. remove nasal crusts
   d. frequent mouth care
   e. maintain tube feedings or hyperalimentation as ordered

f. monitor closely for tracheoesophageal fistula formation
   (1) choking or coughing when drinking sign of fistula
   (2) usually given colored water to drink for first intake so if fistula is present, color is apparent on suctioning
g. medicate for pain frequently
h. Semi-Fowler's position for maximal chest expansion
i. ambulate early and encourage deep breathing to prevent pneumonia
j. monitor wound drainage carefully
k. offer support and encourage client to express grief
l. teach client stoma care
m. teach client to suction self and clean tracheostomy tube as needed
n. clean inner cannula as needed and teach client procedure
o. keep extra tracheostomy tube and obturator at bedside in case of emergency
p. always have two people to change ties on tracheostomy tube
q. teach client to cover stoma when coughing
r. suggest use of light, porous covering over healed stoma
s. teach safety precautions
   (1) shower with care
   (2) wear Medic Alert bracelet stating ''Neck Breather''
t. encourage client to stop cigarette smoking and alcohol consumption
u. encourage client to work on alternate speech method

D. Evaluation

1. Client recovered from surgery without complications
2. Client learned alternate form of communication
3. Client recovered from radiation therapy without complications
4. Client coped with altered body image
5. Client's nutritional status is adequate
6. Client's pain is controlled
7. Client and significant others able to perform therapeutic regimen with assistance
8. Client and significant others cope with potentially terminal prognosis

Cardiopulmonary Resuscitation
I. ASSESSMENT: A, B, C

A. Airway

1. Look and listen for signs of distress
2. Check mouth and throat for obstruction

3. New: check, call, care
   a. check airway
   b. call for assistance
   c. care for client

B. Breathing

1. Listen and feel for breathing
2. Look for chest movement
3. Note rate and quality of respirations

C. Circulation

1. Check for presence and strength of carotid pulse
2. Monitor rate and quality of pulse

D. Level of Consciousness

1. Responsiveness
2. Degree of orientation

II. IMPLEMENTATION

A. Restore Airway

1. Clear mouth and throat
2. Head tilt–chin lift maneuver if no sign of spinal injury: if neck injury suspected, use jaw-thrust maneuver
3. Two full breaths
4. Monitor chest for movement

B. Restore Circulation

1. Compress heart by pressing over lower sternum
2. If single rescuer, compression 15 times at first, then at rate of two breaths to 15 compressions
3. For single rescuer, reassess for pulse after four cycles of compression and breathing
4. If two rescuers, rate of one breath to five compressions
5. With two rescuers, switch as you become tired

III. EVALUATION

A. Stop When Client Returns to Spontaneous Respiration and Heart Beat

B. Stop When Another Rescuer Takes Over

C. Stop When You Are Exhausted

D. Stop When Client Is Pronounced Dead

Fluid and Electrolyte Balance

I. NORMAL FLUID BALANCE

Fluid intake and output should be equal, homeostasis (average intake and output is about 2500 mL/day)

A. Fluid Intake

1. Water in food and beverages makes up about 90% of total intake
   a. drinking water and beverages account for about 60% of intake or 1500 mL
   b. fluids in moist foods account for about 1000 mL or 30% of intake
2. Water metabolism makes up about 10% of intake or 250 mL; result of by-products of oxidative metabolism of various nutrients

B. Fluid Output

Environmental factors, such as temperature, relative humidity, and amount of physical exercise, influence output
1. Fluid loss in urine about 1500 mL/day
2. Fluid loss in water vapor from exhaled air via lungs about 400 mL
3. Fluid loss by perspiration about 400 mL, even if client does not appear to be sweating
4. Fluid loss via feces 400 mL

C. Regulation of Fluid Intake

1. Thirst primary regulator of water intake
2. Thirst center located in hypothalamus
3. Receptors in thirst center sensitive to water loss and cause a person to feel thirsty and seek water; with water loss, osmotic pressure of extracellular fluid increases and osmoreceptors in hypothalamus stimulated

D. Regulation of Fluid Output

1. Some water loss is related to body functions and largely unavoidable
   a. water is lost via skin through vaporization and is a necessary part of the body's temperature control mechanism
   b. water is lost in feces via undigested food wastes

   c. water is lost via evaporation from lungs and diffusion through skin is not easily controlled
   d. insensible water loss maintains body temperature; increased loss with increased perspiration
2. Urine production primary regulator of fluid output
   a. antidiuretic hormone (ADH) from the pituitary controls water loss through urine
      (1) ADH secretion is inhibited with increased fluid intake, leading to increased urine output
      (2) ADH secretion is stimulated when fluid intake is low, leading to decreased urine output
      (3) stimulated by many factors such as stress, pain, hypotension, surgery, and certain medications
   b. aldosterone from adrenal glands controls fluid through sodium regulation
      (1) acts on kidney tubules to increase reabsorption of sodium and decrease reabsorption of potassium
      (2) water moves with sodium
      (3) stimulated by many factors, including levels of sodium and potassium
   c. diuretics may be prescribed to increase urine output
   d. natural diuretics include coffee, tea, and alcohol

E. Distribution of Body Water

1. Intracellular: fluid contained within all cells; represents about 2/3 to 3/4 of total body water; contains large amounts of potassium, phosphate, and protein
2. Extracellular: fluid not contained inside cell; represents 1/4 to 1/3 of total body water; contains large amounts of sodium, chloride, and bicarbonate ions

F. Fluid Dynamics

Movement of fluid from one compartment to another via the following dynamics
1. *Diffusion:* movement of substance from area of high concentration to one of low concentration
2. *Active transport:* transport of substances across membrane from area of low concentration to one of high concentration; requires energy expenditure
3. *Osmosis:* movement of water across semipermeable membrane into solution with high solute concentration
4. *Filtration:* passage of fluid through semipermeable membrane as a result of difference in hydrostatic pressure

5. *Osmolality:* measurement of ratio of water to solutes in a solution

G. Additional Concepts

1. Sodium attracts water; a concentration of sodium anywhere in the body attracts water until sodium is diluted to "normal" concentration
2. If there is a high level of sodium in plasma, blood volume increases because water is drawn into capillaries to dilute sodium
3. If there is a high level of sodium in interstitial fluid, water is attracted to dilute sodium, resulting in edema
4. If concentration of ions in either intracellular or extracellular spaces changes, water shifts from an area of low concentration to an area of high concentration until concentrations are equal; shift shrinks or expands respective spaces

Fluid Imbalances

I. EDEMA—EXTRACELLULAR FLUID EXCESS

A. Assessment

1. Definition/pathophysiology: abnormal accumulation of fluid in interstitial (extracellular) spaces of tissues; third space
2. Incidence: occurs whenever there is shift of fluids to third space
3. Predisposing/precipitating factors: multiple medical or surgical conditions may cause edema, including
   a. renal failure
   b. congestive heart failure
   c. cirrhosis
   d. corticosteroid therapy
   e. excessive salt intake
   f. hypertension
4. Types of edema
   a. pitting edema: tissues hold indentation made by pressure of fingertips for as long as 10 minutes (volume of interstitial fluid increased)
   b. localized edema: fluid drawn to site of injury, insect bite, burn, or other trauma
   c. generalized or dependent edema: affected by gravity
      (1) facial edema develops if client is in a prone position
      (2) sacral and shoulder edema occurs when client is on bed rest in a supine position
      (3) dependent edema of lower extremities occurs when client has been sitting or standing for long periods of time

5. Signs and symptoms
   a. full bounding pulse
   b. tachycardia
   c. jugular vein distention
   d. increased arterial and central venous blood pressure
   e. rapid weight gain
   f. peripheral, dependent edema
   g. tachypnea, dyspnea, or cyanosis
   h. if severe, pulmonary edema
   i. ascites
   j. anasarca
6. Diagnostic tests
   a. CBC
   b. serum electrolytes
   c. daily weights
   d. serum and urine osmolality
7. Usual treatment
   a. correction of underlying problem if possible
   b. diuretics (see Table 7–3)
   c. low-sodium diet (see Table 5–3)

B. Planning, Goals, Expected Outcomes

1. Client complies with treatment plan
2. Client identifies and avoids high-sodium foods
3. Client is free of edema

C. Implementation

1. Monitor intake and output
2. Observe and record signs and symptoms of edema
3. Weigh client daily: same time, same scale, same clothes, and same nurse if possible
4. Instruct client to avoid high-sodium foods
5. Administer diuretics as prescribed, such as furosemide (Lasix) and hydrochlorothiazide (see Table 7–3)
6. Elevate extremities when sitting to decrease edema
7. Assess breath sounds for presence of fluid rales
8. Measure abdominal girth

D. Evaluation

1. Client complied with treatment plan
2. Client identified and avoided high-sodium foods
3. Client free of edema

II. DEHYDRATION—EXTRACELLULAR FLUID DEFICIT

A. Assessment

1. Definition/pathophysiology: excessive loss of water and often sodium from body tissues

2. Predisposing/precipitating factors
   a. decreased intake of water and electrolytes, usually sodium
   b. loss of water and sodium from severe vomiting or diarrhea
   c. hemorrhage
   d. severe burns
3. Signs and symptoms
   a. thirst
   b. loss of skin turgor
   c. cracked lips and dry mucous membranes
   d. decreased urine output (normal output 30 mL/hour)
   e. concentrated urine: dark amber color and odorous
   f. low central venous pressure
   g. orthostatic hypotension
   h. severe dehydration may result in hypotension, stupor, and marked oliguria
4. Diagnostic tests
   a. CBC
   b. serum electrolytes
   c. 24-hour urine output
   d. serum and urine osmolality
5. Usual treatment
   a. oral fluid replacement if dehydration is mild
   b. isotonic intravenous fluids, such as normal saline or Ringer's lactate, if dehydration is more severe

B. Planning, Goals, Expected Outcomes

1. Client recognizes symptoms of dehydration
2. Client maintains adequate oral fluid intake
3. Client remains well hydrated

C. Implementation

1. Administer intravenous fluids as ordered
2. Encourage adequate oral fluid intake
3. Closely monitor intake and output and electrolyte balance
4. Observe, record, and report signs and symptoms of dehydration
5. Attempt to identify cause of dehydration to prevent recurrence

D. Evaluation

1. Client recognized signs and symptoms of dehydration
2. Client maintained adequate oral intake
3. Client remained well hydrated

Electrolyte Imbalances

I. HYPERNATREMIA

A. Assessment

1. Definition/pathophysiology: serum sodium elevated above 145 mEq/L; either an absolute increase of sodium or a loss of water without sodium loss
2. Predisposing/precipitating factors
   a. increased salt intake without increase in water intake
   b. loss of water without loss of sodium
   c. profuse, watery diarrhea
   d. severe burns
   e. dehydration
3. Signs and symptoms
   a. pitting edema
   b. excessive weight gain; more than 2 pounds/day
   c. dyspnea
   d. increased blood pressure
   e. symptoms of dehydration
   f. thirst
   g. flushed skin
   h. dry mucous membranes
   i. low urine output
   j. restlessness and tachycardia
   k. convulsions
4. Diagnostic tests
   a. CBC
   b. serum electrolytes
   c. urinary electrolytes
5. Usual treatment
   a. correct cause of imbalance
   b. limit sodium intake
   c. limit water intake
   d. sodium-wasting diuretics (see Table 7–3)

B. Planning, Goals, Expected Outcomes

1. Client's serum sodium returns to normal
2. Client does not have further problems with excessive sodium

C. Implementation

1. Record intake and output and electrolyte balance
2. Help identify cause of imbalance
3. Restrict sodium intake (see Tables 7–4 and 7–5)
4. Restrict fluids

D. Evaluation

1. Client's serum sodium level returned to normal
2. Client had no further problems with excessive sodium

II. HYPONATREMIA

A. Assessment

1. Definition/pathophysiology: serum sodium less than 135 mEq/L; either absolute loss of sodium and water or addition of water without sodium increase
2. Predisposing/precipitating factors
   a. diuretics, sodium wasting
   b. profuse diaphoresis
   c. excessive water intake without sodium
   d. excessive gastrointestinal losses
3. Signs and symptoms
   a. mental confusion
   b. muscle weakness, fatigue
   c. restlessness
   d. muscle twitching
   e. abdominal cramping
   f. postural hypotension
   g. headache
   h. if severe: convulsions, coma, and death
4. Diagnostic tests
   a. CBC
   b. serum electrolytes
   c. urinary electrolytes
5. Usual treatment
   a. correct cause of imbalance
   b. oral administration of sodium (salt water, salt tablets, or foods high in sodium) with great care to avoid hypervolemia
   c. intravenous administration of isotonic (0.9%) sodium chloride or Ringer's lactate

B. Planning, Goals, Expected Outcomes

1. Client's serum sodium level returns to normal
2. Client does not have further problems with low sodium level

C. Implementation

1. Administer oral sodium as ordered
2. Maintain accurate intake and output
3. Monitor intravenous fluids carefully
4. Monitor client's vital signs and fluid and electrolyte balance when replacing sodium

D. Evaluation

1. Client's serum sodium level has returned to normal
2. Client had no further problems with low sodium

III. HYPERKALEMIA

A. Assessment

1. Definition/pathophysiology: serum potassium more than 5.0 mEq/L
2. Predisposing/precipitating factors
   a. renal failure (unable to excrete potassium)
   b. severe burns or crush injuries (cell destruction releases intracellular potassium)
   c. adrenal insufficiency
   d. overuse of salt substitutes containing potassium
   e. increased intake of potassium orally through foods or medication
3. Signs and symptoms
   a. diarrhea, nausea
   b. muscle weakness, flaccid paralysis
   c. cardiac arrhythmias
   d. if severe and uncorrected: cardiac arrest may occur
4. Diagnostic tests
   a. CBC
   b. serum electrolytes
   c. urinary electrolytes
5. Usual treatment
   a. correct cause of imbalance
   b. decreased potassium intake if mild (see Tables 5–4 and 7–9)
   c. if severe, sodium polystyrene sulfonate (Kayexalate) orally or enemas (cation-exchange resin) or dialysis if life-threatening

B. Planning, Goals, Expected Outcomes

1. Client's serum potassium level returns to normal
2. Client does not have further problems with excessive potassium

C. Implementation

1. Monitor intake and output and electrolyte balance
2. Maintain cardiac monitoring, monitor for arrhythmias
3. Check pulses carefully for arrhythmias
4. Observe character and rate of respirations
5. Administer sodium polystyrene sulfonate (Kayexalate) orally or per enema as ordered

D. Evaluation

1. Client's serum potassium level has returned to normal

2. Client does not have further problems with excessive potassium

IV. HYPOKALEMIA

A. Assessment

1. Definition/pathophysiology: serum potassium less than 3.5 mEq/L
2. Predisposing/precipitating factors
   a. diuretics, potassium wasting
   b. loss of fluid from gastrointestinal tract
      (1) vomiting
      (2) diarrhea
      (3) nasogastric tubes
3. Signs and symptoms
   a. fatigue, weakness
   b. anorexia leading to nausea/vomiting
   c. cardiac arrhythmias
   d. severe hypokalemia may result in hypotension, flaccid paralysis, and death as a result of cardiac arrest
4. Diagnostic tests
   a. CBC
   b. serum electrolytes
   c. urinary electrolytes
5. Usual treatment
   a. correct cause of imbalance
   b. increase oral potassium intake: potassium-rich foods or oral potassium salts (see Tables 5–4 and 7–9)
   c. intravenous administration of potassium salt, such as potassium chloride (KCl); intravenous potassium always given in diluted solution because undiluted injection of KCl would always be fatal

B. Planning, Goals, Expected Outcomes

1. Client's serum potassium level returns to normal
2. Client does not have further problems with low potassium

C. Implementation

1. Administer oral potassium as ordered
2. Maintain accurate intake and output
3. Monitor intravenous fluids and electrolytes carefully
4. Monitor client vital signs and fluid balance when replacing potassium
5. Monitor pulse carefully for arrhythmias
6. Educate client on food sources of potassium

D. Evaluation

1. Client's serum potassium level has returned to normal
2. Client does not have further problems with low potassium level

V. HYPERCALCEMIA

Normal serum calcium, 9–11 mg/dL

A. Assessment

1. Definition/pathophysiology: serum calcium greater than 11 mg/dL
2. Predisposing/precipitating factors
   a. excess doses of vitamin D
   b. prolonged immobilization
   c. hyperparathyroidism
   d. excessive calcium intake
   e. many types of cancer
3. Signs and symptoms
   a. deep bone pain
   b. anorexia, nausea, vomiting
   c. polyuria, polydypsia
   d. mental changes, lethargy
   e. muscle weakness
   f. constipation, abdominal distention
   g. if chronic, may result in kidney stones
4. Diagnostic tests
   a. CBC
   b. serum electrolytes
   c. urine electrolytes
5. Usual treatment
   a. correct cause of imbalance
   b. mild hypercalcemia treated by forcing fluids and limiting oral calcium intake
   c. acute or severe hypercalcemia treated by administering intravenous sodium chloride plus diuretics, such as furosemide, to increase calcium excretion in urine; also calcitonin, gallium nitrate (Ganite)

B. Planning, Goals, Expected Outcomes

1. Client's serum calcium level has returned to normal
2. Client does not have further problems with high calcium

C. Implementation

1. Limit oral calcium intake
2. Monitor intake and output and serum calcium

3. Observe and report mental changes or lethargy
4. Monitor for signs and symptoms of kidney stones
5. Teach client preventive strategies such as ambulation, decreased dairy products

D. Evaluation

1. Client's serum calcium level has returned to normal
2. Client does not have further problems with high calcium level

VI. HYPOCALCEMIA

A. Assessment

1. Definition/pathophysiology: serum calcium less than 9 mg/dL
2. Predisposing/precipitating factors
   a. burns
   b. acute pancreatitis
   c. surgical removal of parathyroid glands
   d. hypoparathyroidism
3. Signs and symptoms
   a. numbness and tingling of fingers and toes and area around mouth (circumoral paresthesia)
   b. muscle and abdominal cramping
   c. carpopedal spasms, tetany—Trousseau's and Chvostek's signs
   d. convulsions
4. Diagnostic tests
   a. CBC
   b. serum electrolytes
   c. urinary electrolytes
5. Usual treatment
   a. correct cause of imbalance
   b. administer calcium orally
   c. administer intravenous calcium salts, such as calcium gluconate

B. Planning, Goals, Expected Outcomes

1. Client's serum calcium level has returned to normal
2. Client does not have further problems with low calcium level

C. Implementation

1. Administer oral or intravenous calcium as ordered
2. Maintain accurate intake and output and serum calcium
3. Observe seizure precautions (padded side rails up, padded tongue blade at bedside) until calcium deficit corrected
4. Check for early signs of tetany

D. Evaluation

1. Client's serum calcium level has returned to normal
2. Client does not have further problems with low calcium level

Acid-Base Imbalances

I. NORMAL VALUES

A. pH 7.35–7.45

B. Po_2 80–100 mm Hg

C. Pco_2 35–45 mm Hg

D. HCO_3^- 23–28 mEq/L

II. IMBALANCES

A. Decreased arterial pH indicates state of acidosis that may be of either metabolic or respiratory origin

1. In metabolic acidosis, serum bicarbonate level below normal
2. In respiratory acidosis, Pco_2 elevated

B. Increased arterial pH indicates state of alkalosis that may be either metabolic or respiratory

1. In metabolic alkalosis, serum bicarbonate level above normal
2. In respiratory alkalosis, Pco_2 decreased

C. The body has many compensatory mechanisms that can help to balance abnormalities in pH, such as retaining H^+ ions to balance the excessive bicarbonate

III. RESPIRATORY ACIDOSIS

A. Assessment

1. Definition/pathophysiology: condition in which arterial blood pH is below 7.35 caused by retention

of CO_2 that combines with H_2O to form carbonic acid (H_2CO_3)

2. Predisposing/precipitating factors
   a. hypoventilation
   b. acute pulmonary edema
   c. aspiration
   d. pneumonia
   e. pneumothorax
   f. oversedation
   g. chronic obstructive pulmonary disease
   h. ascites
3. Signs and symptoms
   a. headache
   b. increased pulse, blood pressure, respirations
   c. mental cloudiness
   d. weakness
   e. symptoms of increased intracranial pressure
   f. cardiac arrhythmias
4. Diagnostic tests
   a. history and physical examination to determine underlying cause
   b. blood gas, pH, and electrolyte levels
      (1) pH below 7.35
      (2) Pco_2 greater than 45 mm Hg
      (3) HCO_3^- normal before compensation, elevated if compensation occurs
5. Usual treatment
   a. reversal of cause
   b. improvement of ventilation
   c. bronchodilators (see Table 7–13)
   d. pulmonary hygiene
   e. oxygen and mechanical ventilation if acute
6. Complications
   a. cardiac arrhythmias from elevated serum potassium
   b. hypotension
   c. congestive heart failure
   d. shock
   e. increased intracranial pressure from vasodilatory effect of CO_2 on cerebral blood vessels

B. Planning, Goals, Expected Outcomes

1. Client has adequate ventilation
2. Client does not have complications from respiratory acidosis
3. Client does not have complications from oxygen therapy

C. Implementation

1. Specific implementations depend on cause of ventilatory impairment; the following are general measures to increase ventilation
   a. establish patent airway
   b. administer mechanical ventilatory aids as prescribed
   c. facilitate removal of tracheobronchial secretions by teaching and encouraging client to cough and deep breathe and to take in adequate fluids
   d. prevent respiratory infections
2. Administer antibiotics or bronchodilators
3. Monitor client's blood gas values and signs and symptoms of worsening hypoventilation and acidosis
4. Administer prescribed drugs, such as sodium bicarbonate, if necessary, to neutralize excess acid
5. Administer oxygen cautiously, especially to clients with chronic obstructive pulmonary disease, to increase tissue oxygenation without causing respiratory depression
   a. monitor for signs of CO_2 narcosis, such as respiratory depression, decreasing level of sensorium, cardiac arrhythmias
   b. monitor for signs of oxygen toxicity, such as pulmonary edema and presence of blood in tracheobronchial secretions

D. Evaluation

1. Client effectively coughed and deep breathed
2. Blood gas analysis normal
3. Client showed no signs of respiratory distress
4. Client had no evidence of CO_2 narcosis, O_2 toxicity, or rebound respiratory alkalosis

IV. RESPIRATORY ALKALOSIS

A. Assessment

1. Definition/pathophysiology: condition in which arterial blood pH greater than 7.45 caused by a decrease in Pco_2 to less than 35 mm Hg secondary to increased alveolar ventilation
2. Predisposing/precipitating factors
   a. hyperventilation
   b. anxiety
   c. hysteria
   d. early salicylate intoxication
   e. gram-negative septicemia
   f. mechanical ventilators
3. Signs and symptoms
   a. lightheadedness
   b. inability to concentrate
   c. numbness and tingling of fingertips and around mouth
   d. tinnitus
   e. fainting

4. Diagnostic tests
   a. history and physical examination to determine underlying cause
   b. blood gas, pH, and electrolyte levels
      (1) pH greater than 7.45
      (2) P_{CO_2} less than 35 mm Hg
      (3) HCO_3^- normal or decreased with compensation
5. Usual treatment
   a. rebreather bag
   b. sedation
6. Complications
   a. tetany, convulsions
   b. hypokalemia
   c. dizziness and fainting

B. Planning, Goals, Expected Outcomes

1. Underlying cause of respiratory alkalosis is identified and eliminated
2. Client's acid-base balance is restored
3. Client is free from complications of treatment for respiratory alkalosis

C. Implementation

1. Specific interventions depend on cause
   a. salicylate abuse: instruct client about appropriate use of aspirin
   b. anxiety reaction: assist client to recognize and cope with situations that provoke anxiety; teach client to take slow deep breaths or temporarily hold breath in situations that precipitate hyperventilation; breathe into paper bag
   c. mechanical ventilation: monitor ventilatory settings and client's blood gases and electrolytes
2. Administer rebreathing mask, prescribed sedatives, or 5% CO_2 for inhalation
3. Maintain seizure precautions
4. Monitor blood gases and electrolytes during treatment to detect overshoot metabolic acidosis

D. Evaluation

1. Underlying cause of client's respiratory alkalosis identified and corrected
2. Client's blood pH, HCO_3^-/CO_2, and electrolytes within normal limits; no signs or symptoms of alkalosis
3. Client did not sustain injuries
4. Client showed no evidence of overshoot metabolic acidosis

V. METABOLIC ACIDOSIS

A. Assessment

1. Definition/pathophysiology: condition in which arterial blood pH below 7.35; caused by either accumulation of fixed (nonvolatile) acid or base deficit
2. Predisposing/precipitating factors
   a. diabetic ketoacidosis
   b. lactic acidosis
   c. late salicylate poisoning
   d. uremia
   e. starvation
   f. diarrhea from intestinal fistula
   g. administration of large quantities of isotonic saline or ammonium chloride
3. Signs and symptoms
   a. headache
   b. confusion
   c. drowsiness
   d. Kussmaul's respiration: rapid and deep breathing
   e. nausea/vomiting
4. Diagnostic tests
   a. history and physical examination to determine underlying cause
   b. blood gas, pH, and electrolyte levels
      (1) pH less than 7.35
      (2) CO_2 normal or low with compensation
      (3) HCO_3^- normal or low then increased with compensation
5. Usual treatment: dependent on cause
   a. correct cause
   b. administer bicarbonate in some instances
   c. administer insulin with ketoacidosis
6. Complications
   a. fluid and electrolyte loss from vomiting and diarrhea
   b. cardiac arrhythmias from elevated serum potassium
   c. hypotension
   d. congestive heart failure

B. Planning, Goals, Expected Outcomes

1. Underlying cause of the client's metabolic acidosis is identified
2. Client's acid-base balance is restored
3. Client does not develop complications from metabolic acidosis
4. Client does not develop complications from the therapy for metabolic acidosis

C. Implementation

1. Specific implementations depend on underlying cause

a. diabetic ketoacidosis: administer prescribed insulin, fluids, and potassium; instruct client on insulin and diet therapy

b. renal tubular disease: replace bicarbonate kidneys unable to reabsorb

c. lactic acidosis: improve tissue perfusion via cardiovascular support

2. If therapy of underlying cause does not reverse acidosis rapidly enough, administer prescribed drugs, such as sodium bicarbonate or sodium lactate, to neutralize acid

3. Monitor input and output; replace fluid and electrolytes lost from vomiting, diarrhea, or osmotic diuresis

4. Monitor client for manifestations of overshoot metabolic alkalosis; monitor for manifestations of hypokalemia because as acidosis is corrected, potassium reenters cells; administer prescribed potassium supplements

D. Evaluation

1. Underlying cause of metabolic acidosis identified

2. Client's blood pH and HCO_3^-/CO_2 and urine pH normal; no signs or symptoms of metabolic acidosis

3. Client had no evidence of fluid or electrolyte imbalance

4. Client had not sustained injuries

VI. METABOLIC ALKALOSIS

A. Assessment

1. Definition/pathophysiology: condition in which arterial blood pH greater than 7.45 caused by either loss of acid or gain of base

2. Predisposing/precipitating factors
   a. vomiting or gastric suctioning
   b. potassium loss
   c. hyperaldosteronism and Cushing's syndrome
   d. excessive ingestion of alkali

3. Signs and symptoms
   a. tingling in fingers and toes
   b. dizziness
   c. hypertonic muscles
   d. depressed respirations

4. Diagnostic tests
   a. history and physical examination to determine underlying causes

b. blood gas, pH, and electrolyte levels
   (1) pH greater than 7.45
   (2) CO_2 low or normal then increased with compensation
   (3) HCO_3^- high or normal then lower with compensation

5. Usual treatment
   a. reverse underlying disorder
   b. administer sodium chloride intravenously

6. Complications
   a. respiratory depression from blunting of respiratory drive caused by H^+ deficiency
   b. tetany, convulsions
   c. hypokalemia

B. Planning, Goals, Expected Outcomes

1. Underlying cause of metabolic alkalosis is identified

2. Client's acid-base balance is restored

3. Client is free from complications from therapy for metabolic alkalosis

C. Implementation

1. Specific implementations depend on the underlying cause
   a. excessive ingestion of sodium bicarbonate: instruct client about appropriate use of sodium bicarbonate–containing drugs
   b. chloride loss: administer prescribed chloride replacements
   c. potassium deficit: administer prescribed potassium supplements; encourage foods high in potassium

2. If treatment of underlying cause does not reverse alkalosis rapidly enough, administer prescribed acidifying drugs, such as ammonium chloride and acetazolamide (Diamox)

3. Observe seizure precautions

4. Monitor blood gases and electrolytes during therapy to detect overshoot metabolic acidosis

D. Evaluation

1. Underlying cause of metabolic alkalosis identified

2. Client's blood pH, HCO_3^-/CO_2 normal

3. No evidence of overshoot metabolic acidosis

4. Client's serum potassium within normal limits

? QUESTIONS

1. Fatty materials deposited within the arteries is termed:

   ① Hypercholesterolemia
   ② Ankylosis
   ③ Atherosclerosis
   ④ Hyperuricemia

2. Mr. Anthony is 60 years old with a 5-year history of emphysema. He is admitted to the hospital for pneumonia, with a chief complaint of shortness of breath and congestion. Using Maslow's Hierarchy of Needs, the most basic need of Mr. Anthony at this point in time would be:

   ① Safety
   ② Oxygen
   ③ Self-esteem
   ④ Food

3. An important nursing diagnosis at this point in the care of a client with chronic obstructive pulmonary disease (COPD) would be:

   ① Altered nutrition: less than body requirements related to inability to swallow
   ② Risk for ineffective coping secondary to chronic illness
   ③ Ineffective breathing pattern related to chronic lung disease
   ④ Impaired circulation secondary to congestive heart failure

4. The wife of your client with COPD reports that he usually sleeps on two or three pillows at home. Which of the following nursing interventions is most appropriate based on this information?

   ① Have him assume the semi-Fowler's position for sleep
   ② Allow him to sit in a chair to sleep
   ③ Ambulate three times a day with breathing exercises
   ④ Apply oxygen as needed for dyspnea

5. Because of the breathing problems, your client with COPD is most likely also to have problems with:

   ① Loss of consciousness
   ② Dehydration
   ③ Fatigue
   ④ Dementia

6. Which of the following would indicate that the COPD client's problems with pneumonia are resolving?

   ① He is able to sleep through the night without nocturia
   ② He sits up at the bedside for meals without distress
   ③ He has resumed normal bowel habits
   ④ He ambulates the length of the hall without dyspnea

7. If your client's condition is diagnosed as both pneumonia and emphysema, the medications most likely to be administered would be:

   ① Digoxin and furosemide
   ② Penicillin and aminophylline
   ③ Digoxin and streptomycin
   ④ Furosemide and theophylline

8. Most leukemias involve changes in the:

   ① Erythrocytes
   ② Platelets
   ③ Monocytes
   ④ Lymphocytes

9. Because of the changes in the white blood cells in leukemia, the nurse knows to expect the client to demonstrate:

   ① Enlargement of the lymph nodes
   ② A lower resistance to infections
   ③ A greater risk of phlebitis
   ④ An increase in clotting activity

10. Thrombocytopenia frequently occurs in leukemia. Nursing interventions to prevent excessive bleeding include:

    ① Using swabs for mouth care
    ② Encouraging dry meals
    ③ Maintaining strict bed rest
    ④ Avoiding people with infections

11. It seems to the nurse that your client with leukemia is often irritable and difficult to please. This is probably an indication that:

    ① She is neurotic
    ② This is typical behavior for women of her age when hospitalized
    ③ This is a symptom of her illness and outside her control
    ④ She has not accepted her illness and needs spiritual help

12. Mr. Hammer was brought in through the emergency department complaining of sudden, severe chest pain while at work. He is now anxious, short of breath, and diaphoretic. The physician orders morphine sulfate to be given intravenously. The nurse knows that the purpose of this is to:

    ① Relieve any nausea and vomiting
    ② Increase the respiratory rate
    ③ Increase the blood circulation
    ④ Relieve the severe pain

13. Your client had a heart attack 2 days ago. He is now stabilized but continues to be apprehensive and states that he feels as if he is going to die. His wife asks the nurse why he is this way and if he is going to die. The nurse should explain that:

    ① People who are dying often feel this way
    ② He is not going to die now, so she can stop worrying
    ③ This is usual after heart attacks and will resolve with continued reassurance
    ④ This is an indication that he may have suffered cerebral hypoxia during the attack

14. The physician has ordered warfarin sodium (Coumadin) to help prevent further occlusions after your client has had a heart attack. Nursing care for this client should include:

    ① Increasing intake of iron-rich foods
    ② Monitoring stools for blood
    ③ Having protamine sulfate on hand
    ④ Monitoring white blood cells

15. To prevent problems from warfarin sodium (Coumadin), your post–heart attack client should be taught to:

    ① Take the apical pulse daily
    ② Avoid sexual intercourse
    ③ Avoid any products containing aspirin
    ④ Increase the intake of potassium

16. Your client is suffering from peripheral arterial disease in his legs. Appropriate teaching would include:

    ① Elevating the legs whenever possible
    ② Wearing support stockings
    ③ Applying a warm water bottle to the lower abdomen
    ④ Avoiding standing for any length of time

17. Mr. Martin is admitted with a diagnosis of congestive heart failure for the last 5 years with increasing symptoms over the last 2 days. Mr. Martin has been experiencing increased edema of the ankles and lower extremities. On the basis of this, the nurse knows that his heart failure is probably:

    ① Right-sided
    ② Left-sided
    ③ Complete
    ④ Cor pulmonale

18. Your client with congestive heart failure is placed on a low-sodium diet to help control the edema. Foods allowed on this diet would include:

    ① Fresh fruits
    ② Canned soups
    ③ Milk and cheese
    ④ Lunch meat

19. Your client with congestive heart failure is to be placed on medication to strengthen his heart and decrease his edema. The most likely combination of drugs would be:

    ① Furosemide and enalapril (Vasotec)
    ② Isoproterenol and digoxin
    ③ Digoxin and hydrochlorothiazide
    ④ Furosemide and hydrochlorothiazide

20. When you are giving a cardiac glycoside and a thiazide diuretic, what problem would predispose the client to drug toxicity?

    ① Hyponatremia
    ② Hypercalcemia
    ③ Hypophosphatemia
    ④ Hypokalemia

21. To prevent drug hypokalemia, you should teach your client to increase the intake of:

    ① Milk
    ② Oranges
    ③ Fresh vegetables
    ④ Cheeses

22. Daily weights are ordered for clients on diuretics to monitor:

    ① Fluid balance
    ② Body fat
    ③ Blood volume
    ④ Appetite

23. Your client with congestive heart failure suddenly exhibits respiratory distress with frothy sputum. The nurse realizes that the client has probably developed:

    ① A pulmonary embolus
    ② Right-sided heart failure
    ③ Pulmonary edema
    ④ Cor pulmonale

24. Your client is scheduled for a chest radiograph. Preparation for this test includes:

    ① Wearing of only a hospital gown
    ② Nothing by mouth for 8 hours
    ③ A cleansing enema before the test
    ④ Injection of a dye into the trachea

25. The physician performs a bronchoscopy on an elderly client who is suffering from increasing respiratory distress. When the client returns from the test, the nurse must:

    ① Realize that the client will not be able to speak for several hours
    ② Suction the client frequently for the next 24 hours
    ③ Provide cool gargles to prevent bleeding
    ④ Withhold food and fluids until the gag reflex returns

26. Which of the following manifestations should be promptly reported if it occurs after the bronchoscopy?

    ① Blood-streaked sputum
    ② Swelling of the neck
    ③ Hoarseness
    ④ Discomfort when swallowing

27. The physician orders that an elderly client with respiratory distress receive oxygen. The nurse's primary responsibility for this includes:

    ① Explaining the dangers of it to the client
    ② Preventing the client from becoming dependent on the oxygen
    ③ Administering the oxygen with the same care as any medication
    ④ Adjusting the flow as needed based on assessments of cyanosis

28. The most accurate way to determine the need for oxygen in a client with COPD is by:

    ① Observing the skin color
    ② Noting changes in the vital signs
    ③ Asking the client how he or she feels
    ④ Blood gas analysis

29. Your client has been diagnosed as having COPD. The physician orders postural drainage. The purpose of this is to:

    ① Increase the blood supply to the lungs
    ② Strengthen the respiratory drive
    ③ Remove fluid from the pleural cavity
    ④ Remove mucus from the bronchial tree and lungs

30. The best time for the postural drainage to be done is:

    ① Before breakfast and dinner
    ② Right before visiting hours
    ③ Only during the night shift
    ④ After breakfast and lunch

31. You are teaching your client with chronic lung disease to cough and deep breathe effectively. Which of the following would *not* be included in your instructions?

    ① Assume a sitting position, leaning forward slightly
    ② Feel the breaths distend your abdomen
    ③ Exhale quickly and cough forcefully
    ④ Splint the chest and abdomen with a pillow

32. Your client with chronic lung disease has sputum that is:

    ① Thick and tenacious
    ② Thin and watery
    ③ Blood-tinged and frothy
    ④ Highly contagious

33. A thoracentesis is done to remove fluids from the:

    ① Spaces around the alveoli
    ② Bronchioles and main bronchi
    ③ Pleural space
    ④ Area between the skin and the pleura

34. The most common symptom of thrombophlebitis in the lower leg is:

    ① Cyanosis of the affected limb
    ② Positive Homans' sign in the affected leg
    ③ Severe ankle edema in the affected leg
    ④ Distention of the affected vessels

35. A nursing intervention contraindicated in thrombophlebitis would be:

    ① Maintaining strict bed rest
    ② Turning the client from side to side
    ③ Applying warm packs to the affected leg as ordered
    ④ Massaging the affected leg

36. You are teaching your client about hypertension. You can tell the client that hypertension is best described as a disease that:

① Can be controlled with treatment
② Can be cured
③ Often disappears without treatment
④ Is usually fatal

37. The treatment for hypertension is usually directed at:

① Lowering the blood pressure to below normal levels
② Repairing the damaged blood vessels
③ Increasing the urine output
④ Preventing further damage to the blood vessels

38. Your client has just returned from an above-the-knee amputation. Immediate postoperative care includes:

① Elevating the stump on several pillows for 12–24 hours
② Positioning the client on the unaffected side
③ Leaving the stump flat on the bed with the head of the bed elevated
④ Having the client lie in a prone position

39. The day after surgery for an above-the-knee amputation, the best position for your client to assume for at least 1 hour out of 4 is:

① Prone with the stump straight
② Supine with the stump elevated
③ Sitting with the stump dependent
④ Semi-Fowler's position with the stump on pillows

40. Mr. Carter has returned from surgery for a left lobectomy for cancer of the lung. The surgeon wrote an order to turn the client to the left side and back only. This was done to:

① Facilitate expansion of the left lung
② Prevent hemorrhage
③ Reduce pain
④ Facilitate drainage from the operative area

41. Your postoperative thoracotomy client had a chest tube inserted. When transferring him from the cart to his bed, the nurse must be careful to:

① Disconnect the tube from the drainage bottle
② Keep the drainage bottle below the level of the chest
③ Clamp the chest tube until the client is stable
④ Wait until the physician is present to prevent displacement

42. If a closed chest drainage tube is disrupted:

① Air will enter the thoracic cavity and collapse the lung
② Air will escape the thoracic cavity and expand the lung
③ Water in the drainage bottle will flow into the pleural cavity
④ Hemorrhage will result

43. Postoperatively following a thoracotomy, frequent coughing and deep-breathing exercises are:

① Prohibited because of the severe pain
② Supervised by the surgeon only
③ Needed for adequate ventilation in the unaffected lung
④ Done only if the client is not in too much pain

ANSWERS AND RATIONALES

Guide to item identification (see pp. 4–5 for further details about each category):
  I, II, III, or IV for the phase of the nursing process
  1, 2, 3, or 4 for the category of client needs
  A, B, C, D, E, F, or G for the category of human functioning
  Specific content category by name; i.e., cholecystectomy

1.
(3)
Atherosclerosis is caused by fatty deposits in the lining of the coronary vessels.
IV, 2, B, Coronary artery disease

2.
(2)
Oxygen is one of the most basic needs for life. This is especially true for clients with COPD.
I & IV, 4, B, Pneumonia

3.
(3)
Oxygenation is always a priority in basic health needs, especially in a client with COPD.
II, 4, B, Pneumonia

4.
(4)
Semi-Fowler's position allows for the best expansion of the lungs and best approximates his sleeping position at home.
III, 2, B, Pneumonia & COPD

5.
(3)
Decreased oxygenation leads to fatigue.
I & IV, 2, B, Pneumonia & COPD

6.
(4)
One way to assess improvement in oxygenation is through increased ability to perform activities without increasing dyspnea.
IV, 2, B, Pneumonia

7.
(2)
Antibiotics are used to treat pneumonia, and bronchodilators are used to treat emphysema.
I & IV, 2, B & D, Pneumonia & COPD

8.
(4)
Most leukemias (about 70%) involve changes in the lymphocytes.
I, 2, B, Leukemia

9.
(2)
The increase in the white blood cells, the leukocytes, in leukemia is misleading because most of them are immature and therefore ineffective. The client, therefore, has a lower resistance to infection.
I, 2, B, Leukemia

10.
(1)
A low platelet count is common. Using soft swabs for mouth care decreases the risk of bleeding from the mucous membranes.
III, 2, B, Leukemia

11.
(3)
It is not unusual for the leukemic client to seem irritable and short-tempered. The nurse should accept that this behavior is a part of the disease process.
I, 2, B & G, Leukemia

12.
(4)
Morphine sulfate is the drug of choice for the pain of a myocardial infarction (MI).
IV, 2, B, MI & medications

13.
(3)
It is common for clients to fear death after a near-death experience, especially after a heart attack. These fears usually resolve with honest reassurance.
III, 2 & 3, B & G, MI

14.
(2)
An adverse effect of Coumadin is abnormal bleeding, which may first appear as blood in the stool.
III, 2, B, MI & medications

15.
(3)
Aspirin is also an anticoagulant, and an irritant to the stomach. A combination of the two can lead to increased anticoagulant effects and gastrointestinal bleeding.
III, 4, B, MI & medications

16.
(3)
Warmth to the lower abdomen can safely cause the pelvic vessels to dilate, thereby increasing the blood flow to the extremities.
III, 4, B, Peripheral arterial disease

17.
(1)
Right-sided heart failure is characterized by a back-up of pressure in the venous return, the periphery.
I, 2, B, Congestive heart failure (CHF)

18.
(1)
Fresh fruits are low in sodium, as are most fresh foods.
III, 2, B & F, CHF

19.
(3)
To strengthen the heart and to decrease the edema, the client will need a cardiac glycoside, digoxin, and a diuretic, hydrochlorothiazide.
IV, 2, B & F, CHF

20.
(4)
Thiazide diuretics cause the loss of potassium.
IV, 2, B & F, CHF

21.
(2)
Oranges are high in potassium.
II, 2, B & G, CHF

22.
(1)
An indirect way to measure a client's fluid balance is to weigh him or her at the same time, on the same scale, and in the same clothes daily.
III, 1 & 2, B, CHF

23. Left-sided heart failure is characterized by an
③ increased pressure in the pulmonary vasculature leading to pulmonary edema.
IV, 2, B, CHF

24. Preparation for a chest radiograph requires only
① that no metal be above the waist.
III, 1, B, COPD

25. Lidocaine (Xylocaine) is sprayed into the back
④ of the throat to inhibit the gag reflex. Food and
fluid must be withheld until the gag reflex returns to prevent aspiration.
III, 1 & 2, B & D, COPD

26. Swelling of the neck might represent subcutane-
② ous emphysema, which would mean that the
integrity of the lung had been interrupted.
III, 2, B, COPD

27. Oxygen has all the same dangers and entails the
③ same responsibilities as any other medication.
II, 1 & 2, B, COPD

28. With a chronic lung disease client, the only accu-
④ rate way to determine hypoxia is through blood
gases.
I, 2, B, COPD

29. Postural drainage is designed to drain excessive
④ secretions from throughout the bronchial tree.
IV, 1, B, COPD

30. The coughing following postural drainage is ex-
① cessive and could trigger vomiting if done after
meals. Be sure to provide good oral care after
postural drainage to improve the client's appetite.
III, 1, B, COPD

31. Forceful coughing is unnecessary and exhaust-
③ ing. Slow exhalation is the objective for the
chronic lung disease client.
III, 2, B, COPD

32. The sputum of a client with COPD is always
① thick and tenacious. It is difficult to increase
hydration because of the fact that many of these
clients also suffer from congestive heart failure
and are on fluid restrictions.
III, 2, B, COPD

33. Fluid is not normal in the pleural space. A thora-
③ centesis is done to remove this abnormal collection of fluid.
III, 2, B, Thoracentesis

34. Homans' sign is pain in the calf when the foot
② is dorsiflexed. It is a characteristic sign of lower
leg thrombophlebitis.
I, 2, B, Thrombophlebitis

35. Massaging the leg can dislodge the clot, leading
④ to an embolus.
III, 2, B, Thrombophlebitis

36. Hypertension is a lifelong problem that can be
① controlled with diet, medication, and other therapies.
I, 2, A & C, Hypertension

37. The purpose of the treatment in hypertension is
④ to minimize the damage to the blood vessels.
Because the disease has no early warning symptoms, some damage is often found at the time
of diagnosis.
IV, 2, B, Hypertension

38. Elevating the stump for 24 hours postopera-
① tively helps to decrease edema. After 24 hours,
it should never be elevated because this could
lead to a flexion contracture.
III, 2, B & F, Peripheral vascular disease/ampu-
tations

39. Flexion contractures occur easily in lower leg
① amputations if the leg is not extended regularly
for stretching.
II, 2, D & E, PVD/amputations

40. Gravity will help facilitate drainage from the
④ operative site. This also allows the remaining
lung to fully expand.
IV, 2, B, Lung cancer

41. The drainage bottle in closed water seal drainage
② should always be kept below the level of the
lungs.
III, 2, B & D, Chest tubes

42. If the closed drainage system is disrupted, the
① pleura loses the negative pressure and the lung
collapses.
I, 2, B & D, Chest tubes

43. The unaffected lung is prone to underinflation,
③ atelectasis, and infection. Coughing and deep-
breathing exercises are vital to a normal return
of respiratory function.
III, 2, B, Thoracotomy

SENSORY/PERCEPTUAL ALTERATIONS

I. NORMAL FUNCTION

A. Communication System in Body

B. Coordinates Sensory and Motor Activities

C. Receives, Interprets, and Relays Messages

D. Composed of Nerve Cells, Which Have Two Properties in Common: Excitability and Conductivity

Disorders of the Cerebral and Central Nervous System

I. INCREASED INTRACRANIAL PRESSURE

A. Assessment

1. Definition/pathophysiology
   a. pressure of brain matter, intracranial blood volume, and cerebrospinal fluid within skull normally is 15 mm Hg.
   b. because the cranium is rigid, an increase in any substance causes an increase in intracranial pressure
2. Predisposing/precipitating factors
   a. head injury with swelling
   b. stroke
   c. brain tumors
   d. infections
   e. intracranial bleeding
3. Signs and symptoms
   a. level of consciousness—varies from:
      (1) alert and oriented to person, place, and time
      (2) confused or disoriented
      (3) lethargic and obtunded
      (4) comatose, various levels
   b. pupillary response—response on affected side ranges from:
      (1) unilateral dilatation
      (2) sluggish reaction to light
      (3) nonreactive
      (4) fixed and dilated
   c. papilledema
   d. blurred vision
   e. vital signs
      (1) increased systolic blood pressure with widened pulse pressure (decreased diastolic pressure)
      (2) decreased pulse
      (3) decreased, irregular respirations
      (4) elevated temperature
   f. motor function
      (1) weakness: flaccid, paresis
      (2) paralysis of limbs, extremities
   g. sensory function
      (1) paresthesia
      (2) absence of feeling
      (3) reflex activity
         (a) corneal: decreased, absent
         (b) gag: decreased, absent
         (c) Babinski: positive, present
         (d) deep tendon: hyperactive/hypoactive
   h. headache
   i. nausea and vomiting
   j. seizure activity
4. Diagnostic test: presence of signs and symptoms and physical examination
5. Usual treatment
   a. dexamethasone (Decadron) to reduce cerebral edema
   b. osmotic diuretics such as mannitol to decrease cerebral edema
   c. treatment of cause of increased pressure

B. Planning, Goals, Expected Outcomes

1. Client does not develop increased intracranial pressure
2. Client does not develop complications of increased intracranial pressure
3. Client recovers from increased intracranial pressure without permanent damage

C. Implementation

1. Observe for signs and symptoms of increased intracranial pressure
2. Administer medications to decrease pressure as ordered
3. Avoid activities that increase pressure (Table 7-14)

TABLE 7-14 Some Do's and Don'ts in the Care of Clients with Increased Intracranial Pressure

Do:
Conduct neurologic checks at least once every hour unless more frequent monitoring indicated.
Report changes immediately.
Maintain a patent airway and adequate ventilation to ensure proper O_2 and CO_2 exchange.
Elevate the head of the bed 15 to 30 degrees to facilitate return of blood from the cerebral veins.
Use measures to maintain normal body temperature. Elevations of temperature raise blood pressure and cerebral blood flow. Shivering also can increase ICP.
Monitor intake and output.
Give passive range-of-motion exercises.

Don't:
Allow client to become constipated or have any reason to perform Valsalva maneuver.
Hyperextend, flex, or rotate client's head.
Flex the client's hips (as in female catheterization).
Place client in Trendelenburg position for any reason.
Allow client to perform isometric exercises.

From Keane, C. B. (1986). *Essentials of medical-surgical nursing,* 2nd ed. Philadelphia, W. B. Saunders Co.
ICP, intracranial pressure.

a. monitor intracranial pressure lines (4–15 mm Hg if client has one)
b. position properly, with head of bed elevated 30 degrees
c. prevent flexion and hyperextension of neck
d. avoid coughing, straining, Valsalva maneuver
e. monitor fluid and electrolyte balance
f. fluid intake limited (1500–1800 mL/24 hours)
4. Control environment
a. quiet atmosphere
b. reassuring touch without startling
5. Administer treatments appropriate to cause as ordered

D. Evaluation

1. Client does not develop increased intracranial pressure
2. Client does not develop complications of increased intracranial pressure
3. Client recovered from increased intracranial pressure without permanent damage

II. INFECTIOUS CONDITIONS

A. Meningitis

1. Assessment
   a. definition: inflammation of membrane covering brain and spinal cord
   b. incidence: occurs at any age
   c. predisposing/precipitating factors
      (1) complication of another bacterial disease
      (2) could follow penetrating head wound
      (3) could result from exposure to virus
   d. signs and symptoms
      (1) severe, persistent headache
      (2) neck pain and stiffness: nuchal rigidity
      (3) photophobia
      (4) irritability
      (5) nausea, vomiting
      (6) signs of upper respiratory infection
      (7) seizures
   e. diagnostic tests
      (1) spinal tap (lumbar puncture)
         (a) needle inserted into arachnoid space between L-3 and L-4
         (b) sterile technique must be used
         (c) nurse responsible for:
            (i) positioning
            (ii) obtaining materials
            (iii) labeling specimens
            (iv) reassuring client
            (v) bed rest with bed flat for 8 hours to reduce headache

(vi) force fluids to replace cerebrospinal fluid
      (2) neurologic check
   f. usual treatments
      (1) specific antibiotics for causative organism
      (2) anticonvulsants
      (3) supportive care
2. Planning, goals, expected outcomes
   a. client experiences relief of headache pain
   b. client does not have increased seizure activity
   c. client does not develop problems of immobility
   d. client and family are supported emotionally
3. Implementation
   a. room darkened and noise-free
   b. anticonvulsants administered on time
   c. client turned frequently
   d. deep breathing encouraged, no coughing
   e. adequate hydration maintained
   f. all procedures explained to client and family
4. Evaluation
   a. client obtained relief from headaches and discomfort
   b. client did not develop increased seizure activity
   c. client did not develop problems of immobility
   d. client and family verbalized understanding of procedures and treatment plan

B. Encephalitis

1. Assessment
   a. definition: infection and inflammation of brain tissue
   b. incidence: anyone
   c. predisposing/precipitating factors
      (1) exposure to virus
      (2) bite of mosquito or tick
   d. signs and symptoms
      (1) sudden or slow onset
      (2) headache
      (3) fever
      (4) restlessness
      (5) lethargy
      (6) muscular weakness
      (7) coma
      (8) mental confusion
      (9) disorientation
   e. diagnostic tests
      (1) lumbar puncture
      (2) electroencephalogram (EEG)
      (3) good history and physical examination
   f. complications: death

g. usual treatment
   (1) supportive care
   (2) anticonvulsants
   (3) intravenous therapy
   (4) sedative for rest
   (5) steroids (dexamethasone) to reduce cerebral edema
   (6) medication to relieve headache pain, non-narcotics

2. Planning, goals, expected outcomes
   a. client is made comfortable
   b. seizures are decreased
   c. client receives supportive care to prevent complications of immobility
   d. emotional support is given to client and family

3. Implementation
   a. room noise-free and darkened
   b. anticonvulsants administered
   c. client turned frequently
   d. adequate hydration maintained
   e. procedures and client activities explained to family and client

4. Evaluation
   a. client's comfort was maintained
   b. client's seizure activity was decreased
   c. client and family were supported emotionally

III. ACUTE DISORDERS

A. Trauma: Head Injury

1. Assessment
   a. definitions
      (1) concussion: closed head injury
      (2) contusion: brain tissue bruised
      (3) subdural hematoma: venous bleeding; blood-filled swelling between arachnoid membrane and dura mater
      (4) epidural hematoma: bleeding from large artery, medical emergency
   b. incidence: most frequent cause of death between age 1 and 35 years
   c. predisposing/precipitating factor: trauma
   d. signs and symptoms
      (1) outward signs
         (a) bruising
         (b) swelling
         (c) laceration
         (d) bleeding
      (2) signs of increasing intracranial pressure (Chart 7–2)
   e. diagnostic tests
      (1) radiograph of skull; no special preparation

   (2) cerebral angiography
      (a) injection of radiopaque dye into carotid artery to visualize arterial system
      (b) series of pictures taken
      (c) client usually on NPO status
      (d) check for allergies to iodine
      (e) after test: check injection site, level of consciousness, and vital signs
   (3) EEG
      (a) records electrical impulses from brain
      (b) wash hair before test to remove oil so electrodes adhere better
      (c) usually no stimulants, coffee, tea, or certain medications, before test
   (4) brain scan, CT scan
      (a) use of computer to obtain three-dimensional picture
      (b) no special preparation
      (c) no pain
   (5) MRI: similar to CT scan
   f. complications
      (1) exacerbation of symptoms
      (2) death
   g. usual treatment
      (1) conservative first
         (a) maintain open airway
         (b) observe for signs of increased intracranial pressure
         (c) check for leakage of cerebrospinal fluid
            (i) check ears, nose
            (ii) fluid tests positive for glucose on Chemstix; mucus does not
            (iii) on white gauze, cerebrospinal fluid looks clear with dark halo surrounding the fluid
      (2) surgical intervention, if necessary, usually to drain hematoma

2. Planning, goals, expected outcomes
   a. client is aware of possible complications of head injury
   b. client understands diagnostic tests to be performed
   c. client is observed for changes in neurologic status

3. Implementation
   a. head injury instructions are given to client and family if client not admitted to hospital (Chart 7–3)
   b. full explanation of diagnostic tests is given
   c. neurologic check is performed
      (1) level of consciousness
      (2) neuromuscular responses
      (3) pupillary reactions
      (4) vital signs

Chart 7–2
Signs of Increasing Intracranial Pressure

Sign

1. Change in level of consciousness	2. Change in vital signs	3. Change in limb movement	4. Change in pupil size

Nursing Assessment

1. Note change in awareness, whether increasing or decreasing; orientation; decreasing response to stimulation	2. Slowing pulse rate; elevated systolic blood pressure with decreased diastolic blood pressure leading to increased pulse pressure; labored breathing; rising body temperature	3. Extreme restlessness; muscle weakness or paralysis	4. Bilateral or unilateral dilation; unilateral dilation may be sign of cerebral hemorrhage with rapid deterioration

4. Evaluation
    a. client and family aware of potential complications and understand need to return to hospital
    b. client verbalizes understanding of diagnostic tests
    c. client's neurologic checks within normal range

B. Cerebrovascular Accident (Stroke)

1. Assessment
    a. definition
        (1) interruption in blood flow to area of brain
        (2) may be caused by
            (a) cerebral thrombosis
            (b) cerebral hemorrhage
            (c) embolism
            (d) pressure on blood vessel
    b. incidence: third most common cause of death in United States; most common cause of neurologic disability
    c. predisposing/precipitating factors
        (1) hypertension
        (2) atherosclerosis
        (3) heart disease
        (4) obesity
        (5) smoking
        (6) diabetes mellitus
    d. signs and symptoms vary with area of brain affected
        (1) aphasia
        (2) weakness or paralysis
        (3) visual disturbances
        (4) dizziness, ataxia
        (5) confusion
        (6) slurred speech
        (7) headache, loss of consciousness
    e. diagnostic tests
        (1) CT scans, brain scans show areas of ischemia
        (2) lumbar puncture
        (3) angiography
        (4) EEG
    f. complications
        (1) paralysis
        (2) aphasia: all types, e.g., receptive, expressive
        (3) visual disturbances
        (4) death

Chart 7–3 Instructions for Home Care After Head Injury

1. Avoid strenuous physical activities for at least 24 hours after injury.

2. Apply icebag to areas of swelling; continue for at least 24 hours after injury.

3. Give light diet for 24 hours after injury.

4. Arouse client every 2 hours day and night for at least 24 hours.

Call physician immediately or return to emergency department if:

1. Client becomes confused, irrational, disoriented, "talks out of head," or doesn't know where he or she is.

2. Unable to arouse client.

3. Client continues to be nauseated or vomits more than once.

4. Client has trouble with balance.

5. Client complains of double or blurred vision.

6. Headache persists or becomes more intense 12 hours after injury.

---

g. usual treatments
  (1) maintain open airway
  (2) surgical intervention if stroke caused by thrombus or embolus; procedure is end-arterectomy (removal of plaques from inner wall of artery)
  (3) medical
    (a) anticonvulsant drug to prevent seizures
    (b) stool softeners to prevent constipation
    (c) corticosteroids to reduce inflammation
    (d) analgesics to reduce pain and headache
2. Planning, goals, expected outcomes
  a. maintain patent airway and oxygen supply
  b. assess vital signs and neurologic status
  c. maintain fluid and electrolyte balance
  d. ensure adequate nutrition
  e. maintain proper gastrointestinal function
  f. maintain good mouth care
  g. prevent problems of immobility
  h. support client and family emotionally
3. Implementation
  a. loosen clothing and position to maintain open airway

b. assess vital signs and perform neurologic check; notify physician of any changes
c. monitor intravenous and oral fluids
d. offer diet as tolerated; check gag reflex before feeding
e. adjust diet to needs of client, to prevent either constipation or diarrhea; include fruits, fluids, and fiber as tolerated
f. cleanse mouth before each meal to enable client to taste food
g. turn client every 2 hours to prevent pressure ulcers
h. encourage active range of motion to unaffected limbs and passive range of motion to affected areas
i. encourage deep breathing and coughing
j. encourage emotional health by
  (1) explaining activities and procedures to client and family
  (2) assist client to communicate, avoiding frustration
  (3) anticipate needs of client
  (4) place materials that client may need near unaffected extremity
  (5) keep family informed of all progress and procedures
4. Evaluation

a. client returned to optimum health for condition
b. client performed basic activities of daily living alone or with assistance, as dictated by extent of disability
c. client and family able to verbalize feelings related to diagnosis
d. used social service agencies as needed

C. Spinal Cord Injuries

1. Assessment
   a. definition
      (1) injury to spinal cord in which cord is severed or compressed, causing decreased function
      (2) classified according to location
         (a) cervical
         (b) thoracic
         (c) lumbar
   b. incidence: most frequently in men between age 20 and 40 years
   c. predisposing/precipitating factors
      (1) most injuries result from trauma
      (2) accidents: automobile, diving, gunshot wounds, falls
      (3) spinal cord tumors
   d. signs and symptoms
      (1) symptoms occur below level of cord affected
      (2) paralysis
      (3) decreased perspiration in paralyzed area
      (4) bowel and bladder dysfunction
      (5) if cervical
         (a) hypotension
         (b) decreased body temperature
         (c) bradycardia
         (d) respiratory complications
   e. diagnostic tests
      (1) complete physical and neurologic examination
      (2) radiographs
   f. complications
      (1) infections: bladder, lung, pressure ulcers
      (2) mental depression
      (3) death
   g. usual treatments
      (1) immediate care
         (a) handle with extreme care at scene of accident
         (b) head and spine stabilized before transfer
      (2) supportive treatment
         (a) prevent shock
         (b) control hemorrhage
      (3) traction
         (a) Crutchfield tongs
         (b) halo ring and fixation pins
      (4) begin rehabilitation to assist client's return to a productive life
2. Planning, goals, expected outcomes
   a. proper anatomic alignment is maintained
   b. infection is prevented
   c. proper fluid intake and output is maintained
   d. constipation is prevented
   e. likelihood of development of pressure ulcers is reduced
   f. client and family deal with emotional aspects of accident and injury
3. Implementation
   a. client maintained in proper traction and correct positions
   b. provide sterile wound and catheter care to prevent infection
   c. encourage deep breathing and coughing
   d. monitor intake and output; force fluids to prevent bladder problems
   e. encourage diet high in fiber and bulk
   f. encourage high-protein diet
   g. begin bowel retraining program
      (1) establish regular time for elimination
      (2) give laxative, stool softeners, or suppositories as ordered
   h. change client's position frequently to prevent pressure ulcers
   i. encourage client and family to verbalize feelings
   j. refer to psychiatrist, social workers, and other members of support team
4. Evaluation
   a. client recovers physically to highest level of functioning possible
   b. client and family adjust emotionally to condition
   c. complications of immobility decreased or prevented
   d. client maintains adequate food and fluid intake

D. Brain Tumors

1. Assessment
   a. definition: new growth of tissue (benign or malignant) within brain; space-occupying lesion
   b. incidence: dependent on type of tumor
      (1) cause unknown
      (2) 2% of yearly cancer deaths
   c. predisposing/precipitating factors
      (1) heredity
      (2) congenital

(3) radiation

(4) secondary to cerebral trauma

(5) metastases from other sites

d. signs and symptoms: depend on location and rate of growth

    (1) headache*

    (2) nausea and vomiting*

    (3) papilledema*

    (4) signs of increased intracranial pressure (see earlier)

    (5) dizziness

    (6) personality changes

    (7) localized clinical manifestations

        (a) seizure activity

        (b) motor deficits

        (c) sensory deficits

        (d) speech deficits

e. diagnostic tests

    (1) history and physical examination

    (2) visual and fundoscopic examination

    (3) skull radiograph

    (4) EEG

    (5) angiogram

    (6) nuclear magnetic resonance imaging (NMRI)

    (7) CT scan

f. complications

    (1) shock

    (2) uncontrolled intracranial pressure

    (3) seizures

    (4) residual paralysis, paresthesia

g. usual treatment: alone or in combination

    (1) surgery

    (2) radiation

    (3) chemotherapy

2. Planning, goals, expected outcomes

a. client has stable vital and neurologic signs

b. client does not develop signs of increased intracranial pressure

c. client does not develop complications of immobility

d. client recovers from craniotomy without complications

3. Implementation

a. establish and maintain patent airway

b. assess vital signs

c. prevent neck flexion

d. turn every 2 hours

e. body position: dependent on type of craniotomy

    (1) supratentorial: elevate head of bed 30 degrees

    (2) infratentorial: position from side to side, not on back

f. establish baseline neurologic assessment

g. monitor, assess, and evaluate neurologic status in terms of baseline data

h. check level of consciousness

i. vital signs

j. monitor and control intracranial pressure

    (1) position properly with head of bed elevated 30 degrees, unaffected side

    (2) prevent flexion and hyperextension of neck

    (3) avoid coughing, straining, Valsalva maneuver

    (4) monitor fluid and electrolyte balance

    (5) fluid intake limited (1500–1800 mL/24 hours)

k. administer appropriate medications as ordered

    (1) dexamethasone (Decadron) to decrease cerebral edema

    (2) osmotic diuretics, intravenous to decrease intracranial pressure

    (3) phenytoin (Dilantin) to prevent seizures

    (4) cimetidine (Tagamet) to prevent stress ulcers

l. assess for pain and administer analgesic

    (1) codeine as needed

    (2) acetaminophen (Tylenol) as needed

    (3) narcotic analgesics (morphine and meperidine) *contraindicated;* mask symptoms of increased intracranial pressure

m. log rolling (if necessary)

n. eye care: patches to prevent corneal ulcerations if blink reflex absent

o. range-of-motion, passive exercises

p. let family participate in care, activities

q. teach client and family activities of daily living, diet, activity, medication, safety measures

4. Evaluation

a. client's vital and neurologic signs stable

b. client did not develop signs of intracranial pressure

c. client did not develop complications of immobility

d. client recovered from craniotomy without complications

IV. CHRONIC DISORDERS

A. Epilepsy

1. Assessment

a. definition

    (1) abnormal electrical activity of brain resulting in seizure activity

    (2) excessive firing at times, other times normal

---

*Classic triad of symptoms for brain tumor.

(3) classification on basis of origin
  (a) idiopathic—cause unknown
  (b) cause known: e.g., blow on head, endocrine disorder
b. incidence: affects 1%–2% of population; occurs in families with history of disease
c. predisposing/precipitating factors
  (1) unknown problem in brain chemistry
  (2) trauma at birth
  (3) infectious diseases
  (4) inherited disorder
  (5) head injury
  (6) metabolic disorders
  (7) cerebrovascular accident
d. classification of seizures
  (1) generalized seizures
    (a) *absence seizure (petit mal):* brief loss of consciousness, "staring" expression with immediate return to alert state; usually affects children
    (b) *tonic-clonic seizure (grand mal):* tonic (stiffening) and clonic (twitching) phases; may be accompanied by aura, loss of consciousness, incontinence; drowsy after seizure; can progress to status epilepticus, a prolonged seizure with no periods of consciousness; a medical emergency
    (c) *myoclonic seizure:* single or repetitive muscle flexion spasms
    (d) *atonic seizure:* brief loss of posture or muscle tone; person conscious during attack
  (2) partial seizures: involve a localized area of cerebral cortex
    (a) *simple partial:* localized motor or sensory disturbance usually without loss of consciousness
    (b) *complex partial:* psychomotor, temporal lobe seizures; often involves tongue, hands, feet, or trunk; may or may not involve loss of consciousness
e. diagnostic examinations
  (1) initially based on symptoms present
  (2) EEG
  (3) skull radiograph
  (4) lumbar puncture
  (5) brain scan
  (6) cerebral angiography
f. complications
  (1) death from status epilepticus
  (2) school failures related to loss of attention
  (3) emotional disorders related to public's intolerance

g. usual treatments
  (1) drug therapy
    (a) phenytoin
      (i) *action:* stabilizes neuronal membranes, limits seizure activity by controlling passage of sodium ions across cell membrane
      (ii) *use:* grand mal and psychomotor seizures
      (iii) *side effects:* ataxia, slurred speech; gingival hyperplasia, thrombocytopenia, nausea and vomiting
      (iv) *nursing implications:* do not stop drug suddenly; call physician if side effects develop; stress importance of good oral hygiene
    (b) phenobarbital
      (i) *action:* depresses monosynaptic and polysynaptic transmission in CNS
      (ii) *use:* all forms of epilepsy
      (iii) *side effects:* drowsiness, lethargy, nausea and vomiting, rash
      (iv) *nursing implications:* do not stop abruptly
2. Planning, goals, expected outcomes
  a. client and family understand condition and ways to keep it under control
  b. client and family become aware of medications, side effects, and responsibilities
  c. client and family become aware of first aid treatment for seizures
3. Implementation
  a. encourage client and family to discuss feelings related to diagnosis
  b. stress need to comply with medication plan
  c. instruct in side effects of medications
  d. warn not to drink alcohol
  e. refer to social agencies that deal with epilepsy
  f. instructions for emergency care
    (1) do not restrain during seizure
    (2) remove harmful objects
    (3) maintain airway
    (4) protect from environmental dangers
4. Evaluation
  a. client and family understand condition and ways to keep it under control
  b. client and family are aware of medications, side effects, and responsibilities
  c. client and family are aware of first aid treatment for seizures

TABLE 7-15 Antiparkinsonian Drugs

Example	Action	Use	Common Side Effects	Nursing Implications
Levodopa and carbidopa (Sinemet)	Increases level of dopamine in CNS	To control symptoms of Parkinson's disease	Nausea/vomiting, anorexia, orthostatic hypotension, dry mouth, ataxia, headache, dysphagia, anxiety, insomnia, urinary retention, hypertension	Use with caution in clients with cardiovascular, respiratory, endocrine, hepatic disease or with ulcers, glaucoma, diabetes, or psychosis

CNS, central nervous system.

B. Parkinson's Disease

1. Assessment
   a. definition/pathophysiology: group of neurologic symptoms, progressive and debilitating, probably related to absolute lack of dopamine in brain
   b. predisposing/precipitating factors
      (1) idiopathic: primary cause unknown
      (2) atherosclerosis
      (3) drug-induced, especially phenothiazine and *Rauwolfia* tranquilizers
      (4) toxic reaction to substances, such as carbon dioxide and mercury poisoning
      (5) trauma
   c. signs and symptoms
      (1) tremors at rest that decrease with movement and are absent while asleep
      (2) tremors more pronounced with stress
      (3) muscle rigidity
      (4) poor balance
      (5) shuffling gait
      (6) decreased salivation and sweating
      (7) constipation
   d. diagnostic tests
      (1) history and physical examination
      (2) presence of symptoms
      (3) no laboratory or diagnostic abnormalities
   e. usual treatment
      (1) drug therapy: dopamine derivatives to control symptoms (Table 7–15) along with anticholinergics (Table 7–16)
      (2) physical therapy: to maintain mobility and function
2. Planning, goals, expected outcomes
   a. client copes with physical changes
   b. client remains as active as possible
   c. client understands and complies with therapeutic regimen
3. Implementation
   a. support client emotionally
   b. assess client closely after medication is started to ensure optimum dose
   c. encourage client independence
4. Evaluation
   a. client adjusts to physical changes
   b. client remains independent
   c. client follows therapeutic regimen

C. Multiple Sclerosis

1. Assessment
   a. definition/pathophysiology: progressive demyelinating disease of CNS characterized by periods of remission and exacerbation; inflammation and resultant demyelination means that no impulses are transmitted to affected muscles
   b. predisposing/precipitating factors
      (1) young white women
      (2) possible viral origin
      (3) currently unknown cause
   c. signs and symptoms
      (1) early symptoms vague
      (2) motor dysfunctions
         (a) diplopia
         (b) muscle weakness and eventual paralysis
         (c) muscle spasticity
      (3) sensory dysfunctions
         (a) patchy or total blindness
         (b) paresthesia

TABLE 7-16 Anticholinergics

Example	Action	Use	Common Side Effects	Nursing Implications
Atropine sulfate	Inhibits the effect of acetylcholine as transmitter for impulses in parasympathetic nervous system at synapses	To treat Parkinson's disease, to decrease saliva and respiratory secretions preoperatively	Dry mouth, blurred vision, acute glaucoma, constipation, dilated pupils, urinary retention, tachycardia	Avoid use in clients with glaucoma, BPH, myasthenia gravis, CHF, and hypertension; monitor vital signs; check for side effects; monitor I & O

BPH, benign prostatic hyperplasia; CHF, congestive heart failure; I & O, intake and output.

(c) neuropathies with pain and burning
(d) tinnitus and deafness
  (4) coordination
    (a) ataxia
    (b) scissors gait
    (c) intention tremors, absent at rest
    (d) nystagmus
    (e) dysphagia
    (f) scanning speech
  (5) mentation
    (a) depression
    (b) labile emotions with inappropriate euphoria
  (6) other
    (a) urinary and bowel incontinence
    (b) sexual dysfunction
    (c) extreme fatigue
  d. diagnostic tests
    (1) no easily available tests
    (2) diagnosis made through analysis of symptoms
    (3) nerve biopsy shows demyelination
    (4) MRI may show demyelination of optic nerve
  e. usual treatment
    (1) symptomatic supportive therapy mainly
    (2) adrenocorticotropic hormone (ACTH) injections to increase client's own cortisol level and induce remissions (Table 7–17)
2. Planning, goals, expected outcomes
  a. client maintains independence and functions as long as possible
  b. client copes with progressive disability
  c. client understands and complies with therapeutic regimen

d. client and family cope with terminal prognosis of disease
3. Implementation
  a. maintain independence
  b. provide emotional support
  c. prevent potential complications associated with decreased mobility
  d. monitor ability to swallow and prevent choking
  e. encourage client to join multiple sclerosis support group
  f. plan with client for discharge and home care
  g. encourage good health practices to keep disease in remission
  h. help client cope with terminal prognosis
4. Evaluation
  a. client maintains independence within limitations of disease
  b. client copes with disability and prognosis
  c. client follows therapeutic regimen

D. Myasthenia Gravis

1. Assessment
  a. definition/pathophysiology: progressive disorder of acetylcholine that inhibits transmission across myoneural junction and produces severe muscle weakness
  b. predisposing/precipitating factors
    (1) probably autoimmune
    (2) no specific risk factors
  c. signs and symptoms
    (1) ptosis
    (2) difficulty chewing and swallowing

TABLE 7-17 Anti-inflammatories

Class	Example	Action	Use	Common Side Effects	Nursing Implications
Steroids	Cortisone acetate	Block inflammatory, allergic and immune responses similar to glucocorticoids	To treat a wide variety of inflammatory, autoimmune, allergic disorders, to replace natural glucocorticoids	Na^+ and water retention, GI ulceration, hypertension, CHF, delayed wound healing, protein breakdown, osteoporosis, cataracts, leukopenia, diabetes, hypokalemia	Advise client to avoid infections; increased needs during stress and illness; monitor for Addison's disease; give with antacids; use low-salt, high-potassium diet; teach client not to stop taking drug without physician's approval
Nonsteroidal drugs	Ibuprofen (Motrin, Advil)	Act by inhibiting prostaglandin synthesis	To reduce inflammation of arthritis and other disorders	Prolonged bleeding time, edema, tinnitus, GI distress, rash	Avoid in clients with ulcers or asthma; teach that it takes weeks to reach full effect; give with food or milk; watch for side effects

CHF, congestive heart failure; GI, gastrointestinal.

(3) severe muscle weakness, gradual at first then increasing

(4) fatigue

(5) eventually, inability to walk

(6) all skeletal muscles weaken, with eventual loss of ability to breathe

d. diagnostic tests

(1) Tensilon test: inject edrophonium (Tensilon), producing immediate increase in muscle strength

(2) inject neostigmine with return of muscle strength

e. usual treatment

(1) if disease is mild, symptomatic treatment with potassium chloride, ephedrine, and guanidine

(2) plasmapheresis

(3) anticholinesterase therapy, neostigmine (Prostigmin) or pyridostigmine (Mestinon), to inactivate acetylcholinesterase and improve muscle strength (Table 7–18)

(4) ACTH and prednisone as immunosuppressive therapy (see Table 7–17)

2. Planning, goals, expected outcomes

a. client maintains independence as long as possible

b. client copes with physical disability

c. client understands and complies with therapeutic regimen

d. client and family cope with terminal diagnosis

3. Implementation

a. monitor for cholinergic crisis from drugs

(1) symptoms of cholinergic crisis

(a) nausea and vomiting

(b) abdominal cramps

(c) diarrhea

(d) blurred vision

(e) pallor

(f) facial muscle twitching

(g) hypotension

(2) have atropine on hand as antidote

b. observe for myasthenic crisis caused by undermedication with cholinergic drugs

(1) symptoms of myasthenic crisis

(a) increased pulse and respiration

(b) increased blood pressure

(c) anoxia, cyanosis

(d) incontinence

(e) decreased urine output

(f) absent cough and swallow reflex

c. provide emotional support

d. teach client to avoid stress

e. educate client about nature of disease

f. teach client correct medication administration and symptoms and treatment of cholinergic crisis

g. avoid drugs that cause dangerous effects, such as CNS depressants, thyroid drugs, "mycin" antibiotics, phenothiazines, and cardiac drugs

h. help client adjust to terminal diagnosis

4. Evaluation

a. client remains independent within physical limitations

b. client accepts diagnosis and nature of disease

c. client follows therapeutic regimen

Eye: Normal Function

I. LOCATION

In protective bony orbit in skull

II. COMPOSITION

Three layers of tissue

A. Sclera

1. Thick, white fibrous tissue

2. Cornea: transparent section over front of eyeball that permits light rays to enter

B. Choroid

1. Middle vascular area

2. Extends to ciliary body, which helps control shape of lens

3. Brings nutrients and oxygen to the eye

4. Front pigment section (iris) gives eye color

5. Pupil lies in center of iris

TABLE 7-18 Cholinergics

Example	Action	Use	Common Side Effects	Nursing Implications
Pyridostigmine bromide (Mestinon)	Inhibits destruction of acetylcholine, promoting stimulation of receptors	To treat myasthenia gravis	Headache, weakness, miosis, bradycardia, abdominal cramps, diarrhea, nausea/vomiting, excess saliva, bronchospasms, hypotension, muscle cramps	Avoid in clients with obstructions, asthma, epilepsy, or ulcers; watch closely for side effects; check vital signs; give before meals

C. Retina

1. Physiology of vision occurs
2. Contains receptors of the optic nerve
3. Neurons shaped like rods and cones
4. Cones permit perception of color, and rods permit perception of light and shade

III. CHAMBERS

A. Anterior

Contains aqueous humor; maintains slight forward curve in cornea

B. Posterior

Contains vitreous humor; keeps eyeball in its spherical shape

IV. CONJUNCTIVA

Mucous membrane that covers eyeball and eyelid; keeps eyeball moist

V. LENS

Transparent structure behind iris that focuses light rays on retina

VI. LACRIMAL APPARATUS

Glands that produce tears to lubricate and cleanse

Visual Disorders

I. CONJUNCTIVITIS

A. Assessment

1. Definition: inflammation of the conjunctiva
2. Predisposing factors: bacteria, viruses, and allergens
3. Signs and symptoms
   a. purulent drainage
   b. itching
   c. eyes erythematous
4. Treatment
   a. ophthalmic antibiotics
   b. antihistamines
   c. baby shampoo lid scrubs

B. Planning, Goals, Expected Outcomes

1. Client administers ophthalmic ointment as prescribed
2. Infection diminishes

C. Implementation

1. Encourage frequent hand washing to prevent transmission to others
2. Cleanse eyelids and remove crusts before administering ophthalmic medications
3. Instruct client how to administer ophthalmic ointment

D. Evaluation

1. No evidence of infection
2. Absence of drainage and itching

II. CATARACT

A. Assessment

1. Definition: transparent crystalline lens becomes clouded and opaque
2. Incidence
   a. higher in clients with diabetes or on steroids
   b. more common in 60s through 80s age group
3. Predisposing factors
   a. congenital
   b. result of diabetes, steroids
   c. senile cataracts as a result of aging process
   d. infections or trauma
   e. radiation therapy to head
   f. overexposure to sun's rays
4. Signs and symptoms
   a. gradual loss of vision
   b. progressive blurring
5. Diagnostic examinations
   a. examination with ophthalmoscope (absence of red reflex)
   b. client history
6. Usual treatments
   a. surgical removal of completely opaque (ripe) lens with or without lens implant
   b. corrective lenses are necessary after surgery unless an artificial lens is implanted at time of surgery

B. Planning, Goals, Expected Outcomes

1. Client verbalizes understanding of usual preoperative and postoperative care and routines

2. Client verbalizes understanding of precautions necessary to prevent infection and dislodgment of implanted lens
3. Client verbalizes understanding of expected effects on vision of cataract extraction and of implantation of lens

C. Implementation

Most done on outpatient basis so that client and significant other must be taught self-care
1. Instruct client to avoid coughing, bending, or rapid head movements
2. Provide bed rest for amount of time prescribed by physician, if at all
3. Maintain client flat in low Fowler's position
4. Have client deep breathe (avoid coughing)
5. Have client avoid straining (give stool softener)
6. Help client avoid vomiting (an antiemetic is usually ordered)
7. Observe and report pain or bleeding
8. Position client on unoperated side
9. Use eyepatch as ordered by physician
10. Insert eye drops as ordered

D. Evaluation

1. Client is free of infection
2. Client's implanted lens is not dislodged

III. GLAUCOMA

A. Assessment

1. Definition: Intraocular pressure increases because of imbalance between production and drainage of aqueous humor as angle of drainage closes
   a. *acute (closed-angle) glaucoma:* dramatic onset of symptoms; immediate treatment is required, usually surgery
   b. *chronic (open-angle) glaucoma:* symptoms develop slowly and may be ignored; if condition is not diagnosed early, there may be permanent loss of vision
2. Incidence
   a. increases over 40 years of age
   b. family history increases risk
3. Signs and symptoms
   a. painless loss of peripheral vision
   b. halos around lights
   c. permanent loss of vision
   d. pain, malaise, nausea and vomiting (late symptoms)

4. Diagnostic examinations
   a. measurement of intraocular pressure
   b. measurement of visual fields
   c. history of symptoms
5. Usual treatments
   a. miotics used to decrease intraocular pressure by constricting pupil and increasing outflow of humor
   b. iridectomy: surgical incision through cornea to remove part of iris to allow for drainage of humor
   c. medications
      (1) agents that decrease the formation of aqueous humor
         (a) carbonic anhydrase inhibitors: acetazolamide (Diamox)
         (b) osmotic diuretics: mannitol (Osmitrol)
         (c) beta-adrenergic blocking agents: timolol (Timoptic)
      (2) direct-acting miotics—parasympathomimetics: carbachol (Isopto Carbachol)

B. Planning, Goals, Expected Outcomes

1. Client is free from pain
2. Client does not suffer permanent loss of vision

C. Implementation

1. Administer eye medications on schedule
2. Inform client that drugs containing atropine should be avoided
3. Inform client that straining and lifting are discouraged

D. Evaluation

1. Client does not experience pain
2. Client's vision loss does not progress

IV. DETACHED RETINA

A. Assessment

1. Definition: sensory layer separates and is unable to receive visual stimuli
2. Incidence: more common among those over age 40 years
3. Predisposing factors
   a. penetrating injury
   b. sudden blow

c. tumors or eye hemorrhage

d. cause frequently unknown

4. Signs and symptoms
   a. spots and flashes of light
   b. floating spots
   c. loss of vision in affected area

5. Preoperative care
   a. client should be on bed rest
   b. cover both eyes with patches to prevent further detachment

6. Surgical treatments
   a. immediate surgery with drainage of fluid from subretinal space so that retina returns to normal position
   b. retinal breaks are sealed by various methods that produce inflammatory reactions
      (1) cryosurgery
      (2) electrodiathermy
      (3) photocoagulation (use of a laser beam)

B. Planning, Goals, Expected Outcomes

1. Client does not develop further loss of vision
2. Client has improved vision after surgery

C. Implementation

1. Postoperative nursing care
   a. physician's orders are specific; provide care individually
   b. client may be kept on complete bed rest for 1 day or longer; sandbags may be ordered on both sides of the head for immobilization
   c. client should not be turned or moved unless movement ordered
   d. both eyes may be covered; client should always have call light within reach
   e. before discharge, client is instructed to avoid jarring or bumping head and not to do any heavy lifting

2. Maintain bed rest preoperatively and postoperatively as ordered

3. Maintain eye patches to prevent further detachment

4. Instructions given to avoid sudden, jarring movements

D. Evaluation

1. Client's vision loss does not progress
2. Client's vision improves following surgery

Hearing: Normal Auditory Function

I. OUTER EAR

Picks up sound waves from environment and takes them to eardrum (tympanic membrane)

II. MIDDLE EAR

Contains the malleus, incus, and stapes bones, which transmit sound waves from the eardrum to the inner ear

III. INNER EAR

Contains the cochlea, which has duct filled with fluid that vibrates when sound waves from stirrup bone strike against it; hair-like cells (organ of Corti) pick up sound waves and transmit them through auditory nerve to hearing center of brain (sense of balance is also located in inner ear)

Auditory Disorders

I. OTOSCLEROSIS

A. Assessment

1. Definition: a result of bony ankylosis of stapes, which interferes with vibration of stapes and transmission of sound to inner ear

2. Incidence
   a. more common among women
   b. hearing loss usually becomes apparent to client during second and third decades of life

3. Predisposing factors: cause unknown, but most clients have family history of disease

4. Signs and symptoms
   a. progressive loss of hearing
   b. tinnitus (ringing or buzzing in the ears)

5. Diagnosis: hearing test

6. Usual treatments
   a. hearing aid
   b. surgery: stapedectomy (removal of diseased bone and replacement with prosthetic implant)

B. Planning, Goals, Expected Outcomes

1. Client verbalizes understanding of usual preoperative and postoperative care and routines

2. Client verbalizes understanding of major precautions necessary to prevent infection and dislodgment of prosthesis

3. Client verbalizes understanding of expected effects of surgery on hearing

C. Implementation

1. Preoperative instructions should include information that movement may cause dizziness for 48–96 hours after surgery
2. Bed rest for 24 hours after surgery is expected to prevent dislodgment of the prosthesis
3. Precautions to avoid dislodgment of prosthesis
   a. avoid blowing nose
   b. avoid coughing and sneezing
   c. if nauseated, request antiemetic agent so that vomiting is avoided
4. reinforce physician's explanation of effects of surgery and explain that edema and accumulation of blood in ear may diminish hearing in operative ear until condition is resolved
5. postoperative care
   a. keep client in supine position or as ordered by physician
   b. do not turn client
   c. have client deep breathe every 2 hours, but do not allow coughing
   d. check for drainage; report excessive bleeding
   e. client may have vertigo when ambulatory; stay with client and advise client to avoid quick movements

D. Evaluation

1. Client is free of infection
   a. afebrile
   b. negative culture specimens of ear drainage
2. Client's prosthesis does not dislodge
   a. improvement in hearing
   b. absence of dizziness and tinnitus

II. ACUTE OTITIS MEDIA

A. Assessment

1. Definition: acute infection of middle ear usually resulting from spread of microorganisms to middle ear through eustachian tube during upper respiratory infections
2. Incidence: more common in young children
3. Signs and symptoms

   a. fever
   b. severe earache
   c. diminished hearing
   d. pus present in auditory canal (if eardrum has perforated)
4. Diagnosis
   a. using otoscope, physician notes that eardrum red and bulging
   b. culture of ear drainage
5. Usual treatments
   a. myringotomy: incision in eardrum that may prevent spontaneous rupture and allow purulent material to escape
   b. antibiotics given to control infection
   c. fluids encouraged
6. Complications
   a. usually occur when otitis media goes untreated
   b. mastoiditis: middle ear connects with mastoid process by complex passages through which infection can travel
   c. scarring or permanent perforation of the eardrum
   d. hearing loss
   e. meningitis
   f. chronic otitis media: chronic discharge from ear, reduction of hearing, and sometimes slight fever

B. Planning, Goals, Expected Outcomes

1. Client is free from earache
2. Client does not experience hearing loss

C. Implementation

1. Client takes medications as prescribed by physician
2. Importance of follow-up ear examination after course of antibiotic therapy stressed
3. Client instructed in symptoms of recurrence of acute otitis media

D. Evaluation

1. Client does not experience earache
2. Client experiences no permanent hearing loss

? QUESTIONS

1. Mr. Daniels is admitted for a neurologic workup. The first test to be performed is a lumbar puncture. He tells you that he does not understand the procedure and does not know what to expect. Your best response to him would be to:

   ① Tell him that you will call the physician to come explain the procedure to him
   ② Explain the proper position for the procedure, tell him to relax and breathe normally, and say that local anesthetic is used to prevent pain
   ③ Explain that the physician will be inserting a large needle into the spinal column and withdrawing some of the fluid from around his spinal cord and brain to test for an infection
   ④ Tell him that someone will explain the procedure when it is time and that there is no need to worry about being hurt or paralyzed by the test

2. The most effective way to help relieve a client's anxiety over a test such as a lumbar puncture is to:

   ① Give the client a brief explanation of the exact procedure
   ② Reassure the client that the physician is experienced in this procedure
   ③ Ask the client exactly what he or she is anxious about and listen to him or her
   ④ Ask the client to write down questions to give to the physician before the test

3. After a lumbar puncture is completed, the client should be:

   ① Encouraged to ambulate
   ② Placed in Trendelenburg position for 2 hours to equalize the pressure
   ③ Encouraged to lie flat for 6–12 hours
   ④ Placed on strict bed rest for at least 48 hours

4. Your client is scheduled for an EEG. The main reason for an EEG is to:

   ① Identify the location of a brain tumor
   ② Diagnose epilepsy
   ③ Administer small shocks and record brain response
   ④ Record the normal electrical activity of brain cells

5. In preparing a client for an EEG, the nurse should:

   ① Sedate the client with phenobarbital
   ② Withhold all medications
   ③ Keep the client awake for 48 hours before the test
   ④ Shampoo the client's hair

6. The nurse is trying to determine a client's level of consciousness. Which of the following is the most appropriate description of a client's level of consciousness?

   ① Alert and able to state name and time
   ② Seems to be comatose
   ③ Remains unable to respond
   ④ Somewhat stuporous and does not know location

7. Which of the following could the nurse chart to give the most objective observation concerning neuromuscular status?

   ① Paralysis of lower extremities
   ② Unable to grip nurse's hand with left hand but strong grip with right
   ③ Weak and lethargic most of the time; confused at frequent intervals
   ④ Poor response to painful stimuli

8. You are to check the client's pupillary response. This is best done:

   ① In a well-lighted room with a flashlight
   ② In a darkened room with a penlight
   ③ After the client has received a mydriatic
   ④ After the client has received a miotic

9. When caring for a client who suffers from dysarthria, it is important for the nurse to:

   ① Administer tube feedings accurately
   ② Maintain adequate fluid intake
   ③ Face the client when speaking so he or she can lip read
   ④ Speak slowly and clearly and allow time for response

10. Which of the following statements regarding meningitis is true? It:

   ① Is simply an inflammation of brain tissue
   ② Can be caused by a tick bite
   ③ Occasionally follows a cerebrovascular accident or cerebral bleed
   ④ Can be caused by a bacterial or viral infection

11. When a client has meningitis, it is important that the nurse:

① Provide a quiet, dimly lit environment for the client
② Ventilate the room properly and provide sufficient sunlight
③ Eliminate strong odors and unpleasant sights to prevent vomiting
④ Allow frequent visits from family to prevent depression from isolation

12. Your client is scheduled for a cerebral CT scan. You can best prepare the client by:

① Premedicating the client for pain
② Keeping the client on NPO status for at least 12 hours before the test
③ Protecting the client from overexposure to radiation
④ Assuring the client that this is a safe and painless test

13. After which of the following operations must vomiting be absolutely prevented?

① A prostatectomy
② A cholecystectomy
③ A colon resection
④ A cataract extraction

14. A high fever often accompanies meningitis. A nursing intervention most helpful in relieving the febrile delirium would be:

① Restraining the client to prevent self-injury
② Applying a warm water bottle to the back of the neck
③ Increasing fluid intake to prevent dehydration
④ Application of cool compresses or an icebag to the head

15. When a client is admitted with a head injury, one of the most important aspects of nursing care would be:

① Restraining the client to prevent self-injury
② Administering phenobarbital to prevent convulsions
③ Carefully monitoring the client's vital signs
④ Turning the client frequently to prevent paralysis

16. Clients with head injuries are not given sedatives because these drugs may:

① Produce coma
② Mask the client's symptoms
③ Increase the client's blood pressure
④ Lead to cerebral hemorrhage

17. If the client has suffered a head injury, there is a risk that cerebrospinal fluid leakage may occur. It should be suspected in head-injured clients with:

① Bleeding from the nose or mouth
② Purulent, thick drainage from the nose or ears
③ Clear yellow or pink-tinged fluid from the nose or ears
④ Watering of the eyes and drainage of mucus from the nose

18. To confirm the presence of cerebrospinal fluid drainage, the nurse should:

① Test the fluid for the presence of glucose
② Send a specimen to the laboratory for diagnosis
③ Test for the presence of albumin
④ Send a culture for sensitivity

19. If there is confirmed leakage of cerebrospinal fluid, the client should be:

① Cautioned against blowing or picking the nose
② Positioned with the head lower than the rest of the body
③ Cautioned against moving the head
④ Encouraged to blow the nose to remove secretions

20. Which of the following is not considered a cause of stroke?

① Cerebral thrombosis
② Cerebral hemorrhage
③ Cerebral encephalitis
④ Cerebral atherosclerosis

21. A client who has had a stroke should have range-of-motion exercises done regularly. This is an important nursing intervention because the:

① Muscles have been damaged by the interruption of blood flow
② Bone and joints have been affected and contractures may occur
③ Part of the brain controlling muscles has been destroyed and will never function normally
④ Use of the muscles may return if complications involving the musculoskeletal system have been prevented

22. When a stroke has been caused by a hemorrhage, the nurse should:

    ① Position the client flat in bed
    ② Have the client cough and deep breathe hourly
    ③ Position the client in semi-Fowler's position
    ④ Administer Coumadin as ordered

23. Approximately half of epileptics who experience grand mal seizures experience a warning sign referred to as a(n):

    ① Prodromal symptom
    ② Aura
    ③ Sequela
    ④ Icteric

24. If the nurse comes on a client having a seizure, the nurse should:

    ① Protect the head from injury and turn the client to the side if possible
    ② Restrain the client to prevent injury
    ③ Place an object between the teeth and move the client to an upright position
    ④ Move the client to the floor and hold the client down

25. When "log rolling" a client to the side, it is important for the nurse to:

    ① Elevate the head of the bed slightly to avoid pressure on the back
    ② Raise the knees slightly to avoid pressure on the hips
    ③ Support the back with pillows and place a pillow between the legs to avoid back strain
    ④ Remove the pillow from under the client's head and place it under the shoulders

ANSWERS AND RATIONALES

Guide to item identification (see pp. 4–5 for further details about each category):

I, II, III, or IV for the phase of the nursing process
1, 2, 3, or 4 for the category of client needs
A, B, C, D, E, F, or G for the category of human functioning
Specific content category by name; i.e., cholecystectomy

1. ② The nurse should explain the procedure in broad terms without interjecting information that will needlessly frighten the client.
III, 1, A & C, Lumbar puncture

2. ③ The best way to reassure a client is first to find out exactly what that client is anxious about.
III, 1, A & C, Lumbar puncture

3. ③ Lying flat for 6 to 12 hours allows the pressure to return to normal and decreases the risk of spinal headache.
III, 1, C, Lumbar puncture

4. ④ An EEG simply records the electrical activity of the brain. It is used to diagnose conditions such as epilepsy.
I, 1, C, EEG

5. ④ The electrodes need to make good contact with oil-free skin.
III, 1, C, EEG

6. ① When collecting and recording data, the most objective description should always be used.
I & II, 2, C, Neurologic assessment

7. ② The statements charted should be as objective and descriptive as possible.
I & II, 2, C, Neurologic assessment

8. ② To see the change in the pupils, the room should be dimly lit and a focused light source used to test the pupils.
I & II, 2, C, Neurologic assessment

9. ④ Dysarthria means that the client has difficulty speaking, so the nurse should speak slowly and clearly and allow time for response.
III, 2, C, Neurologic assessment

10. ④ Meningitis is an inflammation of the membranes covering the brain and spinal cord caused by a virus or bacteria.
I, 2, C & D, Meningitis

11. ① With the photosensitivity and irritability exhibited in clients with meningitis, the environment should be as calm and controlled as possible.
III, 2, C & D, Meningitis

12. ④ The CT scan is a simple, painless test with a variety of uses.
III, 1, C, CT scan

13. ④ The client with a cataract extraction must avoid any activity that would increase intraocular pressure and precipitate acute glaucoma.
II, 2, C, Cataract

14. ④ Cool compresses or icebags applied to the forehead help relieve the febrile delirium.
II, 2, C & F, Meningitis

15. ③ Clients with head injuries may develop increased intracranial pressure, and a widening pulse pressure (the difference between the systolic and diastolic blood pressures) is an early sign of this.
III, 2, A & C, Head injury

16. ② Decrease in the level of consciousness is an important sign in clients with head injuries, and sedatives themselves alter the consciousness.
IV, 2, C, Head injury

17. ① Cerebrospinal fluid is clear, yellowish fluid and often leaks from the nose or ears with severe head injuries.
I, 2, C, Head injury

18. ① Cerebrospinal fluid contains glucose, whereas normal nasal drainage does not.
III, 2, C & D, Head injury

19. ① If the integrity of the skull is disrupted in the nasal region, bacteria from the nose can easily migrate into the cerebrospinal fluid.
II, 2, C & D, Head injury

20. ④ Encephalitis does not cause a stroke.
I, 2, C, Cerebrovascular accident (CVA)

21. ④ A stroke may cause only temporary loss of function, so it is important to prevent contractures so that the client has the opportunity to regain maximal function.
III, 2, C & E, CVA

22. Positioning in semi-Fowler's position allows for
③ increased venous return. Also, intracranial pressure is lessened.
III, 2, C, CVA

23. An aura is the set of symptoms that precede a
② grand mal seizure.
IV, 2, C, Seizures

24. Protecting the head from trauma and decreasing
① the risk of aspiration are the priorities for client safety.
III, 2, C, Seizures

25. Supporting the back and body as an immovable
③ whole is the principle of "log rolling."
III, 1, C & E, Laminectomy

PROTECTIVE FUNCTIONS

Sexually Transmitted Diseases (Table 7–19)

I. CHLAMYDIAL INFECTIONS

A. Assessment

1. Definition/pathophysiology: most common type of sexually transmitted disease; includes spectrum of genital infections caused by *Chlamydia trachomatis*
   a. men—nongonococcal urethritis
   b. women—mucopurulent cervicitis
   c. frequently co-infection of gonorrhea
2. Predisposing/precipitating factors
   a. highest rate in young men and women under age 20
   b. sexually transmitted disease
   c. transmission to neonates of infected mothers during passage through birth canal
3. Signs and symptoms
   a. women
      (1) asymptomatic 70% of time
      (2) burning on urination
      (3) vaginal discharge
   b. men
      (1) asymptomatic 25% of time
      (2) burning on urination
      (3) penile discharge
      (4) swelling of testicles
4. Diagnostic tests
   a. cell cultures most reliable but expensive
   b. antigen detection from genital tract specimen
5. Usual treatment
   a. doxycycline 100 mg orally twice a day for 7 days
   b. tetracycline 500 mg orally four times a day for 7 days
6. Complications
   a. transmission to newborns
   b. reinfection if partner not treated
   c. can lead to cervicitis, salpingitis, and endometritis in women
   d. can lead to prostatitis, epididymitis, and proctitis in men

B. Planning, Goals, Expected Outcomes

1. Client understands how disease is transmitted and how to avoid contact
2. Client understands and complies with therapy
3. Client recovers without permanent complications

C. Implementation

1. Make sure client understands how disease is transmitted and risks of reinfection if sexual behavior not modified
2. Teach client importance of taking full course of medication exactly as directed
3. Encourage client to have sexual partner receive treatment to decrease risk of reinfection
4. Advise client to avoid sex until client and partner cured
5. Discuss use of condoms and spermicide to decrease risk of future infections
6. Explain risk to unborn child to pregnant client

D. Evaluation

1. Client understands how disease is transmitted and how to avoid contact
2. Client understood and complied with therapy
3. Client recovered without permanent complications

II. GONORRHEA

A. Assessment

1. Definition/pathophysiology: common sexually transmitted disease and major public health problem, caused by *Neisseria gonorrhoeae* and easily transmitted from one person to another; most commonly reported disease in United States, although numbers have decreased

TABLE 7-19 Common Sexually Transmitted Diseases (STDs)

Disease	Cause/Incubation Period	Diagnosis	Signs and Symptoms	Complications	Treatment
Chlamydial infections	*Chlamydia trachomatis;* 5 to 10 days or longer	Cell cultures best; antigen detection from genital tract specimens	Women: 50% asymptomatic, dysuria, vaginal discharge Men: dysuria, watery, mucoid penile discharge	Women: mucopurulent cervicitis, salpingitis, endometritis Men: epididymitis, prostatitis, proctitis Newborns: conjunctivitis, pneumonia	Tetracycline or doxycycline
Gonorrhea	*Neisseria gonorrhoeae;* 3 to 6 days	Culture from cervix, rectum, urethra, or pharynx	Women: dysuria, mucopurulent discharge Men: burning on urination, purulent, profuse discharge from urethra	Women: pelvic inflammatory disease progressing to sterility Men: prostatitis, epididymitis, proctitis Neonates: eye infections	Ceftriaxone followed by doxycycline
Genital herpes	Herpes simplex virus type 1 (HSV-1) or type 2 (HSV-2); 3 to 7 days	Isolation of virus in tissue culture; Papanicolaou or Tzanck smears	Vesicular lesions on cervix or penis; systemic including headache, malaise, low-grade fever	Biggest risk to neonate; may be localized or disseminated, seriously compromising infant's chances for survival	Treat symptomatically; oral acyclovir helps, but does not cure
Syphilis	*Treponema pallidum;* 10 to 90 days Primary stage: 2 to 12 weeks Secondary stage: 8 to 30 weeks Latency stage: approximately 10 weeks Tertiary stage: ~5 years	Blood tests: FTA-ABS; VDRL	Primary: chancre on genitals, mouth, or rectum Secondary: skin rash, malaise, fever, sore throat, generalized lymphadenopathy Latency: no symptoms Tertiary: cardiovascular, neurologic and skin changes	Blindness, deafness, brain damage, paralysis, heart disease Newborn: death in utero or after delivery if not treated	Penicillin, tetracycline, doxycycline
HIV infection/AIDS	HIV 7 to 10 years	Blood tests: ELISA; Western blot; history and clinical evaluation; presence of clinical condition as defined by CDC	Fatigue, low-grade fever, weight loss, night sweats, thrush, lymphadenopathy, cough, shortness of breath	Depression of immune system puts client at risk for opportunistic infections; *Pneumocystis carinii* pneumonia and Kaposi's sarcoma are most common	Treat secondary infections; antivirus include zidovudine (AZT), ddI, ddC

Universal Concepts of STDs

Transmission: All STDs are spread via sexual contact. The greater the number of sexual partners, the greater the likelihood of developing an STD.

Latency: Many STDs have a latency period when there are no symptoms—for example, for syphilis, AIDS, and genital herpes—but disease can still be transmitted during intercourse.

Effect on newborn: The presence of an STD during pregnancy will impact on the health of the fetus.

Co-infections: It is common to have more than one STD simultaneously—for example, AIDS and genital herpes, gonorrhea and *Chlamydia.*

Modified from Matassarin-Jacobs, E. (1994). *Saunders review for NCLEX-RN,* 2nd ed. Philadelphia: W.B. Saunders Co., pp. 220–221.
Abbreviations: HIV, human immunodeficiency virus; AIDS, acquired immunodeficiency syndrome; ELISA, enzyme-linked immunosorbent assay; CDC, Centers for Disease Control and Prevention; FTA-ABS, fluorescent treponemal antibody absorption test; VDRL, Venereal Disease Research Laboratory; AZT, azidothymidine (zidovudine); ddI, dideoxyinosine; ddC, dideoxycytidine.

2. Predisposing/precipitating factors
   a. sexually active individuals with multiple partners at greater risk
   b. exposure to microorganism
   c. newborns can contract disease from infected mothers
   d. more common in men than women
   e. often co-infection with *Chlamydia* or syphilis
3. Signs and symptoms
   a. women
      (1) vaginal discharge
      (2) pain in lower abdomen
      (3) burning on urination
      (4) may involve ovaries and tubes, causing sterility
   b. men
      (1) burning on urination
      (2) whitish or yellowish pus discharge from penis
      (3) inflammation of prostate and testes, leading to sterility
   c. both
      (1) may be asymptomatic or symptoms may appear 1–2 weeks after contact
      (2) septic arthritis
      (3) meningitis
      (4) peritonitis
      (5) endocarditis
4. Diagnostic test: culture of organisms from discharge
5. Usual treatment
   a. ceftriaxone (Rocephin) 250 mg intramuscularly given one time
   b. follow with doxycycline (Vibramycin) 100 mg orally twice a day for 7 days
   c. avoid further sexual contact until cultures are negative

B. Planning, Goals, Expected Outcomes

1. Client does not contract gonorrhea
2. Client understands and complies with therapy
3. Client recovers without permanent complications

C. Implementation

1. Teach client about risk to others until infection is cured
2. Ask client about sexual contacts because they all must receive treatment
3. Teach client that successful treatment does not bring immunity
4. Avoid self-contamination through use of gloves and good hand washing
5. Administer medications as ordered

D. Evaluation

1. Client did not develop gonorrhea
2. Client complied with therapy and gonorrhea cured
3. Client recovered without permanent complications

III. SYPHILIS

A. Assessment

1. Definition/pathophysiology: generalized infection caused by spirochete, *Treponema pallidum*, and transmitted mainly through sexual contact, but also through any contact with body fluids
2. Predisposing/precipitating factors
   a. sexual contact with infected persons
   b. multiple sexual contacts increase risk
   c. infants born of infected mothers
   d. contact with infected bodily fluids
3. Signs and symptoms
   a. primary stage
      (1) chancre—hard, painless sore on mucous membranes of mouth or genitalia
      (2) often unnoticed in women because it is in vagina
      (3) sore highly infectious in this stage
      (4) enters blood stream within 3 days
      (5) headache
      (6) enlarged lymph nodes near chancre
      (7) symptoms disappear in 3–8 weeks
   b. secondary stage
      (1) slight malaise and headache
      (2) some clients asymptomatic
      (3) skin rash or sore throat
      (4) loss of patches of hair
      (5) arthritis, neuritis, retinitis
      (6) symptoms eventually subside when disease enters latent period
   c. tertiary stage
      (1) begins 1 year after infection, but serious symptoms may not occur for 4–5 years
      (2) invasion of all body tissues by spirochetes
      (3) CNS involvement common
      (4) may damage cardiovascular system
4. Diagnostic tests
   a. Venereal Disease Research Laboratory (VDRL) blood serum test for primary and secondary stages
   b. examination of cerebrospinal fluid from lumbar puncture for tertiary stage
   c. fluorescent treponema antibody absorption test (FTA-ABS) for all stages
   d. rapid plasma reagin (RPR) may be used

5. Usual treatment
   a. penicillin antibiotic of choice, in one massive, injectable long-acting dose, such as benzanthine penicillin G 2.4 million units intramuscularly in a single dose
   b. if client is penicillin-sensitive, use tetracycline or erythromycin (see Table 7–19)
   c. contact and treatment of sexual contacts

B. Planning, Goals, Expected Outcomes

1. Client does not contract syphilis
2. Client complies with therapy to treat disease
3. Client recovers without long-term or life-threatening complications

C. Implementation

1. Teach client to avoid casual sexual contact to avoid exposure to disease
2. Encourage compliance with therapy
3. Be nonjudgmental
4. Teach client that treatment offers no immunity to further disease
5. Discuss safe sexual practices with clients, such as use of condoms

D. Evaluation

1. Client did not contract disease
2. Client complied with therapy and disease successfully treated
3. No permanent complications occurred

IV. ACQUIRED IMMUNODEFICIENCY SYNDROME (AIDS)

A. Assessment

1. Definition/pathophysiology: severe, life-threatening clinical condition caused by the human immunodeficiency virus (HIV), which suppresses the immune system and damages other organ systems; AIDS is the clinical end-point of HIV infection; mortality rate approaches 100%; although first identified in homosexual men, the largest number of new infections are now in women and teens
2. Predisposing/precipitating factors
   a. transmission of virus possible through contact with infected persons' bodily fluids
   b. unprotected oral, anal, or vaginal intercourse with an infected partner
   c. injectable drug use with contaminated and shared needles
   d. infants born of HIV-positive mothers have about 30% chance of developing disease at birth or shortly after
   e. exposure to infected blood or blood products
   f. health care workers have low rate of exposure if universal precautions used consistently
3. Signs and symptoms
   a. progression of symptoms
      (1) initial acute HIV infection may last 1–2 weeks and cause flu-like symptoms
      (2) some cases asymptomatic with no signs or symptoms for months to years
      (3) symptomatic HIV infection referred to as AIDS-related complex (ARC)
         (a) persistent generalized lymphadenopathy
         (b) chronic diarrhea
         (c) fever of 38° C (100.5° F) or higher for 2 or more months
         (d) drenching night sweats
         (e) fatigue
         (f) unexplained weight loss
      (4) AIDS final clinical stage of HIV infection—current definition includes
         (a) opportunistic infections
         (b) several cancers, including lymphoma and Kaposi's sarcoma
         (c) extrapulmonary tuberculosis
         (d) wasting syndrome
         (e) HIV dementia or sensory neuropathy
   b. clinical categories
      (1) category A: one or more of the following in HIV-infected adult or adolescent. No conditions from category B or C present
         (a) asymptomatic HIV infection
         (b) persistent generalized lymphadenopathy
         (c) acute HIV infection or history of acute HIV infection
      (2) category B: symptomatic conditions in HIV-infected adult or adolescent that are not included in category C and that meet at least one of the following criteria
         (a) conditions attributed to HIV or indicative of defect in cell-mediated immunity
         (b) conditions considered to have clinical course or management complicated by HIV infection
      (3) category C: any condition arising from 1987 definitions for AIDS in adult or adolescent HIV-infected client classified on the basis of both

(a) lowest accurate CD4$^+$ determination

(b) most severe clinical condition diagnosed regardless of client's current condition

4. Diagnostic tests
   a. positive serologic test (enzyme-linked immunosorbent assay or enzyme immunoassay and Western blot)
   b. history and physical examination
   c. presence of clinical condition as defined by Centers for Disease Control case definitions
   d. CD4$^+$ levels
      (1) category I: $\geq$500 CD4$^+$ cells
      (2) category II: 200–499 CD4$^+$ cells
      (3) category III: <200 CD4$^+$ cells
5. Usual treatment
   a. antivirals
      (1) zidovudine (AZT)
      (2) other experimental antiviral agents also used
   b. prophylaxis for *Pneumocystis carinii* pneumonia
      (1) sulfamethoxazole (Bactrim)
      (2) pentamidine (Pentam)

B. Planning, Goals, Expected Outcomes

1. Client develops strategies for coping with changes in function and health status
2. Client understands disease and its transmission
3. Client does not develop infection because of lowered immunity
4. Client understands and complies with treatment regimen
5. Client maintains adequate nutritional intake
6. Client understands how to prevent the transmission of HIV to others and not to engage in unsafe behaviors
7. Client and significant others cope with terminal prognosis

C. Implementation

1. Assist client to express concerns and fears associated with disease
2. Help client cope with changes in health status through support groups or other means
3. Teach client signs and symptoms of disease, and encourage client to report any changes in health immediately to health care provider
4. Help client identify risks to own health and ways to avoid exposure to those risks, such as avoiding people with infections

5. Identify client's need for information concerning transmission of HIV and living successfully with diagnosis
6. Explain need for universal precautions to prevent spread of disease
7. Encourage client to eat nutritious meals and suggest methods for controlling symptoms such as nausea
8. Review with client ways of preventing spread of HIV through sexual abstinence and avoiding sharing of needles and drug equipment
9. Explain the need for HIV testing before pregnancy
10. Suggest counseling and recommend appropriate community agencies for emotional and other types of support

D. Evaluation

1. Client developed strategies for coping with changes in function and health status
2. Client understood disease and its transmission
3. Client does not develop infection because of lowered immunity
4. Client understood and complied with treatment regimen
5. Client maintained adequate nutritional intake
6. Client understood how to prevent the transmission of HIV to others and did not engage in unsafe behaviors
7. Client and significant others accepted terminal prognosis

Skin Disorders

I. BURNS

A. Assessment

1. Definition/pathophysiology: burns are injuries to skin caused by agents such as heat, electricity, chemicals, or radiation
2. Classification
   a. amount of body surface
      (1) "rule of nines," a way of expressing portions of body surface burned
         (a) head and neck: 9%
         (b) anterior trunk: 18%
         (c) posterior trunk: 18%
         (d) each arm: 9%
         (e) each leg: 18%
         (f) genitalia and perineum: 1%
   b. depth of burn, old method
      (1) first-degree: involves epidural layer only
      (2) second-degree: involves superficial to deep dermis

(3) third-degree: involves all layers of dermis, extends into subcutaneous tissues

(4) fourth-degree: includes muscle and bone

c. depth of burn, new method

(1) partial-thickness: epidermal appendages (sweat and oil glands and hair follicles) intact and wound heals itself if no further injury occurs

(2) full-thickness: involves all layers of skin and destruction of epidermal appendages and requires grafting for healing to occur

3. Signs and symptoms

a. first-degree: red, dry skin and pain

b. second-degree: mottled white to cherry-red, skin moist with or without blisters, and extreme pain

c. third-degree: white and leathery to charred dry skin without elasticity and little or no pain

d. fourth-degree: skin charred to dead white, without pain

e. pulmonary involvement: respiratory wheezing or distress, redness of face and neck, or cough and sooty sputum

4. Usual treatment

a. depth of wound assessed

b. intravenous Ringer's lactate to maintain fluid balance and prevent shock

c. pain medication: often intravenous morphine for severe pain

d. continuous replacement of lost fluids with care to prevent fluid overload

e. monitor respiratory status if upper respiratory tract burned

f. open method

(1) wounds left open to air in sterile settings

(2) wet compresses or soaks used to debride burn

g. closed method

(1) occlusive dressings with silver sulfadiazine antibiotic cream to control infection

(2) debridement of wound

h. skin grafting

(1) split-thickness for less severe and shallow burns

(2) full-thickness for severe and deep burns

B. Planning, Goals, Expected Outcomes

1. Client recovers from burns without permanent impairment

2. Client does not develop infection

3. Client maintains positive nitrogen balance and fluid balance so healing can occur

4. Client does not develop contractures

5. Client copes with emotional aspects of burn injury

6. Client understands and complies with therapy for burns after discharge

C. Implementation

1. Emergency treatment

a. minor burns treated with immersion in cold water and application of cold compresses

b. never apply salves or any greasy substance

c. smother burns immediately

d. remove clothes and jewelry that might be holding in heat if not adherent to skin

e. for severe burns, simply cover area with clean occlusive bandage and transfer client to hospital immediately; never try to remove clothes stuck to burn

f. irrigate chemical burns with water

2. Nursing interventions

a. prevention of infection a top priority

b. application of topical medications

c. strict aseptic technique when caring for burns

d. assess scar tissue and prevent contractures

e. encourage prescribed exercises to prevent contractures and maintain function

f. maintain adequate fluid intake

g. monitor intake and output carefully

h. maintain adequate body temperature

i. encourage diet high in protein, vitamin C, iron, and calcium (see Chapter 5)

j. provide emotional support to client and family, especially if burns are disfiguring

k. teach client and family home care for discharge

l. refer to support groups as appropriate

D. Evaluation

1. Client recovered without complications

2. Client did not develop infection

3. Client maintained positive nitrogen balance and good fluid balance

4. Client did not develop contractures

5. Client coped with altered body image caused by burns

6. Client able to care for burns at home

Perioperative Care

I. PREOPERATIVE PERIOD

A. Assessment

1. Laboratory data

a. ECG

b. CBC; make sure hemoglobin at least 10 g/mL and no elevated white blood cells

c. urinalysis
d. liver function studies for clotting factors, albumin, and function
e. chest radiograph
2. Vital signs for baseline normal
3. Allergies
4. Current medications
5. Nutritional status
   a. obesity increases risk in many ways
      (1) venipuncture and intubation harder
      (2) effect of general anesthesia prolonged because agents bind to fat
      (3) more respiratory complications
      (4) time of surgery prolonged
      (5) slowed healing time and more risk of wound disruption
      (6) more easily dehydrated
   b. malnourishment
      (1) protein depletion means poorer healing
      (2) fewer defensive cells to fight infections
      (3) postoperatively, always in catabolic state
6. Chronic health problems that increase risk of surgical problems
   a. heart disease
   b. diabetes
   c. circulatory impairment
   d. respiratory problems such as chronic obstructive pulmonary disease and asthma
   e. circulatory problems
   f. smoking
   g. liver disease
   h. drug or alcohol abuse
7. Psychological readiness
   a. fear of unknown greatest fear
   b. need adequate explanation of procedures and what to expect
   c. assess specific fears of client
8. Spiritual needs
   a. fear of not waking up
   b. often need to speak to clergy
   c. use available resources to meet spiritual needs, such as anointment for Catholics
9. Learning needs
   a. teaching now being done in physician's office or outpatient setting because clients usually not admitted until day of surgery
   b. postoperative exercises
   c. knowledge of surgery and outcome
   d. discharge and home care needs in light of earlier discharge
   e. pharmacologic and nonpharmacologic pain control methods
10. Clients should be told about possibility of predonation of blood for possible use

B. Planning, Goals, Expected Outcomes

1. Client is adequately physically prepared for surgery
2. Client is adequately psychologically prepared for surgery

C. Implementation

1. Client teaching
   a. general information about surgery
   b. coughing and deep breathing
   c. leg exercises
   d. turning
   e. ambulation
   f. pain control
2. Preparation of skin per hospital policy
3. Restriction of oral intake
   a. NPO after midnight
   b. sometimes have intravenous line started for hydration
4. Elimination
   a. GoLYTELY often used to clear bowel before surgery of lower intestine
   b. rarely catheterized before surgery
5. Rest
   a. need good night's sleep, so sedative often given night before surgery
   b. need to remain quiet and rested day of surgery
6. Consent for surgery signed and on chart before any narcotics or sedatives given
7. Immediate preoperative care
   a. surgical gown and cap
   b. all hairpins and metal objects removed
   c. wedding ring may be taped on
   d. all valuables off and safely stored
   e. dentures out and other prostheses removed
   f. identification or allergy bracelet on and correct
   g. have client void before surgery
   h. medication given about 30 minutes before surgery or in holding area to
      (1) reduce anxiety and promote rest
         (a) pentobarbital sodium or secobarbital sodium: sedatives
         (b) hydroxyzine hydrochloride: mild tranquilizer
         (c) meperidine or morphine sulfate: narcotics
      (2) decrease secretion of mucus and other body fluids: atropine sulfate or glycopyrrolate (Robinul)
      (3) reduce nausea and vomiting with hydroxyzine or promethazine hydrochloride

(4) enhance effects of anesthesia, sedatives, narcotics, and tranquilizers
    i. do not allow client up after preoperative medications, raise side rails, lower lights

D. Evaluation

1. Client is physically prepared for surgery
2. Client is psychologically prepared for surgery

II. INTRAOPERATIVE PERIOD

A. Anesthesia

1. Inhalation or general anesthesia—causes total loss of sensation, loss of consciousness, and loss of certain reflexes
2. Intravenous agents
3. Regional anesthesia—reduces all painful sensation to specific area of body without loss of consciousness
    a. topical
    b. rectal
    c. spinal
    d. nerve blocks

B. Safety

1. Verify client identity
2. Position so no pressure on bony prominences
3. Hypothermia induced
    a. slows metabolic rate
    b. slows oxygen consumption
    c. slows bleeding
4. Sponge and instrument counts
5. Precautions against transmission of HIV and other agents—double gloving and goggles to protect mucous membranes
6. Grounding client to prevent electrical burns

III. POSTOPERATIVE PERIOD

A. Immediate Postoperative Period

1. Assessment
    a. level of consciousness
    b. patent airway
    c. vital signs
    d. intravenous fluids
    e. operative site
    f. type of anesthesia
    g. return of movement and sensation with spinal anesthesia
    h. dressing, drains, and other devices

2. Planning, goals, expected outcomes
    a. client recovers from anesthesia without difficulty
    b. client airway remains patent
    c. client does not develop postoperative complications
3. Implementation
    a. position for safety and to maintain patent airway
    b. administer oxygen as ordered
    c. maintain intravenous flow rate
    d. assist in client comfort—administer pain medications as needed
    e. provide warm blankets
    f. have emesis basin available if nausea and vomiting occur
    g. monitor urine output: at least 30 mL/hour
    h. monitor dressing, drainage, wounds
    i. provide emotional support
4. Evaluation
    a. client recovered from anesthesia without difficulty
    b. client airway remained patent
    c. client did not develop postoperative complications

B. General Postoperative Period

1. Assessment
    a. vital signs
    b. symptoms of shock or hemorrhage
    c. dressings
    d. respiratory status
    e. tubes and drains
    f. wound
        (1) infection: presence of any redness or purulent drainage
        (2) dehiscence: any wound separation
        (3) evisceration: protrusion of abdominal contents
    g. elimination
        (1) adequate urinary output; at least 30 mL/hour
        (2) return of peristalsis
        (3) hiccoughs
    h. pain
    i. lower extremities for presence of deep vein thrombosis
    j. emotional reaction to surgery
2. Planning, goals, expected outcomes
    a. client does not develop any complications
    b. client recovers from surgery
3. Implementation
    a. vital signs: compare with preoperative levels
    b. dressings

(1) check hourly first day

(2) reinforce as needed

(3) change using sterile technique as ordered

(4) accurately describe wound and amount, color, and consistency of drainage

c. respiratory status

(1) cough and deep breathe hourly; use incentive spirometer

(2) ambulate

(3) auscultate breath sounds for abnormalities

d. wound care (Table 7–20)

(1) clean wound as ordered using sterile technique

(2) monitor for wound infection, usually 5–7 days after surgery

(3) teach client home care of wound

(4) prevent dehiscence with binder; never apply if wound has already separated

(a) treat dehiscence with bed rest in (semi-Fowler's position with knees gatched), clean dressing, and notification of physician

(b) treat evisceration with bed rest, moist sterile dressing, and preparation of client for return to surgery for reclosure of wound; medical emergency

e. elimination

(1) encourage ambulation

(2) use nasogastric tube to treat nausea, vomiting, and severe distention

(3) increase diet as peristalsis returns (see Chapter 5)

(a) clear liquid

(b) full liquid

(c) soft diet

(d) regular diet

(4) ensure that client voids at least 30 mL/hour and within 8–12 hours after surgery

f. peripheral circulation

(1) use antiembolic hose or sequential pressure boots to prevent phlebitis

(2) encourage early ambulation and leg exercises

TABLE 7-20 Nutrients Influencing Wound Healing

Nutrient	Specific Component	Contribution to Wound Healing
Proteins	Amino acids	Needed for neovascularization, lymphocyte formation, fibroblast proliferation, collagen synthesis, and wound remodeling
		Required for certain cell-mediated responses including phagocytosis and intracellular killing of bacteria
	Albumin	Prevents wound edema secondary to low serum oncotic pressure
Carbohydrates	Glucose	Needed for energy requirement of leukocytes and fibroblasts to function in inhibiting activities of wound infection
Fats	Essential unsaturated fatty acids a. Linoleic b. Linolenic c. Arachidonic	Serve as building blocks for prostaglandins that regulate cellular metabolism, inflammation, and circulation Constituents of triglycerides and fatty acids contained in cellular and subcellular membranes
Vitamins	Ascorbic acid	Hydroxylates proline and lysine in collagen synthesis Enhances capillary formation and decreases capillary fragility A necessary component of complement that functions in immune reactions and increases defenses to infection
	B complex	Serve as cofactors of enzyme systems
	Pyridoxine (B_6), pantothenic and folic acid	Required for antibody formation and white blood cell function
	A	Enhances epithelialization of cell membranes Enhances rate of collagen synthesis and cross-linking of newly formed collagen Antagonizes the inhibitory effects of glucocorticoids on cell membranes
	D	Necessary for absorption, transport, and metabolism of calcium Indirectly affects phosphorus metabolism
	E	No special role known; may be important if there is a fatty acid deficiency
	K	Needed for synthesis of prothrombin and clotting factors VII, IX, and X Required for synthesis of calcium-binding protein
Minerals	Zinc	Stabilizes cell membranes Needed for cell mitosis and cell proliferation in wound repair
	Iron	Needed for hydroxylation of proline and lysine in collagen synthesis Enhances bactericidal activity of leukocytes Secondarily, deficiency may cause decrease in oxygen transport to wound
	Copper	An integral part of the enzyme, lysyloxidase, that catalyzes formation of stable collagen cross-links

Modified from Schumann, D. (1979). Preoperative measures to promote wound healing. *Nurs Clin North Am* 14:683.

(3) assess for Homans' sign, redness, tenderness, or swelling in extremities

g. pain

(1) medicate client with narcotics, anti-inflammatory medications, or use patient-controlled analgesia (PCA) pump for client control

(2) promote comfort through back rubs, repositioning, distraction, and other non-invasive measures

h. provide emotional support as needed

i. discharge teaching

(1) teach normal restrictions such as no lifting, driving, or intercourse, usually for 4–6 weeks

(2) teach care specific to surgery

(3) arrange for visiting nurses or other help as needed after discharge

4. Evaluation

a. client recovered from surgery

b. client did not develop postoperative complications

Immune/Autoimmune Disorders

I. CANCER

A. Assessment

1. Definition

a. abnormal growth of cells, with alteration in cell's DNA that causes cell to multiply rapidly and spread (metastasize) to other parts of body

b. cancer cells take over normal cells' nourishment and space

2. Incidence

a. occurs at any age; some age-specific cancers

b. incidence increases with age

c. often associated with exposure to "carcinogens" (substances in environment that can add to likelihood of cancer development)

3. Predisposing/precipitating factors

a. major risk factors for cancer (Table 7–21)

b. age

c. exposure to chemical carcinogens

d. obesity

e. cigarette smoking

4. Signs and symptoms

a. seven warning signals of cancer (*caution*)

(1) *c*hange in bowel or bladder habits

(2) *a* sore that does not heal

(3) *u*nusual bleeding or discharge

(4) *t*hickening or lump in breast or elsewhere

(5) *i*ndigestion or difficulty swallowing

TABLE 7-21 Major Risk Factors for Cancer

Lung	Heavy smoker over age 50 years Smoked a pack a day for 20 years Cigarette cough Started smoking at age 15 years or before
Breast	Lump or nipple discharge History of breast cancer Close relatives with history of breast cancer Age over 35 years; especially over 50 years Never had children; first child after age 30 years
Colorectal	History of rectal polyps Rectal polyps run in family History of ulcerative colitis Blood in stool Over age 40 years
Uterine cervical	Unusual bleeding or discharge Frequent sex in early teens or with many partners Low-income background Poor care during or following pregnancy Age 40 to 49 years
Uterine endometrial	Unusual bleeding or discharge Late menopause (after age 55 years) Diabetes, high blood pressure, and obesity Age 50 to 64 years
Skin	Excessive exposure to sun Fair complexion Work with coal tar, pitch, or creosote
Oral	Heavy smoker and drinker Poor oral hygiene Chewing tobacco
Ovary	History of ovarian cancer among close relatives Age 50 to 59 years
Prostate	Over age 65 years
Stomach	History of stomach cancer among close relatives Diet heavy in smoked, pickled, or salted foods Some link with blood group A

(6) *o*bvious change in wart or mole

(7) *n*agging cough or hoarseness

b. others specific to site of cancer

5. Diagnostic tests

a. biopsy: surgically taking piece of tissue to examine microscopically

b. radiographs

(1) use of radiopaque liquids; e.g., barium for gastrointestinal tract

(a) nurse needs to be sure ordered preparation given before examination; usually cleansing enemas or NPO or clear liquid diet only

(b) after examination, nurse needs to check for laxative order to aid in elimination of barium

    (2) use of radioactive materials to "scan" body; radioactive material concentrates in tumor areas, creating "hot spots"; no special preparation; client not radioactive

    (3) CT scan

        (a) uses computer and low radiation to obtain three-dimensional picture

        (b) possibly enemas for abdominal scan; explain procedure to client

    (4) MRI

        (a) uses magnetic fields, no radiation

        (b) some clients experience claustrophobia during test

        (c) no preparation except explanation

  c. blood tests, such as PSA level for prostate, carcinoembryonic antigen (CEA) for adenocarcinomas, and CA-125 for ovarian cancer

  d. endoscopy: use of fiberoptic flexible scope to examine internal gastrointestinal system

6. Usual treatment

  a. surgical excision of tumor and surrounding tissues

  b. chemotherapy: use of drugs that interfere with cell metabolism and inhibit tumor growth and spread (Table 7–22)

  c. radiation therapy: use of radiation from x-rays, radium, and other sources to destroy tumor with minimal damage to normal tissue; can be internal or external (Table 7–23)

B. Planning, Goals, Expected Outcomes

1. Client can identify risk factors related to cancer
2. Client knows seven warning signals of cancer
3. Client follows prescribed treatment plan
4. Client is assisted in dealing with side effects of treatment
5. Client participates in continued check-ups for cancer recurrence or prevention
6. Client is assisted to deal with emotional aspects of diagnosis

C. Implementation

1. Assist client to learn side effects of carcinogens such as sun, chemicals, and smoking
2. Modify diet by reducing fat intake and increasing fiber intake (see Chapter 5)
3. Encourage client to use early detection practices, such as breast or testicular self-examination, mammography, or screening tests
4. Identify seven warning signs of cancer

5. Encourage client to participate in treatment process

  a. identify social support system

  b. refer to social service agencies, such as American Cancer Society, Ostomy Association, I Can Cope, for assistance

6. Assist client to take measures to reduce side effects of treatments
7. Make outpatient appointments, arrange follow-up visits, and schedule continued monitoring
8. Help client verbalize feelings concerning diagnosis
9. Make referrals to appropriate resources and people as needed, such as American Cancer Society, Reach for Recovery, psychiatrist, social worker

D. Evaluation

1. Client recovered from treatment of primary cancer
2. Client avoided sun, smoking, and other carcinogens
3. Client modified diet
4. Client kept follow-up appointments
5. Side effects of cancer treatments reduced or coped with
6. Client discussed feelings concerning diagnosis and learned ways to cope
7. Support systems identified and used effectively by client

II. SYSTEMIC LUPUS ERYTHEMATOSUS

A. Assessment

1. Definition/pathophysiology: chronic, systemic, inflammatory disease involving connective tissue and multiple body systems; probably autoimmune in nature; characterized by remissions and exacerbations; variable course of disease
2. Incidence

  a. women more than men

  b. nonwhite women more than white

  c. women most often during childbearing years

3. Predisposing/precipitating factors

  a. drug-induced syndrome: hydralazine (Apresoline) and procainamide (Pronestyl)

  b. stress

  c. genetic predisposition

4. Signs and symptoms

  a. joint inflammation, arthritis-like

  b. insidious onset

  c. extreme fatigue, generalized weakness, and anorexia

TABLE 7-22 Chemotherapeutic Agents (Antineoplastics)

Class	Example	Action	Use	Common Side Effects	Nursing Implications
Alkylating agents	Cyclophosphamide (Cytoxan)	Wide variety of drugs that act to destroy rapidly dividing cells; classified as cell-cycle specific (those that attack cells at a specific point in the process of cell division) or cell-cycle nonspecific (those that act at any time during cell division)	To treat a wide variety of cancers including leukemia, lymphoma multiple myeloma, breast, lung, ovarian	Bone marrow depression in 7 to 14 days, nausea and vomiting, anorexia, alopecia, hemorrhagic cystitis, amenorrhea, sterility	Monitor blood counts closely; teach client safety precautions about low blood counts; use antiemetics preventively; increase fluid intake; administer IV slowly
	Cisplatin (Platinol)		To treat testicular, lung, ovarian, head and neck cancer	Severe nausea and vomiting, anorexia, nephrotoxicity, peripheral neuropathy, ototoxicity, moderate bone marrow depression at 14 to 21 days with high-dose therapy, potassium and magnesium wasting, hypersensitivity	Hydrate well with IV fluids and mannitol before therapy; monitor hearing; assess motor and sensory function; check weight daily; use antiemetics preventively; monitor for allergic reactions; monitor renal function, potassium, magnesium, and CBC
Antimetabolites	Methotrexate (Mexate)		To treat leukemia, lymphoma, ovarian, breast	GI ulceration, severe stomatitis, bone marrow depression in 10 to 14 days, nephrotoxicity, diarrhea, hepatotoxicity, pulmonary toxicity, neurologic symptoms with intrathecal use, photosensitivity	With high-dose therapy, give leucovorin to prevent toxicity, hydrate well, and maintain alkaline urine; monitor CBC and renal function closely; oral hygiene and comfort measures; avoid sun exposure, use sunblock
Antibiotics	Doxorubicin (Adriamycin)		To treat breast, lung, head and neck, pancreas, soft tissue sarcoma, ovarian	Bone marrow depression 10 to 14 days, severe tissue necrosis with extravasation, nausea and vomiting, anorexia, cardiotoxicity, alopecia, stomatitis, diarrhea, red discoloration of urine	Avoid extravasation; monitor cardiovascular function; warn about red urine; provide antiemetic therapy; warn about alopecia; monitor CBC; treat stomatitis
Plant alkaloids	Vincristine (Oncovin)		To treat testicular, neuroblastoma, leukemia, lymphoma, breast lung, multiple myeloma	Neurotoxicity, constipation, peripheral neuropathies, abdominal pain, rare and mild bone marrow depression, alopecia, tissue necrosis with extravasation	Monitor for sensory or motor changes; administer stool softeners; avoid extravasation; observe for neurotoxicity; administer IV slowly
Hormones Androgens	Testosterone propionate	Growth of certain tumors (breast, thyroid, prostate, uterine) depends on specific hormonal environment; altering this environment impairs/arrests tumor growth	Replacement therapy for males; to treat dysmenorrhea and menopause in women; to treat inoperable breast cancer in women	Males: impotence, gynecomastia, epididymitis, bladder irritation; females: hirsutism, amenorrhea, masculinization; both: nausea and vomiting, fluid retention, hypercalcemia with bone metastases	Warn about possible changes in sexual characteristics; use with caution in clients on oral anticoagulants; monitor I & O; check for edema; monitor calcium levels
Antiandrogens	Flutamide (Eulexin)	Antagonizes androgen effects at cellular level; decreases growth in androgen-sensitive tumor	To treat metastatic prostate cancer; used with leuprolide	Diarrhea, nausea, vomiting, loss of libido, impotence, gynecomastia, hot flashes, edema, hypertension	Monitor for GI side effects, warn about side effects concerning sexuality; encourage compliance

Table continued on following page

TABLE 7-22 Chemotherapeutic Agents (Antineoplastics) *Continued*

Class	Example	Action	Use	Common Side Effects	Nursing Implications
Estrogens	Diethylstilbestrol (DES)		Postmenopausal syndrome, amenorrhea due to ovarian failure, suppression of lactation; prostatic cancer; breast cancer	Nausea and vomiting, anorexia, abdominal distention and bloating, spotting, menstrual changes, fluid retention, depression, hypercalcemia, migraines, breast tenderness and enlargement, reduced glucose tolerance, possible uterine cancer, thromboemboli, increased incidence of cardiovascular-associated deaths; males: similar but also development of female secondary sexual characteristics (impotence, loss of libido)	Contraindicated in pregnancy, some breast cancers, thrombophlebitis, thyroid and liver disease; use cautiously in clients with hypertension, migraines, diabetes, and asthma; monitor for edema and congestive heart failure; watch for depression; monitor serum calcium; counsel about sexual dysfunction
Antiestrogens	Tamoxifen (Nolvadex)		To treat estrogen receptor positive breast cancer	Rare transient bone marrow depression, nausea, menstrual irregularity, hot flashes, "flare" reaction (bone and tumor pain), hypercalcemia in women with bone metastases, induces ovulation in premenopausal women	Monitor menstrual function; advise premenopausal women to use birth control; monitor serum calcium level; reassure that flare reaction will subside—not an indication of disease progression; rather, drug effectiveness
Synthetic luteinizing hormone	Leuprolide (Lupron)	Lowers testosterone level with continuous use	To treat advanced prostate cancer; used with flutamide; used in clients who cannot tolerate an orchiectomy or estrogen therapy	Dizziness, headache, decreased libido, impotence, anorexia, increased bone pain, hot flashes, paresthesias	Monitor for increase in bone pain; with vertebral metastasis, watch for loss of function; monitor acid phosphatase for response to therapy; teach client about side effects

Modified from Matassarin-Jacobs, E. (1994). *Saunders review for NCLEX-RN*, 2nd ed. Philadelphia: W.B. Saunders Co.

IV, intravenous; CBC, complete blood count; GI, gastrointestinal; I & O, intake and output.

TABLE 7-23 Radiation Treatment of Cancer

Area Irradiated	Effect	Nursing Management
Abdomen/ pelvis	Cramps, diarrhea	Opium tincture, camphorated diphenoxylate with atropine (Lomotil), low residue diet, maintain fluid and electrolyte balance
Head	Alopecia	Encourage patient to wear wig or head covering
	Mucositis	Mouthwash with viscous lidocaine, cool carbonated drinks, ice pops, soft, nonirritating diet
	Monilial infection	Nystatin mouthwash, avoidance of commercial mouthwash
	Dental caries	Fluoride applied to teeth prophylactically, provide gingival care
Chest	Lung tissue devitalization	No smoking, avoidance of people with upper respiratory infections, provide humidifier, if necessary
	Pericarditis	Control arrhythmias with appropriate agents (procainamide, disopyramide phosphate), monitor for heart failure
Kidneys	Nephritis, lassitude, headache, edema, dyspnea on exertion, hypertensive nephropathy, azotemia, secondary anemia	Maintain fluid and electrolyte balance, watch for signs of renal failure

    d. weight loss
    e. fever—cardinal symptom of exacerbation
    f. "butterfly rash"—raised rash across cheeks and bridge of nose
    g. generalized rash
    h. polymyositis
    i. vasculitis—often direct cause of death
        (1) renal
        (2) CNS
        (3) cardiac
    j. hypertension
    k. peripheral vascular disease
    l. gastrointestinal problems
        (1) pain
        (2) cramping
        (3) nausea and vomiting

    m. pneumonitis
    n. Raynaud's phenomenon
5. Diagnostic tests
    a. CBC
    b. antinuclear antibodies
    c. assessments of affected organ systems
6. Complications
    a. peripheral vascular disease, loss of limbs
    b. hypertension
    c. stroke
    d. renal failure
    e. congestive heart failure
    f. chronic obstructive pulmonary disease
7. Usual treatments
    a. anti-inflammatory drugs
        (1) steroids (see Table 7–17)
        (2) nonsteroidal agents (see Table 7–17)
    b. hydroxychloroquine (Plaquenil), antimalarial for skin lesions
    c. topical steroids
    d. symptomatic treatment to each affected body system; i.e., antihypertensives

B. Planning, Goals, Expected Outcomes

1. Client's skin integrity is maintained
2. Client's pain and discomfort are decreased
3. Client's symptoms are controlled
4. Client copes with altered body image
5. Client develops minimal complications
6. Client maintains maximal level of independence
7. Client understands and complies with medical regimen

C. Implementation

1. Maintain skin integrity
    a. use cool baths
    b. avoid soaps and powders
    c. apply topical steroids as ordered
2. Administer medication as ordered
3. Avoid things that exacerbate disease
    a. sunlight
    b. stress
    c. pregnancy
4. Provide frequent rest periods
5. Encourage maximal independence
6. Provide diet high in protein (unless renal involvement), vitamins, and iron
7. Monitor for easy bruising and injury
8. Educate client about hair care because alopecia may occur
9. Educate client to report fever immediately to health care provider because this is cardinal symptom of disease exacerbation
10. Refer female clients to medical cosmetologist for help with makeup

11. Allow grieving over potential terminal nature of disease

D. Evaluation

1. Client's skin remained intact
2. Client stated relief or control of pain and discomfort
3. Client coped with altered body image
4. Client's symptoms were controlled
5. Client understood and complied with medical regimen
6. Client maintained maximal independence

QUESTIONS

1. A malignant tumor differs from a benign tumor in that the malignant tumor:

   ① Grows more slowly
   ② Spreads more easily
   ③ Is easily removed by surgery
   ④ Is encapsulated

2. The term "metastasis" is best defined as:

   ① The spread of malignant cells to another part of the body
   ② A second primary tumor in a new location
   ③ The presence of malignant cells in a tumor
   ④ Contamination of the tumor with bacteria

3. Cancer is spread in many ways. One way it is *not* spread is:

   ① Through the circulatory system
   ② On surgical instruments and gloves during surgery
   ③ Through sexual intercourse with a person with cancer
   ④ Through the lymphatic system

4. Which of the following would *not* be risk factors for the development of cancer?

   ① Smoking
   ② Asbestos
   ③ Testosterone
   ④ Sunlight

5. Which of the following is *no longer* recommended by the American Cancer Society as a test for early detection of cancer?

   ① Monthly breast self-examination and a yearly mammogram for women over age 50 years
   ② Yearly stools tested for guaiac in all people over age 50 years
   ③ Digital rectal examination for men over age 40 years
   ④ Annual sputum analysis and yearly chest radiograph for smokers

6. To prevent cancer and to screen for its early detection, the nurse must know:

   ① Those at greatest risk for each cancer
   ② The cause of all cancers
   ③ The prognosis for the treatment of all cancers
   ④ The current treatment protocol for each cancer

7. If a person is a heavy smoker and a heavy drinker for years, he or she is at greatest risk for:

   ① Lung cancer
   ② Laryngeal cancer
   ③ Stomach cancer
   ④ Oral cancer

8. A client with cancer is often described as being in remission. This means that the client is:

   ① Cured of the cancer permanently
   ② Free of the cancer for at least 5 years
   ③ Free of the cancer for an undetermined time
   ④ Currently having active disease and in need of treatment

9. Cancer in general is most correctly diagnosed by:

   ① A culture
   ② A biopsy
   ③ Laboratory analysis of blood
   ④ Diagnostic radiographs

10. Side effects of external radiation are usually:

    ① Generalized to all body systems
    ② Localized to the area tested
    ③ Minimal if the dose is given all at once
    ④ Serious and potentially life-threatening

11. When caring for the client receiving external radiation, the nurse should take extra precautions with the skin over the site of the therapy. Care of this area should include:

    ① Cleansing with soap and water daily
    ② Applying lotion to prevent drying
    ③ Avoiding tight clothing over the site
    ④ Avoiding any contact with the area

12. When radiation therapy is given to the mouth and upper neck, which of the following side effects is likely to develop?

    ① Stomatitis
    ② Alopecia
    ③ Thrombocytopenia
    ④ Leukopenia

13. If the above-listed side effect does develop, the most appropriate nursing intervention to treat it is:

    ① Avoid intramuscular injections
    ② Place the client in reverse isolation
    ③ Encourage the client to wear a wig or scarf
    ④ Administer lidocaine (Xylocaine) gargle before meals as ordered

14. Before caring for the client with cancer, the nurse should know:

① The usual treatment for that cancer
② The client's social support system
③ Whether the client knows the diagnosis
④ The most recent experimental therapy available

15. Gonorrhea is a venereal disease that:

① Is incurable in women
② Can be contracted only once, then the person has immunity
③ Is not highly infectious
④ Can be cured with antibiotics such as penicillin

16. It is difficult to control the spread of gonorrhea because:

① Women with the disease are often misdiagnosed
② Few women have symptoms severe enough to seek treatment
③ The symptoms are similar to those of syphilis
④ Men have so few symptoms of the disease

17. The client receiving chemotherapeutic agents in the treatment of cancer may suffer from numerous side effects, including leukopenia, thrombocytopenia, anemia, and gastrointestinal distress and bleeding. The nurse knows that these side effects occur because:

① Chemotherapeutic agents are toxins
② Both normal and abnormal rapidly dividing cells are destroyed
③ The dosages of chemotherapy are usually higher than they should be to ensure cure
④ Chemotherapeutic agents are lethal to all cells

18. Nursing interventions for the client suffering from leukopenia secondary to chemotherapy would include:

① Protecting the client from infections
② Avoiding venipunctures for blood work
③ Providing for periods of rest
④ Administering antiemetics before meals

19. Nursing interventions for the client with thrombocytopenia secondary to chemotherapy would include:

① Protecting the client from infections
② Avoiding venipunctures for blood work
③ Providing for periods of rest
④ Administering antiemetics before meals

20. Nursing interventions for the client with anemia secondary to chemotherapy would include:

① Protecting the client from infections
② Avoiding venipunctures for blood work
③ Providing for periods of rest
④ Administering antiemetics before meals

21. Nursing interventions for the client suffering from gastrointestinal distress secondary to chemotherapy would include:

① Protecting the client from infections
② Avoiding venipunctures for blood work
③ Providing for periods of rest
④ Administering antiemetics before meals

22. If the client is suspected of suffering from gastrointestinal bleeding secondary to chemotherapy, the nurse should:

① Test all stools and urine for blood
② Administer only cold liquids
③ Avoid venipunctures that could increase blood loss
④ Place the client on complete bed rest

ANSWERS AND RATIONALES

Guide to item identification (see pp. 4–5 for further details about each category):

I, II, III, or IV for the phase of the nursing process
1, 2, 3, or 4 for the category of client needs
A, B, C, D, E, F, or G for the category of human functioning
Specific content category by name; i.e., cholecystectomy

1. The major characteristic of a malignant tumor is its
② ability to spread beyond the limits of normal cells.
I, 2, D & F, Cancer

2. Metastasis involves the spread of a malignant
① cell from its point of origin to another part of the body.
I, 2, D & F, Cancer

3. Cancer cannot be spread through personal contact.
① I, 2, D & F, Cancer

4. All are risk factors except the male hormone
③ testosterone. The nurse should be aware of risk factors to teach and protect clients.
I, 2, D & F, Cancer

5. All are routine screening examinations except
④ the sputum analysis and chest radiograph, which were dropped because they did nothing to improve the early detection of cancer.
I & III, 2 & 4, D & F, Cancer

6. Knowing the risk factors for each type of cancer
① allows the nurse to screen and do health promotion with the correct populations.
I & III, 2 & 4, D, Cancer

7. The combination increases a person's risk for
② cancer of the larynx.
I, 2, D & F, Cancer

8. Remission means that the disease is temporarily
③ under control, but the time it lasts is undetermined.
I, 2, D & F, Cancer

9. A biopsy is the only absolute way to diagnose
② cancer.
I, 2, D, Cancer

10. Side effects from radiation are more likely to be
② localized to the area exposed, although some systemic effects may occur.
I, 2, D, Cancer/radiation therapy

11. The nurse should teach the client to avoid any
③ irritation of the irradiated skin, which may increase the breakdown of the skin.
III, 2, D, Cancer/radiation therapy

12. Stomatitis is the irritation of the mucous membranes caused by either radiation or chemotherapy.
① III, 2, D, Cancer/radiation therapy

13. The mouth is sore with stomatitis, and local anesthesia must be administered before meals or mouth care.
④ III, 2, D, Cancer/radiation therapy

14. Before the nurse cares for the client with cancer,
③ it is important to determine exactly what the client has been told about the condition.
III, 2, D & G, Cancer

15. Gonorrhea can be treated with antibiotics.
④ IV, 4, A & D, Sexually transmitted diseases

16. Only about 20% of women exhibit symptoms of
② gonorrhea, making it difficult to diagnose because most women do not know they have it.
IV, 4, A, Sexually transmitted diseases

17. The side effects of chemotherapy and radiation
② therapy occur because both malignant and normal rapidly dividing cells are destroyed. The cells of the bone marrow and the mucous lining of the gastrointestinal tract are some of the most rapidly dividing cells in the body.
I, 2, D, Cancer/chemotherapy

18. A lowered white blood cell count increases the
① client's risk of contracting an infection.
III, 2, D, Cancer/chemotherapy

19. A low platelet count predisposes the client to
② bleeding. Venipunctures or any injections can lead to subcutaneous bleeding and should be avoided.
III, 2, D, Cancer/chemotherapy

20. Red blood cells are also destroyed by chemo-
③ therapy, leaving the client anemic and fatigued.
III, 2, C & D, Cancer/chemotherapy

21. Gastrointestinal distress occurs because of de-
④ struction of the mucous membrane lining of the tract, which often leads to nausea, vomiting, diarrhea, and anorexia. Antiemetics before meals may help the client to eat.
III, 2, D & F, Cancer/chemotherapy

22. Testing the urine and stools for blood confirms
① the presence of gastrointestinal and urinary tract bleeding.
III, 2, D, Cancer/chemotherapy

MOBILITY, ACTIVITY, COMFORT

Hazards of Immobility

I. GENERALIZED

A. Survival

Adults need mobility to survive

B. Duration

Many and varied problems arise if a client is immobilized for even 24 hours, and problems increase with length of immobilization

C. Avoidance

Most problems can be avoided with proper nursing care

D. Extent

Immobility affects all body systems

II. CARDIOVASCULAR SYSTEM

A. Assessment

1. Blood vessels
   a. muscular activity aids in movement of blood
   b. with no activity, blood flow is sluggish
   c. inadequate nourishment to all cells
   d. decreased flow predisposes to clot formation
2. Workload of heart
   a. heart works harder when body at rest and supine
   b. more frequent use of Valsalva maneuver every time client moves up in bed
3. Blood pressure
   a. orthostatic changes occur within hours
   b. client at risk for fainting or falling

B. Nursing Interventions

1. Exercises to maintain adequate circulation, within limits of client's condition
   a. passive range of motion
   b. active range of motion
   c. isometric exercises
2. Positioning
   a. teach client to change position without using Valsalva maneuver
   b. change position minimally at least every hour and completely every 2 hours
   c. elevate head of bed at intervals
   d. encourage client to move extremities, even a little, as much as possible

III. RESPIRATORY SYSTEM

A. Assessment

1. Pulmonary stasis and accumulation of secretions
   a. wheezing
   b. productive cough
   c. altered respiratory depth and rate
2. Inadequate aeration of lungs
   a. shortness of breath
   b. pain
   c. feeling of tightness in chest

B. Nursing Interventions

1. Have client cough and deep breathe every 2 hours
2. Turn client at least every 2 hours
3. Maintain adequate hydration of at least 2000–3000 mL/24 hours
4. Change position to include semi-Fowler's to Fowler's
5. Support incision or painful area during coughing
6. Medicate as needed to encourage coughing
7. Avoid codeine and other cough suppressants
8. Provide rest periods
9. Give frequent mouth care

IV. GASTROINTESTINAL SYSTEM

A. Assessment

1. Ingestion
   a. decreased appetite
   b. emotions often low so less willing to eat
   c. usually low protein intake
2. Elimination
   a. constipation related to:
      (1) decreased peristalsis
      (2) physical inactivity
      (3) inability to use bedpan
      (4) decreased muscle tone
      (5) embarrassment over using bedpan and asking for help
      (6) amount and type of food eaten
      (7) fluid intake

b. impaction
    (1) absence of stools for 3 days
    (2) may have diarrhea as liquid seeps around impaction

B. Nursing Interventions

1. Check client's dietary intake
    a. provide adequate liquids, 2000–3000 mL/24 hours
    b. increase bulk and roughage in diet (see Chapter 5)
2. Provide privacy for defecation
3. Use bedside commode if at all possible
4. Position client sitting on bedpan if client must remain in bed
5. Encourage client to follow normal bowel habits, must heed urge to defecate
6. Administer stool softeners such as docusate sodium or bulk laxatives such as psyllium (Metamucil) as ordered
7. Institute bowel training program
8. Avoid cathartics or enemas unless absolutely necessary

V. MUSCULOSKELETAL SYSTEM

A. Assessment

1. Range of motion (see Chapter 3)
    a. muscle activity maintains range of motion
    b. without joint motion, muscles lose elasticity and shorten
    c. fibrous tissue develops
    d. contractures may occur and cause permanent damage
2. Osteoporosis
    a. new bone formed because of stress and strain placed on bones by walking and standing
    b. inactivity causes depletion of calcium, phosphorus, and nitrogen in bone
    c. demineralization causes increased bone porosity and increased risk factors

B. Nursing Interventions

1. Prevent footdrop with foot board
2. Use supportive devices to prevent contractures and deformities
3. Active and passive range-of-motion exercises
4. Stand and allow weight bearing if possible
5. Increase calcium in diet through foods such as yogurt, sardines, greens, milk, or cheese (see Table 5–7)

VI. INTEGUMENTARY SYSTEM

A. Assessment

1. Decubitus ulcers: lesions produced by sloughing of inflamed and necrosed tissue
    a. caused by pressure, especially over bony prominence (Fig. 7–2)
    b. caused by shearing force
2. Erythema begins within 1–2 hours of pressure and congestion because of impaired blood flow
3. Breakdown most likely to occur if individual is malnourished, obese, or elderly or has circulatory impairment
4. Other risk factors include warm, moist skin subjected to irritating substances, such as urine, feces, sweat, or other discharges
5. Classification
    a. stage I
        (1) skin is deep pink, red, or mottled
        (2) skin is warm and firm or tightly stretched
        (3) reversible; no permanent skin damage
    b. stage II
        (1) skin blistered, cracked, or abraded
        (2) skin integrity disrupted
        (3) skin around area red and warm
    c. stage III
        (1) skin ulcerated with crater-like sore
        (2) underlying tissues involved
        (3) usually infected
        (4) infection causes continued erosion and copious secretions
    d. stage IV
        (1) deep ulceration and necrosis involving deep underlying muscle and maybe bone
        (2) extensively infected
        (3) ulcer either dry and covered with thick necrotic tissue or wet and oozing

B. Nursing Interventions

1. Prevention of ulcers is much easier than treatment
    a. frequent position changes
    b. pad all bony prominences
    c. support extremities
    d. turn at least every 2 hours or more frequently
    e. use special devices such as egg crate mattress, foam pads, flotation pad, sheepskin, Clinitron bed, or other therapeutic devices to distribute pressure and help prevent breakdown
    f. keep client and all linens clean and dry
    g. use lotion to moisturize skin
    h. massage all potential breakdown areas; do not massage areas once redness has occurred
    i. maintain adequate nutrition and hydration

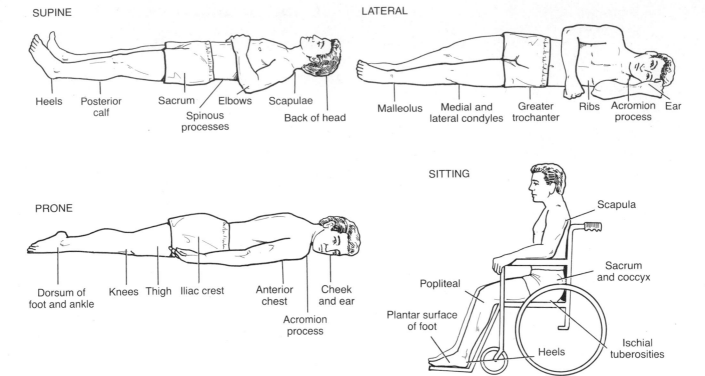

SUPINE

Heels   Posterior calf   Sacrum   Spinous processes   Elbows   Scapulae   Back of head

LATERAL

Malleolus   Medial and lateral condyles   Greater trochanter   Ribs   Acromion process   Ear

PRONE

Dorsum of foot and ankle   Knees   Thigh   Iliac crest   Anterior chest   Acromion process   Cheek and ear

SITTING

Scapula   Sacrum and coccyx   Popliteal   Plantar surface of foot   Heels   Ischial tuberosities

FIGURE 7-2 Bony prominences most susceptible to skin breakdown, according to position. (From Linton, A.D., Matteson, M.A., & Maebius, N.K. (1995). *Introductory nursing care of adults.* Philadelphia: W.B. Saunders Co., p. 259.)

    j. reposition to avoid shearing force of sliding clients

2. Treatment of pressure sores varies by institution
    a. keep ulcer clean and dry
    b. care required constantly to prevent further damage
    c. use protocol established by institution for treatment

VII. URINARY SYSTEM

A. Assessment

1. Stasis common when client is not in upright position
2. When client is supine, urine flow is sluggish and pooling occurs
3. Calculi and infections are common with stasis
4. Loss of bladder tone from distention
5. Lose control of urinary sphincters because of excessive pressure
6. Retention with overflow and incontinence is common

B. Nursing Interventions

1. Encourage adequate fluid intake, at least 2–3 L/day
2. Have client void regularly
3. Restrict calcium intake
4. Encourage acid-ash foods, such as cranberry juice, cereals, fish, meats, and vitamin C, to acidify urine
5. Have women sit and men stand to void to facilitate bladder emptying
6. Use appropriate methods to encourage voiding (see Chapter 3)
7. Catheterize as a last resort; physician's order necessary

VIII. PSYCHOLOGICAL ASPECTS

A. Assessment

1. Loss of independence
2. Sense of hopelessness is common
3. Feelings of isolation and depression
4. Worry over family and financial matters

B. Nursing Interventions

1. Allow maximum independence and decision making on part of client
2. Help client set realistic goals
3. Help client see own worth and maintain dignity
4. Arrange consultations with social services or clergy as needed

Musculoskeletal Disorders
I. TRAUMATIC DISORDERS

A. Casts

1. Assessment
   a. types of casts
      (1) long or short leg casts
      (2) walking casts with extra support for weight bearing
      (3) spica casts cover trunk and one or two extremities
   b. observe closely for pressure on nerves or blood vessels
      (1) monitor "5 Ps":
         (a) pulselessness
         (b) pallor
         (c) pain
         (d) paresthesia
         (e) paralysis
      (2) observe for numbness, tingling, or increased pain
      (3) observe distal tissues for impaired circulation; assess color and warmth by checking blanching
      (4) monitor for signs of infection: elevated temperature, presence of foul odor
      (5) check for warmth or "hot spots" under cast, which could signal inflammation
2. Nursing interventions
   a. allow cast to dry completely before moving it
   b. if moving wet cast, use palms, not fingertips
   c. support cast on pillows
   d. leave cast exposed to air until dry
   e. do not use hair dryer or heat source on cast
   f. cast takes at least 24 hours to dry or longer in higher humidity
   g. keep cast clean, dry, and free from bodily secretions
   h. tape edges of cast to prevent irritation
   i. continually monitor circulation and sensation under cast
   j. monitor for complications
   k. teach client home cast care, especially not to stick objects under cast
   l. elevate casted extremities to decrease normal swelling

B. Traction

1. Assessment
   a. traction: application of mechanical pull to a body part to
      (1) reduce and set a fracture
      (2) immobilize a part
      (3) relieve pain
   b. types of traction (Fig. 7–3)
      (1) skeletal: traction applied directly to bone
      (2) skin: traction applied directly to skin
         (a) Buck's extension: lower extremity, usually to treat fractured hip
         (b) Russell's: for fractured hip or knee
         (c) cervical or pelvic: for cervical or lumbar strain
   c. be sure weights hang free
   d. observe all skin areas for possible pressure sores
   e. monitor pin sites for possible infection
   f. assess for impaired circulation or undue pressure on nerves
2. Nursing interventions
   a. maintain proper body alignment for traction and countertraction
   b. turn and position client as allowed by type of traction
   c. clean pin sites daily and dress per institutional policy
   d. provide diversional activities
   e. use fracture bedpan

C. Fractures

1. Assessment
   a. types of fractures (Fig. 7–4)
      (1) complete: bone broken in two parts with complete separation of parts
      (2) incomplete: bone broken into two parts that do not separate
      (3) comminuted: bone shattered into more than two fragments
      (4) closed or simple: skin not broken
      (5) open or compound: break in skin with protrusion of bone fragments
      (6) greenstick: common in children when bone is partially bent and partially broken
      (7) other types include pathologic, longitudinal, spiral, transverse, and oblique
   b. predisposing/precipitating factors
      (1) old age
      (2) osteoporosis; greatest in postmenopausal women
      (3) trauma
      (4) cancer
   c. signs and symptoms
      (1) pain
      (2) swelling
      (3) deformities
      (4) of fractured hip: leg shortened, abducted, and externally rotated
      (5) inappropriate movement, grating sound on movement

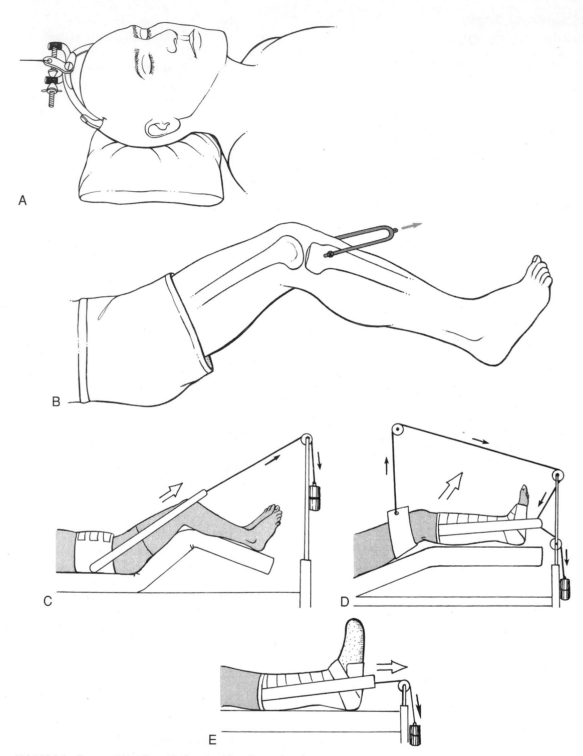

FIGURE 7-3 Types of traction. *A,* Cervical traction using tongs. *B,* Skeletal traction. (*A* and *B* from Monohan, F.D., Drake, T., & Neighbors, M. (1994). *Nursing care of adults.* Philadelphia: W.B. Saunders Co., p. 1363.) *C,* Pelvic traction. *D,* Russell traction, which may be used in the treatment of the shaft of the femur. *E,* Buck's extension. (*C–E,* from Matassarin-Jacobs, E. (1994). *Saunders review for NCLEX-RN,* 2nd ed. Philadelphia: W.B. Saunders Co., p. 277.)

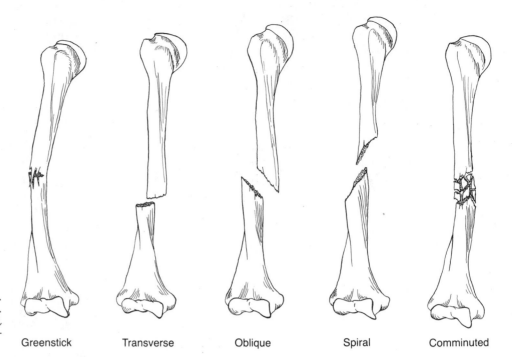

FIGURE 7-4 Types of fractures. (From Matassarin-Jacobs, E. (1994). *Saunders review for NCLEX-RN,* 2nd ed. Philadelphia: W.B. Saunders Co., p. 278.)

Greenstick   Transverse   Oblique   Spiral   Comminuted

d. diagnostic tests
   (1) history of injury
   (2) radiographic examination
   (3) physical examination
e. usual treatment
   (1) goal is to reunite bone fragments in as close to normal alignment as possible, so that bone can heal normally; healing occurs in four stages:
      (a) blood from trauma clots and forms hematoma between broken ends of bone
      (b) granulation tissue forms that becomes firm and becomes link between pieces of broken bone
      (c) new bone tissue enters area, forming woven bone; ends have begun to knit
      (d) immature cells replaced by mature cells, callus formed, tissue resembles normal bone
   (2) closed reduction
      (a) bones realigned without surgery
      (b) once bones are in alignment, cast is usually applied to hold bones in alignment
   (3) open reduction
      (a) surgical realignment of bone fragments
      (b) cast or traction usually applied postoperatively
   (4) internal fixation

      (a) follows open reduction
      (b) application of screws, plates, pins, nails, and so on to hold fragments in alignment
      (c) may also involve removal of damaged bone and replacement with prosthesis
      (d) used for the elderly because it provides immediate bone strength
      (e) increased risk of infection
   (5) external fixation
      (a) sturdy external frame with multiple pins through bone
      (b) used with extensive open fractures with soft tissue damage
      (c) if infected, fractures do not heal properly
      (d) with multiple traumas
      (e) more freedom of movement than with traction
      (f) greater risk of infection with multiple open pin sites
2. Planning, goals, expected outcomes
   a. client has fracture treated and heals without complications
   b. client does not develop problems of immobility
   c. client understands and complies with home care instructions
3. Implementation
   a. monitor circulation and sensation distal to fracture

b. usual postoperative care

c. meticulous care of pin site and incision to prevent infection

d. monitor for pulmonary embolus or with fractures of long bones, fat embolus
   (1) stabbing chest pain
   (2) shortness of breath
   (3) frothy, blood-tinged sputum
   (4) moderate-to-severe respiratory distress
   (5) with fat embolus, petechiae across the chest wall

e. prevent complications of immobility

f. teach client and family home care for discharge

g. for hip pinning
   (1) turn client to unaffected side
   (2) partial weight bearing for affected hip 3–6 months
   (3) out of bed day after surgery
   (4) keep leg abducted with pillows

4. Evaluation

a. fracture healed without complications

b. no complications of immobility occurred

c. client and family understood and followed discharge instructions

II. CHRONIC DISORDERS

A. Arthritis: Rheumatoid Arthritis and Osteoarthritis (Chart 7–4)

1. Assessment

a. definition/pathophysiology
   (1) rheumatoid arthritis
       (a) systemic inflammatory collagen disease causing pathologic changes within joint, leading to permanent deformity
       (b) chronic inflammation of synovial membranes and formation of pannus
   (2) osteoarthritis
       (a) nonsystemic, progressive degenerative joint disease
       (b) degeneration of cartilage with wear and tear with formation of bony buildup, Heberden's nodes

b. predisposing/precipitating factors
   (1) rheumatoid arthritis
       (a) unknown; probably autoimmune in nature
       (b) onset age 30 to 40 years; some instances of juvenile arthritis
   (2) osteoarthritis
       (a) joints of wear and tear
       (b) highly stressed joints
       (c) obesity
       (d) onset rare before age 40 years

c. signs and symptoms
   (1) rheumatoid arthritis
       (a) redness and swelling of joints
       (b) deformity and displacement of proximal joints
       (c) pain on motion
       (d) underweight
       (e) anemia
       (f) chronic low-grade fever, slight leukocytosis
       (g) presence of rheumatoid factors
       (h) muscle atrophy
       (i) morning stiffness
   (2) osteoarthritis
       (a) pain and stiffness on movement
       (b) distal joint enlargement
       (c) presence of Heberden's nodes
       (d) symptoms aggravated by humidity and temperature changes
       (e) weight-bearing joint involvement
       (f) localized, nonsystemic symptoms

d. diagnostic tests
   (1) CBC
   (2) rheumatoid factor
   (3) radiographs

e. usual treatment
   (1) anti-inflammatory agents (see Table 7–17)
       (a) nonsteroidal anti-inflammatories
       (b) steroids
   (2) remissive agents
       (a) gold
       (b) D-penicillamine
       (c) hydroxychloroquine
   (3) orthopedic splints during acute inflammation to prevent deformity
   (4) total joint replacement

2. Planning, goals, expected outcomes

a. client maintains functional abilities as long as possible

b. client copes with diagnosis of chronic disease

c. client understands and complies with therapy

d. client recovers from surgery without complications

3. Implementation

a. balance rest and activity

b. exercise only to point of pain

c. apply heat and cold to control pain

d. administer medications as ordered

e. encourage well-balanced diet

f. assist with discharge planning, including need for home assistance

g. after total hip replacement
   (1) monitor immediately for shock and hemorrhage
   (2) keep leg widely abducted (four pillows) and prevent flexion or external or internal rotation

Chart 7-4
Comparison of Rheumatoid Arthritis and Osteoarthritis

Characteristic	Rheumatoid Arthritis	Osteoarthritis
Definition	A systemic disease, but pathologic changes and disability result from chronic inflammation of the joints	A progressive degenerative joint disease
Pathology	Chronic inflammation of synovial membranes and formation of chronic granulation tissue (pannus) in the joint. Pannus capable of eroding cartilage in joints, and spreading to bone, ligaments, and tendons	Microscopic changes in the cartilage in the joint. Eventually there is loss of cartilage, bony enlargement, and malalignment of joints
Etiology	Unknown. Evidence that the pathologic changes are immunologic	Unknown. May be due to "wear and tear" of aging
Rheumatoid factors (autoantibodies)	Usually present	Usually absent
Age at onset	30 to 40 years	50 to 60 years; rarely before 40
Weight	Normal or underweight	Usually overweight
General state of health	Usually anemic, "chronically ill." Low-grade fever and slight leukocytosis	Well nourished
Appearance of joints	Early: soft tissue swelling Late: ankylosis: extreme deformity Joint involvement usually symmetric and generalized	Early: slight joint enlargement Late: enlargement more pronounced, slight limitation of motion Joints usually involved are weight bearing: spine, hips, knees
Muscles	Pronounced muscular atrophy, particularly in later stages	Usually not affected
Other	Morning stiffness, pain on motion, swelling and tenderness of joints Subcutaneous nodules Typical rheumatoid changes seen on radiograph	Stiffness, relieved by moderate motion; joint malalignment Symptoms increase in cold, wet weather

From de Wit, S.C. (1992). *Keane's Essentials of medical-surgical nursing,* 3rd ed. Philadelphia: W.B. Saunders Co.

(3) prevent infection
(4) teach client home care
  (a) do not lie on operative side
  (b) do not adduct legs, including crossing legs for 1 year
  (c) do not bend or flex hip more than 90 degrees for 1 year
  (d) partial weight bearing for 3 months
4. Evaluation
  a. client remained functional
  b. client coped with diagnosis of chronic disease
  c. client understood and followed therapeutic regimen
  d. client recovered from total joint surgery without complications

B. Ruptured Intervertebral Disc

1. Assessment
  a. definition/pathophysiology: protrusion of disc outside of normal intervertebral space causing pressure on adjacent nerves and nerve roots
  b. predisposing/precipitating factors
    (1) poor body mechanics
    (2) heavy lifting
    (3) prolonged sitting, such as that experienced by long-distance truck drivers
    (4) sudden strenuous exercise
  c. signs and symptoms
    (1) 95% occur in lumbar spine
    (2) pain in lower back radiating down back of leg to foot
    (3) pain increases with walking, sneezing, coughing, or straining
    (4) pain in arm and hand if cervical injury
  d. diagnostic tests
    (1) myelogram: radiopaque dye injected into spinal column to visualize patency of column
      (a) client assumes side-lying, knee-chest position for lumbar puncture
      (b) force fluids after test to decrease risk of spinal headache
      (c) keep client flat for 6–12 hours after test
    (2) radiographs
    (3) electromyogram (EMG)
    (4) CT scan or MRI of spine
  e. usual treatment
    (1) conservative therapy
      (a) bed rest
      (b) cervical or pelvic traction
      (c) hot packs
      (d) medication: muscle relaxants, such as methocarbamol (Robaxin) or diazepam (Valium) (Table 7–24)
      (e) back braces
      (f) special exercises after acute episode
    (2) laminectomy: removal of a portion of vertebra to decrease pressure
    (3) spinal fusion: fusion of two or more vertebrae when multiple vertebrae involved
    (4) chemolysis: chymopapain injections to dissolve affected disc
2. Planning, goals, expected outcomes
  a. client does not develop ruptured intervertebral disc
  b. client recovers without surgery
  c. client recovers from surgery without complications
  d. client understands and complies with therapeutic regimen and exercises to prevent recurrence
3. Implementation
  a. maintain bed rest with client in semi-Fowler's position with knees slightly raised to decrease pressure on spine
  b. administer medications and treatments as ordered
  c. postoperative care
    (1) log-roll client
    (2) use fracture bedpan
    (3) allow men to stand to void
    (4) encourage client to avoid sitting
    (5) prevent constipation
  d. teach client discharge care
  e. encourage client to follow exercises and other instructions

TABLE 7-24 Muscle Relaxants

Example	Action	Use	Common Side Effects	Nursing Implications
Methocarbamol (Robaxin)	Reduces transmission of impulses from spinal cord to skeletal muscles	To treat painful skeletal muscle spasms or other disorders	Drowsiness, lightheadedness, headache, hypotension, gastrointestinal distress, rash	Watch for sensitivity, warn client about impaired mental functioning, avoid alcohol or other depressants, give with food or milk, watch for hypotension

    f. teach client good body mechanics

4. Evaluation

    a. ruptured disc did not occur

    b. client recovered without surgery

    c. client recovered from surgery without complications

    d. client understood and followed therapeutic regimen

?QUESTIONS

1. Mrs. Masters is an elderly woman admitted for a fractured left hip. She had a pinning done yesterday. You know that because of her age and diagnosis, she is at risk for developing decubitus ulcers. Which of the following would *not* be a risk factor for skin breakdown?

   ① Emaciation or obesity
   ② Adequate hydration
   ③ Wrinkles in the sheets
   ④ Urinary incontinence

2. When bathing your elderly client with a fractured hip, you want to prevent skin breakdown on her shoulder of the unaffected side. To prevent skin impairment, the nurse should:

   ① Place a rubber ring under the shoulder
   ② Rub the area vigorously with the fingertips
   ③ Gently massage around the area
   ④ Keep the client positioned only on the back to decrease the pressure on the shoulder

3. A problem your elderly client with a fractured hip is likely to develop because of her age and her diagnosis would be constipation. The most appropriate nursing measure to treat this would be:

   ① Get her up to the bathroom three times daily
   ② Give her milk of magnesia three times a day
   ③ Administer enemas till clear
   ④ Add prune juice and fiber to her diet

4. Andy, age 20 years, fractured his leg while skiing. He is placed in skeletal traction. The primary purpose of skeletal traction is to:

   ① Maintain the client on bed rest
   ② Prevent shifting of the bone fragments
   ③ Reduce and set the fracture
   ④ Relieve the painful muscle spasms

5. Nursing care for a client in skeletal traction must include:

   ① Inspecting and cleaning of pin sites each shift
   ② Turning the client to the unaffected side each shift
   ③ Getting the client up in the chair for meals
   ④ Encouraging the client to exercise both legs

6. After a fracture has begun to heal, a long leg cast is applied. Your client complains that he is now having pain. The most appropriate initial action would be to:

   ① Call the physician
   ② Medicate with the ordered analgesics
   ③ Elevate the casted leg
   ④ Check the circulation of the toes on the casted leg

7. Your client with a long leg cast is complaining that the skin under the cast is itching. Your best intervention to relieve the itching would be to:

   ① Tell the client not to put anything down the cast to scratch it
   ② Ask the physician to order an antipruritic
   ③ Pour some alcohol down the cast
   ④ Tell the client this means that the leg is healing and the cast will be removed soon

8. Betty Olson, age 40 years, is admitted with severe rheumatoid arthritis. The treatment regimen prescribed for Mrs. Olson would most likely be:

   ① Bed rest until all symptoms subside
   ② Daily bicycle riding
   ③ A balance between rest and exercise
   ④ Vigorous exercise followed by complete rest

9. The drug of choice to treat rheumatoid arthritis is:

   ① Aspirin
   ② Acetaminophen
   ③ Codeine
   ④ Copper

10. Side effects of nonsteroidal anti-inflammatories can be avoided if the client takes the drug:

   ① Only at bedtime
   ② With food
   ③ Before arising in the morning
   ④ With at least three glasses of water

11. The type of arthritis seen most commonly in the elderly is:

   ① Acute rheumatoid arthritis
   ② Gouty arthritis
   ③ Osteoarthritis
   ④ Traumatic arthritis

ANSWERS AND RATIONALES

Guide to item identification (see pp. 4–5 for further details about each category):
  I, II, III, or IV for the phase of the nursing process
  1, 2, 3, or 4 for the category of client needs
  A, B, C, D, E, F, or G for the category of human functioning
  Specific content category by name, i.e., cholecystectomy

1. ② Adequate hydration helps to prevent tissue breakdown.
I, 2, E, Immobility

2. ③ Gentle massage helps to restore circulation without causing tissue trauma. Potential breakdown should always be reported and charted.
III, 2, E, Immobility

3. ④ Constipation is associated with decreased mobility and with the decreased peristalsis of age. It is preferable to treat it with dietary measures rather than medications.
III, 2, E, Immobility

4. ③ Skeletal traction actually reduces and sets fractures by direct pull on the bone.
IV, 2, E, Traction

5. ① When a client is in skeletal traction, the pin sites must be cleaned and inspected each shift.
III, 2, D & E, Traction

6. ④ The first action is to check the circulation in the toes and, if it is impaired, to call the physician.
III, 2, E, Fracture/cast

7. ② Never put anything down a cast. Antipruritics such as diphenhydramine (Benadryl) or hydroxyzine (Atarax) help the itching.
III, 2, B, Fracture/cast

8. ③ It is important for the arthritic client to balance rest and activity to maintain function and reduce deformity.
II, 2, E, Rheumatoid arthritis

9. ① Aspirin, a nonsteroidal anti-inflammatory agent, is the drug of choice for arthritis.
III, 2, F, Rheumatoid arthritis

10 ② Aspirin causes gastrointestinal distress and possible gastrointestinal bleeding if taken on an empty stomach. Food helps to decrease this side effect.
III, 2, E, Rheumatoid arthritis

11. ③ Osteoarthritis is a result of the degeneration of the bones that occurs with aging.
I, 2, E, Osteoarthritis

METABOLISM AND ELIMINATION

Endocrine Disorders

Normal endocrine function is shown in Chart 7–5.

I. THYROID

A. Hyperthyroidism

1. Assessment
   a. definition/pathophysiology: disease in which thyroid secretes excessive amounts of triiodothyronine (T_3) and thyroxine (T_4)
   b. predisposing/precipitating factors
      (1) women between age 30 and 50 years
      (2) family history of hyperthyroidism
      (3) may be autoimmune
   c. signs and symptoms
      (1) hypermetabolic symptoms, such as increased metabolic rate and heat production
      (2) weakness and fatigue
      (3) weight loss with increased appetite
      (4) insomnia
      (5) tachycardia and palpitations
      (6) dyspnea
      (7) exophthalmos (protrusion of eyeballs), not reversible with treatment of disease
      (8) goiter
      (9) diaphoresis
      (10) tremors
      (11) premature graying with increased hair loss
   d. diagnostic tests
      (1) T_3 and T_4
      (2) elevated thyroid-stimulating hormone if secondary hyperthyroidism
      (3) client history and physical examination
      (4) thyroid scan
      (5) protein-bound iodine and serum cholesterol
   e. usual treatments
      (1) radioactive iodine 131 (^{131}I)

Chart 7-5
Functions of Endocrine Glands

Gland	Hormone	Action on Target Tissue
Pituitary Anterior lobe	Thyroid-stimulating hormone (TSH); also called thyrotropin	Controls all known activities of thyroid glandular cells; influences body's metabolic processes
	Growth hormone (GH); also called somatotropic hormone (SH) and somatotropin	Causes growth of all tissues capable of growing; enhances protein synthesis, increases utilization of fats, and conserves carbohydrate by decreasing use of glucose
	Follicle-stimulating hormone (FSH)	Stimulates development of ovarian follicles and estrogen secretion; stimulates production of sperm
	Luteinizing hormone (LH)	Affects maturation of ovarian follicles, ovulation, and progesterone secretion; stimulates Leydig cells of testes and testosterone secretion
	Prolactin (PRL)	Maintains corpus luteum and secretion of progesterone; promotes lactation
	Adrenocorticotropic hormone (ACTH); also called adrenocorticotropin and corticotropin	Controls secretion of some of the hormones of the adrenal cortex; e.g., the glucocorticoids (chiefly cortisol and, to some extent, aldosterone and adrenal sex hormones)
Posterior lobe	Vasopressin (VP); also called antidiuretic hormone (ADH)	Elevates blood pressure in relatively high doses; conserves water by decreasing urinary output
	Oxytocin (OT)	Activates uterine contraction and in response to sexual stimulation, transports sperm during coitus; increases secretion of milk
Intermediate part	Melanocyte-stimulating hormone (MSH)	Increases pigmentation of skin
Thyroid	Thyroxine (T_4); also called tetraiodothyronine and levothyroxine; triiodothyronine (T_3); also called liothyronine	Stimulate metabolism (catabolic phase); e.g., increase respiratory rate and utilization of oxygen, production of body heat, gluconeogenesis, strength and force of heart rate, and enhance muscle tone

Chart 7–5
Functions of Endocrine Glands
Continued

Gland	Hormone	Action on Target Tissues
Parathyroid	Calcitonin	Decreases serum calcium
	Parathyroid hormone (PTH); also called parathormone	Maintains constant serum level of calcium
Adrenal cortex	Glucocorticoids (chiefly cortisol)	Increase protein breakdown, impair utilization of glucose, and increase hepatic output of glucose, hence are called diabetogenic hormones; essential for survival under stress
	Mineralocorticoids (chiefly aldosterone)	Promote retention of sodium and loss of potassium and hydrogen in urine
	Androgens and estrogens	See under testes and ovaries
Medulla	Epinephrine, norepinephrine (to a much smaller extent)	Increase cardiac output, elevate blood glucose and blood lipids, raise blood pressure
Ovaries	Estrogens: beta-estradiol, estrone, and estriol	Cause proliferation and growth of sexual organs and other reproductive tissues; induce proliferative phase of the menstrual cycle
	Progesterone	Prepares endometrium for implantation of the fertilized ovum, decreases frequency of uterine contractions, promotes secretory changes in mucosal lining of uterine tubes for nutrition of fertilized ovum, prepares mammary tissue for lactation
Placenta	Human chorionic gonadotropin (hCG)	Maintains the corpus luteum and stimulates progesterone secretion
	Human placental lactogen (hPL)	Acts in combination with prolactin to induce lactation; also promotes growth and acts as an insulin antagonist

Chart continued on following page

Chart 7–5
Functions of Endocrine Glands
Continued

Gland	Hormone	Action on Target Tissues
Testes	Androgens: testosterone, dihydrotestosterone, androstenedione	Promote development of male sex characteristics in fetus, stimulate descent of testes into scrotum, stimulate protein production, responsible for masculinization
Islets of Langerhans of pancreas Beta cells	Insulin	Promotes uptake, storage, and use of glucose, particularly by liver, muscles, and fat tissue, increases transport of glucose into cells and their usage of glucose, causes active transport of many amino acids into cells, promotes protein synthesis and inhibits catabolism of proteins, depresses rate of gluconeogenesis, and has synergistic effect with GH
Alpha cells	Glucagon	Causes glycogenolysis in liver and release of glucose, which raises blood glucose level; increases rate of gluconeogenesis, which causes continued hyperglycemia
Delta cells	Somatostatin	Inhibits secretion of both insulin and glucagon; also secreted by hypothalamus as growth hormone inhibiting hormone
Thymus	Thymosin	Induces differentiation of T-lymphocytes involved in cell-mediated immunity

From Miller, B.F., & Keane, C.B. (1992). *Encyclopedia and dictionary of medicine, nursing, and allied health,* 5th ed. Philadelphia: W.B. Saunders Co. (pp. 494–495).

TABLE 7-25 Antithyroid Agents

Example	Action	Use	Common Side Effects	Nursing Implications
Iodine (SSKI, saturated solution of potassium iodide)	Inhibits thyroid hormone formation, blocks thyroid hormone release	To treat hyperthyroidism	Nausea, metallic taste, rash, hyperemia, fever, headache	Dilute in water or juice, give after meals, store in light-resistant bottles, give with other antithyroid agents
Propylthiouracil (PTU)	Inhibits oxygenation of iodine, blocking iodine's ability to bind with thyroid to form thyroxine	To treat hyperthyroidism	Agranulocytosis, headache, vertigo, nausea and vomiting, rash, arthralgia, loss of taste	Use carefully in pregnancy, watch for signs of hypothyroidism, monitor complete blood count, avoid use of iodine, store in light-resistant container, give with meals

     (2) antithyroid drugs (Table 7–25): drugs must be given several months before surgery to produce euthyroid state
     (3) subtotal thyroidectomy
2. Planning, goals, expected outcomes
  a. client has hyperthyroidism diagnosed and treated before permanent damage occurs
  b. client understands and complies with therapeutic regimen
  c. client recovers from partial thyroidectomy without complications
3. Implementation
  a. preoperative care
     (1) keep client calm and quiet to decrease metabolic rate
     (2) prepare client adequately for tests
     (3) maintain weight through high-calorie diet: 3000–4000 cal/day
     (4) weigh daily
     (5) explain condition, diagnostic procedures, medications, and treatment
     (6) maintain cool environment
     (7) check vital signs regularly
     (8) assist with comfort measures
     (9) monitor for symptoms of thyroid storm and be prepared to act if it occurs
    (10) administer medications as ordered
    (11) prepare client emotionally for surgery
  b. postoperative care
     (1) place client in semi-Fowler's position to facilitate breathing
     (2) monitor for signs and symptoms of parathyroid deficit
      (a) check for hypocalcemia with Chvostek's and Trousseau's signs
      (b) monitor for other signs of tetany, such as numbness and tingling around lips or in extremities
      (c) have calcium gluconate on hand in case symptoms of hypoparathyroidism occur

     (3) have tracheostomy set at bedside and monitor for respiratory distress because of possible laryngeal nerve damage
     (4) monitor for symptoms of thyroid storm, a condition of severe hypermetabolism with severe tachycardia, fever, tachypnea, and possible death from heart failure
     (5) check dressing frequently for tightness and drainage, especially sides and underneath neck
     (6) report difficulty swallowing or talking
     (7) make sure client understands medication usage on discharge; may need lifelong thyroid replacement
     (8) teach client signs of hypothyroidism
4. Evaluation
  a. client diagnosed and treated for hyperthyroidism without permanent complications
  b. client understood and followed therapeutic regimen preoperatively and postoperatively
  c. client recovered from thyroidectomy without complications
  d. client can explain disease, treatment, home care management, and follow-up care

B. Hypothyroidism

1. Assessment
  a. definition/pathophysiology: inadequate production of thyroid hormones leading to hypometabolic state; cretinism is hypothyroidism in childhood; myxedema is hypothyroidism in adulthood
  b. predisposing/precipitating factors
     (1) thyroidectomy
     (2) thyroid treatment
     (3) prenatal thyroid treatment
     (4) inflammation

c. signs and symptoms
   (1) goiter
   (2) symptoms of hypometabolism
   (3) decreased appetite with increased weight gain
   (4) constipation
   (5) slowed mentation
   (6) excessive sleep
   (7) dry, scaly skin and dry hair
   (8) depression
   (9) edema
   (10) accelerated cardiovascular disease with increased serum cholesterol and slowed pulse
   (11) fatigue
   (12) forgetfulness
   (13) sensitivity to cold
   (14) muscle stiffness and pain
   (15) intention tremor
d. diagnostic tests
   (1) high serum cholesterol
   (2) low levels of thyroid hormones
   (3) low thyroid-stimulating hormone secondary to pituitary disease
e. usual treatment
   (1) thyroid medication: levothyroxine (Synthroid), thyroid
   (2) partial thyroidectomy if goiter does not decrease with medications

2. Planning, goals, expected outcomes
   a. client has hypothyroidism diagnosed and treated before irreversible damage occurs
   b. client understands and complies with therapeutic regimen
   c. client knows signs of hyperthyroidism to report
3. Implementation
   a. keep client comfortable and safe
   b. provide protection for skin
   c. provide emotional support
   d. treat constipation with fluids and diet
   e. provide extra warmth for client
   f. teach client lifelong medication regimen
   g. monitor and report changes in vital signs
   h. encourage activity and diet to lose weight
   i. monitor thought process for improvement after treatment begun
4. Evaluation
   a. client did not develop complications of hypothyroidism
   b. client followed therapeutic regimen
   c. client understood signs of hyperthyroidism and when to report them

II. PARATHYROID

A. Hypoparathyroidism

1. Assessment
   a. definition/pathophysiology: drop in parathormone that results in drop in serum calcium level by increasing its excretion in renal tubules
   b. predisposing/precipitating factors
      (1) accidental removal with thyroidectomy
      (2) irradiation of thyroid
      (3) idiopathic atrophy
   c. signs and symptoms
      (1) numbness and tingling around mouth and fingertips
      (2) muscle tetany
      (3) convulsions
      (4) cardiac arrhythmias
      (5) laryngeal spasms
      (6) arrhythmias
      (7) congestive heart failure
      (8) dry, scaly skin
      (9) confusion
      (10) headache
      (11) visual problems, photophobia
      (12) abdominal pain and cramping
   d. diagnostic tests
      (1) serum calcium, decreased
      (2) serum parathormone, decreased
      (3) serum phosphorus, increased
   e. usual treatments
      (1) intravenous calcium gluconate; immediate treatment
      (2) with chronic disease, calcium and vitamin D along with parathyroid hormone replacement
2. Planning, goals, expected outcomes
   a. client is diagnosed and treated for disease before life-threatening complications occur
   b. client understands and complies with therapeutic regimen
3. Implementation
   a. monitor for early signs of tetany
   b. monitor calcium levels
   c. assess, report, and record vital signs and symptoms
   d. deep intravenous calcium and emergency equipment available
   e. institute seizure precautions
   f. provide client teaching for discharge, including correct medication regimen for discharge
4. Evaluation
   a. client did not develop complications of hypoparathyroidism
   b. client followed therapeutic regimen
   c. client understood home care

B. Hyperparathyroidism (von Recklinghausen's Disease)

1. Assessment
   a. definition/pathophysiology: excessive synthesis and excretion of parathormone leading to excessively high levels of calcium in blood
   b. predisposing/precipitating factors
      (1) postmenopausal women
      (2) renal failure
   c. signs and symptoms
      (1) osteoporosis
      (2) pathologic fractures with bone pain and tenderness
      (3) anorexia
      (4) constipation, abdominal pain
      (5) renal stones
      (6) renal failure
      (7) increased myocardial contractility and sensitivity to digitalis
      (8) decreased reflexes
      (9) fatigue and muscle flaccidity, weakness, atrophy
      (10) depression
      (11) decreased mentation
      (12) chronic low back pain
      (13) hypertension
   d. diagnostic tests
      (1) serum calcium, increased
      (2) serum parathormone, increased
      (3) serum phosphorus, decreased
      (4) urine calcium, increased
      (5) history and physical examination
   e. usual treatments
      (1) infusion of isotonic saline plus large dose of diuretic such as furosemide to promote diuresis of calcium (see Table 7-3)
      (2) administration of oral phosphorus
      (3) administration of mithramycin to inhibit skeletal release of calcium
      (4) administration of calcitonin to decrease rate of skeletal breakdown
      (5) surgical removal of all but small portion of one parathyroid gland
2. Planning, goals, expected outcomes
   a. client is diagnosed and treated for condition before life-threatening complications occur
   b. client understands and complies with therapeutic regimen
   c. client recovers from surgery without complications
3. Implementation
   a. monitor vital signs
   b. monitor for life-threatening complications
   c. monitor output carefully
   d. monitor electrolytes
   e. care for client postoperatively as for thyroidectomy client
   f. teach client and family long-term care
   g. provide safe environment, such as preventing fractures
   h. teach client correct diet and measures to prevent constipation
4. Evaluation
   a. client received prompt treatment
   b. client followed therapeutic regimen
   c. client recovered from surgery without complications

III. ADRENALS

A. Cushing's Syndrome—Excess Adrenocortical Hormone

1. Assessment
   a. definition/pathophysiology: group of symptoms caused by excessive amounts of cortisol; caused by
      (1) excessive secretion of ACTH
      (2) functional tumor of adrenal cortex
      (3) ectopic production of ACTH by tumor commonly associated with lung cancer
      (4) iatrogenic; steroid therapy most common cause
   b. predisposing/precipitating factors
      (1) lung cancer
      (2) adrenal cortical tumors
      (3) steroid therapy
   c. signs and symptoms
      (1) altered metabolism
         (a) protein catabolism and muscle wasting
         (b) increased fat deposits around shoulders, face, and trunk
         (c) increased blood glucose levels and increased resistance to insulin
         (d) calcium release from bones and osteoporosis
      (2) fluid and electrolyte imbalances
         (a) sodium retention
         (b) fluid retention
         (c) potassium loss
      (3) immunosuppression and increased susceptibility to infection
      (4) decreased collagen tissue formation
         (a) striae
         (b) increased bruising
         (c) decreased wound healing
      (5) hypertension
      (6) gastric hyperacidity and decrease of gastric mucosa leading to peptic ulcers
      (7) hirsutism

(8) inability to withstand stress
(9) altered libido
(10) emotional lability and irritability
(11) insomnia
(12) bone pain and pathologic fractures
d. diagnostic tests
(1) serum cortisol level: normally diurnal secretion pattern, constant level with Cushing's syndrome
(2) serum electrolytes
(3) vital signs
(4) blood glucose
(5) CBC
(6) serum protein levels
(7) history and physical examination
(8) increased urinary calcium levels
e. usual treatments
(1) regulate cortisone therapy carefully
(2) administer diuretics to control edema and hypertension (see Table 7–3)
(3) bilateral adrenalectomy for adrenal tumors
2. Planning, goals, expected outcomes
a. client has symptoms of Cushing's syndrome controlled as much as possible
b. client recovers from surgery for adrenal tumor without complications
c. client understands and complies with therapeutic regimen
3. Implementation
a. monitor vital signs
b. monitor intake and output
c. daily weights
d. protect from infections and monitor closely for the development of infections
e. maintain low-calorie, low-sodium, low-fat, high-potassium, high-protein, high-calcium diet (see Chapter 5)
f. administer antacids or histamine receptor antagonists to control hyperacidity
g. administer medications as ordered
h. teach client symptoms of hyperglycemia
i. assess, report, and record signs and symptoms
j. warn client not to vary medication dosage without specific physician's orders
k. teach client to avoid stress and promote rest
l. teach client to avoid trauma
m. provide emotional support
n. prepare client and significant others for surgery
o. teach client self-care for discharge, including steroid replacement
4. Evaluation
a. client develops minimal side effects
b. client recovers from surgery without complications
c. client follows therapeutic regimen

B. Addison's Disease—Adrenocortical Insufficiency

1. Assessment
a. definition/pathophysiology: deficiency of adrenocortical hormones, glucocorticoids, and mineralocorticoids, which leads to death if not treated promptly; caused by
(1) nonfunctioning adrenal tumor
(2) pituitary malfunction
(3) atrophy of adrenals secondary to cortisone therapy
b. predisposing/precipitating factors
(1) adrenal tumor
(2) pituitary tumor
(3) steroid therapy
(4) infections
(5) trauma
c. signs and symptoms
(1) vague symptoms early in disease
(2) electrolyte imbalance
(a) hyponatremia
(b) hyperkalemia
(c) hypovolemia and hypotension
(3) hypoglycemia
(4) inability to withstand stress
(5) bronzing of skin with areas of absent pigmentation
(6) cardiac arrhythmias
(7) anorexia, nausea, weakness, and fatigue
(8) decreased mentation
(9) depression
(10) decreased ability to withstand stress
(11) weight loss
(12) coma and death if untreated or from acute addisonian crisis
d. diagnostic tests
(1) plasma cortisol levels
(2) serum electrolytes
(3) history and physical examination
e. usual treatment
(1) removal of tumor
(2) replacement of hormones with steroid therapy
2. Planning, goals, expected outcomes
a. client does not develop life-threatening complications of Addison's disease
b. client understands and complies with lifelong steroid therapy
3. Implementation
a. assess, report, and record symptoms and reactions to treatment
b. monitor vital signs
c. protect from stress
d. observe for hypoglycemia
e. monitor for signs of shock

f. teach client about lifelong steroid therapy, home care, and self-care

g. provide care for client receiving steroids

4. Evaluation

a. client did not develop life-threatening complications

b. client understood and followed life-long steroid therapy

IV. DIABETES MELLITUS

A. Assessment

1. Definition/pathophysiology: deficiency of insulin leading to problems in oxidation and metabolism of glucose and complex syndrome of disorders

a. categories

(1) type I, insulin-dependent diabetes mellitus (IDDM)

(a) little or no insulin produced

(b) insulin required daily

(c) prescribed diet therapy and exercise program must be followed

(d) potential renal, retinal, cardiovascular, and neurologic problems

(e) potential for hyperglycemia and hypoglycemia

(2) type II, non–insulin-dependent diabetes mellitus (NIDDM)

(a) controlled by diet or oral hypoglycemic agents

(b) most clients obese

(c) ketosis or hypoglycemia rarely develops

2. Predisposing/precipitating factors

a. genetic predisposition

b. obesity

c. possibly viral origin

d. possibly immunologic, autoimmune factors

e. incidence increasing; more than 10 million in United States

3. Signs and symptoms

a. polyuria

b. polyphagia

c. polydipsia

d. weight loss with IDDM

e. fatigue and lack of energy

f. weight gain with NIDDM

g. infections

h. symptoms of complications in renal, retinal, cardiovascular, and neurologic systems

4. Diagnostic tests

a. fasting blood sugar

b. glucose tolerance tests

c. urinalysis

d. urinary function studies

5. Usual treatments

a. insulin or oral hypoglycemic agents (Table 7–26) and insulin (Fig. 7–5)

b. diet modification, diabetic exchange list (see Chapter 5)

c. prescribe regular exercise regimen

B. Planning, Goals, Expected Outcomes

1. Client is diagnosed with diabetes before permanent complications occur

2. Client does not develop complications of diabetes

TABLE 7-26 Oral Hypoglycemics

Generic Name (Trade Name)	Onset (hr)	Duration (hr)	Dosage*
FIRST-GENERATION AGENTS			
Tolbutamide			Initial: 1–2 g/day in 1 to 3 doses
(Orinase)	1	6–12	Maximum: 2–3 g/day in 1 to 3 doses
Acetohexamide			Initial: 0.25–1.5 g/day in 1 or 2 doses
(Dymelor)	1	12–24	Maximum: 1.5 g/day in 1 or 2 doses
Tolazamide			Initial: 100–200 mg/day with breakfast
(Tolinase)	4–6	12–24	Maximum: 0.75–1 g in 2 divided doses
Chlorpropamide			Initial: 250 mg once a day
(Diabinese)	1	24–72	Maximum: 750 mg once a day
SECOND-GENERATION AGENTS			
Glipizide			Initial: 5 mg once a day with breakfast
(Glucotrol)	1	12–24	Maximum: 40 mg/day in 2 divided doses
Glyburide Nonmicronized			
(DiaBeta, Micronase)	2–4	12–24	Initial: 2.5–5 mg/day with breakfast / Maximum: 20 mg/day in 1 or 2 doses
Micronized			Initial: 1.5–3 mg/day with breakfast
(Glynase PresTab)	1	24	Maximum: 12 mg/day in 1 or 2 doses

Modified from Lehne, R.A., Moore, L., Crosby, L., & Hamilton, D. (1994). *Pharmacology for nursing care*, 2nd ed. Philadelphia: W.B. Saunders Co.
*The dosages listed are for nonelderly clients. Elderly clients should use smaller doses.

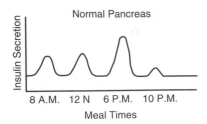

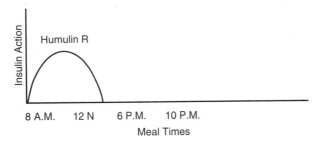

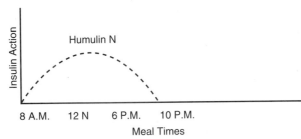

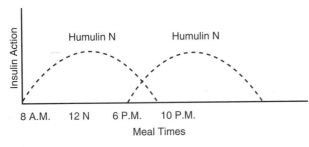

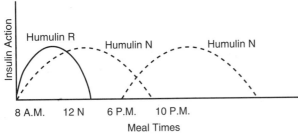

FIGURE 7-5 Relationship between food intake and the onset, peak, and duration of different patterns of insulin injections and preparations. (From Monohan, F.D., Drake, T., & Neighbors, M. (1994). *Nursing care of adults.* Philadelphia: W.B. Saunders Co., p. 1231.)

3. Client maintains blood glucose within specified limits
4. Client understands and complies with therapeutic regimen of insulin administration, foot care, home glucose monitoring, diet modification, exercise, and regular health care
5. Client and family cope with diagnosis of chronic disease

C. Implementation

1. Client and family education
    a. insulin administration
        (1) injection techniques
        (2) sites (Fig. 7–6)
        (3) types of insulin
        (4) storage of insulin
        (5) mixing of insulins
    b. pathophysiology of diabetes
    c. complications of diabetes
        (1) neuropathy: death of peripheral nerves, leading to paresthesias and eventually anesthesia
        (2) retinopathy: vascular leakage in retina and eventual loss of vision
        (3) nephropathy: renal vascular damage eventually leading to renal failure
        (4) vascular damage: peripheral vascular degeneration, accelerated atherosclerosis, coronary heart disease
    d. home glucose testing
        (1) urine testing for glucose and ketone bodies (acetone)
        (2) home glucose monitor of blood from finger stick
        (3) may be difficult for elderly to measure own glucose because of dexterity and visual problems
    e. exercise regimen
    f. diet teaching
        (1) six food exchanges (see Table 5–9)
        (2) do not skip meals
        (3) follow prescribed meal plan
        (4) do not eat foods other than those in meal plan
        (5) check with physician before altering diet
    g. foot care
        (1) do not go barefoot
        (2) wash and dry feet daily and carefully
        (3) wear white cotton socks to absorb perspiration
        (4) examine feet daily for sores
        (5) wear well-fitting shoes, leather or canvas
        (6) do not cut nails or corns; see a podiatrist
        (7) do not burn feet with hot bath water
        (8) monitor for and treat all injuries, cuts, and blisters
        (9) see physician immediately for any foot trauma that does not heal quickly or is severe
    h. teach client signs of hyperglycemia and hypoglycemia and what to do if either occurs (Chart 7–6)
    i. encourage client to express feelings

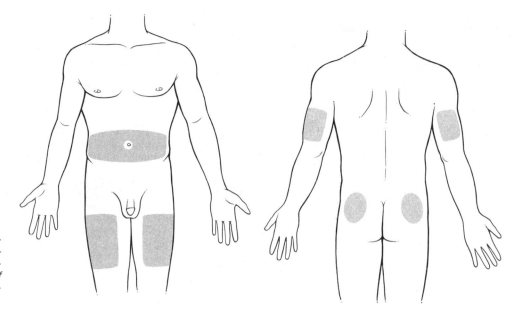

FIGURE 7-6 Rotation sites for injection of insulin. (From Monohan, F.D., Drake, T., & Neighbors, M. (1994). *Nursing care of adults.* Philadelphia: W.B. Saunders Co., p. 1233.)

j. encourage client to seek other resources, such as dietitians and social service, as needed

k. help client achieve self-care competency

D. Evaluation

1. Client diagnosed with diabetes early
2. Client did not develop complications
3. Client's blood glucose remained within specified limits
4. Client followed diabetic therapeutic regimen
5. Client and family accepted diagnosis of chronic disease

Digestive Disorders

I. PEPTIC ULCER DISEASE

A. Assessment

1. Definition/pathophysiology: ulceration of mucous lining of lower esophagus, stomach, and duodenum that may involve submucosal and muscular layers (Fig. 7–7)
2. Incidence
   a. gastric
      (1) two times more common in men
      (2) age over 50 years
      (3) often malnourished
      (4) familial tendency
      (5) lower socioeconomic class
   b. duodenal
      (1) four times more common in men
      (2) between ages 25 and 50 years
      (3) highly stressed individuals

      (4) over 80% of all ulcers
      (5) blood type O
3. Predisposing/precipitating factors
   a. smoking
   b. diet not clearly documented
   c. economic and social status
   d. presence of *Helicobacter pylori*
   e. ulcerogenic drugs, such as aspirin, corticosteroids, and nonsteroidal anti-inflammatories
   f. alcohol consumption
   g. chronic stress
   h. physiologic stress, e.g., burns, major trauma
4. Signs and symptoms
   a. epigastric pain that may be burning, gnawing, or aching
   b. feeling of distention followed by nausea and vomiting more often in gastric ulcers
   c. weight loss with gastric ulcers and may exhibit weight gain with duodenal ulcers
   d. anorexia
   e. eructations
   f. pain less in early morning and just after eating with duodenal ulcers; greater at those times with gastric ulcers
   g. pain worse on empty stomach and 2–3 hours after eating, when gastric acid level high with duodenal ulcer
   h. pain less when stomach empty with gastric ulcers
   i. melena with duodenal ulcers
   j. hematemesis with gastric ulcers
5. Diagnostic tests
   a. history and physical examination
   b. CBC
   c. upper gastrointestinal radiographic series (barium swallow); PN responsibilities

Chart 7–6
Comparison of Hypoglycemic (Insulin) Reaction and Hyperglycemia (Diabetic Ketoacidosis)

Characteristic	Hypoglycemic Reaction	Diabetic Ketoacidosis
Definition	Blood glucose less than 60 mg/dL	Acidosis due to excessive production of ketone bodies; blood sugar over 300 mg/dL
Etiology	Too much insulin for food intake	Insufficient insulin for food intake
Predisposing/precipitating factors	Increased physical work or exercise, stress	Decreased exercise, stress, infection, diarrhea and vomiting, injury, surgery, pregnancy
Onset	Sudden if regular insulin, slower if modified insulin, or hypoglycemics given orally	Slow (days, probably because somatostatin suppresses high glucagon level for 48 hours)
Clinical manifestations	Diaphoretic and pale skin, feels cold; looks weak; nervous; trembling; neuroglycopenia; blurred vision; hunger; headache; shallow rapid respirations; numbness, tingling lips, fingers; confusion, slurred speech; glycosuria not usually present, depends on time of last voiding, tachycardia	Hot, dry, flushed skin; dehydration; polydipsia; polyuria; ketonuria; looks very ill; headache; abdominal pain; Kussmaul's respirations, deep and gasping sweetish odor due to acetone, acidosis, hyperglycemia; glycosuria
Client goal	Client will recognize the signs and symptoms of hypoglycemia and will seek help appropriately	Client will recognize the signs and symptoms of diabetic ketoacidosis and will seek help appropriately

Chart 7–6
Comparison of Hypoglycemic (Insulin) Reaction and Hyperglycemia (Diabetic Ketoacidosis)
Continued

Characteristic	Hypoglycemic Reaction	Diabetic Ketoacidosis
Implementation	Give client a glass of orange juice, soft drink, or hard candy; offer complex carbohydrate and protein to prevent another hypoglycemic reaction; give glucagon parenterally if necessary; investigate cause of hypoglycemic reaction, and teach client to make necessary adjustments in lifestyle or diet, to prevent recurrence	Insert IV and Foley catheter; take blood and urine samples to examine for glucose, ketone bodies, and hypokalemia or hyperkalemia; administer insulin (regular) IV; observe cardiac monitor for hypokalemic arrhythmias as acidosis subsides; replace fluid and electrolytes; treat cause of acidosis; teach client how to avoid a recurrence of ketoacidosis by compliance with health regimen and monitoring for hyperglycemia
Evaluation	Client remains free from further hypoglycemic reactions	Client remains free from further episodes of diabetic ketoacidosis

From Matassarin-Jacobs, E. (1994). *Saunders review for NCLEX-RN*, 2nd ed. Philadelphia: W.B. Saunders Co.

    (1) client education: explain procedure
    (2) administer cathartics and enemas as ordered night before
    (3) keep client on NPO status after midnight
    (4) administer cathartics or enemas after procedures as ordered
  d. endoscopic examination of esophagus, stomach, duodenum; direct visualization with a flexible scope; PN responsibilities
    (1) client education
    (2) administer cathartics and enemas as ordered
    (3) keep client on NPO status after midnight
    (4) administer preprocedure medications as ordered

    (5) monitor for return of swallowing reflex in postprocedure period; NPO status until then
    (6) monitor vital signs in postprocedure period
  e. test stools for occult blood
  f. gastric analysis
  g. observe vomitus for "coffee-ground" appearance or bright red blood; test for occult blood
6. Complications
  a. hemorrhage
  b. perforation
  c. obstruction
  d. after surgery: "dumping syndrome," which consists of nausea, weakness, palpitations,

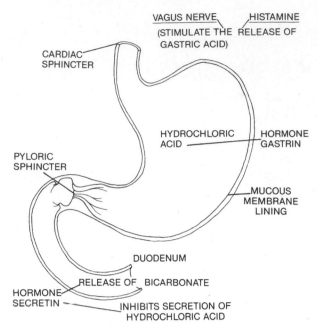

FIGURE 7-7 The stomach.

sweating, syncope, and diarrhea about 30 minutes after ingestion of food

7. Usual treatments
   a. pharmacologic (Table 7–27); primary treatment
      (1) histamine receptor antagonists
      (2) antacids
      (3) anticholinergics
      (4) analgesics, sedatives
      (5) antibiotics to treat *H. pylori*
   b. dietary modification possible, particularly reduction in caffeine and alcohol (Table 7–28)
   c. reduction of stress, quiet environment
   d. stop smoking
   e. assess signs and symptoms and reactions to or effects of prescribed treatments, including side effects of drugs
   f. surgical intervention; done only if medication fails or for complications
      (1) subtotal gastrectomy: removal of ulcerated portion of stomach (Fig. 7–8)
      (2) vagotomy: division of branch of tenth cranial nerve, vagus, that sends cerebral stimuli to stomach muscles and glands, thereby reducing gastric motility and secretions
      (3) total gastrectomy: removal of stomach (see "Gastric Cancer," further on)
      (4) closure if perforation has occurred
      (5) pyloroplasty for obstruction of duodenum: plastic surgery of pylorus to provide larger opening; done with vagotomy
   g. nasogastric tube to decompress the gastrointestinal tract and remove gastric acid

B. Planning, Goals, Expected Outcomes

1. Client identifies and alleviates risk factors
2. Client is free from pain
3. Client does not develop complications from peptic ulcer
4. Client maintains adequate nutrition

C. Implementation

1. Assist client to identify presence of risk or precipitating factors in life
2. Modify diet to eliminate ulcerogenic substances, such as caffeine, alcohol, and medications
3. Modify time frame of diet to include regular meals or possibly six small meals a day
4. Stop smoking
5. Monitor vital signs and stool for occult blood to detect early signs of hemorrhage
6. Administer medications as ordered (see Table 7–27); may require transfusions if hemorrhage occurs
7. Help client to identify signs and symptoms of complications and to notify nurse and physician
8. Monitor client for signs and symptoms of perforation, hemorrhage, obstruction; notify team leader immediately
9. Ensure intake of adequate fluids and nutrients
10. Help client comply with pharmacologic treatment of nausea, vomiting, diarrhea, or constipation (Table 7–29)
11. Help client understand and comply with surgical intervention
12. Assist RN to educate client in preoperative phase regarding
    a. surgical procedure
    b. need to cough and deep breathe
    c. early ambulation
    d. possible presence of drainage tubes
13. Assist RN in postoperative period to monitor
    a. vital functions
    b. intake and output; list each drainage tube separately
    c. early ambulation, cough and deep breathe
    d. medicate for pain as ordered
14. Prevent or treat "dumping syndrome"
    a. small, frequent meals
    b. low-carbohydrate, high-protein, moderate-fat diet to slow gastric emptying
    c. drink liquids only between meals, not with meals
    d. lie down on left side for 1 hour after meals

TABLE 7-27 Pharmacologic Treatment of Peptic Ulcer

Class	Example	Action	Use	Common Side Effects	Nursing Implications
Histamine receptor antagonists	Cimetidine (Tagamet), ranitidine (Zantax)	Inhibit histamine at receptor sites on parietal cells	Decrease gastric acid secretion	Agranulocytosis Mental confusion Dizziness Bradycardia Mild diarrhea Impotence Interstitial nephritis Lower sperm count	Monitor BUN; antacids should not be given at same time (1 h before or 2 h after)
Antacids: nonsystemic, systemic	Nonsystemic: Mylanta, Riopan Systemic: bicarbonate of soda (baking soda)	Elevate gastric acid pH	Weaken gastric acidity	Anorexia Constipation (aluminum) or diarrhea (magnesium)	Can interfere with absorption of cartain medications, such as tetracycline; do not give together Systemic antacids can cause alkalosis
Anticholinergics	Clidinium bromide (Quarzan)	Block acetylcholine	Decrease GI motility and inhibit gastric acid secretion	Headache Confusion Excitability Palpitations Blurred vision Urinary retention	Contraindicated in narrow-angle glaucoma Obstructive uropathy; obstruction of GI tract Paralytic ileus Monitor vital signs, intake and output
Analgesics	Oxycodone hydrochloride (Percodan)	Binds with opiate receptors in CNS	Control moderate to severe pain	Sedation Clouded sensorium Hypotension Bradycardia Depressed respirations Nausea Vomiting Constipation	Monitor vital signs, particularly respirations

BUN, blood urea nitrogen; CNS, central nervous system; GI, gastrointestinal.

15. If total gastrectomy, client needs to receive bi-weekly vitamin B₁₂ injections

D. Evaluation

1. Peptic ulcer healed
2. Client had no pain

TABLE 7-28 Bland Diet

Foods Allowed	Foods Prohibited
Milk	Preserved meats
Cheeses	Smoked fish
Butter or margarine	Raw vegetables
Beef and lamb, roasted or broiled	Raw fruits
Chicken, roasted or broiled	Pastries
Fish, broiled or poached	Preserves
Cream soups	Candies
Cooked vegetables	Alcoholic beverages
Bananas	Caffeine
Baked apples without skins	Carbonated beverages
Stewed fruits	High-fiber foods
Applesauce	Spices or condiments
Bread	Acidic foods
Custard	Fried foods
Ice cream	Fatty foods
Pudding	Smoked meats
Plain cakes	

3. Client recovered from ulcer or surgery without complications
4. Client achieved adequate nutrition

II. HIATAL HERNIA

A. Assessment

1. Definition/pathophysiology: protrusion of part of stomach, often proximal area, through esophageal hiatus in diaphragm upward into mediastinal cavity; reflux of acid gastric contents, often causing gastritis in herniated portion and causing bleeding and anemia
2. Incidence: small, asymptomatic hiatal hernias appear in many people, as shown by upper gastrointestinal series
3. Predisposing/precipitating factors
   a. congenital weakness
   b. trauma
   c. increased intra-abdominal pressure
   d. relaxation of gastric sphincter and musculature
   e. obesity

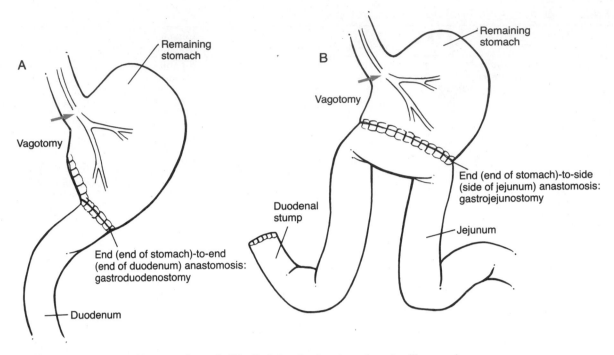

FIGURE 7-8 Subtotal gastric resection. *A,* Billroth I (gastroduodenostomy) with vagotomy. *B,* Billroth II (gastrojejunostomy) with vagotomy. (From Monohan, F.D., Drake, T., & Neighbors, M. (1994). *Nursing care of adults.* Philadelphia: W.B. Saunders Co., p. 932.)

TABLE 7-29 Pharmacologic Treatment of Nausea, Vomiting, Diarrhea, or Constipation

Class	Example	Action	Use	Common Side Effects	Nursing Implications
Antiemetics: phenothiazines anticholinergics antihistamines	Phenothiazine: prochlorperazine maleate (Compazine)	Act on the chemoreceptor trigger zone in the medulla	Inhibit nausea and vomiting	Agranulocytosis Orthostatic hypotension Blurred vision Urinary retention Cholestatic jaundice	Do not give with antacids Monitor for CNS depression Monitor vital signs Monitor for alkalosis from loss of acidity
Laxatives: irritant saline bulk-forming lubricant stool softeners	Irritant: castor oil	Stimulate intestinal mucosa	Increase motility and secretion	Abdominal cramps Fluid depletion Hypokalemia Hypotension	May interfere with absorption of food and medication
Antidiarrheals: demulcents protectants adsorbents astringents opiates	Opiate: diphenoxylate (Lomotil)	Inhibit motility and propulsion, diminish digestive secretions	Slow down or stop diarrheal stool	Sedation Lethargy Tachycardia Paralytic ileus Dry mouth	Treat the cause as well as the symptom; if diarrhea caused by a poison, do not treat diarrhea until poison is eliminated Monitor for hypovolemia and hypokalemia Monitor for acidosis Contains atropine, so contraindicated in glaucoma

CNS, central nervous system.

f. anorexia nervosa, bulimia

g. smoking

h. alcohol caffeine ingestion

4. Signs and symptoms

    a. heartburn

    b. regurgitation

    c. dysphagia

    d. sternal pain; may mimic angina after a heavy meal

    e. difficulty in breathing, dyspnea

    f. esophagitis from acid gastric contents pushed up on esophageal mucous membrane

5. Diagnostic tests

    a. history and physical examination

    b. chest and abdominal radiograph

    c. upper gastrointestinal radiographic examination

    d. esophagoscopy

6. Complications

    a. esophageal ulcer

    b. stenosis of distal portion of esophagus

    c. esophagitis

    d. occult bleeding, melena

    e. anemia

    f. gastritis

7. Usual treatments

    a. weight reduction

    b. positioning

        (1) avoid lying down after meals for 1 hour

        (2) sleep with head of bed elevated

    c. antacids

    d. small, frequent meals

    e. surgical repair

B. Planning, Goals, Expected Outcomes

1. Client identifies and alleviates risk factors

2. Client is free from pain

3. Client does not develop complications of hiatal hernia

4. Client understands and complies with therapeutic regimen

C. Implementation

1. Assist client to identify presence of risk and precipitating factors—avoid alcohol, caffeine, and smoking

2. Assist client to increase exercise and decrease caloric intake to decrease obesity

3. Administer antacids to weaken gastric acidity; histamine receptor antagonists sometimes used

4. Teach client to use positioning to prevent increase in herniation

5. Teach client to use positioning to prevent gastric reflux

6. Encourage client to avoid heavy meals

7. Teach client hazards of esophagitis

8. Teach client to avoid activities that increase intra-abdominal pressure, such as lifting heavy objects, bending over, or wearing tight clothes

9. Prepare client for surgery

10. Provide postoperative care for client as per ulcer surgery—know that if thoracic approach used, client may have chest tube in place

D. Evaluation

1. Client remains asymptomatic

2. Client had no pain

3. Client recovered from surgical repair without complications

III. GASTRIC CANCER

A. Assessment

1. Definition/pathophysiology: cancerous growth in stomach usually carcinoma; cause unknown; most start in lesser curvature, causing no symptoms until it spreads to sphincters

2. Incidence: declining in United States but still accounts for about 15,000 deaths per year

3. Predisposing/precipitating factors

    a. chronic gastric ulcers

    b. chronic gastritis

    c. familial tendency

    d. presence of *H. pylori*

4. Signs and symptoms

    a. early, usually vague

    b. late in disease, decrease in gastric motility

    c. anorexia

    d. weight loss

    e. weakness

    f. anemia

    g. pain

    h. melena

    i. hematemesis

    j. dysphagia

    k. constipation

    l. vomiting, possibly "coffee-ground" material from old blood

5. Diagnostic tests

    a. history and physical examination

    b. CBC and electrolytes

    c. upper and lower gastrointestinal radiographic studies

    d. gastroscopy with biopsy: PN responsibilities (see "Peptic Ulcer Disease")

e. gastric analysis: nasogastric tube passed, stimulant such as histamine given, then stomach contents removed; contents analyzed for free and total acid, occult blood, and lactic acid; client on NPO status after midnight

6. Complications
    a. metastasis, often to liver
    b. obstruction of pyloric or cardiac sphincter
    c. malnutrition
    d. malabsorption
    e. hemorrhage
    f. perforation with peritonitis
    g. shock
    h. after surgery: "dumping syndrome" (see "Peptic Ulcer Disease")
    i. vitamin B_{12} deficiency: pernicious anemia

7. Usual treatments
    a. surgical treatment
        (1) radical subtotal gastrectomy: resection of tumor plus ridge of healthy tissue, with anastomosis of stump of stomach to jejunum
        (2) total gastrectomy with removal of stomach; anastomosis between ends of esophagus and jejunum
        (3) less radical subtotal gastrectomy if tumor metastasized
    b. radiation and chemotherapy if client not surgical candidate
    c. radiation and chemotherapy after surgery if metastasis known or suspected; radiation and chemotherapy in combination for cancer of stomach to slow down growth of tumor

B. Planning, Goals, Expected Outcomes

1. Client is prepared for surgery
2. Client is free of pain
3. Client has no complications of surgery
4. Client maintains adequate nutrition
5. Client has controlled side effects from usage of radiation and chemotherapy
6. Client copes with diagnosis and prognosis

C. Implementation

1. Assist RN to provide preoperative care
    a. explain diagnostic procedures
    b. explain surgical procedure
    c. explain radiation and chemotherapy
    d. monitor intravenous therapy; intake and output
    e. monitor nasogastric tube for contents, pressure, output, placement; keep nares lubricated with water-soluble lubricant
    f. provide support for client and significant others

2. Assist RN to provide postoperative care
    a. monitor vital functions
    b. monitor intake and output, including nasogastric tube output
    c. monitor intravenous therapy and blood
    d. monitor hyperalimentation feeding if appropriate
    e. turn, cough, and deep breathe hourly
    f. administer pain medication as ordered
    g. give nose and mouth care
    h. when ordered, provide multiple small, dry meals
    i. administer vitamin B_{12} intramuscularly to treat pernicious anemia every 2 weeks

3. Administer pain medication as ordered

4. Monitor or assist RN to assess for postoperative complications
    a. monitor vital signs
    b. monitor for blood in nasogastric drainage; some old blood normal first few days
    c. monitor for increased abdominal pain and distention
    d. auscultate for bowel sounds
    e. monitor intake and output for overhydration or dehydration
    f. monitor for signs and symptoms of infections, especially respiratory
    g. if client on parenteral hyperalimentation, monitor blood glucose regularly, usually every 6 hours

5. Assist RN to monitor hyperalimentation feeding, blood administration, intravenous therapy, or enteral tube feeding as appropriate

6. Assist client to eat frequent, small, bland, dry meals with vitamin supplements

7. Assist client to understand and comply with the function of radiation and chemotherapy (see Table 7–22)

8. Monitor for bone marrow suppression, radiation burns on skin; be sure radiation markings on skin not removed

9. Assist client to comply with pharmacologic treatment for nausea, vomiting, diarrhea, or constipation (see Table 7–29)

10. Assist client and significant others with feelings about malignant disease and altered body image

11. Assist client to contact clergy as appropriate

12. Assist with J-tube feedings for clients who are poor surgical risks

13. Provide palliative care, including analgesia, for inoperable clients

D. Evaluation

[handwritten note in Cyrillic, partially covering text:]

Присутствие одного или многих углублений образованию воспалива слизистой оболочки через дефект в мышечной оболочке кишки; симптомы *anastomosis* — Едешие двух полов отделов *colostomy* — наложение свища на ободочную кишку

b. diverticulitis: inflammation of one or multiple diverticula of colon; caused by bacteria or other irritating substances collected in blind pouches of diverticula

c. Meckel's diverticulum: congenital condition

2. Incidence: approximately 10% of population over 50 years of age, 40% over 70 years of age

3. Predisposing/precipitating factors
   a. chronic constipation from stress and low-fiber diet
   b. congenital weakness of colon
   c. constipation from spastic colon syndrome

4. Signs and symptoms
   a. crampy pain in left lower quadrant of abdomen
   b. bowel irregularity with diarrhea
   c. generalized abdominal cramps
   d. narrow stools from fibrotic strictures
   e. melena possible
   f. occult bleeding
   g. low-grade fever
   h. elevated white blood cell count
   i. signs of complete or incomplete bowel obstruction

5. Diagnostic tests
   a. history and physical examination
   b. sigmoidoscopy: direct visualization of sigmoid colon
   c. barium enema: lower gastrointestinal radiographic series
   d. colonoscopy: endoscopic examination of entire colon by means of colonoscope admitted transanally; PN responsibilities
      (1) client education concerning examination
      (2) administer cathartics and enemas as ordered night before examination
      (3) keep client on NPO status after midnight
      (4) monitor for rectal bleeding after examination
      (5) monitor for signs and symptoms of bowel perforation after examination
      (6) monitor vital signs
   e. check stools for occult blood
   f. laboratory studies: CBC, erythrocyte sedimentation rate

6. Complications
   a. anemia
   b. abscess
   c. peritonitis
   d. hemorrhage through erosion of arterial blood vessel

7. Usual treatments
   a. pharmacologic treatment to reduce bacterial flora and soften fecal mass (Table 7–30)
      (1) antispasmodics
      (2) tranquilizers
      (3) sedatives
      (4) bowel antimicrobials such as neomycin
      (5) stool softeners
      (6) evacuant suppositories
   b. intravenous fluids
   c. surgical treatment if untreatable medically
      (1) primary resection with end-to-end anastomosis: removal of area of disease and inflammation and reconnection of both ends of colon
      (2) "double-barrel" colostomy if complications such as perforation, fistula, or obstruction; this is two-stage procedure; in first stage, diseased part of colon resected, but two ends of colon brought out to abdominal wall as stomas; allows inflammation process to subside while fecal flow diverted to proximal stoma; after 6–8 weeks, second stage involves closure of colostomy and anastomosis of two ends of colon for normal fecal flow
   d. soft, low-carbohydrate diet, with low residue gradually progressing to high-fiber diet over several weeks

B. Planning, Goals, Expected Outcomes

1. Assist client to identify and alleviate risk factors
2. Client is free of pain
3. Client maintains normal bowel elimination
4. Client is prepared for surgery
5. Client develops no complications of surgery
6. Client maintains integrity of the skin

TABLE 7-30 Pharmacologic Treatment of Diverticulitis

Class	Example	Action	Use	Common Side Effects	Nursing Implications
Antispasmodics	Dicyclomine hydrochloride (Bentyl)	Direct spasmolytic action on smooth muscle	Spastic colon	Headache Dizziness Palpitations Urinary retention Paralytic ileus	Monitor I & O Monitor vital signs
Tranquilizers, sedatives	Diazepam (Valium)	Depress CNS in limbic system	Antianxiety	Drowsiness Hypotension Cardiovascular collapse Abdominal discomfort	Possible addiction Dosage should be reduced in elderly clients Do not withdraw abruptly
Bowel antimicrobials	Neomycin sulfate	Inhibit protein synthesis in bacterial cell	"Sterilize colon" for surgery	Headache Ototoxity Nephrotoxicity	Ask client about drug allergies Monitor I & O Hydrate well to avoid renal toxicity
Stool softeners	Docusate sodium (Colace)	Reduce surface tension of liquid content of bowel	Incorporate more liquid in stool	Bitter taste Mild abdominal cramping Diarrhea	—
Evacuant suppositories	Bisacodyl (Dulcolax)	Direct action on smooth muscle at colon	Increase peristalsis	Nausea Vomiting Abdominal cramps Diarrhea	Monitor for laxative dependence, particularly in elderly

CNS, central nervous system; I & O, intake and output.

7. Client adjusts to altered body image
8. Client is able to care for colostomy if appropriate
9. Client and significant others cope with disease and surgery

C. Implementation

1. Identify presence of risk or precipitating factors in life
2. Assess, report, and record symptoms and response to medical regimen
3. Assist client to identify and use high-residue foods such as bran and fruits (Table 7–31)
4. Assist client to understand and comply with pharmacologic regimen
5. In acute phase
   a. client kept on NPO status
   b. provide oral care and analgesia
   c. administer antibiotics as ordered
   d. advance diet as tolerated when acute symptoms subside
   e. maintain quiet, low-stress environment
   f. observe and report stools
   g. closely monitor intake and output

TABLE 7-31 High-Residue Foods

Milk	Raw vegetables	Fried foods
Whole grains	Nuts	Cheese
Bran	Tough meats	Cooked corn
Fruits with seeds or skin	Pork	Popcorn
Raw fruits except bananas		

h. administer intravenous fluids while client takes nothing by mouth
6. Assist RN to prepare client for surgery as appropriate
   a. client education about procedure
   b. let client express fears and anxieties
   c. teach to turn, cough, and deep breathe
   d. explain possibility of drainage tubes
   e. explain possibility, appearance, and care of stoma as appropriate
   f. ensure that client knows whether colostomy is permanent or temporary
   g. monitor intravenous therapy
   h. monitor intake and output
7. Monitor client and assist RN in postoperative care
   a. turn, cough, and deep breathe hourly
   b. monitor vital functions
   c. measure intake and output; record each drainage tube separately
   d. provide stoma care with skin care
   e. auscultate for bowel sounds
   f. monitor for signs and symptoms of hemorrhage, perforation, or peritonitis
8. Provide pouch to fit snugly around stoma to prevent leakage of intestinal contents onto skin, which can cause chemical burn; use skin barrier
9. Wash skin well, and dry well
10. Administer enemas into proximal stoma as ordered by physician

11. Administer enemas to distal stoma and rectum as ordered by physician before closure of colostomy and reanastomosis
12. Assist client to watch stoma care, then gradually to become involved in self-care or involve family member in care
13. Allow client to express feelings concerning altered body image
14. Encourage use of "ostomy" visitor

D. Evaluation

1. Client's diverticulitis healed without complications
2. Client's diverticulitis did not recur
3. Client had pain controlled
4. Client recovered from surgery without complications
5. Client learned ostomy self-care
6. Client went through reanastomosis without complications

II. ULCERATIVE COLITIS

A. Assessment

1. Definition/pathophysiology: inflammation of large intestine that contains ulcerations of mucosa of colon; disease tends to begin in rectum and sigmoid colon, then ascends upward possibly to include entire colon; ulcerations may develop into an abscess; increases risk for development of colon cancer
2. Incidence: associated with persons under high stress; young adults, genetic predisposition; increasing in women and upper socioeconomic groups
3. Predisposing/precipitating factors
   a. cause unknown
   b. stress
   c. autoimmune factors
   d. repeated intestinal infections
   e. family tendency
4. Signs and symptoms
   a. diarrhea, can be bloody
   b. abdominal pain
   c. rectal bleeding
   d. nausea
   e. weight loss
   f. dehydration
   g. anemia
   h. body wasting, cachexia
5. Diagnostic tests
   a. history and physical examination
   b. stool examination for ova and parasites
   c. sigmoidoscopy
   d. barium enema
      (1) done less frequently
      (2) do not use enemas or laxative as preparation because megacolon or perforation can result
      (3) clear liquids for 24 hours should be sufficient to clear bowel
   e. colonoscopy with biopsy
   f. CBC and electrolytes
6. Complications
   a. carcinoma of colon
   b. megacolon with perforation of colon
   c. peritonitis
   d. hemorrhage
   e. hypokalemia, hypocalcemia, iron deficiency
   f. volume depletion
   g. malabsorption with loss of elasticity of colon
   h. stricture formation
   i. arthritis
   j. nephrolithiasis
7. Usual treatments
   a. pharmacologic (Table 7–32)
      (1) antidiarrheal medication
      (2) sedation
      (3) antibiotics, particularly sulfonamides (see Table 7–10)
      (4) steroids (see Table 7–17)
      (5) anticholinergics (see Table 7–16)
      (6) analgesics (see Table 7–8)
   b. rest, particularly after meals
   c. hydration: intravenous, oral
   d. intake and output
   e. psychotherapy
   f. well-balanced, low-residue, high-protein diet (Table 7–33; see also Chapter 5)
   g. vitamin and mineral supplements
   h. avoidance of milk and milk products if lactose intolerance present
   i. surgical (fewer than 20% require this): total colectomy with ileostomy
   j. parenteral hyperalimentation possible

B. Planning, Goals, Expected Outcomes

1. Client identifies and alleviates risk factors
2. Client maintains fluid and electrolyte balance
3. Client maintains adequate nutrition
4. Client maintains integrity of skin

C. Implementation

1. Assist client to reduce stress and avoid intestinal infections

TABLE 7-32 Pharmacologic Treatment of Ulcerative Colitis

Class	Example	Action	Use	Common Side Effects	Nursing Implications
Corticotropic hormones	ACTH (corticotropin)	Stimulate adrenal gland	Stimulate whole endocrine system	Sodium and fluid retention Convulsions Dizziness Hemorrhage Euphoria	Watch for overstimulation of endocrine system Side effects of Cushing's syndrome
Corticosteroids	Prednisone	Suppress immune response	Decrease inflammation	Euphoria Congestive heart failure Hypertension Edema	Medication must be stepped down Monitor for glucosuria
Antibiotics	Sulfasalazine	Decrease bacterial folic acid synthesis	Treat infectious process in colon or secondary infection	Leukopenia Nausea Vomiting Diarrhea Toxic nephrosis	Check for allergies Push fluids to prevent crystallization in renal tubules
Antidiarrheals			(see Table 7–29)		
Anticholinergics	Atropine sulfate	Inhibit acetylcholine	Slow diarrhea	Headache Restlessness Ataxia Hallucinations	Watch for tachycardia and urinary retention Contraindicated in acute glaucoma
Analgesics			(see Table 7–27)		

2. Assist client to understand and comply with pharmacologic treatment to decrease diarrhea and pain (see Table 7–32)
3. Monitor and chart number and character of stools, intake and output, including diarrheal stools
4. Provide good skin care to all bony prominences or pressure areas
5. Assist client to understand and comply with need to increase fluids and electrolytes through oral route or intravenous route
6. Assist client to understand and comply with di-

TABLE 7-33 High-Calorie, High-Protein, Low-Residue, Bland Diet for Inflammatory Bowel Disease

Type	Reason	Examples	Foods to Avoid
High-protein	Healing of mucosal tissue Replacement for malabsorbed protein in diet	Eggs Meat Cheese	Milk in early stages or if client is sensitive to milk
High-calorie	Spare protein Energy production Restore nutritional deficits	Pastas Desserts Meat Poultry Bread products Sugar Honey Hard candy	Ice cream Very cold foods High-fat foods
Low-residue, bland	Avoid irritation of mucosal lining	Eggs, except fried Small amounts of cheese Tender meat, not fried Small amounts of margarine, butter Cooked or canned vegetables and fruits Strained fruit juice Cooked, nonwhole grain cereals Gelatin desserts Sponge cake Plain custard Ices Hard candy Gumdrops Plain gravy Salt	Heavy roughage Alcohol Raw vegetables Highly spiced foods Raw fruits Whole grain breads and cereals Fried foods Nuts Popcorn Milk Pepper

etary modification to decrease intestinal irritation (see "Regional Enteritis [Crohn's Disease]")

7. Maintain medical asepsis by cleaning perianal area after each diarrheal stool to prevent excoriation of the perianal area
8. Provide care for client receiving steroids
9. Prepare client for surgery if appropriate
10. Assist client to have uncomplicated surgical recovery (see "Regional Enteritis [Crohn's Disease]")
11. Assist client not to develop complications of colectomy with ileostomy (see "Regional Enteritis [Crohn's Disease]")

D. Evaluation

1. Client's ulcerative colitis is in remission
2. Client had no recurrence
3. Client's pain controlled
4. Client's fluid and electrolyte balance maintained
5. Client maintained adequate nutrition
6. Client's skin integrity maintained

III. REGIONAL ENTERITIS (CROHN'S DISEASE)

A. Assessment

1. Definition/pathophysiology: inflammatory process of unknown origin; affects primarily terminal portion of ileum but can affect any portion of small or large intestine; inflammatory segments can be separated by normal intestine; chronic disease with relapses of acute inflammatory symptoms
2. Incidence
   a. occurs in both sexes about equally
   b. higher occurrence in persons of Eastern European Jewish origin
   c. highest occurrence in persons age 15–35 years
3. Predisposing/precipitating factors
   a. familial tendency
   b. abnormal immune response
4. Signs and symptoms
   a. early signs are insidious
   b. abdominal cramping and pain unrelieved by defecation, severe because of thickening and narrowing of bowel wall
   c. diarrhea
   d. scar tissue with constriction of intestinal lumen
   e. crampy abdominal pain, particularly after meals
   f. anorexia, anemia

g. weight loss, malnutrition
h. constant irritating discharge, causing chronic diarrhea
i. fever if abscess present
j. abdominal tenderness
k. ulcerations may perforate or lead to fistula formation, especially perianal fistulas
l. constriction of parts of intestine, particularly distal ileum on gastrointestinal radiographic examinations, may lead to obstruction in small bowel
m. melena

5. Diagnostic tests
   a. history and physical examination
   b. proctosigmoidoscopic examination with biopsy to rule out ulcerative colitis (colitis ruled out if rectosigmoid is normal)
   c. upper gastrointestinal radiographic examination (barium swallow)—do not use strong laxatives or enemas
   d. lower gastrointestinal radiographic examination (barium enema)—do not use strong laxatives or enemas
   e. endoscopic examination
   f. colonoscopy; PN responsibilities
      (1) educate client about procedures
      (2) cleanse bowel carefully, usually small enema to prevent perforation
      (3) keep client in NPO status
      (4) monitor and report bleeding or signs and symptoms of perforation
      (5) monitor vital signs
   g. CBC, electrolytes, clotting time

6. Complications
   a. strictures of the intestinal lumen
   b. malabsorption syndrome
   c. abscesses
   d. fistulas
   e. perianal ulcerations
   f. transmural penetration with perforation
   g. hemorrhage
   h. peritonitis

7. Usual treatments
   a. pharmacologic (see Table 7–32)
   b. high-calorie, high-protein, low-residue, bland diet with vitamin and iron supplements (see Table 7–33 and Chapter 5)
   c. hydration by intravenous route
   d. blood transfusion possible
   e. surgical interventions
      (1) resection of colon with end-to-end anastomosis if limited to particular area
      (2) permanent colostomy depending on area of inflammation: removal of diseased portion of large intestine, with remaining end of colon brought to

surface of abdomen through artificial opening called a stoma; anus sutured closed

    (3) permanent ileostomy: removal of diseased portion of colon and ileum, with remaining end of ileum brought to surface of abdomen through artificial opening called stoma; anus sutured closed

    (4) continent ileostomy or ileoanal anastomosis for continence; client must learn correct way to drain pouch or control diarrhea

  f. total parenteral hyperalimentation nutrition may be required

B. Planning, Goals, Expected Outcomes

Same as for ulcerative colitis

C. Implementation

1–3. Same as ulcerative colitis

4. Assist client to understand and comply with dietary modifications to decrease intestinal irritation (see Table 7–33)

5. Maintain medical asepsis by cleaning perianal area after each diarrheal stool and using a skin protection cream

6. Assist RN to prepare client for surgery as appropriate (see "Diverticulosis/Diverticulitis")

7. Provide emotional support for client and significant others to prepare mentally for surgery

8. Monitor client and assist RN in postoperative care

  a. similar to diverticulosis/diverticulitis except stoma permanent

  b. ileostomy drains diarrheal stool frequently, about 1200 mL/day; report to physician if >1500 mL/day

  c. drainage pouch must be emptied frequently

  d. drainage pouch must fit snugly around stoma to avoid spilling ileal contents onto skin, causing chemical burn

  e. pouch must be changed immediately if leakage occurs: use skin barrier such as Stomahesive or karaya

  f. monitor vital signs; hemoglobin and hematocrit; intake and output; record each drainage bag separately

  g. monitor for growth of yeast or fungus around stoma; use nystatin (Mycostatin) powder to treat

  h. assist client to look at surgical site and slowly begin to involve client in care of appliance

  i. provide emotional support for client and significant others to accept ostomy and altered body image

  j. allow client to express feelings, anxieties, and fears about surgical procedure

  k. encourage "ostomy" visitor

  l. comply with instructions given by enterostomal therapist

  m. be sure that client and significant others prepared to care for stoma before discharge or arrange for visiting nurse or enterostomal therapist to see client after discharge

9. Assist client to understand dietary restrictions and comply with avoiding foods that produce gas or malodors, such as asparagus, beans, and nuts

D. Evaluation

1. Client's regional enteritis was in remission
2. Client's disease did not recur
3. Client's pain was controlled
4. Client's fluid and electrolyte balance maintained
5. Client maintained adequate nutrition
6. Client's skin integrity maintained
7. Client learned and practiced self-care of ileostomy

IV. HERNIA

A. Assessment

1. Definition/pathophysiology: protrusion of intestine contained in hernial sac occurring in groin where abdominal area meets thighs; increased abdominal pressure from lifting, coughing, sneezing, or an accident often cause

  a. *direct:* hernia sac pushes directly outward through weakest point in abdomen

  b. *indirect:* hernia sac pushes downward into inguinal canal

  c. *femoral:* protrusion of loop of intestine into femoral canal

  d. *incisional:* protrusion of an organ at the site of the incision

2. Incidence: direct and indirect hernias more common in males, femoral hernia more common in females

3. Predisposing/precipitating factors

  a. congenital weakness of abdominal wall

  b. acquired weakness of abdominal wall related to straining or the aging process or secondary to previous incision

   c. trauma
   d. obesity
   e. pregnancy
4. Types
   a. *reducible:* the hernial sac can be placed back into abdominal cavity
   b. *irreducible or incarcerated:* hernia cannot be reduced
   c. *strangulated:* irreducible plus obstruction of blood and intestinal flow
5. Signs and symptoms
   a. outpouching of the hernia sac when client is upright or straining
   b. pain may be present in certain circumstances
   c. if the herniation becomes obstructed, there is:
      (1) colicky abdominal pain
      (2) vomiting
      (3) distention of the hernial sac
   d. auscultation of bowel sounds from outpouching
6. Diagnostic tests: history and physical examination
7. Complications
   a. strangulation
   b. peritonitis
8. Usual treatments
   a. surgery
      (1) herniorrhaphy: removal of hernial sac
      (2) hernioplasty: reinforcement of suture line with overlay of synthetic sutures or mesh
   b. manual reduction with or without truss

B. Planning, Goals, Expected Outcomes

1. Client identifies and alleviates risk factors
2. Client is prepared for surgery
3. Client has no complications of surgery
4. Client is free of pain

C. Implementation

1. Teach client dangers of poor body mechanics, obesity, and prolonged coughing from allergies or heavy smoking
2. Encourage client to lose weight, practice good body mechanics, stop smoking, and treat allergies as appropriate
3. Give preoperative explanations and teaching similar to that for other surgeries of abdominal area
4. Monitor in the postoperative period in manner similar to that for other surgeries of abdomen
5. Medicate for pain as ordered by physician
6. Teach client to support incisional area with hands or pillow during coughing, sneezing, or performing other activities that increase abdominal pressure
7. Teach client that driving can usually be resumed in 6 weeks, activity should be increased gradually, no heavy lifting for at least 6 weeks
8. Remind client to follow physician's instructions to prevent recurrence

D. Evaluation

1. Client verbalizes knowledge of risk factors
2. Client's hernia did not recur
3. Client recovered from surgery without complications
4. Client's pain controlled

V. HEMORRHOIDS

A. Assessment

1. Definition/pathophysiology: enlarged varicose veins in rectal and anal area; may be internal or external; caused by prolonged, increased abdominal pressure and prolonged pressure on rectal, anal area
2. Incidence: fairly common; more common in women than in men
3. Predisposing/precipitating factors
   a. pregnancy
   b. prolonged sitting
   c. chronic constipation
   d. hard, dry stools
   e. obesity
   f. heredity
   g. coughing, sneezing
   h. right-sided congestive heart failure
   i. anything that increases intra-abdominal pressure, such as cirrhosis or ascites
4. Signs and symptoms
   a. may be asymptomatic
   b. pain
   c. burning
   d. itching
   e. bright red blood on stool
   f. visible or palpable mass in anal area
5. Diagnostic tests
   a. history and physical examination
   b. digital examination (rectal examination)
   c. proctoscopic examination to rule out tumors
6. Complications
   a. anal fissure
   b. thrombosis of hemorrhoid
   c. strangulation of varicosity
7. Usual treatments
   a. symptomatic

(1) maintain cleanliness of area
(2) astringent topical medication to shrink mucous membrane
(3) stool softeners and laxatives
(4) high-fiber and high-fluid diet to keep stool soft
(5) sitz baths

b. surgical
(1) hemorrhoidectomy: removal of hemorrhoids by excision, clamp, cautery, laser, or cryosurgery
(2) conservative surgical treatment, Barron's ligation (rubber band ligation): hemorrhoids bound with rubber ligatures to produce necrosis, then sloughing of ligated portion

B. Planning, Goals, Expected Outcomes

1. Client identifies and alleviates risk factors
2. Client is free of pain
3. Client does not develop complications of hemorrhoids
4. Client is prepared for surgery
5. Client does not develop complications of hemorrhoidectomy

C. Implementation

1. Assist client to identify presence of risk or precipitating factors
2. Teach client to use symptomatic treatments
3. Teach client signs and symptoms of complications and notify nurse or physician; record and report any such signs
4. Provide privacy to decrease straining
5. Teach client appropriate diet and prevention
6. Give preoperative education
7. Monitor postoperatively for vital functions, intake and output
8. Turn, cough, deep breathe, early ambulation
9. Medicate for pain as ordered by physician, pain severe with first bowel movement
10. Monitor closely for first bowel movement
    a. use stool softeners and mineral oil to soften feces
    b. warn client that pain is often severe with first bowel movement; provide adequate pain relief
    c. warn client that fainting may occur at first bowel movement so provide safety precautions
11. Monitor for signs and symptoms of complications, such as hemorrhage, perforation of colon

D. Evaluation

1. Client's hemorrhoids remained asymptomatic
2. Client did not develop complications of hemorrhoids
3. Client's surgery was uneventful and without complications

VI. COLON/RECTAL CANCER

A. Assessment

1. Definition/pathophysiology: cancerous process in intestine that is relatively rare in small intestine and relatively common in large intestine; most colorectal cancers arise from preexisting polyps; polyp is growth, protruding from mucous membrane; polyps can be benign or malignant, but all need to be removed from colon; polyps may be attached by stalk or have broad base
2. Incidence: colorectal cancer most common intestinal cancer in United States; age of affected persons usually over 40 years
3. Predisposing/precipitating factors
   a. exact cause unknown
   b. polyps in colon and rectum
   c. chronic inflammation, such as ulcerative colitis
   d. diverticula
   e. lesions; pathologic discontinuity of tissue-like mucous membrane
   f. familial history
   g. diet high in animal fat and low in fiber
4. Signs and symptoms
   a. initially vague
   b. blood in feces
   c. abdominal pain
   d. anemia, weakness, and fatigue
   e. changes in bowel patterns; constipation alternating with diarrhea
   f. changes in stool shape as a result of strictures
   g. obstruction in colon from polyps or tumorous growth
   h. weight loss, anorexia
   i. abdominal pain, rectal pain
   j. abdominal distention
   k. signs of obstructions
5. Diagnostic tests
   a. history and physical examination
   b. proctosigmoidoscopy with biopsy
   c. upper gastrointestinal radiographic examination (barium swallow)
   d. lower gastrointestinal radiographic examination (barium enema)
   e. colonoscopy with biopsy

f. CBC and electrolytes
g. stool for occult blood
6. Complications
    a. obstruction of the colon
    b. hemorrhage
    c. metastasis within digestive system
    d. metastasis beyond digestive system
    e. malnutrition
    f. malabsorption
7. Usual treatments
    a. cancer chemotherapy (see "Cancer")
    b. radiation therapy (see "Cancer")
    c. surgery: depends on location and presence of metastasis
        (1) colon resection with end-to-end anastomosis for localized tumor polyp with no metastasis
        (2) colon resection with end-to-end anastomosis may be done as palliative treatment for metastatic cancer
        (3) abdominal perineal resection for cancer of rectum: involves cutting of colon above tumor, removal of affected portion of colon through perineal incision; remaining end of colon brought out to abdomen through opening called stoma
        (4) colostomy may be performed for inoperable tumors or in presence of partial or complete obstruction to allow emptying of colon through stoma
        (5) NPO order and nasogastric tube before surgery to decompress and rest the gastrointestinal tract
        (6) cathartics and enemas before surgery
        (7) intestinal anti-infectives, such as neomycin, before surgery to kill intestinal bacteria
        (8) drainage tubes in surgical area postoperatively to remove excess body fluids that collect in areas of inflammation
        (9) indwelling catheter possible
        (10) intravenous therapy
        (11) blood transfusion possible
        (12) total parenteral hyperalimentation nutrition possible
        (13) pain medication

B. Planning, Goals, Expected Outcomes

1. Client identifies and alleviates risk factors
2. Client does not develop complications
3. Client understands and complies with cancer chemotherapy or radiation
4. Client is prepared for surgery
5. Client has uncomplicated recovery from surgery
6. Client maintains skin integrity
7. Client adjusts to altered body image
8. Client is able to perform self-care with ostomy appliances
9. Client copes with diagnosis and prognosis

C. Implementation

1. Assist client to understand and comply with early detection through rectal examination, proctoscopic examination, stool guaiac examination after age 40 years
2. Assist client to comply with need for removal of rectal and colon polyps
3. Teach client signs of complications, such as increased abdominal pain and bleeding, and to report these to physician or nurse immediately
4. Teach client action, adverse effects, and treatment of adverse effects of cancer chemotherapy and radiation therapy (see Tables 7–22 and 7–23)
5. Assist client to comply with protocol for cancer chemotherapy or radiation therapy
6. Assist RN to prepare client for surgery (see "Diverticulosis/Diverticulitis")
7. Monitor client and assist RN in postoperative care of client (similar to diverticulosis/diverticulitis except there is only one stoma; because colostomy is permanent, anus sutured closed)
    a. auscultate for bowel sounds
    b. monitor for type and consistency of stool; closer the colostomy to ileum, more watery the stool; closer the colostomy to rectum, more normal the consistency of stool because of normal reabsorption of fluid in large intestine
    c. assist client to understand, if appropriate, means to help control regularity of bowel movements through diet and colonic irrigations; closer the colostomy to rectum, greater the chance of bowel regularity through bowel training regimen
    d. monitor drainage tubes, including perineal drain, if present after abdominal perineal resection
    e. notify physician of signs and symptoms of complications, such as frank blood draining from or around stoma, paralytic ileus, melena, changes in bowel pattern, extensive skin excoriation, hypotension, fluid and electrolyte abnormalities, acid-base abnormalities
    f. replace fluids and blood as ordered
8. Have enterostomal therapist assist client; contact ostomy association
9. Assist client to look at surgical site and gradually assist in own care

10. Educate client and significant others in care of stoma and ostomy appliances
11. Teach client need for continued follow-up care to monitor cancer
12. Allow client to ventilate fears, anxieties, anger, and depression
13. Provide emotional and spiritual support to client and significant others
14. Assist client to contact clergy as appropriate

D. Evaluation

1. Client's tumor successfully treated with no recurrence
2. Client recovered from treatment without complications
3. Client received successful palliative treatment
4. Client's skin remained intact
5. Client adjusted to altered body image
6. Client assumed self-care
7. Client's spiritual needs met; client coped with diagnosis and prognosis

Liver and Biliary Disorders

I. HEPATITIS

A. Assessment (Table 7–34)

1. Definition/pathophysiology: inflammation of liver; inflammation causes necrosis of hepatocytes; if liver heals with no scar tissue, it is termed acute; if scar tissue and nodules occur, it is termed chronic; liver has immense capability for regeneration, thereby producing resistance to permanent damage
2. Incidence: 85% of viral hepatitis attributed to hepatitis A virus (HAV) or hepatitis B virus (HBV)
3. Predisposing/precipitating factors
   a. amebiasis of *Entamoeba histolytica* type: leading to amebic abscess; results from ingestion of contaminated food and water
   b. anicteric, viral hepatitis primarily of infants and children that produces no jaundice
   c. viral type called cholangiolitic or cholestatic: associated with obstructive jaundice in biliary tract
   d. *HAV:* infectious, usually transmitted by oral-fecal route; especially prevalent in environments with overcrowding and poor sanitation; contaminated seafood or other food contaminated with fecal material; higher incidence among children and young adults; when HAV antibody detected in serum, it usually coincides with disappearance of HAV in stool, usually 1–2 months after onset

of disease; HAV antibody seems to confer long-term, even lifelong, immunity to HAV
   e. *HBV:* transmitted in blood, blood products, contaminated needles, and body fluids such as tears, saliva, and semen; infant can be infected by its mother during pregnancy; great risk exists in commercially prepared clotting concentrates obtained from commercial donors because testing for hepatitis B surface antigen (HB$_s$Ag) concentrates not as reliable in commercial clotting concentrates as in whole blood; six different antigens detectable in serum; onset and progression of HBV differs from HAV in that HBV has more insidious onset and longer course because it is more difficult to rid body of HBV than HAV; higher mortality rate than HAV
   f. *hepatitis C virus (HCV):* similar to hepatitis B with shorter incubation period; can lead to chronic hepatitis
   g. *hepatitis D (delta agent):* co-infects with hepatitis B and similar to hepatitis B in most respects; endemic in Mediterranean
   h. *hepatitis E:* epidemic in parts of Asia, Africa, and Mexico with poor sanitation; fecal-oral contamination route therefore similar to hepatitis A; self-limiting disease; mortality rate 10%–20% in pregnant women
   i. fulminant, acute hepatitis: client lapses into coma as result of extensive necrosis to liver by poisonous chemicals, medication overdosages, and virus
4. Signs and symptoms
   a. amebic: severe diarrhea, gastrointestinal upset, anorexia, abdominal pain
   b. anicteric: gastrointestinal upset, anorexia, low-grade fever, absence of jaundice
   c. cholestatic or cholangiolitic: jaundice, fatigue, hepatomegaly, bilious vomit, pruritus
   d. HAV: symptoms usually occur 2–7 weeks after ingestion of contaminated food; includes gastrointestinal and respiratory disturbances with sudden-onset jaundice, hepatomegaly, tenderness of liver, pruritus, muscular aches and pains, weight loss
   e. HBV: may be asymptomatic or more usually has an insidious onset 6 weeks to 6 months after contact with contaminated product; includes sudden onset of fever, chills, severe headache, gastrointestinal upset, jaundice, pruritus, hepatomegaly, tenderness of liver, splenomegaly
   f. hepatitis C and D similar to B; hepatitis E similar to A
   g. fulminant: sudden onset of high fever, gastrointestinal upset, convulsions, coma, death, usually within 10 to 14 days

TABLE 7-34 Comparison of Five Types of Hepatitis

Factor	Hepatitis A	Hepatitis B	Hepatitis C	Hepatitis D (delta agent)	Hepatitis E
Incidence	Endemic in areas of poor sanitation; common in fall and early winter	Worldwide, especially in drug addicts, homosexuals, clients and others exposed to blood and blood products; occurs all year	Post-transfusion, those working around blood and blood products; occurs all year	Causes hepatitis only in association with hepatitis B and only in presence of HB$_s$Ag; endemic in Mediterranean	Parts of Asia, Africa, and Mexico where there is poor sanitation
Incubation period	2–6 weeks	6 weeks–6 months (12–14 weeks average)	6–7 weeks	Same as hepatitis B	2–9 weeks
Risk factors	Close personal contact or by handling feces, contaminated wastes	Health care workers in contact with body secretions, blood, and blood products; hemodialysis and post-transfusion clients; homosexually active males and drug abusers	Similar to hepatitis B	Same as hepatitis B	Individuals traveling or living in areas where incidence is high
Transmission	Infected feces, fecal-oral route; may be airborne if copious secretions; shellfish from contaminated water; also rarely parenteral	Parenteral, sexual contact, and fecal-oral route; carrier state	Contact with blood and body fluids; source of infection uncertain in many clients; carrier state	Co-infects with hepatitis B, close personal contact; carrier state	Fecal-oral route, food or water-borne; no carrier state
Severity	Mortality low; rarely causes fulminating hepatic failure	More serious, may be fatal; mortality rate up to 60%	Can lead to chronic hepatitis	Similar to hepatitis B; more severe if it occurs with chronic active hepatitis B	Illness self-limiting; mortality rate in pregnant women 10%–20%
Diagnostic tests	Anti-HAV; IgM positive in acute; IgG positive after infection	HB$_s$AG or anti HB$_c$-IgM	Anti-HCV or anti-HDV; recombinant immunoblot assay (RIBAII)	HD Ag-positive	Anti-HEV
Prophylaxis and active or passive immunity	Hygiene; immune serum globulin (passive); vaccine under development (active)	Hygiene, avoidance of risk factors; immune serum globulin (passive); hepatitis B vaccine (active)	Hygiene; immune serum globulin (passive)	Hygiene; hepatitis B vaccine (active)	Hygiene, sanitation; no immunity

From Black, J., & Matassarin-Jacobs, E. (1993). *Luckmann's medical/surgical nursing: A psychophysiologic approach,* 4th ed. Philadelphia: W.B. Saunders Co.

5. Diagnostic tests
   a. history and physical examination
   b. blood work
      (1) CBC
      (2) prothrombin time
      (3) liver enzymes, including SGOT, serum glutamic-pyruvic transaminase (SGPT), to indicate amount of liver damage
      (4) serum bilirubin
      (5) serum for antigens for HAV, HBV, HCV, HDV, and HEV
      (6) other tests include IgM and IgG, which elevate with HAV, HB$_s$AG plus similar tests for C, D, and E
   c. urinalysis
      (1) color: dark yellow to brown could indicate presence of bilirubin
      (2) urobilirubin: indicator of abnormal levels of bilirubin waste
      (3) presence of red blood cells; white blood cells, protein, indicating poor renal filtration

d. stool examination
  (1) presence of HAV
  (2) clay color: too little bilirubin
  (3) dark color: too much bilirubin
  (4) melena: blood in stool
e. liver biopsy: cells to assist with diagnosis, indicator of extent of liver damage
  (1) explain procedure
  (2) position client on right side after procedure to apply pressure to puncture site
  (3) instruct client to remain on bed rest
  (4) obtain baseline vital signs before procedure and frequent vital signs after procedure
  (5) observe for bleeding at puncture site
  (6) maintain blood and body fluid precautions
  (7) maintain pressure on biopsy site
f. CT scan of liver

7. Complications
  a. acute becomes chronic with extensive necrosis of hepatocytes
  b. opportunistic pathogenic organism invasion
  c. impaired clotting ability, increased bleeding time because of impaired metabolism or splenomegaly
  d. hepatic encephalopathy
  e. hepatic coma
  f. altered metabolism of digestion
  g. altered detoxification of medications

8. Usual treatments
  a. bed rest with bathroom privileges as needed
  b. diet depends on client's needs and metabolism; may range from diet as tolerated to diet high in protein, carbohydrate, and calories and low in fat for tissue repair with little need of fat metabolism (protein restricted only if blood ammonia level increased)
  c. isolation precautions: universal precautions covering all body fluids
  d. passive immunity such as human gamma globulin
  e. high-risk individuals including health care workers should be immunized against HBV

B. Planning, Goals, Expected Outcomes

1. Client understands and complies with need for bed rest
2. Client complies with dietary regimen
3. Client does not develop complications for hepatitis
4. Client's skin remains intact
5. Client complies with isolation regulations
6. Client complies with medication regimen

C. Implementation

1. Explain to client that reason for fatigue is decreased metabolism by the liver
2. Assist client with activities of daily living
3. Client needs rest in protected, quiet environment so liver can heal and regenerate
4. Assist client in finding and using acceptable diversional activities
5. Explain reason for prescribed diet and assist client to make choices that are acceptable
6. Monitor vital signs, intake and output, hematuria, melena, and changes in neurologic signs, such as decreased state of consciousness
7. Assist client to change position every 2 hours; watch for reddened areas, particularly over bony prominences; clean skin with nonirritants, particularly if pruritus is present because of bile salt accumulation
8. Explain disease process and need for isolation techniques; assist client with compliance
9. Assist client to comply with pharmacologic treatment (Table 7–35)
10. Provide comfort measures
11. Measure intake and output, daily weights; ensure that client maintains adequate caloric intake
12. Avoid all drugs that are detoxified in liver
13. Increase fluid levels by intravenous and oral routes
14. Vitamin K preparations as ordered
15. Monitor laboratory values for liver function
16. Use warm water, baking soda, and lotion for bath for pruritus; avoid soap
17. Maintain bleeding precautions

D. Evaluation

1. Client's energy levels returned to normal
2. Adequate nutrition achieved
3. Client recovers without complications
4. Client's skin remained intact
5. Disease not transmitted to others
6. Client's liver healed
7. Client's pain controlled

II. CIRRHOSIS

A. Assessment

1. Definition/pathophysiology: chronic inflammatory disease of liver, characterized by abnormal formation of fibrous connective tissue (scar tissue), which causes abnormal partitioning of liver into irregular nodules, degenerative changes of parenchymal cells, and fatty infiltration

TABLE 7-35 Pharmacologic Treatment of Hepatitis

Drug	Action	Use	Side Effects	Nursing Implications
Human immune globulin	Antiviral drug that contains antibodies against various diseases	Bolsters immune system	Urticaria Local pain Headache Malaise Anaphylaxis	Obtain history of allergy or reaction to immunization
Hepatitis B immune globulin	Antiviral drug that contains antibodies against hepatitis B virus	Bolsters immune system	Anaphylaxis	Obtain history of allergy or reaction to immunization
Hepatitis B vaccine	Causes body to produce antibodies against hepatitis B	Immunization of high-risk populations	Pain at injection site Slight fever Malaise	The vaccine will *not* prevent hepatitis B in clients who are incubating the virus before vaccination
Vitamin K	Improved clotting ability in the presence of depressed prothrombin time	Replacement of vitamin K in liver disease	Transient hypotension Nausea Vomiting Dizziness Sweating Flushing Bronchospasms Anaphylaxis	Monitor prothrombin time
Antiemetics such as Emete-con (benzquinamide hydrochloride)	Prevent or treat nausea due to impaired metabolism	May be given 1/2 hour before meals or to treat nausea	May cause drowsiness	Avoid phenothiazines, such as Compazine, which is detoxified in liver
Antacids such as Mylanta	Counteract gastric acidity	After meals to help neutralize gastric acidity	Diarrhea	Systemic antacids should be avoided to prevent alkalosis

2. Incidence: approximately 20% of chronic alcoholics who are also malnourished develop cirrhosis
3. Predisposing/precipitating factors: disease has long latency period; can be due to multiple factors
   a. alcoholism (Laennec's cirrhosis) with progressive destruction of hepatocytes, fatty infiltration, and resultant portal hypertension
   b. nutritional deficiencies, particularly of protein, kwashiorkor; alcoholics often have nutritional deficiencies
   c. biliary disorders from chronic inflammation of bile ducts and retention of bile from obstructive pathology
   d. toxic results from chemical poisons, such as carbon tetrachloride, or overdosage of certain medications, such as chlorpromazine
   e. metabolic disorders, such as those of amino acid metabolism
   f. secondary to severe congestive heart failure
   g. following hepatitis if liver stress before complete healing occurs
   h. can occur following use of halothane anesthetic agents
4. Signs and symptoms: lengthy latency period tends to be followed by rapid onset of abdominal pain, abdominal swelling, hematemesis, edema, and possibly jaundice; signs and symptoms related to failure of liver's normal functions

   a. fluid retention from abnormal fluid and electrolyte balance, leading in advanced stages to ascites with increased abdominal girth leading to decreased circulation in lower extremities
   b. bleeding from abnormal clotting factors
   c. malnutrition from abnormal metabolism
   d. toxic effects from many medications as a result of abnormal detoxification
   e. fever and dehydration from poor nutrition and inadequate fluid intake
   f. spider angiomas from abnormal clotting factors and capillary fragility
   g. delirium tremens from withdrawal of alcohol
   h. hypoglycemia and hypoproteinemia caused by poor nutrition and abnormal metabolism
   i. hypertension from congestion in the portal system
   j. abnormal neurologic symptoms from poor metabolism of chemicals, particularly ammonia (NH_3), which is formed from nitrogen in protein joined to hydrogen
   k. fatigue and weight loss from abnormal metabolism
   l. esophageal varices from portal hypertension
   m. anorexia, nausea and vomiting
   n. respiratory distress with severe ascites

o. pruritus
p. development of hemorrhoids secondary to portal hypertension
5. Diagnostic tests
  a. history and physical examination
  b. liver biopsy: PN responsibilities
    (1) explain procedure
    (2) obtain baseline vital signs before procedure, frequent vital signs after procedure
    (3) position client on right side after biopsy
    (4) monitor for bleeding at puncture site
    (5) keep client on bed rest per physician's order with pressure on puncture site
  c. liver enzymes
  d. CBC
  e. liver scan
  f. glucose tolerance test
6. Complications
  a. *ascites:* late symptom, abnormal accumulation of serous fluid in peritoneal cavity secondary to portal hypertension and hypoproteinemia
  b. *portal hypertension:* abnormally increased pressure in portal system caused by scar tissue obstruction in portal venous system
  c. *esophageal varices:* varicosities in esophagus secondary to prolonged portal hypertension; varices large, fragile, and bleed easily
  d. *hepatic encephalopathy (coma):* changes in neurologic status secondary to abnormal detoxification and retention of ammonia in blood; marked changes in state of consciousness, progressing to coma, flapping tremors (asterixis)
  e. hemorrhage from abnormal clotting factors
7. Usual treatments: supportive in nature
  a. rest to decrease energy expenditure
  b. restriction of alcohol—absolutely no alcohol

c. diet
  (1) early in disease, can be diet as tolerated to high in protein, high in calories for tissue repair, with supplemental vitamins and minerals
  (2) late in the disease as serum ammonia level elevates, restricted proteins to limit hepatic encephalopathy, high in calories to use carbohydrates and fats as tolerated, plus supplemental vitamins and minerals (see Table 5–10)
d. assessment for signs of bleeding, such as spider angioma, hematemesis, guaiac-positive stool and urine, vital signs
e. neurologic signs to monitor for abnormalities
f. paracentesis to relieve symptoms of ascites
g. monitor laboratory values for liver status
h. fluid restriction to decrease edema
i. pharmacologic treatment
  (1) antibiotics (see Table 7–10)
  (2) vitamin K
  (3) diuretics
  (4) lactulose laxative

B. Planning, Goals, Expected Outcomes

1. Client identifies and alleviates risk factors
2. Client improves nutritional status
3. Client decreases energy expenditure
4. Early signs of complications are not undetected
5. Client has decreased anxiety

C. Implementation

1. Assist client to identify presence of risk or precipitating factors, such as alcoholism

TABLE 7-36 Medications Used in Cirrhosis

Drug	Action	Use	Common Side Effects	Nursing Implications
Broad-spectrum antibiotics, e.g., neomycin	Disinfect the bowel	Decrease the production of ammonia in colon	Headache Lethargy Ototoxicity Nephrotoxicity	Watch for oliguria, elevation of BUN
Vitamin K	Improve clotting ability	Replacement of vitamin K	Transient hypotension Nausea Vomiting Dizziness Sweating Bronchospasms Anaphylaxis	Monitor prothrombin time
Diuretics such as Lasix (furosemide)	Reduce blood volume	Decrease edema	Fluid and electrolyte depletion	Monitor I & O, vital signs, K$^+$ level

BUN, blood urea nitrogen; I & O, intake and output; K$^+$, potassium.

2. Administer medications as ordered (Table 7–36)
3. Assist client to understand reason for restrictions in diet, such as for salt and protein, and assist client in selection of choices acceptable to him or her (Table 7–37; see also Table 5–10)
4. Assist client to rest; assist with and provide diversional activities
5. Monitor client's vital signs, intake and output, neurologic signs, signs of bleeding, weight, electrolytes
6. Check skin, gums, stools, and urine for bleeding; apply extra pressure to injection sites
7. Measure abdominal girth daily
8. Provide meticulous skin care; cut client's nails to prevent scratching
9. Provide emotional support to client and significant others; assist with spiritual needs as appropriate

D. Evaluation

1. Progression of client's disease slowed
2. Adequate nutrition achieved as tolerated by client
3. Client's energy level increased
4. Complications in client's condition prevented or detected and treated
5. Client's anxiety decreased; spiritual needs met

III. CHOLELITHIASIS/CHOLECYSTITIS

A. Assessment

1. Definition/pathophysiology
   a. cholelithiasis: presence of gallstones in the gallbladder
   b. cholecystitis: inflammation of the gallbladder
2. Incidence: more common in women than in men; more common in obese clients
3. Predisposing/precipitating factors
   a. most frequently caused by presence of gallstones
   b. other factors include chemical irritants; medications, such as erythromycin estolate (Ilosone); bacteria, such as *Staphylococcus* and *Streptococcus*; and obstruction in biliary tract from stones or tumor
   c. phrase "fair, fat, forty, fertile, and female" used in reference to high-risk group
   d. increasingly documented after pregnancy and delivery
   e. sluggishness of gallbladder
4. Signs and symptoms
   a. acute cholecystitis
      (1) may be gradual onset or sudden; moderate amount of pain and tenderness in abdomen, particularly in right upper quadrant
      (2) nausea and vomiting, malaise, and low-grade fever
      (3) abdominal pain may radiate to back and right shoulder area
      (4) if complete obstruction occurs, pain becomes excruciating with high-grade fever and more pronounced nausea and vomiting
      (5) visible jaundice present in about 25% of clients; clients with obstruction
      (6) may have clay-colored stools and dark urine if obstruction present
   b. chronic cholecystitis
      (1) symptoms less pronounced and progress more slowly than in acute
      (2) most common symptoms: discomfort after eating, nausea, and flatulence
      (3) if particularly large meal or high-fat meal has been ingested, symptoms become more pronounced and include regurgitation, eructation, and vomiting
      (4) may be mild right upper quadrant pain
      (5) untreated chronic cholecystitis can lead to damage of gallbladder and liver
5. Diagnostic tests
   a. history and physical examination
   b. CBC, watching for elevated white blood count
   c. liver enzymes as indicators of inflammation
   d. cholecystography: radiopaque dye in form of tablets administered night before test; ex-

TABLE 7-37 High- and Low-Protein Foods

Low-Protein Foods	High-Protein Foods
Fruits, fresh or canned	Meats
Green vegetables	Eggs
Carrots	Fish
Potatoes	Milk
Margarine	Soybeans
Prepared low-protein items such as breads	Gelatin
	Protein supplements
Farina	Yogurt
Sherbet	Peanut butter
Corn starch	Cheeses
Wheat starch	Legumes
	Protein-fortified cereals

Low-Protein Diet

RESTRICTIONS	REASON
Milk	Restrict the exogenous source of nitrogen in amino acids; NH_3 = ammonia; ammonia buildup = hepatic encephalopathy
Milk products	
Eggs	
Cheese	
Meat	
Fish	
Fowl	
Legumes	
Meat extracts, such as gravies, soups	

amination done to evaluate capacity of gallbladder to fill, concentrate bile, and empty;
PN responsibilities
  (1) explain procedure to client
  (2) administer cathartics and enemas as or-
      dered night before
  (3) administer tablets as ordered after fat-
      free supper
  (4) keep client on NPO status as ordered
      by physician
  e. intravenous cholangiography: radiopaque
     dye as contrast medium, administered intra-
     venously by physician, to determine patency
     of hepatic and common bile ducts
  f. CT scan; PN responsibilities
    (1) explain test to client
    (2) restriction of fluids per physician's or-
        der to concentrate dye
    (3) administer cathartics and enemas per
        physician's order
6. Complications
  a. cholelithiasis becomes cholecystitis by stones
     moving into bile ducts
  b. rupture of gallbladder
  c. tear in bile ducts
  d. hepatitis secondary to obstruction in bili-
     ary tract
  e. jaundice
  f. disturbance of clotting mechanism because
     of vitamin K absorption interference
7. Usual treatments
  a. preferred treatment in acute cholecystitis is
     cholecystectomy after acute episode sub-
     sides
  b. if cholecystectomy not possible, then chole-
     cystotomy, which is draining of gallbladder
     with removal of stones, followed by chole-
     cystectomy at future time
  c. in chronic cholecystitis, preferred treat-
     ment is cholecystectomy if stones are
     present
  d. if stones not present, preferred treatment
     rest, antibiotics, antispasmodics, analgesics,
     low-fat diet, and hydration by intravenous
     or oral route

B. Planning, Goals, Expected Outcomes

1. In acute cholecystitis
  a. client is free from pain
  b. client has an uncomplicated recovery from
     surgery
2. In chronic cholecystitis
  a. client identifies the presence of risk or precip-
     itating factors in life

  b. client complies with diet modification to
     low-fat diet, avoidance of heavy meals
  c. client is free of complications

C. Implementation

1. In acute cholecystitis
  a. assist client to understand pathology of cho-
     lecystitis and reason cholecystectomy is pre-
     ferred treatment
  b. assist client in preoperative period by
    (1) explaining diagnostic tests
    (2) explaining surgical procedure
    (3) teaching coughing and deep breathing
        procedure, possible presence and care
        of drainage tubes, pain medication,
        early ambulation
    (4) maintaining fluid balance
    (5) monitoring for signs and symptoms of
        complications
    (6) reporting abnormalities to RN
  c. assist client in the postoperative period by
    (1) monitoring vital functions
    (2) monitoring for bleeding
    (3) monitoring drainage of tubes
    (4) helping client cough and deep breathe,
        ambulate frequently
    (5) medicating for pain per physician's
        orders
    (6) administering intravenous therapy
    (7) educating client and significant others
        about T-tube, diet, activity
    (8) administering prescribed diet when al-
        lowed
    (9) reporting abnormalities to RN
2. In chronic cholecystitis
  a. assist client to identify risk factors and pre-
     cipitating factors in life
  b. assist client to comply with low-fat diet (Ta-
     ble 7–38; see also Table 5–6)
  c. assist client to comply with pharmacologic
     regimen (Table 7–39)
  d. assist client to identify signs and symptoms
     of complications and report them to phy-
     sician

D. Evaluation

1. Client's pain alleviated
2. Client recovered from surgery without complications
3. Acute cholecystitis prevented
4. Client complied with diet modification
5. Client recovered without complication

TABLE 7-38 Low-Fat Diet

Contents	Reason
Foods are prepared with the avoidance of added fat	Fat is the main stimulator of the gallbladder to contract in order to release bile; the contractions cause pain in the inflamed gallbladder, particularly in the presence of stones; during contraction, small stones can be expelled into the bile ducts, blocking them and causing acute pain
Foods to be avoided include:	
1. Meats, particularly fatty cuts	
2. Meat gravies, creams	
3. Lard	
4. Oils	
5. Dairy products of cream, butter, eggs	
6. Nuts	
7. Avocados	
Food substitutions include:	
1. Lean meats, such as veal, liver, lamb	
2. Lean meats that are broiled, baked, or roasted	
3. Dairy products of skim milk, cottage cheese, margarine	
4. All kinds of breads and cereals	
5. All kinds of vegetables	
6. Three eggs per week, not fried	

IV. PANCREATITIS

A. Assessment

1. Definition/pathophysiology: inflammatory condition of pancreas that can be acute or chronic; primarily exogenous functions of pancreas diminished, with endogenous functions of islets of Langerhans possibly affected in later stages; digestive enzymes of pancreas released into pancreatic tissue, producing autodigestion

2. Incidence: higher in alcoholics (men) and persons with cholelithiasis (women)

3. Predisposing/precipitating factors
   a. alcoholism
   b. drug toxicity, such as acetaminophen overdose
   c. obstruction in biliary tract
   d. viral infection
   e. nutritional deficiencies
   f. trauma
   g. peptic ulcer disease
   h. cause often unknown

4. Signs and symptoms
   a. in acute pancreatitis: signs and symptoms related to rapid onset of necrosis, suppuration, gangrene, and hemorrhage in the pancreas
      (1) moderate-to-severe epigastric pain radiating straight through to back
      (2) nausea and vomiting
      (3) malaise and fever
      (4) eructation, hiccoughing
      (5) collapse from pain, fluid and electrolyte loss
      (6) rigid abdomen over umbilicus
      (7) jaundice if due to biliary obstruction
   b. in chronic pancreatitis: signs and symptoms related to loss of exogenous functions with diminished production of pancreatic en-

TABLE 7-39 Medications Used in Cholelithiasis/Cholecystitis

Drug	Action	Use	Common Side Effects	Nursing Implications
Antibiotics such as ampicillin	Bactericidal agent	Kill pathogenic organisms, causing or contributing to cholecystitis	Nausea Vomiting Diarrhea Stomatitis Yeast infection Anemia Thrombocytopenia Leukopenia	Question client about allergy to penicillin or any antibiotics before administration
Antispasmodics such as Pro-Banthine (propantheline bromide)	Smooth muscle relaxants	Treat spasms in bile ducts	Headache Insomnia Palpitations Blurred vision Constipation	Over-dose can cause curare-like symptoms
Analgesics such as meperidine	Central-acting analgesic	Treat pain of cholecystitis	Sedation Euphoria Hypotension Nausea Vomiting Constipation Urinary retention	Controlled substance, watch for respiratory depression Morphine not used, since it increases spasms of the duct
Chenodiol	Suppressor of hepatic synthesis of cholesterol	Gradual dissolution of gallstones through biliary cholesterol desaturation	Diarrhea Cramps Nausea Vomiting Liver toxicity	Watch for hepatic enzyme elevations

zymes; in long-standing chronic pancreatitis, symptoms of deficiency of endogenous islets of Langerhans may be present
    (1) bulky, fatty, foul-smelling stool because of malabsorption of protein, carbohydrate, fats
    (2) weight loss
    (3) malaise
    (4) nausea and vomiting
    (5) fever
    (6) wasting of muscle tissue
    (7) easy bruising because of malabsorption of fat-soluble vitamins A, D, E, and K
    (8) signs and symptoms of diabetes mellitus
    (9) increased white blood cell count, altered bilirubin and blood glucose
5. Diagnostic tests
    a. history and physical examination
    b. CT scan of pancreas
    c. abdominal radiographs
    d. fiberoptic endoscopy to visualize head of the pancreas
    e. pancreatography: radiographic examination performed during surgery in which contrast medium is injected into pancreatic duct
    f. liver enzymes, amylase, lipase
    g. CBC
6. Complications
    a. acute hemorrhagic pancreatitis
    b. malabsorption with malnutrition
    c. diabetes mellitus
7. Usual treatments
    a. in acute pancreatitis
        (1) maintain bed rest with bathroom privileges
        (2) analgesics for pain—meperidine never morphine
        (3) maintain hydration with intravenous fluids
        (4) keep client NPO
        (5) possible gastrointestinal decompression with nasogastric tube to intermittent suction
        (6) administer antibiotics if appropriate
        (7) administer steroids if appropriate
        (8) when eating, may require supplemental pancreatic extracts
    b. in chronic pancreatitis
        (1) encourage rest
        (2) give supplemental pancreatic enzymes with each meal
        (3) give analgesics
        (4) ensure adequate nutrition

B. Planning, Goals, Expected Outcomes

1. Client identifies and alleviates risk factors, especially alcohol
2. Client is free of pain
3. Client maintains adequate hydration
4. Client maintains adequate nutrition
5. Client does not develop complications

C. Implementation

1. Assist client to identify presence of risk or precipitating factors in life, such as alcoholism
2. Assist client in compliance with bed rest with bathroom privileges; assist client with diversional activities, position to relieve pain
3. Educate client about the pharmacologic regimen; administer medications as ordered (Table 7–40)
4. Monitor intake and output; administer intravenous hydration as appropriate; monitor for signs and symptoms of overhydration or dehydration
5. Educate client to need for pancreatic enzymes with meals and patterns of adequate nutrition
6. Monitor client's vital functions; report abnormalities to team leader
7. Monitor for signs and symptoms of diabetes mellitus
8. Maintain client NPO; provide mouth care
9. Assist with intravenous therapy
10. Monitor respiratory status
11. Provide emotional support to client and significant others
12. Teach client importance of no further alcohol consumption, adequate nutrition, home care, and follow-up

D. Evaluation

1. Pain free or pain controlled
2. Client's hydration and nutrition was maintained
3. Client did not develop complications or received early treatment for complications

Renal/Urinary Disorders

I. URINARY TRACT DISORDERS

A. Cystitis

1. Assessment
    a. definition/pathophysiology: inflammation of urinary bladder; may be primary or secondary to ascending urethritis or secondary to descending nephritis or ureteritis; pathogenic organism usually bacteria, often *Escherichia coli* in women

TABLE 7-40 Medications Used in Pancreatitis

Drug	Action	Use	Common Side Effects	Nursing Implications
Analgesics such as meperidine			See Table 7–8	
Antibiotics such as ampicillin			See Table 7–10	
Steroids such as prednisone	Decrease inflammation	Treat inflammatory symptoms	Euphoria Hypertension Edema Gastrointestinal irritation Peptic ulcer (See Table 7–17)	Can produce symptoms of diabetes mellitus Can cause pancreatitis Drug dosage must be reduced slowly
Pancreatic extract such as pancreatin (Viokase)	Supplemental replacement of pancreatic enzymes	Aids digestion of starches, fats, proteins	Nausea Vomiting	Antacids may negate the effect

   b. incidence: more common in women than in men
   c. predisposing/precipitating factors
       (1) infection in another part of urinary system
       (2) poor perineal hygiene
       (3) dehydration
       (4) urinary catheterization
       (5) tight clothing around groin
       (6) obstruction in urethra or bladder, such as prostatic hyperplasia or urethritis
       (7) vaginal infections
       (8) sexual intercourse (women)
   d. signs and symptoms
       (1) dysuria
       (2) hematuria
       (3) frequency and urgency of urination, nocturia
       (4) chills and fever if infection in other parts of urinary system as well as bladder
       (5) cramps/bladder spasms
       (6) suprapubic or low back pain
   e. diagnostic tests
       (1) history and physical examination
       (2) urine culture and sensitivity
       (3) urinalysis
       (4) CBC
       (5) cystoscopy
   f. complications
       (1) acute cystitis becomes chronic
       (2) involvement in other parts of urinary tract, such as ureteritis and pyelonephritis
   g. usual treatment
       (1) pharmacologic (Table 7–41)
           (a) antibiotics
           (b) urinary antiseptics
           (c) urinary analgesics
           (d) analgesics (antispasmodics)
       (2) treat obstruction if present

           (a) removal of hypertrophy of prostate (see "Benign Prostatic Hyperplasia")
           (b) dilation of urethra
   2. Planning, goals, expected outcomes
       a. client identifies and alleviates risk factors in life
       b. client is free of pain
       c. client is free of infection
       d. client does not experience complications
       e. client does not develop further infections
   3. Implementation
       a. assist client in carrying out good personal hygiene, selecting clothes not binding in groin area, avoiding irritant soaps, avoiding physical irritations such as prolonged bike riding, sexual intercourse
       b. assist client to understand and comply with pharmacologic regimen; push fluids, particularly acid-ash fruit juices, such as cranberry juice
       c. administer smooth muscle antispasmodics, such as dicyclomine hydrochloride
       d. obtain culture and sensitivity specimens, sterile technique with catheters
       e. monitor client for signs and symptoms of extending infection; notify team leader
       f. force fluids to at least 3 L/day
       g. monitor intake and output
       h. ensure client takes full course of antibiotics
       i. educate female clients on ways to prevent future infections
           (1) avoid tub baths
           (2) wear cotton underpants
           (3) void after intercourse
           (4) do not wear pantyhose with slacks
           (5) wipe after urination from front to back
   4. Evaluation
       a. client's cystitis cured, bladder mucosa healed
       b. client complied with pharmacologic regimen
       c. client's pain controlled

TABLE 7-41 Medications Used in Urinary Tract Infections

Drug	Action	Use	Common Side Effects	Nursing Implications
Antibiotics, particularly penicillin-like, oxacillin	Inhibit pathogenic cell wall synthesis	Treat systemic infections	Anaphylaxis Thrombocytopenia Neuropathy Hepatitis Interstitial nephritis	Resists penicillinase Ask client about medication allergy, particularly to penicillin, before administration
Urinary tract antibiotics such as cotrimoxazole (sulfamethoxazole-trimethoprim)	A sulfonamide bacteriostatic agent	Decrease bacterial folic acid synthesis	Aplastic anemia Nausea Vomiting Headache Toxic nephrosis	Must push fluids to prevent crystalluria Check for sulfa allergy
Urinary tract antiseptics such as nalidixic acid (NegGram)	Inhibit microbial DNA synthesis	In acute and chronic urinary tract infections caused by gram-negative pathogens	Drowsiness Weakness Headache Abdominal pain Diarrhea Photosensitivity	Needs renal and liver function studies for long-term therapy Resistant bacteria may develop early
Urinary tract analgesics such as phenazopyridine hydrochloride (Pyridium)	Local anesthetic	Anesthetic effect on urinary mucosa	Headache Nausea	Urine turns reddish orange May alter Clinistix; use Clinitest for accuracy
Analgesics such as Demerol	Narcotic analgesic	Central pain reliever	Nausea Vomiting Hypotension	May cause urinary retention, constipation, respiratory depression
Steroids such as prednisone	Anti-inflammatory	Treat inflammation; try to limit autoimmune response	Euphoria Fluid retention Congestive heart failure	Dose must be tapered when stopping treatment to prevent addisonian crisis
Quinolones, ciprofloxacin (Cipro), norfloxacin (Noroxin)	Exhibit a bactericidal effect by interfering with bacterial DNA gyrase to prevent bacterial DNA synthesis	Treat gram-negative and gram-positive infections	Dizziness Insomnia Nausea Vomiting Diarrhea Rash Joint or back pain	Antacids impair absorption; use with caution in clients with a history of CNS disease; avoid alkalinization of urine; safe use during pregnancy or lactation has not been established; maintain good hydration; teach client to take complete course of medication even if symptoms disappear

CNS, central nervous system; DNA, deoxyribonucleic acid.

d. client's urine culture grew no bacteria
e. client recovered without complications
f. client did not develop another infection

B. Urethritis

1. Assessment
   a. definition/pathophysiology: inflammation of urethra, causing mucous membrane to swell; can impede flow of urine
   b. incidence: high in cases of gonorrhea, particularly in men
   c. predisposing/precipitating factors
      (1) gonorrhea
      (2) prostatitis
      (3) catheterization
      (4) sexually transmitted nonspecific pathogen

   d. signs and symptoms
      (1) frequency and urgency
      (2) burning on urination, dysuria
      (3) purulent discharge
      (4) systemic symptoms such as fever
      (5) women with gonorrhea may be asymptomatic
   e. diagnostic tests
      (1) history and physical examination
      (2) urine culture and sensitivity
      (3) culture and sensitivity of discharge
      (4) cystoscopy
   f. complications
      (1) cystitis
      (2) hydronephrosis
      (3) pyelonephritis
      (4) uremia
      (5) renal failure
   g. usual treatment

(1) antibiotics
(2) analgesics
(3) dilation of stricture of urethra
2. Planning, goals, expected outcomes
   a. client identifies and alleviates risk factors in life
   b. client understands and complies with treatment
   c. client is free of pain
   d. client experiences no recurrence
3. Implementation
   a. assist client to identify personal risk factors and accept treatment for causes such as gonorrhea, nonspecific sexually transmitted pathogen, or stricture
   b. assist client to comply with pharmacologic therapy or dilation
   c. provide pain medication as ordered
   d. instruct client to avoid recurrence, such as being careful with sexual partners (make sure partner is treated and use latex barriers during intercourse); have early signs of gonorrhea treated quickly
   e. same teaching as with cystitis
   f. force fluids, acidify urine
4. Evaluation
   a. client's urethritis healed
   b. client complied with treatment
   c. client's pain controlled
   d. client recovered without complications
   e. client's condition did not recur

C. Pyelonephritis

1. Assessment
   a. definition/pathophysiology: inflammation of kidney and renal pelvis; can be acute or chronic; can involve glomerulus, tubules, or interstitial renal tissue; damage to glomeruli results in impairment of filtration process; kidney becomes enlarged, inflammation in mucosa present, abscesses can form
   b. incidence: occurs most frequently in children and young people; persons with recent sore throat, scarlet fever, or streptococcal infections; and persons with previous infection in lower urinary tract
   c. predisposing/precipitating factors
      (1) previous sore throat, scarlet fever
      (2) previous streptococcal infection that may cause autoimmune response
      (3) infection in lower genitourinary tract that ascends to kidney
      (4) presence of indwelling urinary catheter
      (5) pregnancy with vesicoureteral reflux

   d. signs and symptoms
      (1) in acute pyelonephritis
         (a) dull pain in flank, costovertebral angle tenderness
         (b) chills and fever
         (c) headache
         (d) malaise
         (e) hematuria, pyuria
         (f) wine-colored urine
         (g) frequency and urgency
         (h) cloudy urine from albuminuria, white blood cells
         (i) edema secondary to protein loss
         (j) hypertension
      (2) in chronic nephritis (nephrosis)
         (a) may occur right after acute attack or appear after long interval that was asymptomatic
         (b) may occur with no history of acute attack
         (c) in early stages
            (i) malaise
            (ii) albuminuria
            (iii) hematuria
            (iv) possibly anemia
         (d) in second stage (follows latent stage that is usually asymptomatic): edema, particularly in face, legs, and arms
         (e) in final stage:
            (i) uremia
            (ii) kidney failure
   e. diagnostic tests
      (1) history and physical examination
      (2) urinalysis
      (3) urine for culture and sensitivity
      (4) intravenous pyelogram
      (5) kidney, ureter, and bladder (KUB) radiograph
      (6) cystoscopy
      (7) CT scan
      (8) BUN and creatinine levels
   f. complications
      (1) uremia
      (2) renal failure
      (3) septicemia
      (4) hypertension
      (5) opportunistic secondary infections
   g. usual treatment
      (1) bed rest
      (2) antibiotics
      (3) urinary antiseptics
      (4) analgesics
      (5) high-protein, low-sodium diet (Table 7–42; see also Chapter 5)
      (6) hydration by intravenous method and orally as long as output maintained

TABLE 7-42 High-Protein, Low-Sodium Diet*

High-Protein Foods	Reason
Milk	Replace protein lost in urine
Eggs	Protein needed for tissue
Lean meat, fish, poultry	repair
Vegetables	Provide adequate calories for
Fruits	energy
Whole grain, enriched bread and cereal	
Butter, margarine	

Foods High in Sodium to Be Avoided†	Reason
Salt at the table	Prevent or limit edema, thereby decrease hypertension
Salt, preserved foods such as hot dogs, cold cuts	
Kosher meats	Less sodium causes less fluid retention, therefore increased urinary output
Salted snack foods like chips, peanuts, popcorn	
Spices and condiments such as bouillon cubes, meat tenderizers, pickles, soy sauce	
Cheeses	
Peanut butter	

*Used in presence of edema, hypertension, or oliguria.
†May be 500–1000 mg/day.

    (7) steroid hormones possible
    (8) hemodialysis possible
    (9) kidney transplant drastic method

2. Planning, goals, expected outcomes
  a. client is free of infection
  b. client is free of pain
  c. client does not develop secondary infection
  d. client does not develop recurrence
  e. client maintains adequate nutrition and hydration
3. Implementation
  a. assist client to understand and comply with pharmacologic regimen (see Table 7–40)
  b. assist client to comply with bed rest; provide diversional activities
  c. administer pain medication as ordered
  d. assist client to understand need to avoid persons with infections and to avoid becoming overly fatigued and undernourished
  e. assist client to take full regimen of antibiotics and steroids as appropriate
  f. assist client to understand and comply with high-protein, low-sodium diet plus hydration at levels prescribed by physician (see Table 7–42); appetite usually poor so need encouragement to eat
  g. provide skin and mouth care for client comfort
4. Evaluation
  a. client's infection cleared
  b. client did not develop secondary infection
  c. client did not suffer recurrence
  d. client maintained adequate nutrition and hydration

II. URINARY CALCULI (NEPHROLITHIASIS)

A. Assessment

1. Definition/pathophysiology: presence of calculi in kidney and urinary tract; caused by abnormal precipitation of chemicals out of urine; majority of kidney stones composed of calcium and magnesium in combination with phosphate or oxalate; calculi range from large to as small as grains of sand; smaller stones can be passed from kidney into ureters to bladder and down urethra; some stones mainly composed of uric acid (urate)
2. Incidence: occurrence higher in men than women, particularly in those between ages of 30 and 50 years, with sedentary occupations
3. Predisposing/precipitating factors
  a. persistent urinary tract infections
  b. obstruction of flow of urine, such as with benign prostatic hyperplasia
  c. stasis of urine due to immobility
  d. abnormalities in metabolism of certain chemicals
  e. diet high in calcium, phosphates, purines, oxalates
  f. insufficient fluid intake
  g. overusage of sodium bicarbonate (alkaline urine leads to increased precipitation of calcium)
4. Signs and symptoms
  a. may produce no symptoms unless dislodged from renal pelvis into ureter
  b. colicky pain in flank region of the costovertebral angle (costovertebral angle tenderness)
  c. pain may radiate around to abdomen and down to genitalia
  d. colicky pain may not be controllable by medication or position change
  e. nausea and vomiting
  f. hematuria
  g. fever
  h. pain on urination
  i. frequency and urgency
  j. pyuria
  k. diaphoresis
  l. pain may stop spontaneously once stone passes either into bladder or out urethra
5. Diagnostic tests
  a. history and physical examination
  b. urinalysis
  c. CBC
  d. cystoscopy: surgical placement of scope through urethra into bladder for direct visualization; PN responsibilities
    (1) teach client what to expect from procedure, depending on whether per-

formed under local anesthesia or general anesthesia
    (2) intake and output
    (3) vital signs
    (4) strain urine for stones
    (5) monitor for voiding after procedure
  e. urine culture and sensitivity
  f. KUB radiographs
  g. intravenous pyelogram
6. Complications
  a. stone lodged in ureter or urethra
  b. hydronephrosis secondary to obstruction
  c. pyelonephritis
  d. perforation of ureter, with development of septic shock
  e. peritonitis from perforation
  f. stone moved to bladder, blocks urethra
  g. cystitis, urethritis
7. Usual treatment
  a. antibiotics
  b. analgesics
  c. hydration, intravenous or oral
  d. cystoscopy with passage of ureteral catheter and stone basket to remove stone
  e. cystoscopy with passage of instrumentation to crush stone in ureter or bladder and remove (lithotripsy)
  f. *nephrolithotomy:* surgical removal of stone from kidney
  g. *pyelolithotomy:* surgical removal of stone from renal pelvis
  h. *ureterolithotomy:* surgical removal of stone from ureter

B. Planning, Goals, Expected Outcomes

1. Client identifies and alleviates risk factors
2. Client is free from pain
3. Client does not develop complications

C. Implementation

1. Assist client to identify foods high in calcium and phosphorus to be avoided (Table 7–43)

TABLE 7-43 Foods to Be Avoided in Clients with Renal Calculi

Foods High in Calcium	Foods High in Phosphorus
Milk	Milk
Milk products	Milk products
Leafy vegetables	Whole grain cereals
Whole grains	Rye and whole grain breads
	Dried fruits
	Fish, shellfish
	Chocolate, nuts
	Cream sauces

2. Assist client during diagnostic studies and surgical procedures
  a. PN responsibilities: preoperative
    (1) client education about procedures
    (2) teach client to cough and deep breathe
    (3) teach client about early ambulation and pain medication
    (4) strain urine for stones
  b. PN responsibilities: postoperative
    (1) monitor vital functions
    (2) intake and output
    (3) cough and deep breathe
    (4) early ambulation
    (5) pain medication as ordered
3. Monitor intake and output; monitor vital signs
4. Monitor for signs and symptoms of infection
5. Monitor for signs and symptoms of peritonitis

D. Evaluation

1. Client's stones removed
2. Client's infection cleared
3. Client's pain was controlled
4. Client's stones did not recur
5. Client recovered without complications

III. HYDRONEPHROSIS

A. Assessment

1. Definition/pathophysiology: renal pelvis and calices of kidney distend with urine as outflow obstructed; as disease progresses, nephrons destroyed; as distention progresses and pressure builds, muscular walls of renal pelvis and calices stretch; replaced by fibrous tissue progressing to functionless sac
2. Incidence: higher in men than women
3. Predisposing/precipitating factors
  a. obstruction of urinary tract, such as
    (1) ureteral tumors
    (2) calculi
    (3) benign or malignant prostatic hyperplasia
    (4) cancer of bladder and urethra
    (5) edema from urinary tract infections affecting ureters or urethra
  b. atrophy of urinary tract
4. Signs and symptoms
  a. dull and nagging pain in kidney area (costovertebral angle tenderness)
  b. sharp pain in kidney area
  c. hematuria
  d. pyuria

e. elevated white blood count if infection develops
f. fever
5. Diagnostic tests
    a. history and physical examination
    b. urinalysis
    c. culture and sensitivity of urine
    d. pyelography
    e. cystoscopy
    f. intravenous pyelogram
    g. CT scan
6. Complications
    a. uremia if both kidneys involved
    b. renal failure
    c. pyelonephritis
7. Usual treatment
    a. treat cause
    b. bladder catheterization to drain urine
    c. prostatectomy
    d. nephrostomy tube to drain pelvis of kidney
    e. antibiotics (see Table 7–10)
    f. analgesics (see Table 7–8)
    g. antipyretics

B. Planning, Goals, Expected Outcomes

1. Client understands and complies with treatment
2. Client has adequate intake and output
3. Client is free of pain
4. Client does not develop complications

C. Implementation

1. Assist client to understand need for treatments and comply with treatments
    a. help client to recognize that this can occur with any obstruction of urinary flow
    b. urinary antiseptics and antibiotics: to reduce edema by decreasing infection in urinary tract (see Table 7–41)
    c. intravenous pyelogram
    d. nephrostomy with placement of drainage tubes: PN responsibilities
        (1) teach client about procedure
        (2) usual preoperative teaching
        (3) postoperative care with coughing and deep breathing, monitoring vital functions, using sterile technique for tube care, recording intake and output
    e. urinary catheter: PN responsibilities
        (1) urinary catheter care
        (2) intake and output
        (3) assess for blood and pus
    f. prostatectomy (see ''Benign Prostatic Hyperplasia'')

2. Monitor intake and output
3. Hydration by intravenous route or oral route
4. Administer pain medications as ordered
5. Use sterile technique to prevent further infection
6. Monitor vital functions for signs of infection; administer antibiotics as ordered

D. Evaluation

1. Client's hydronephrosis reversed
2. Client's infection cleared
3. Client maintained adequate fluid levels and adequate output
4. Client's pain controlled
5. Client recovered without complications

IV. RENAL FAILURE: ACUTE AND CHRONIC

A. Assessment

1. Definition/pathophysiology: inability of kidney to carry on normal function; can be caused by multiple factors; kidney failure affects multiple body functions, including fluid and electrolyte balance, acid-base balance, excretion of waste products, control of blood pressure; renal failure can be acute with recovery or can become chronic
2. Incidence: higher in men than women
3. Predisposing/precipitating factors
    a. prerenal causes—problems occurring before the kidney itself
        (1) circulatory collapse with decreased blood flow to kidney
        (2) severe dehydration
        (3) prolonged hypotension
        (4) physical trauma
    b. renal causes—problems within the kidney itself
        (1) infection or inflammation
        (2) toxic chemicals, such as mercury
        (3) nephrotoxic medications, such as multiple antibiotics
        (4) electrolyte imbalances, such as hyperkalemia
        (5) diabetes mellitus
        (6) blood transfusion reaction
        (7) lupus erythematosus
        (8) polycystic kidneys
    c. postrenal causes—obstructed urinary flow beyond the kidneys
        (1) benign prostatic hyperplasia
        (2) urinary calculi
        (3) lower urinary tract obstruction

4. Signs and symptoms
   a. acute renal failure
      (1) nausea, vomiting, loss of appetite
      (2) diarrhea
      (3) oliguria (decreased output), which may progress to anuria (no output)
      (4) headache, drowsiness, disorientation, lethargy from retained waste products (urea)
      (5) possibly hypertension and edema from retained fluids
      (6) possibly hypertension secondary to circulatory collapse or severe dehydration
      (7) signs and symptoms of electrolyte imbalances and metabolic acidosis
      (8) elevated BUN, creatinine levels
   b. chronic renal failure (end stage) (Fig. 7–9)
      (1) high serum BUN and creatinine levels because of tubular necrosis
      (2) hyperkalemia
      (3) cardiac arrest from hyperkalemia
      (4) hypertension may become malignant
      (5) susceptibility to infection
      (6) gastrointestinal problems
      (7) anorexia with nausea and vomiting
      (8) uremic breath
      (9) anemia with weakness
      (10) bleeding tendencies
      (11) oliguria to anuria
      (12) pruritus from uremic frost
      (13) fluid and electrolyte imbalances
      (14) acid-base imbalances
      (15) anasarca (severe generalized edema)
      (16) neurologic signs and symptoms progressing to convulsions, coma, and death

5. Diagnostic tests
   a. history and physical examination
   b. BUN and creatinine levels
   c. kidney function tests
   d. CT scan
   e. intravenous pyelogram: PN responsibilities
      (1) teach client about procedure
      (2) keep client NPO before examination
      (3) administer cathartics or enemas night before as ordered
      (4) ask client if allergic to any iodine dyes
      (5) vital signs before and after procedure
      (6) monitor intake and output
      (7) watch for allergic reaction
   f. urinalysis for presence of blood, protein, white blood cells, glucose
   g. radiograph of kidney to assess for size, urinary tract obstruction: KUB

6. Complications
   a. hypertension
   b. fluid and electrolyte abnormalities
   c. acid-base imbalances
   d. hemorrhage
   e. anasarca
   f. convulsions
   g. coma
   h. death

7. Usual treatment
   a. treat cause if possible
   b. peritoneal dialysis: sterile catheter placed in peritoneal space to allow input of dialysate solution; solution left in for prescribed period of time then drained out; principle involves diffusion of fluid through semipermeable membrane, in this case, peritoneal membrane; fluid toxins and waste products pulled into hypertonic dialysate solution and then drained out; output should be more than input (see Fig. 7–9)
   c. hemodialysis: surgical arteriovenous shunt created to allow arterial blood to be tapped and then channeled to hemodialysis machine, which uses external physical semipermeable membranes for diffusion; blood that has had fluids and chemicals removed then returned to venous circulation (Figs. 7–10 and 7–11)
   d. renal transplant: if appropriate, diseased kidney removed and donor kidney surgically implanted; danger of rejection present

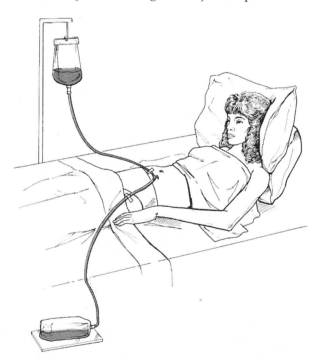

FIGURE 7-9 Peritoneal dialysis. (From Linton, A.D., Matteson, M.A., & Maebius, N.K. (1995). *Introductory nursing care of adults*. Philadelphia: W.B. Saunders Co., p. 771.)

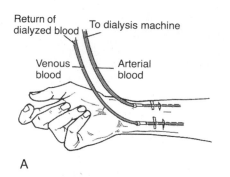

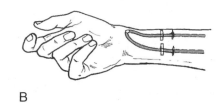

FIGURE 7-10 An arteriovenous shunt in use for dialysis (*A*) and not in use (*B*). (From Linton, A.D., Matteson, M.A., & Maebius, N.K. (1995). *Introductory nursing care of adults.* Philadelphia: W.B. Saunders Co., p. 771.)

A   B

B. Planning, Goals, Expected Outcomes

1. Client identifies reason for and complies with fluid restrictions
2. Client maintains fluid, electrolyte, and acid-base balance
3. Client identifies need for alternate form of removal of waste products normally performed by kidney
4. Client complies with needs of alternate form of removal of waste products
5. Client is free of complications for renal failure
6. Client is free of pain

C. Implementation

1. Assist client to understand and comply with fluid restrictions; maintain intake and output
2. Monitor for signs and symptoms of fluid, electrolyte, or acid-base balance; report abnormalities to team leader
3. Assist client to understand need for alternative form of removal of wastes
4. In peritoneal dialysis: monitor intake and output, vital signs, signs of peritonitis, infection, fluid overload
5. In hemodialysis: monitor intake and output, vital

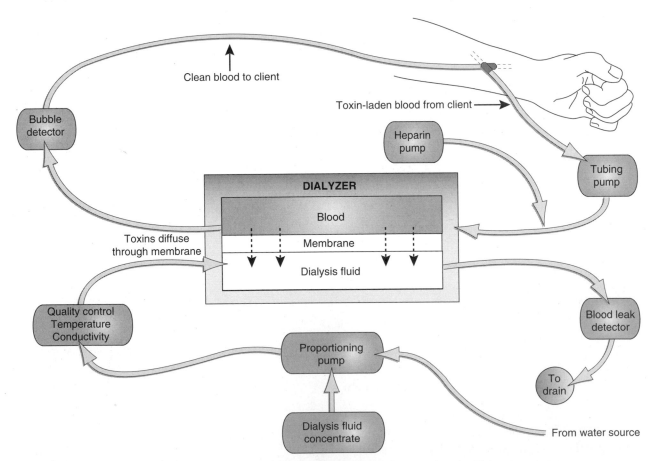

FIGURE 7-11 Schematic diagram of hemodialysis. (From Linton, A.D., Matteson, M.A., & Maebius, N.K. (1995). *Introductory nursing care of adults.* Philadelphia: W.B. Saunders Co., p. 770.)

signs, signs of infection at site of shunt or systemic; monitor for circulation through shunt by listening with stethoscope for "whooshing" sound at shunt site

6. In renal transplant: monitor intake and output, vital signs, signs of transplant rejection, fever, malaise, increased white blood cell count, hypertension; report abnormalities to team leader

7. Teach client signs and symptoms of complications and to report them to nurse and physician; monitor for signs and symptoms of complications and report to team leader

8. Administer pain medications as ordered; monitor for complications; provide symptomatic treatment as needed

9. Provide emotional support for a difficult time

D. Evaluation

1. Client maintained adequate fluid balance
2. Client maintained normal fluid and electrolyte balance, acid-base balance
3. Client complied with treatment
4. Client experienced no complications or had early treatment of complications
5. Client recovered from transplant surgery without complications

V. KIDNEY TUMORS

A. Assessment

1. Definition/pathophysiology: tumor in kidney that can be primary or secondary ascending from tumor lower in genitourinary system or as metastasis from another part of body; all malignant with no early signs and symptoms
2. Incidence: higher in males than females
3. Predisposing/precipitating factors
   a. unknown etiology
   b. tumor elsewhere in genitourinary system
   c. tumor metastasis elsewhere in body
4. Signs and symptoms
   a. in early stage usually none, often discovered secondary to radiograph for another reason
   b. in later stages
      (1) hematuria without pain
      (2) symptoms from metastatic process, depending on sites of invasion
      (3) weight loss
      (4) anemia
      (5) low-grade fever
      (6) elevated blood pressure
5. Diagnostic tests
   a. history and physical examination
   b. intravenous pyelogram

   c. KUB radiograph
   d. CT scan
   e. renal biopsy: PN responsibilities
      (1) teach client about procedure
      (2) vital signs preoperative and postoperative
      (3) intake and output
      (4) monitor for bleeding at incision site
      (5) position lying on biopsy site to apply pressure
      (6) blood-tinged urine is normal
      (7) no heavy lifting, exertion, hot baths for 2 weeks after biopsy
   f. CBC
   g. urinalysis
6. Complications
   a. kidney failure
   b. hemorrhage
   c. hypertension
   d. fluid and electrolyte imbalances
   e. acid-base imbalances
   f. metastasis
7. Usual treatment
   a. cancer chemotherapy (see Table 7–22)
   b. radiation therapy (see Table 7–23)
   c. nephrectomy
   d. radical nephrectomy: kidney plus adjacent tissue and lymphatics
   e. peritoneal dialysis possible
   f. hemodialysis, as appropriate, particularly if both kidneys are affected
   g. intravenous therapy for hydration
   h. hyperalimentation feeding possible

B. Planning, Goals, Expected Outcomes

1. Client identifies need for and complies with treatment
2. Client maintains fluid, electrolyte, and acid-base balances
3. Client maintains energy levels
4. Client is free of pain
5. Client does not develop complications of renal tumor

C. Implementation

1. Assist client to understand purpose of surgery, chemotherapy, or radiation
2. Assist client with activities of daily living while receiving treatments
3. Monitor intake and output, particularly drains after surgery, vital signs
4. Monitor for signs and symptoms of fluid and electrolyte balance, acid-base balance; daily weights; report abnormalities to team leader

5. Provide medication for nausea, vomiting, and diarrhea as ordered (see Table 7–29)
6. Assist client to rest; provide diversional activities, space activities
7. Provide small, frequent meals; maintain intravenous therapy; assist RN with monitoring of hyperalimentation feeding
8. Provide emotional support to client and significant others during diagnosis, treatment, and possible death
9. Administer pain medication as ordered (see Table 7–8)
10. Monitor vital functions; monitor for hemorrhage; report abnormalities to team leader

D. Evaluation

1. Client complied with treatment
2. Client had tumor removed or diminished
3. Client's fluid and electrolyte balance and acid-base balance maintained
4. Client's energy levels maintained at optimum
5. Client had no pain or pain controlled
6. Client developed no complications
7. Client and family coped with terminal prognosis

VI. BLADDER TUMORS

A. Assessment

1. Definition/pathophysiology: malignant tumors can range from no penetration beyond the bladder mucosa to metastasis beyond the pelvis; benign tumors always premalignant
2. Incidence: more common in men than women, particularly in those over age 50 years
3. Predisposing/precipitating factors
   a. aging process
   b. cigarette smoking, from toxins in smoke
   c. exposure to industrial dyes, particularly aniline dyes
4. Signs and symptoms
   a. painless hematuria that may come and go in early stages
   b. urinary frequency from diminished bladder capacity as a result of space-occupying tumor
   c. dysuria
   d. urgency
   e. in later stages gross hematuria may occur
   f. signs and symptoms of metastasis, such as weight loss and pain, depending on area of metastasis
   g. anemia

5. Diagnostic tests
   a. history and physical examination
   b. urinalysis
   c. urine culture and sensitivity
   d. CBC
   e. CT scan
   f. KUB radiograph
   g. intravenous pyelogram
   h. cystometrography: a sterile catheter is placed in the client, then volumes and pressures are recorded systematically: PN responsibilities
      (1) teach client about test
      (2) monitor for hematuria
      (3) monitor for signs of infection
      (4) catheter care if indwelling catheter in place
   i. cystoscopy with or without biopsy: PN responsibilities
      (1) teach client about test
      (2) client and significant other support during diagnostic phase
      (3) cathartics and enemas night before per physician's order
      (4) NPO after midnight
      (5) monitor for hematuria, infection
      (6) symptomatic treatment of bladder spasms, such as warm baths if permitted
6. Complications
   a. obstruction of flow of urine
   b. hemorrhage
   c. anemia
   d. atonic bladder
   e. metastasis to other parts of urinary tract
   f. metastasis to other parts of body
7. Usual treatment
   a. in premalignant stage, electrocauterization of tumor via cystoscope
   b. segmental resection (partial resection) of bladder, particularly near trigone region of bladder or near sections where ureters enter bladder
   c. radical cystectomy: total removal of bladder and pelvic lymph nodes, resulting in impotence in men, combined with urinary diversion
   d. urinary diversion (Fig. 7–12): surgical rerouting of urinary output
      (1) ileal conduit: surgical resection of ileal segment of intestine, with blood supply and nerve endings left intact; proximal end sutured into pouch and ureters sutured into ileal segment while distal end brought to outside of abdominal wall in right lower quadrant stoma; urine from kidneys drains down ureters into surgical pouch and

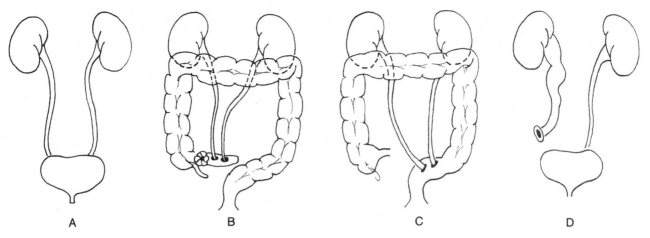

FIGURE 7-12 Urinary diversion. *A,* Normal urinary system. *B,* Ileal conduit. *C,* Ureterosigmoidos-tomy. *D,* Cutaneous ureterostomy.

spills out of stoma into collection pouch

(2) continent urinary diversion (Indiana pouch): internal pouch created with cecal area, ureters anastomosed to pouch; sphincter created rather than true stoma; client taught to self-catheterize every 2–3 hours during day; continent diversion, no external collection device needed

(3) ureterosigmoidoscopy: surgical implantation of ureters into sigmoid colon; urine drains right into sigmoid, liquefying stool and often producing incontinence; common danger is contamination, by *E. coli,* of kidneys via ureters; rarely done now

(4) cutaneous ureterostomy: surgical procedure in which one or both ureters brought to surface of abdominal wall in stoma; urine drains from kidney, down ureters, and out stoma to drainage pouch; complications include infection and scar tissue that causes constriction of surgical opening; flow of urine onto skin can cause chemical burn; usually palliative procedure

(5) bilateral nephrostomy tubes: palliative procedure; catheters inserted directly into kidney pelvis to drain urine if bladder becomes obstructed by tumor; catheters attached to leg bags so client can get around

B. Planning, Goals, Expected Outcomes

1. Client identifies and alleviates risk factors
2. Client understands the need for surgical procedure

3. Client has an uncomplicated surgical procedure and recovery
4. Client maintains skin integrity
5. Client maintains adequate intake and output
6. Client learns to care for own appliances
7. Client adjusts to altered body image and impotence (men)

C. Implementation

1. Assist client to stop smoking and avoid industrial dyes that can be toxic to bladder
2. Assist client to understand need to treat irritating or obstructing conditions of bladder and other parts of urinary system
3. Assist client to understand surgical procedure, including altered body image after surgery
4. Preoperative period
   a. teach client to cough and deep breathe
   b. monitor intake and output
   c. monitor for hematuria, vital signs
   d. assist with diagnostic procedures
   e. provide emotional support for client and significant others; refer men for sexual counseling
   f. administer cathartic, enemas night before surgery as ordered
   g. administer preoperative medications as ordered
5. Postoperative period
   a. monitor vital functions, especially intake and output
   b. monitor for bleeding, infection
   c. scrupulous skin care around stoma or rectal
   d. monitor intravenous hydration
   e. change disposable drainage pouches as needed; prevent fluid buildup
   f. ambulate early
   g. sterile technique for dressing change

h. drainage pouches around stoma need to fit snugly to prevent urine drainage onto skin; change pouches immediately, preventing leakage onto skin

i. monitor for bleeding, infection, scarring of the stoma

j. change drainage pouch opening size appropriately as stoma shrinks

k. monitor intake and output; do not give enemas or rectal suppositories with ureterosigmoidostomy

l. assist RN in teaching client and significant others to care for appliances

m. provide emotional support to client and significant others

n. if acceptable to physician and client, have person with urostomy visit client; make contact with American Cancer Society Ostomy Association

o. refer to enterostomal therapist as appropriate

p. assess client's ability to perform self-care and refer for visiting nurse as appropriate

D. Evaluation

1. Client eliminated risk factors
2. Client complied with treatment
3. Client recovered from surgery without complication
4. Client's skin and mucous membrane intact
5. Client able to care for self
6. Client adjusted psychologically to altered body image

BIBLIOGRAPHY

Baird, S.B., McCorkle, R., & Grant, M. (1991). *Cancer nursing: A comprehensive textbook.* Philadelphia: W.B. Saunders Co.

Black, J., & Matassarin-Jacobs, E. (1993). *Luckmann and Sorensen's medical/surgical nursing: A psychophysiologic approach,* 4th ed. Philadelphia: W.B. Saunders Co.

Bolander, V.R. (1994). *Sorensen and Luckmann's basic nursing: A psychophysiologic approach,* 3rd ed. Philadelphia: W.B. Saunders Co.

Davis, J., & Sherer, K. (1994). *Applied nutrition and diet therapy for nurses,* 2nd ed. Philadelphia: W.B. Saunders Co.

Keane, C. B. (1992). *Essentials of medical-surgical nursing.* Philadelphia: W. B. Saunders Co.

Lehne, R.A., Moore, L., Crosby, L., & Hamilton, D. (1994). *Pharmacology for nursing care,* 2nd ed. Philadelphia: W.B. Saunders Co.

Linton, A.D., Matteson, M.A., & Maebius, N.K. (1995). *Introductory nursing care of adults.* Philadelphia: W.B. Saunders Co.

Matassarin-Jacobs, E. (1994). *Saunders review for NCLEX-RN,* 2nd ed. Philadelphia: W.B. Saunders Co.

Monohan, F.D., Drake, T., & Neighbors, M. (1994). *Nursing care of adults.* Philadelphia: W.B. Saunders Co.

The Nurses' Reference Library: Diseases. (1990). Springhouse, PA: Nursing 90 Books. Intermed Communications.

The Nurses' Reference Library: Drugs. (1990). Springhouse, PA: Nursing 90 Books. Intermed Communications.

? QUESTIONS

1. Mr. Andrews is admitted to your unit with a diagnosis of acute gastroenteritis. He has had nausea, vomiting, and diarrhea for the last 48 hours. One of the most important areas to assess Mr. Andrews for initially is:

   ① His knowledge of the hospital environment
   ② Fluid and electrolyte balance
   ③ Presence of a viral infection
   ④ His ability to withstand the stress of hospitalization

2. A priority of your ongoing assessment of Mr. Andrews, your client with acute gastroenteritis with nausea and vomiting, would be:

   ① Activity tolerance level
   ② Respiratory rate and breath sounds
   ③ Level of consciousness
   ④ Character and frequency of all stools

3. Your goal for Mr. Andrews, your client with acute gastroenteritis with nausea and vomiting, is to have him return to a normal elimination pattern. Which of the following would best reflect this goal in a measurable manner?

   ① The client will have less frequent stools
   ② Diarrhea will be controlled and not recur
   ③ The client will have no more than one stool per day
   ④ The client will return to his normal bowel pattern

4. To have your client with acute gastroenteritis return to a normal bowel pattern once the nausea has resolved, an appropriate intervention would be to:

   ① Allow food and fluids as desired
   ② Limit all fluids until diarrhea disappears
   ③ Administer liberal fluids and a bland diet
   ④ Give unlimited quantities of milk and fruit juice

5. You discover that Mr. Andrews, your client with acute gastroenteritis with nausea and vomiting, has been admitted three times before for the same problem. An important assessment for the LPN to make would be:

   ① His usual bowel habits
   ② If anyone else in his family has the same symptoms
   ③ His usual eating pattern
   ④ Whether or not his wife does the cooking

6. The most common early sign of bladder cancer is:

   ① Painless hematuria
   ② Frequent urinary tract infections
   ③ Frequency and urgency without infection
   ④ Incontinence

7. Besides assessing for the character and number of stools in your client with acute gastroenteritis, another important area to assess would be:

   ① Total intake and output from all sources
   ② The client's ability to sleep through the night
   ③ The amount of intravenous fluid received each 24 hours
   ④ The client's former eating and elimination habits

8. Sara Miles is an obese 40-year-old mother of three who is admitted with a history of chronic cholecystitis. She is ordered to receive vitamin K preoperatively. The reason for this drug is to improve:

   ① Digestion of fats
   ② Healing of tissues
   ③ Elimination of bile
   ④ Clotting of blood

9. Postoperatively the best position for a cholecystectomy client is:

   ① Side lying to prevent aspiration
   ② Semi-Fowler's to facilitate breathing
   ③ Supine to decrease strain on the incision line
   ④ On her abdomen to reduce nausea

10. Your client has a T-tube in place after a cholecystectomy and choledocholithotomy. The purpose of the T-tube is to:

    ① Remove leaking bile from the incision
    ② Provide a means of irrigating the wound
    ③ Provide for drainage of bile from the common bile duct
    ④ Prevent rupture of the inflamed gallbladder

11. Your client with cholecystitis was exhibiting some signs of a jaundice preoperatively. Common signs of jaundice include:

    ① Ascites
    ② Blood-tinged urine
    ③ Icteric sclera
    ④ Dark-colored stools

12. Before a paracentesis, the client must:

① Void to empty the bladder
② Receive cleansing enemas
③ Receive sedation
④ Be in NPO status for 8 hours

13. Diabetes mellitus is a deficiency condition with impaired ability to use:

① Fats
② Glucose
③ Protein
④ Minerals

14. Which of the following would *not* be a risk factor for cystitis?

① Being female
② Emptying the bladder every 8 hours
③ Drinking 2000 mL of fluid daily
④ Pregnancy

15. In teaching your female client to avoid recurrence of her chronic urinary tract infections, the most helpful instruction would be to:

① Decrease her sexual activity for a while
② Wipe carefully from front to back after voiding
③ Restrict her intake of fluids in the evening
④ Take all of the medication that is prescribed

16. One of the first tests ordered to diagnose diabetes is a glucose tolerance test. Preparation for this requires the client to:

① Fast for 24 hours before the test
② Have no foods for 12 hours before the test
③ Take in approximately 100 g of glucose 2 hours before the test
④ No carbohydrates for 24 hours before the test

17. Ellen Marks is a 42-year-old law student who has been complaining of fatigue, weight loss, thirst, and excessive urination. She is admitted by her physician to be worked up for possible diabetes mellitus. Miss Marks is diagnosed as having type II diabetes mellitus. Diabetes is best defined as:

① An absence of insulin in the system
② Failure of the body to metabolize carbohydrates successfully
③ A complex condition related to the control of carbohydrate metabolism
④ A disease affecting the pancreas causing a lack of insulin

18. Ellen has type II diabetes. It is decided to control Ellen's condition with diet, exercise, and medication. The diabetic diet can be described as one that:

① Provides a well-balanced meal using an exchange list
② Severely limits carbohydrates but allows fats and protein
③ Limits the intake of carbohydrates slightly
④ Helps the client lose excess weight

19. Diabetics are much more prone to cardiovascular disease than the normal population. The most likely reason for this is:

① Diabetics have difficulty metabolizing fats and proteins, with the end-products of these accumulating in the vessels
② Diabetics are usually overweight, increasing the workload on the heart and blood vessels
③ Most diabetics are elderly persons who are more likely to have degenerative cardiovascular disease
④ Atherosclerotic changes occur in the blood vessels because of the high levels of glucose and fat with poor control

20. An exercise regimen would be helpful for a type II diabetic because it would:

① Increase the rate of insulin secretion
② Lower the blood glucose by oxidizing carbohydrates
③ Prevent obesity
④ Help the insulin circulate in the body

21. It is important to teach your type II diabetic proper foot care and methods of maintaining and improving circulation to the lower extremities because the client:

① Is more prone to gangrene if an infection develops in the foot
② Has no resistance to infection and can develop septicemia
③ Is a student and will therefore not take the time needed to do foot care
④ Has a lowered resistance to infection and increased bleeding tendencies

22. Before an upper intestinal tract radiograph, the nurse should:

① Administer a strong laxative
② Administer enemas until clear
③ Withhold food and fluids for 8 hours
④ Give a high-fat dinner

23. A tubeless gastric analysis requires that the nurse:

① Obtain a urine specimen for testing
② Withhold food and fluids for 24 hours
③ Insert a nasogastric tube
④ Allow the client to eat normally

24. Ulcerative colitis is best described as:

① Chronic constipation and spastic colon
② Chronic diarrhea caused by improper diet
③ Inflammation and ulceration of the lining of the colon
④ Irritation of the small intestine

25. The cause of ulcerative colitis is unknown, but which of the following is thought to be a risk factor?

① Excessive bulk in the diet
② Stress and emotional tension
③ Overuse of laxatives
④ Excessive use of enemas

26. Mary Weeks is a 34-year-old who has been diagnosed with ulcerative colitis for about 5 years. She is admitted with severe diarrhea and fatigue. The chronic fatigue that Mary is experiencing is probably due to:

① Her lack of interest in activities outside her home
② Lack of appetite related to diarrhea
③ Failure to follow the prescribed diet
④ Anemia and malnutrition because of malabsorption and bleeding

27. The diet most usually recommended for people with active ulcerative colitis is:

① High bulk and residue
② High protein, high vitamin
③ Bland, high fat
④ Low in fluids to decrease diarrhea

28. Your client with ulcerative colitis is scheduled for an ileostomy. This is done to:

① Prevent possible perforation from the colitis
② Decrease the liquid feces
③ Control the odor from the diarrhea
④ Prevent intestinal obstruction

29. Which of the following would *not* be included in the preparation for an ileostomy in a client with ulcerative colitis?

① Administration of antibiotics to lower the bacteria in the bowel
② Enemas until clear

③ Psychologic preparation concerning the stoma
④ Fluids and electrolytes to restore balance

30. Teaching that must be included in the discharge preparation of your client with a new ileostomy done to treat ulcerative colitis would include:

① Information on stoma irrigation
② The need for sexual counseling
③ Care of the skin around the stoma
④ The need to restrict fluids

31. Your client with a new ileostomy must know the symptoms that would require notification of the physician. One of the most important signs of complication you should teach this client would be:

① Diarrhea or liquid stools for 3 days
② Daily output from the stoma of more than 1500 mL/day for several days
③ Intolerance to high-residue foods
④ A decrease in the size of the stoma over the first months after surgery

32. Your client has been diagnosed with Crohn's disease. A characteristic symptom of this condition would be:

① Chronic constipation
② Abdominal cramping before and after defecation
③ Rectal bleeding
④ Jaundice

33. Both ulcerative colitis and Crohn's disease are considered autoimmune diseases. The medications most commonly used to treat this would be:

① Antibiotics
② Nonsteroidal anti-inflammatory agents
③ Steroids
④ Antiparasitic agents

34. Your client is suffering from a deficiency of parathormone. The nurse knows to monitor the client closely for:

① Muscular weakness
② An increase in blood glucose
③ Muscle twitching and spasms of the voluntary muscles
④ Renal calculi

35. Parathormone regulates:

① Acid-base balance
② Potassium secretion
③ Thyroid metabolism
④ Calcium metabolism

36. Cushing's syndrome is often associated with:

① Steroid therapy
② Adrenal atrophy
③ Hyperthyroidism
④ Decreased ACTH secretion

37. Nursing care for a client with Cushing's syndrome would include:

① Giving a high-carbohydrate, low-protein diet
② Teaching the client the signs of hypoglycemia
③ Helping the client learn to avoid infections
④ Maintaining the client on complete bed rest

38. Mrs. Baker is a 50-year-old mother of two admitted with a diagnosis of chronic glomerulonephritis and impending renal failure. On admission, the physician orders a BUN to be done. This is done to measure the:

① Concentration of urine
② Amount of nitrogenous waste products accumulating in the urine
③ Waste products left in the blood as a result of renal failure
④ Amount of bacteria in the blood

39. Mrs. Baker, a client with chronic glomerulonephritis and impending renal failure, begins to experience some muscle twitching. The nurse should be alert for:

① Other neurologic changes
② The need to increase her fluid intake
③ The presence of circulatory changes
④ An increase in her need for calcium

40. Treatment of chronic renal failure is aimed at:

① Increasing the urine output
② Preventing the loss of electrolytes
③ Increasing the concentration of electrolytes in the urine
④ Reducing the workload on the kidneys

41. A client with acute glomerulonephritis is deteriorating and has begun to exhibit signs of renal failure and uremia. To help decrease the discomfort from the uremic frost on the skin, the nurse should:

① Provide cool alcohol baths and lotion
② Wash with diluted vinegar and apply lanolin lotion
③ Apply calamine or steroid cream
④ Wash with soap and apply mineral oil

42. Mr. Lane is admitted with a diagnosis of possible cancer of the colon. The diagnostic test most helpful in diagnosing cancer of the colon would be a:

① Barium enema
② Stool for guaiac
③ CBC
④ Colonoscopy and biopsy

43. A symptom that Mr. Lane, a client with possible colon cancer, may have noticed that led him to suspect colon cancer would be:

① Rectal bleeding and pain
② A change in bowel habits
③ Persistent nausea and vomiting
④ Clay-colored stools

44. Mr. Lane is scheduled for a colon resection and a colostomy. Which of the following would be *inappropriate* teaching for Mr. Lane?

① Sexual counseling about inevitable impotence
② Care of the stoma
③ Irrigation and regulation of the bowel
④ Potential changes in his body image

45. In teaching the postoperative end colostomy client to irrigate his colostomy, the nurse should instruct the client to:

① Use at least 1500 mL of warm tap water
② Stop irrigation and call the physician if cramping occurs
③ Never irrigate if diarrhea is present
④ Irrigate at least twice a day, morning and night

46. After a hemorrhoidectomy, which of the following is most effective for the postoperative pain?

① Tylenol #3
② A sitz bath
③ Laxatives
④ Stool softeners

47. Mrs. Mayer is a 50-year-old type I diabetic client on insulin. She has had diabetes for a number of years and is well controlled on insulin. Recently Mrs. Mayer has been having marital difficulties that leave her emotionally upset. As a result of this stress, it is possible that she will exhibit:

① An insulin reaction more readily than usual
② An increase in her blood glucose
③ A need for less daily insulin
④ A need for more carbohydrates

48. Stress in diabetic clients leads to the increased production of glucocorticoids, which would tend to:

① Decrease the production of fatty acids and lower the blood glucose
② Increase the secretion of insulin and lower the blood glucose
③ Counteract the effects of insulin and raise the blood glucose
④ Increase the production of fatty acids and raise the blood glucose

49. Your type I diabetic is receiving 40 U regular insulin at 7:30 A.M. daily. On the basis of this, you know that the most likely time for her to experience an insulin reaction is:

① By 8 A.M.
② At 4 P.M.
③ During the night
④ Around 11 A.M.

50. Your type I diabetic received NPH insulin at 7:30 A.M.; the most likely time for the reaction to occur would be:

① By 8 A.M.
② At 4 P.M.
③ During the night
④ Around 11 A.M.

51. A characteristic symptom of insulin shock that should alert the nurse to an early insulin reaction would be:

① Diaphoresis
② Drowsiness
③ Severe thirst
④ Coma

52. The physician has scheduled your client with a history of gastric ulcers for a series of diagnostic tests, including radiographs. You know that these studies are:

① Usually not done preoperatively
② Ordered only if the physician is not familiar with the client and his or her history
③ Done preoperatively to confirm a diagnosis
④ Not useful in diagnosing gastric ulcers

53. Your client with gastric ulcers is scheduled for surgery. In preparing the client for a gastric resection, which of the following would *not* be appropriate to teach the client?

① That a nasogastric tube will be in place several days after surgery
② To cough and deep breathe 10 times an hour after surgery
③ To exercise the legs hourly after surgery
④ That a Foley catheter will be in place for 1 week after surgery

54. On the night before surgery, your client with a gastric ulcer wants a "midnight snack," stating that he always has one when he is nervous. Your best response would be to tell him that:

① The kitchen has already closed for the night
② Food or fluids after midnight can lead to aspiration during surgery
③ Food or fluids increase the risk of vomiting after surgery
④ Food or fluids cause improper absorption of the anesthesia during surgery

55. Your client going to surgery for a gastric resection does not want to remove his wedding band before surgery. Your best action in this case would be to:

① Wrap tape around it once to secure it to his finger
② Tell him the surgery cannot be done if he does not remove it
③ Place a note on the chart stating that he refused to remove it
④ Remind the client that the hospital will not be liable for any loss if he insists

56. The anesthesiologist has requested that your client's dental plate be left in when he is sent to surgery for his gastric resection. The most likely reason for this request is that:

① The client has requested it because he is vain
② Dental plates do not have to be removed routinely for general anesthesia
③ Some forms of anesthesia are administered more easily if the dental plates are left in place
④ There is less danger that the dentures will be misplaced if they are not removed during hospitalization

57. While the client is under general anesthesia, there is loss of voluntary control of the sphincter muscles. For this reason, the nurse should:

① Insert a urinary catheter before the client goes to surgery
② Withhold all fluids for 12–24 hours to decrease the amount of urine output
③ Awaken the client frequently the night before surgery to empty his bladder
④ Have the client void immediately before he leaves for surgery

58. Your postoperative gastric resection client is complaining of nausea in the recovery room after his gastric resection. Your best priority action is to:

   ① Irrigate the client's nasogastric tube
   ② Notify the physician
   ③ Put the client in semi-Fowler's position to prevent aspiration
   ④ Medicate the client with a narcotic analgesic

59. Your postoperative gastric resection client, although awake and alert, complains of feeling cold on return to the room. The nurse should:

   ① Apply a heating pad to the client's back for warmth
   ② Recognize that this is a symptom of shock and notify the physician
   ③ Realize that the client is bleeding internally and call the physician
   ④ Apply several blankets to maintain body temperature at a normal level

60. On the first postoperative day, it is important that the postoperative gastric resection client be out of bed and ambulate to a chair. The nurse knows that this is done to prevent the early postoperative complication of:

   ① Atelectasis
   ② Thrombophlebitis
   ③ Nausea and vomiting
   ④ Constipation

61. On the third postoperative day, your postoperative gastric resection client's nasogastric tube is draining bile-colored liquid containing coffee-ground material. Your most appropriate action would be to:

   ① Continue simply to monitor the amount of drainage
   ② Irrigate the nasogastric tube with iced saline
   ③ Call the physician
   ④ Chart the information and ask the RN to irrigate the tube

62. When the client with a gastric resection for a gastric ulcer is discharged, the client will probably be placed on medication to prevent recurrence of the ulcer. Which of the following medications has this action?

   ① Ranitidine
   ② Chlordiazepoxide hydrochloride
   ③ Diazepam hydrochloride
   ④ Milk of magnesia

63. Because your client had a gastric resection and a partial gastrectomy, several potential problems other than recurrence exist. If the client developed symptoms of nausea, diaphoresis, and diarrhea about 1/2 hour after eating, the most likely cause would be:

   ① Pernicious anemia
   ② Pyloric obstruction
   ③ Dumping syndrome
   ④ Hyperemesis

64. The best treatment for dumping treatment would be:

   ① Weekly vitamin B_{12} injections
   ② High-carbohydrate, small meals
   ③ Dry meals with liquids between meals
   ④ Antiemetics before meals

ANSWERS AND RATIONALES

Guide to item identification (see pp. 4–5 for further details about each category):

I, II, III, or IV for the phase of the nursing process
1, 2, 3, or 4 for the category of client needs
A, B, C, D, E, F, or G for the category of human functioning
Specific content category by name; i.e., cholecystectomy

1. (2) Because of the prolonged nausea and vomiting, the most important area to assess is the fluid and electrolyte balance. This is the most potentially life-threatening area.
I, 2, F, Gastrointestinal

2. (4) Because his presenting symptom is diarrhea, the number and consistency of stools are the most important factors to assess for this client.
I, 2, F, Gastrointestinal

3. (4) Goal setting is an important part of client care planning. Goals should be specific and measurable and relate directly to the individual client. Returning to his normal bowel pattern is the most appropriate goal and is measurable for each individual client.
II, 2, F, Gastrointestinal

4. (3) A bland diet helps prevent further nausea, and the fluids are needed to replace those lost. Milk and fruit juice could increase the diarrhea.
III, 2, F, Gastrointestinal

5. (2) Because this is a recurrent problem, it would be helpful to know if anyone else in the family also had the problem. This could help to determine if something in the environment is contributing to the problem.
I, 2 & 4, F, Gastrointestinal

6. (1) The only early symptom of bladder cancer is painless blood in the urine.
I, 2, F, Bladder cancer

7. (1) With nausea, vomiting, and diarrhea, fluid imbalance is one of the next most important assessments.
I, 2, F, Gastrointestinal

8. (4) Vitamin K increases blood clotting. Cholecystitis can decrease the absorption of vitamin K.
I, 2, F, Cholecystitis & medications

9. (2) Semi-Fowler's increases lung expansion after a cholecystectomy.
III, 2, F & B, Cholecystectomy

10. (3) A T-tube is used after a common bile duct exploration to maintain patency of the duct until healing can occur.
IV, 2, F, Cholecystectomy

11. (3) Jaundice can occur if the common bile duct is obstructed with stones. Yellowish coloring around the eyes is a common symptom of jaundice.
I, 2, F, Cholecystitis

12. (1) The bladder can be punctured during a paracentesis if it is distended.
III, 2, F, Ascites

13. (2) Insulin is necessary for the utilization of glucose.
III, 2, F, Nutrition/diabetes

14. (3) Increased fluid intake helps to prevent, not cause, cystitis. All of the others are risk factors.
I, 2, C, Cystitis

15. (2) A common cause of urinary tract infections in women is contamination from the large intestine. Careful wiping can help to control this contamination.
III, 1, F, Cystitis

16. (2) The client must be NPO for 12 hours and is then given a high-carbohydrate source and tested for glucose in the blood and urine.
III, 1, F, Diabetes

17. (3) Diabetes is a complex condition affecting carbohydrate metabolism.
I, 2, F, Diabetes

18. (1) The diabetic diet is a well-balanced diet with controlled amounts of food in the various exchange categories. It is becoming closer to a normal well-balanced diet.
II, 2, F, Diabetes

19. (4) With poor control of diabetes, levels of fat and glucose are high and cause atherosclerosis.
IV, 2, F, Diabetes.

20. (2) Exercise acts to increase oxidation of carbohydrates without increases in insulin.
III, 2, F, Diabetes

21. Diabetics have a decrease in the microcircula-
① tion, especially that of the lower extremities. If
they suffer an injury, it is more likely to become
gangrenous.
III, 4, F, Diabetes

22. For an upper gastrointestinal study, food and
③ fluid are withheld for 8–12 hours before the test
so the stomach and small intestine are empty.
III, 1, F, Upper gastrointestinal

23. A tubeless test requires the urine to be tested
① for the presence of a dye, Diagnex blue, indicating the absence of hydrochloric acid in the
stomach.
III, 1, F, Peptic ulcer

24. Ulcerative colitis is characterized by inflamma-
③ tion and ulceration of the colon.
I, 2, F, Ulcerative colitis

25. Stress and emotional factors are thought to be
② a predisposing factor in ulcerative colitis.
I, 2, F, Ulcerative colitis

26. Anemia and malabsorption leading to malnutri-
④ tion are common problems in ulcerative colitis,
both of which predispose to fatigue.
IV, 2, F, Ulcerative colitis

27. High protein levels are needed for healing and
② high vitamin levels for combating the malabsorption. The diet is also usually high calorie,
high potassium, and low residue. It is also usually a bland diet without gastrointestinal stimulants.
III, 2, F, Ulcerative colitis

28. Colitis can eventually lead to perforation of the
① colon. To prevent it, if conservative medical
therapy has failed, an ileostomy is done and the
entire colon is removed.
IV, 2, F, Ulcerative colitis

29. Enemas in a client with ulcerative colitis can
② lead to megacolon or perforation. The bowel
preparation for this client usually is a single,
gentle enema if needed.
III, 1, F, Ulcerative colitis

30. Care of the skin around the stoma is the most
③ important aspect of care because skin excoriation is a real risk and leads to breakdown and
further problems.
III, 1, F, Ulcerative colitis

31. The client's stools always have a liquid consis-
② tency. The only way to determine diarrhea is
the amount of drainage. The usual amount of
drainage is 1200 mL/day.
III, 1 & 2, F, Ulcerative colitis

32. Abdominal cramping before and after defeca-
② tion is common with Crohn's disease because
the small intestine is swollen with granulomatous tissue.
II, 1, F, Crohn's disease

33. Steroids are commonly used to treat both condi-
③ tions to induce remission. There is no cure for
either disease.
II, 1, F, Crohn's disease

34. Parathormone controls calcium metabolism,
③ and a decrease leads to hypocalcemia, which
can cause muscle tetany.
III, 2, F, Endocrine disorders

35. Parathormone controls calcium metabolism.
④ I, 2, F, Endocrine disorders

36. Clients receiving steroids can develop Cushing's
① syndrome from the excessive amounts of cortisone
required to control the autoimmune process.
I & IV, 2, F, Cushing's syndrome

37. Steroids are immunosuppressants, and the cli-
③ ent is more prone to infections.
III, 2, F, Cushing's syndrome

38. Normally the urea nitrogen is filtered out
③ through the kidneys. With renal failure, it accu-
mulates in the blood.
I, 2, F, Glomerulonephritis

39. As the toxic waste products build up in the
① blood, CNS changes can begin to occur. The
nurse should monitor closely for other neurologic changes.
I, 2, C & F, Glomerulonephritis

40. The goal in chronic renal failure is to prevent
④ acute failure and maintain whatever function is
left. This is best done by minimizing stress and
workload on the kidneys.
IV, 2, F, Glomerulonephritis

41. Diluted vinegar helps to neutralize the urea, and
② the lanolin softens the skin.
III, 2, B, D, & F, Glomerulonephritis

42. Colonoscopy to visualize the lesion and a biopsy
④ of that lesion are the only accurate diagnostic
tests for colon cancer.
I, 2, F, Colon cancer

43. A change in bowel habits is one of the major
② early symptoms of colon cancer.
IV, 2, F, Colon cancer

44. Impotence does not occur after an abdominal-
① perineal resection and a sigmoid colostomy for
physiologic reasons. If the client does experience
sexual problems, they are probably psychological as a result of altered body image.
III, 2 & 4, F & G, Colon cancer

45. The client should never irrigate and cause fur-
③ ther irritation when diarrhea is present.
III, 2 & 4, F, Colon cancer

46. A sitz bath is the most helpful for the pain of a
② hemorrhoidectomy.
III, 2, F, Hemorrhoidectomy

47. Stress causes the adrenals to secrete more corti-
② sol, leading to gluconeogenesis and insulin antagonism and raising the blood glucose.
IV, 2, F, Diabetes

48. Glucocorticoids are also insulin antagonists.
③ IV, 2, F, Diabetes

49. The peak of regular insulin is about 4 hours.
④ I, 2, F, Diabetes

50. The peak for NPH is about 8 hours, and her
② blood glucose would also be low before dinner.
I, 2, F, Diabetes

51. Diaphoresis and a shaky feeling are early signs
① of hypoglycemia.
I, 2, F, Diabetes

52. Radiographs are a common tool used by the
③ physician to confirm a diagnosis before the client
goes to surgery.
IV, 1, F, Gastric ulcers

53. A Foley catheter is not a routine part of gastric
④ surgery. Even if one is inserted in surgery to
monitor output, it would not be left in for a
week. The others are routine with this type of
surgery.
III, 4, F, Gastric surgery

54. A client receiving general anesthesia must be
② NPO for 8–12 hours to prevent vomiting and
aspiration during surgery.
III, 1, F, Gastrectomy

55. Dislodgment during surgery is the risk. If a cli-
① ent absolutely refuses to remove a band, it must
be safely and securely held in place.
III, 1, F, Gastrectomy

56. It is easier and safer to administer the anesthesia
③ with certain types of dentures in place, especially dental plates.
IV, 1, D & F, Gastrectomy

57. To decrease the risk of accidental voiding, have
④ the client void immediately before the preoperative medication is given.
III, 1, D & F, Gastrectomy

58. The nasogastric tube should never be irrigated
② by the nurse following a gastric resection, only
by the physician. The only proper action is to
notify the physician that the tube probably
needs irrigation.
III, 2, F & D, Gastrectomy

59. Chilling is normal after surgery because the tem-
④ perature of the operating rooms is cool. Simply
apply blankets to maintain the client's body temperature.
III, 2, D, Gastrectomy

60. Atelectasis is the most common early postopera-
① tive problem in clients with high abdominal inci-
sions and general anesthesia. To facilitate lung
expansion, the client needs to be moved and
gotten out of bed.
II, 2, D & F, Gastrectomy

61. Coffee-ground material is old blood. This is per-
① fectly normal on the third postoperative day.
III, 2, F, Gastrectomy

62. Ranitidine blocks the release of gastric acid,
① thereby preventing the recurrence of ulcers.
II, 2, F, Gastrectomy

63. Dumping syndrome is a physiologic problem
③ associated with too rapid movement of food
through the remaining stomach. When this undigested hypertonic mass reaches the intestine,
fluids are drawn to dilute it, resulting in hypotension.
I, 2, D & F, Postgastrectomy/dumping syndrome

64. Eating only dry, small meals, lying down after
③ meals, and low carbohydrate intake all help decrease the symptoms of dumping syndrome.
III, 2, D & F, Postgastrectomy/dumping syndrome

The Pediatric Patient

GROWTH AND DEVELOPMENT: LIFE STAGES

I. THE INFANT (1 MONTH TO 1 YEAR)

A. Normal Physical Development

1. Appearance
   a. lifts head when prone by first month
   b. gains 2/3 ounce/day for first 5 months, 1/2 ounce/day for next 7; birth weight doubles by 5 to 6 months and triples by 1 year
   c. head size is 15.75 inches (38 cm) at 12 weeks, 16.5 inches (41 cm) at 20 weeks, 17 inches (42 cm) at 30 weeks, and 2/3 adult size by 1 year
   d. baby grows 1 foot first year
2. Nervous system
   a. under 4 months, objects are not followed out of line of vision
   b. by 7 to 8 weeks, eyes coordinated
   c. by 12 weeks, attends to and prefers novel stimuli
   d. full depth perception by 9 months
   e. touch important to help develop body image
3. Vital signs: by 1 year, pulse is 100–110; blood pressure, 96/66; respirations, 20–40; temperature, 99.7° F
4. Respiratory system
   a. increased susceptibility to infection, respiratory problems
   b. new alveoli developing up to 6 years of age
5. Gastrointestinal system
   a. matures to a degree after 2 to 3 months
   b. stomach emptying time slows
   c. level of hydrochloric acid in stomach reaches adult level by age 1 year
   d. teeth erupt at about 6 months
   e. peristalsis is more adult-like at about 8 months
6. Skin
   a. more prone to skin disorders
   b. sebaceous and sweat glands hypoactive
   c. ineffective for thermal regulation
7. Renal system
   a. reaches adult proportions in size by 5 months
   b. mature functional level at 1 year
   c. cannot handle excessive protein or phosphorus of cow's milk too early in life
8. Hematopoietic system
   a. inflammatory response immature
   b. ability to produce antibodies limited
   c. hemoglobin drops after 2 to 3 months, then gradually increases
   d. white blood cells reach adult level by 1 year

B. Nutritional Needs

1. Breast milk or formula all that is needed first 6 months
2. Solid foods added at varying times after 3 to 4 months
3. Iron stores may be low after 6 months
4. Self-feeding starts about 6 months
5. Food allergies common, so foods added one at a time

C. Sleep

1. By 6 weeks, infant has a nocturnal sleep pattern
2. By 7 to 8 months, infant sleeps through night without waking
3. By 1 year, infant sleeps 12 to 14 hours/night and 1 to 4 hours/day

D. Play

1. Solitary, with body parts
2. Touch, sight, and sound important
3. Way of learning about self and environment and way of developing motor skills

E. Psychosocial/Cognitive Development

1. Erikson's stage of trust versus mistrust
   a. feelings of comfort, safety, and security
   b. sense of trust in primary caregiver

TABLE 8-1 Summary of Toddler Growth and Development and Health Maintenance

Physical Competency	Intellectual Competency	Emotional-Social Competency

General: from 1 to 3 years
Gains 5 kg (11 lb)
Grows 20.3 cm (8 inches)
12 teeth erupt
Nutritional requirements
  Energy: 100 kcal/kg/day
  Fluid: 115–125 mL/kg/day
  Protein: 1.8 g/kg/day
	Learns by exploring and experimenting. Learns by imitating. Progresses from a vocabulary of three to four words at 12 months to about 900 words at 36 months.	Central crisis: to gain a sense of autonomy versus doubt and shame. Demonstrates independent behaviors. Exhibits attachment behavior strongly and regularly until third birthday. Fears persist of strange people, objects, and places and of aloneness and being abandoned. Egocentric in play (parallel play). Imitation of parents in household tasks and activities of daily living.

15 Months Legs appear bowed. Walks alone, climbs, slides down stairs backwards. Stacks 2 blocks. Scribbles spontaneously. Grasps spoon but rotates it, holds cup with both hands. Takes off socks and shoes.	Trial and error method of learning. Experiments to see what will happen. Says at least three words. Uses expressive jargon.	Shows independence by trying to feed self and helps in undressing.
18 Months Runs but still falls. Walks upstairs with help. Slides down stairs backwards. Stack 3 to 4 blocks. Clumsily throws a ball. Unzips a large zipper. Takes off simple garments.	Begins to retain a mental image of an absent object. Concept of object permanence fully develops. Has vocabulary of ten or more words. Holophrastic speech (one word used to communicate whole ideas).	Fears the water. Temper tantrums may begin. Negativism and dawdling predominate. Bedtime rituals begin. Awareness of gender identity begins. Helps with undressing.
24 Months Runs quickly and with fewer falls. Pulls toys and walks sideways. Walks downstairs hanging on a rail (does not alternate feet). Stacks 6 blocks. Turns pages of a book. Imitates vertical and circular strokes. Uses spoon with little spilling. Can feed self. Puts on simple garments. Can turn door knobs.	Enters into preconceptual phase of preoperational period: symbolic thinking and symbolic play. Egocentric thinking, imagination, and pretending are common. Has vocabulary of about 300 words. Uses two-word sentences (telegraphic speech). Engages in monologue.	Fears the dark and animals. Temper tantrums may continue. Negativism and dawdling continue. Bedtime rituals continue. Sleep resisted overtly. Usually shows readiness to begin bowel and bladder control. Explores genitalia. Brushes teeth with help. Helps with dressing and undressing.
36 Months Has set of deciduous teeth at about 30 months. Walks downstairs alternating feet. Rides tricycle. Walks with balance and runs well. Stacks 8 to 10 blocks. Can pour from a pitcher. Feeds self completely. Dresses self almost completely (does not know front from back). Cannot tie shoes.	Preconceptual phase of preoperational period as for 24 months. Uses around 900 words. Constructs complete sentences and uses all parts of speech.	Temper tantrums subside. Negativism and dawdling subside. Bedtime rituals subside. Self-care in feeding, elimination, and dressing enhances self-esteem.

2. Piaget's stages of cognitive development
  a. neonate in reflex stage
  b. at 1 to 4 months, primary circular reactions
    (1) follows objects with eyes and follows sounds
    (2) response to objects varies
    (3) recognizes faces
  c. at 4 to 8 months, secondary circular reactions
    (1) beginning object permanence
    (2) imitates others
    (3) more oriented to environment
    (4) memory traces being developed
  d. at 8 to 12 months, coordination of secondary schemata
    (1) actions show intelligence and experimentation
    (2) increased sense of separateness
    (3) finds hidden objects
    (4) can attain small goals

F. Speech

1. Neonate cry undifferentiated
2. Cry differentiates at about 2 to 3 months
3. By 9 months, all universal sounds can be made
4. By 1 year, several words are spoken

G. Social Development

1. At 1 month, early recognition of faces
2. At 2 months, smiles in response to specific stimuli
3. At 4 months, recognizes primary caregiver

TABLE 8-1 Summary of Toddler Growth and Development and Health Maintenance *Continued*

Nutrition	Play	Safety
General: from 1 to 3 years Milk 16–24 oz. Appetite decreases. Wants to feed self. Has food jags. Never force food; give nutritious snacks. Give iron and vitamin supplementation only if poor intake.	Books at all ages. Needs physical and quiet activities, does not need expensive toys.	Never leave alone in tub. Keep poisons, including detergents and cleaning products, out of reach. Use car seat. Have ipecac in house.
15 Months Vulnerable to iron deficiency anemia. Give table foods except for tough meat and hard vegetables. Wants to feed self.	Stuffed animals, dolls, music toys. Peek-a-boo, hide and seek. Water and sand play. Stacking toys. Roll ball on floor. Push toys on floor. Read to toddler.	Keep small items off floor (pins, buttons, clips). Child may choke on hard food. Cords and table cloths are a danger. Keep electrical outlets plugged and poisons locked away. Risk of kitchen accidents with toddler underfoot.
18 Months Negativism may interfere with eating. Encourage self-feeding. Is easily distracted while eating. May play with food. High activity level interferes with eating.	Rocking horse. Nesting toys. Shape-sorting cube. Pencil or crayon. Pull toys. Four-wheeled toy to ride. Throw ball. Running and chasing games. Rough-housing. Puzzles. Blocks. Hammer and peg board.	Falls: From riding toy In bathtub From running too fast Climbs up to get dangerous objects. Keep dangerous things out of the wastebasket.
24 Months Requests certain foods, therefore snacks should be controlled. Imitates eating habits of others. May still play with food and especially with utensils and dish (pouring, stacking).	Clay and Play-Doh. Finger paint. Brush paint. Cassette player with cassette and story book and song to sing along. Toys to take apart. Toy tea sets. Puppets. Puzzles.	May fall from outdoor large play equipment. Can reach farther than expected (knives, razors, and matches must be kept out of reach).
36 Months Sits in booster seat rather than highchair. Verbal about likes and dislikes.	Likes playing with other children, building toys, drawing and painting, doing puzzles. Imitation household objects for doll play. Nurse and doctor kits. Carpenter kits.	Protect from: turning on hot water falling from tricycle striking matches.

Modified from Foster, R.I., Hunsberger, M.M., & Anderson, J.J. (1989). *Family-centered nursing care of children.* Philadelphia: W.B. Saunders Co.

4. At 7 to 8 months, is shy with strangers
5. At 9 to 10 months, experiences separation anxiety

II. THE TODDLER (1 TO 3 YEARS)
(Tables 8–1 and 8–2)

A. Normal Physical Development

1. Appearance
   a. slower growth rate, but still cephalocaudal, proximal-distal, and general to specific
   b. all teeth in by 2 1/2 to 3 years
   c. chest circumference surpasses head
   d. birth weight quadrupled at 2 years
   e. approximately half of adult height by 2 years
   f. gross motor coordination improves, but still clumsy with fine motor coordination
   g. at 2 to 3 years, can pedal tricycle
2. Elimination
   a. toilet training at 2 to 3 years
   b. renal system functions normally

3. Other systems reach adult functions by 3 years

B. Nutritional Needs

1. 1000 calories/day daily by 1 year; 1300–1500 calories/day daily by 3 years
2. Is capable of and desires to self-feed
3. Likes and dislikes become obvious

C. Sleep

1. Needs 10 to 12 hours sleep at night plus nap
2. Nighttime rituals important

D. Play

1. How toddlers learn about the world
2. Solitary, but positioned parallel to others
3. Likes imitative activities
4. Loves to be read to

TABLE 8-2 Developmental Needs and Nursing Strategies: Toddlers

Physical Needs

To explore and develop muscle skill within a safe environment
Assess prehospitalization exploratory activities.
Provide small manipulative toys (boxes with lids; stack toys; nesting toys; large beads; large puzzles; equipment to color, paint, and scribble).
Provide a crib with an enclosed see-through top when a child attempts to explore by reaching for dangerous objects or crawling out of the crib.
Permit supervised activities in a playroom to explore new toys and the unfamiliar environment.
Allow exploration in child's room under supervision.

To have opportunity to engage in large muscle activity within safe limits
Assess degree of mobility attained.
Provide for supervised out-of-bed activities consistent with patterns at home as the child's condition permits.
Keep floors free of small objects.
Enforce rules about wearing of shoes or nonskid slippers when child is out of bed.
Provide toys for the large muscles (rocking horse, soft ball, indoor slide, push-and-pull toys).

To maintain physiologic function through development of self-care skills
Assess level of self-care attained (eating, elimination, dressing, hygiene, bedtime care).
Provide opportunities for participation in self-care activities:
Eating: Provide highchair or small table and chair, bib, and usual types of food; allow child to feed self in usual manner.
Elimination: Provide a potty chair or diapers according to usual elimination patterns. Reinforce routine as established prehospitalization.
Dressing: Permit child to assist with those activities he or she is capable of doing.
Hygiene: Allow child to participate in handwashing, brushing teeth, manipulating own wash cloth in tub.

Intellectual Needs

To have opportunity to learn via sensorimotor experience and express self through imitation and pretending

To engage in conversation with adults and children to enhance language development; to hear proper language and be encouraged to express self through language

Provide toys that encourage exploration and manipulation.
For older toddler, provide toys and equipment that can be used to reenact hospital experience.
Assess extent of child's vocabulary, especially key phrases and words pertaining to daily activities.
Allow child to complete sentences; avoid speaking for the child.
Reinforce words child has mastered and introduce new words.
Encourage group activities (play and eating) to encourage use of language among children.

To receive explanations about procedures (toddlers can understand more than they can say)
Avoid speaking about children without explanations to them as well.
Explain procedures before doing them.

Emotional-Social Needs

To develop sense of autonomy
Allow child to do things alone pertaining to own care.
Allow child to participate in the bedtime story, and preparation for bed according to home routines.
Give child control over some of own life: allow choices, restrain as little as possible, and praise for completed tasks.

To learn to separate from parent(s)
Encourage care by parents.
Assist family in coping with behaviors in response to hospitalization and separation.
Encourage parents to visit often even though child resists their leaving.
Provide primary nurse when parents cannot be present.
Keep image of parent in child's mind with a picture, personal belongings, or a tape recording.

To learn to adapt socially
Reinforce those socially acceptable behaviors mastered by the child before hospitalization (eating, elimination, play).
Provide play opportunities with other children.

To maintain usual routines and rituals for sense of security
Assess important rituals and routines, especially regarding bedtime (provide security objects and maintain routine; reading story, hugging, use of night light, and other rituals).
Ask parents and child about preferences in foods, toys, routines regarding daily hygiene, elimination, and dressing.
Maintain as many home routines as possible.

Data adapted and compiled from Foster, R.L., Hunsberger, M.M., & Anderson, J.J. (1989). *Family-centered nursing care of children.* Philadelphia: W.B. Saunders Co.

E. Psychosocial/Cognitive Development

1. Erikson's stage of autonomy versus shame and doubt
   a. ability to gain self-control is main goal
   b. if unable to gain self-control or if too controlled, shame and doubt develop
2. Piaget's stages of cognitive development
   a. by 12 to 18 months, fifth stage
      (1) begins to see space and time in new ways
      (2) finds hidden objects
      (3) manipulates new objects to learn
   b. by 18 to 24 months, sixth stage ends sensorimotor period and begins preoperational period
      (1) uses memory and imitation rather than trial and error
      (2) egocentric in thought and behavior

   c. by 2 to 7 years, preoperational stage
      (1) arrives at answers mentally instead of physically
      (2) uses symbolism
      (3) understands simple abstractions
      (4) increases attention span
      (5) begins to understand cause and effect

F. Speech

1. Understands simple commands
2. Begins to put words together, and by age 3 years is speaking in sentences
3. Language development requires feeling of security

TABLE 8-3 Growth, Development, and Health Promotion for Preschoolers

Physical Competency	Intellectual Competency	Emotional-Social Competency
General: 3 to 5 years		
Gains 4.5 kg (10 lb)	Becomes increasingly aware of self and others	Freud's phallic stage
Grows 15 cm (6 inches)		Oedipus complex—boy
20 teeth present	Vocabulary increases from 900 to 2100 words	Electra complex—girl
Nutritional requirements:		Erikson's stage of initiative versus guilt
Energy: 1250–1600 cal/day (or 90–100 kcal/kg/day)	Piaget's preoperational/intuitive period	
Fluid: 100–125 mL/kg/day		
Protein: 30 g/day (or 3 g/kg/day)		
Iron: 10 mg/day		
3 Years		
Runs, stops suddenly	Knows own sex	Shifts between reality and imagination
Walks backward	Desires to please	Bedtime rituals
Climbs steps	Sense of humor	Negativism decreases
Jumps	Language—900 words	Animism and realism: anything that moves is alive
Pedals tricycle	Follows simple direction	
Undresses self	Uses plurals	
Unbuttons front buttons	Names figure in picture	
Feeds self well	Uses adjectives/adverbs	
4 Years		
Runs well, skips clumsily	More aware of others	Focuses on present
Hops on one foot	Uses alibis to excuse behavior	Egocentrism/unable to see the viewpoint of others, unable to understand another's inability to see own viewpoint
Heel-toe walks	Bossy	
Up and down steps without holding rail	Language—1500 words	
Jumps well	Talks in sentences	Does not comprehend anticipatory explanation
Dresses and undresses	Knows nursery rhymes	Sexual curiosity
Buttons well, needs help with zippers, bows	Counts to five	Oedipus complex
Brushes teeth	Highly imaginative	Electra complex
Bathes self	Name calling	
Draws with some form and meaning		
5 Years		
Runs skillfully	Aware of cultural differences	Continues in egocentrism
Jumps 3–4 steps	Knows name and address	Fantasy and daydreams
Jumps rope, hops, skips	More independent	Resolution of Oedipus/Electra complex; girls identify with mother, boys with father
Begins dance	More sensible/less imaginative	
Roller skates	Copies triangle, draws rectangle	
Dresses without assistance	Knows four or more colors	Body image and body boundary especially important in illness
Ties shoelaces	Language—2100 words, meaningful sentences	
Hits nail on head with hammer		Shows tension in nail-biting, nose-picking, whining, snuffling
Draws person—6 parts	Understands kinship	
Prints first name	Counts to 10	

Nutrition	Play	Safety
General: 3 to 5 years		
Carbohydrate intake approximately 40%–50% of calories	Reading books is important at all ages	Never leave alone in bath or swimming pool
Good food sources of essential vitamins and minerals	Balance highly physical activities with quiet times	Keep poisons in locked cupboard; learn what household things are poisonous
Regular tooth brushing	Quiet rest period takes the place of nap time	Use car seats and seatbelts
Parents are seen as examples; if parent won't eat it, child won't	Provide sturdy play materials	Never leave child alone in car
		Remove doors from abandoned freezers and refrigerators
3 Years		
1250 cal/day	Participates in simple games	Teach safety habits early
Because of increased sex identity and imitation, copies parents at table and will eat what they eat	Cooperates, takes turns	Let water out of bathtub; don't stand in tub
	Plays with group	
	Uses scissors, paper	Caution against climbing in unsafe areas, onto or under cars, unsafe buildings, drainage pipes
Different colors and shapes of foods can increase interest	Likes crayons, coloring books	
	Enjoys being read to and "reading"	Insist on seatbelts worn at all times in cars
	Plays "dress-up" and "house"	
	Likes fire engines	
4 Years		
Good nutrition	Longer attention span with group activities	Teach to stay out of streets, alleys
1400 cal/day	"Dress-up" with more dramatic play	Continually teach safety; child understands
Nutritious between-meal snacks essential	Draws, pounds, paints	Teach how to handle scissors
Emphasis on quality, not quantity, of food eaten	Likes to make paper chains, sewing cards	Teach what are poisons and why to avoid
	Scrapbooks	Never allow child to stand in moving car

Table continued on following page

TABLE 8-3 Growth, Development, and Health Promotion for Preschoolers *Continued*

Nutrition	Play	Safety
Mealtime should be enjoyable, not for criticism	Likes being read to, listening to records or tapes, and rhythmic play	
As dexterity improves, neatness increases	"Helps" adults	
5 Years		
Good nutrition	Plays with trucks, cars, soldiers, dolls	Teach child how to cross streets safely
1600 cal/day	Likes simple games with letters or numbers	Teach child not to speak to strangers or get into cars of strangers
Encourage regular tooth brushing	Much gross motor activity: water, mud, snow, leaves, rocks	Insist on seatbelts
Encourage quiet time before meals	Matching picture games	Teach child to swim
Can learn to cut own meat		
Frequent illnesses from increased exposure increases nutritional needs		

From Foster, R.L., Hunsberger, M.M., & Anderson, J.J. (1989). *Family-centered nursing care of children.* Philadelphia: W.B. Saunders Co.

G. Social Development

1. Vacillates between need to be cuddled and need to show independence; tantrums are common
2. After 18 months, imitates parents' behavior (plays house)
3. At 18 to 24 months, learns to undress self
4. By 2 to 3 years, learns to dress self with help
5. Territorial with belongings

III. THE PRESCHOOLER (3 TO 5 YEARS)
(Tables 8–3 and 8–4)

A. Normal Physical Development

1. Appearance
   a. becomes taller and thinner
   b. blood pressure, 90/60 pulse, 80–110; respirations, 30
   c. coordination and balance improve
   d. climbs and jumps rope by 5 years
2. Elimination
   a. toilet-trained except for rare accidents by 3 years
   b. independent in toileting by 4 years
   c. in complete charge of needs by 5 years

B. Nutritional Needs

1. Growth slower; needs about 1700 calories/day
2. Need basic nutritional diet (see Chapter 5)
3. Eating habits simple
4. Definite food preferences

C. Sleep

1. Naps become less needed
2. 9 to 11 hours sleep required each night
3. Nightmares and fears of dark may occur

D. Play

1. Cooperative
2. Imitative and dramatic in play
3. Likes creative toys that allow for imagination

E. Psychosocial/Cognitive Development

1. Erikson's stage of initiative versus guilt
   a. increasing independence from parents
   b. self-assertion outside home
   c. involved in mastering new skills and tasks
2. Piaget's preconceptual and intuitive thought stages
   a. time, such as "tomorrow," has meaning
   b. decreased egocentricity
   c. cause and effect has magical quality
   d. more social
   e. thinks more without acting out

F. Speech

1. At 3 years, constantly asks how and why
2. By 5 years, uses adult-length sentences
3. Learns to read
4. Language has logic

G. Social Development

1. Is socially capable of independence
2. Is verbose even with strangers
3. Can share with others
4. May be more physical and aggressive

IV. THE SCHOOL-AGED CHILD (5 TO 12 YEARS) (Tables 8–5 and 8–6)

A. Normal Physical Development

TABLE 8-4 Developmental Needs and Nursing Strategies: Preschoolers

Physical Needs

To maintain control of body functions
Assess prehospitalization level of control and patterns for eating, elimination, and sleep. Assess words used to describe functions.
Allow normal patterns as much as possible.
Reassure when accidents in elimination occur; do not reprimand or punish.
Praise successes in self-control.
Provide age-appropriate motor stimulation.

To maintain physiologic function through increased development of self-care skills
Assess prehospitalization self-care tasks.
Allow continued self-care when possible; provide some opportunities for decisions on care, especially in aspects of care in which condition or treatment prohibits self-care.
Allow usual eating practices: provide foods child is used to, finger foods, favorite foods, and eating utensils from home; allow family members to eat with child if isolated or to feed if child must be fed; if not isolated, allow eating at child-sized table with hospitalized peers; follow child's usual rituals, such as prayer before eating.
Allow usual elimination practices: provide potty chair (from home if preferred) or regular toilet as child is accustomed to; if mobility is restricted, offer to assist child to toilet or bedpan at usual eliminating times. Keep call bell near so child may get prompt assistance at other times. (Preschoolers still have difficulty "holding off" elimination processes.) Stay with child or provide privacy as child is accustomed.
Allow usual rest and sleep practices. Allow night light if child is used to one or requests one; provide quiet, uninterrupted period during child's usual nap or rest time, if nap still taken; allow usual sleep time attire to be worn; if not contraindicated, allow usual sleep position and amount of cover and pillows used at home; bring any special sleep items (blanket, pacifier, toy) from home.
Permit child to dress at least partially in own clothing during daytime.

Intellectual Needs

To be protected from sense of guilt, which can occur as a result of egocentric thinking
Reassure repeatedly that no one is to blame for the condition or hospitalization.
Reassure that only necessary treatments will be done, and they will not be done without telling the child first.
Provide activities (play, arts and crafts, stories) that stimulate intellectual development.

To be protected from fears created by preoperational thinking (intuitive, magical thoughts)
Explain all procedures, especially describing what child can expect to experience through the senses, before doing them.
Provide for dramatic and therapeutic play; make available safe procedural equipment and dolls during education sessions, in playroom, at bedside.
Do not talk about the child unless child is included in the conversation.

To have opportunity to use expressive language
Encourage questions and ask questions to learn fears, fantasies, and misperceptions (correct these when possible). Give opportunity for verbal expressions during stress.
Encourage child to tell stories about drawings or to tell you a "story" about hospital procedures or experiences.
Teach new words related to simple anatomy and physiology, the disease or treatment, and hospital equipment and personnel.

Emotional-Social Needs

To master control of the environment and develop independence
Encourage self-care in hygiene and participation in medical care and treatments. (The preschooler can cooperate if given adequate instruction and permission to participate.)

Observe safety precautions.
Promptly remove offensive smells and preserve orderliness. As a result of having mastered toilet functions, the preschooler is keenly aware of smells and disorder and is upset by them.
Permit and encourage child's own decision making regarding care and treatments when choices exist.
Praise evidence of competence in all areas of development (self-care, learning new words, helping with a treatment, cooperation during stressful procedures).
Solicit and respect child's suggestions regarding care, room environment changes, toys in room, and so on.

To experience limits within environment to feel security
Enforce safety rules; give simple explanations for rules (child must be in crib or bed with rails up even if used to big bed without rails at home).
Define limits on activity due to illness (isolation from other children while disease is communicable). Since time concept is undeveloped, give idea of how long the limitation will be by associating it with concrete things ("You can go to the playroom Saturday. That is the day that cartoons are on television all morning" or "You can drink water and other drinks again when Nurse Smith comes to care for you this afternoon").
Learn during admission interview if parents want any home rules continued during hospitalization (only certain television shows may be watched or television is allowed only so many hours a day, teeth are to be brushed after each meal, limited beverages are allowed after suppertime) and enforce those not in conflict with treatment regimen.
Explain to parents reasons for any limits that cannot be enforced.

To engage in rituals to feel secure
Assess usual routines and rituals during interview. Integrate rituals into care plan as possible.
Encourage parents or other family members acquainted with the rituals to be present and help child carry out mealtime, bedtime, and other significant rituals.
Ask parents to bring from home those objects related to child's rituals and other security items.

To learn to separate without conflict
Provide for a primary nurse for each shift.
Permit and encourage unlimited parental visits and participation in planning and giving care.
Allow parents to remain and to comfort child, if desired, during treatments or procedures. Primary nurse is present as parent surrogate to stay with and comfort child.
Let parents do as many of the "caretaking" tasks as possible.
Ask parents to bring in familiar toys, family photos, personal belongings that can be left with child as reminders of them during their absence.
During care, make up pleasant stories about home activities, including names of family members in the stories, or encourage child to tell stories about home and family activities.
Provide opportunities for child to become acquainted with other children and parents who may "fill in" as sources of comfort during parental and sibling separations.
Help parents identify ways to keep child in contact with siblings or peers who cannot visit (phone call, tape recordings, notes, pictures).

To achieve sexual identity and comfort with sexual sensations and feelings
Give thorough explanations and continued reassurance about what will happen to the child's body as a result of a treatment or procedure; it is especially important to reassure of continued presence and intactness of genitals when these body parts are involved.
Handle genitalia as little as possible and use gentleness when handling is necessary. Some children respond better if their hand is used with the nurse's in handling the genitalia.
Avoid use of intrusive procedures or treatments whenever possible (preschoolers cope with axillary or oral thermometers better than rectal).

Data adapted and compiled from Foster, R.L., Hunsberger, M.M., & Anderson, J.J. (1989). *Family-centered nursing care of children*. Philadelphia: W.B. Saunders Co.

TABLE 8-5 Competency Development of the School-Aged Child

Physical Competency	Intellectual Competency	Emotional-Social Competency
General: 6 to 12 Years		
Gains an average of 2.5–3.2 kg/year (5 1/2– 7 lb/year). Overall height gains of 5.5 cm (2 inches) per year; growth occurs in spurts and is mainly in trunk and extremities. Loses deciduous teeth; most of permanent teeth erupt. Progressively more coordinated in both gross and fine motor skills. Caloric needs increase with growth spurts.	Masters contrete operations. Moves from egocentrism; learns he or she is not always right. Learns grammar and expression of emotions and thoughts. Vocabulary increases to 3000 words or more; handles complex sentences.	Central crisis; industry versus inferiority; wants to do and make things. Progressive sex education needed. Wants to be like friends; competition important. Fears body mutilation, alterations in body image; earlier phobias may recur, nightmares; fears death. Nervous habits common.
6 to 7 Years		
Gross motor skill exceeds fine motor coordination. Balance and rhythm are good—runs, skips, jumps, climbs, gallops. Throws and catches ball. Dresses self with little or no help.	Vocabulary of 2500 words. Learning to read and print; beginning concrete concepts of numbers, general classification of items. Knows concepts of right and left; morning, afternoon, and evening; coinage. Intuitive thought process. Verbally aggressive, bossy, opinionated; argumentative. Likes simple games with basic rules.	Boisterous, outgoing, and a know-it-all, whiney; parents should sidestep power struggles, offer choices. Becomes quiet and reflective during seventh year; very sensitive. Can use telephone. Likes to make things: starts many, finishes few. Give some responsibility for household duties.
8 to 10 Years		
Myopia may appear. Secondary sex characteristics begin in girls. Hand-eye coordination and fine motor skills, well established. Movements are graceful, coordinated. Cares for own physical needs completely. Constantly on move; plays and works hard; enforce balance in rest and activity.	Learning correct grammar and to express feelings in words. Likes books he or she can read alone; will read funny papers, scan newspaper. Enjoys making detailed drawings. Mastering classification, seriation, spatial and temporal, numerical concepts. Uses language as a tool; likes riddles, jokes, chants, word games. Rules guiding force in life now. Very interested in how things work, what and how weather, seasons, etc., are made.	Strong preference for same-sex peers; antagonizes opposite-sex peers. Self-assured and pragmatic at home; questions parental values and ideas. Has a strong sense of humor. Enjoys clubs, group projects, outings, large groups, camp. Modesty about own body increases over time; sex conscious. Works diligently to perfect skills he or she does best. Happy, cooperative, relaxed and casual in relationships. Increasingly courteous and well-mannered with adults. "Gang" stage at a peak; secret codes and rituals prevail. Responds better to suggestion than dictatorial approach.
11 to 12 Years		
Vital signs approximate adult norms. Growth spurt for girls; inequalities between sexes are increasingly noticeable; boys greater physical strength. Eruption of permanent teeth complete except for third molars. Secondary sex characteristics begin in boys. Menstruation may begin.	Able to think about social problems and prejudices; sees others' points of view. Enjoys reading mysteries, love stories. Begins playing with abstract ideas. Interested in whys of health measures and understands human reproduction. Very moralistic; religious commitment often made during this time.	Intense team loyalty; boys begin teasing girls and girls flirt with boys for attention; best friend period. Wants unreasonable independence. Rebellious about routines; wide mood swings; needs some times daily for privacy. Very critical of own work. Hero worship prevails. "Facts of life" chats with friends prevail; masturbation increases. Appears under constant tension.

1. Appearance
   a. growth rate slow and steady, gaining 1 to 2 feet by 12 years
   b. weight gain of about 10% per year
   c. by 12 years, about 84 pounds and 59 inches tall
   d. growth spurt just before puberty for boys
   e. by 12 years, brain essentially adult size, with head circumference about 21 inches
   f. jaw expands so permanent teeth can erupt, usually all but third molar in by 12 years

2. Vital signs
   a. temperature, 98.6° F; pulse, 60–76; blood pressure, 94/56 to 112/60
   b. heart grows more slowly; is more easily stressed because it is smaller in proportion to body size

3. General considerations
   a. maturation of most body systems occurs by 12 years
   b. at 10 to 12 years, restless energy present

TABLE 8-5 Competency Development of the School-Aged Child *Continued*

Nutrition	Play	Safety
General: 6 to 12 Years Fluctuations in appetite due to uneven growth pattern and tendency to get involved in activities. Tendency to neglect breakfast due to rush of getting to school. Although school lunch is provided in most schools, child does not always eat it.	Plays in groups, mostly of same sex; "gang" activities predominate. Books for all ages. Bicycles important. Sports equipment. Cards, board and table games. Most of play is active games requiring little or no equipment.	Enforce continued use of safety belts during car travel. Bicycle safety must be taught and enforced. Teach safety related to hobbies, handicrafts, mechanical equipment.
6 to 7 Years Preschool food dislikes persist. Tendency for deficiencies in iron, vitamin A, and riboflavin. 100 mL/kg of water/day. 3 g/kg protein daily.	Still enjoys dolls, cars, and trucks. Plays well alone but enjoys small groups of both sexes; begins to prefer same sex peer during 7th year. Ready to learn how to ride a bicycle. Prefers imaginary, dramatic play with real costumes. Begins collecting for quantity, not quality. Enjoys active games such as hide-and-seek, tag, jump-rope, roller skating, kickball. Ready for lessons in dancing, gymnastics, music. Restrict television time to 1–2 hours/day.	Teach and reinforce traffic safety. Still needs adult supervision of play. Teach to avoid strangers, never take anything from strangers. Teach illness prevention and reinforce continued practice of other health habits. Restrict bicycle use to home ground; no traffic areas; teach bicycle safety. Teach and set examples about harmful use of drugs, alcohol, smoking.
8 to 10 Years Needs about 2100 cal/day; nutritious snacks. Tends to be too busy to bother to eat. Tendency for deficiencies in calcium, iron, and thiamine. Problem of obesity may begin now. Good table manners. Able to help with food preparation.	Likes hiking, sports. Enjoys cooking, woodworking, crafts. Enjoys cards and table games. Likes radio and records. Begins qualitative collecting now. Continue restriction on television time.	Stress safety with firearms. Keep them out of reach and allow use only with adult supervision. Know who the child's friends are; parents should still have some control over friend selection. Teach water safety; swimming should be supervised by an adult.
11 to 12 Years Male needs 2500 cal/day; female needs 2250 (70 cal/kg/day). 75 mL/kg of water/day. 2 g/kg protein daily.	Enjoys projects and working with hands. Likes to do errands and jobs to earn money. Very involved in sports, dancing, talking on phone. Enjoys all aspects of acting and drama.	Continue monitoring friends. Stress bicycle safety on streets and in traffic.

Modified from Foster, R.L., Hunsberger, M.M., & Anderson, J.J. (1989). *Family-centered nursing care of children.* Philadelphia: W.B. Saunders Co.

   c. secondary sexual characteristics develop at 10 to 12 years in girls and 12 to 14 years in boys

B. Nutritional Needs

1. Needs 1600 to 2200 cal/day
2. Protein, vitamins, and minerals needed for growth
3. Becomes more influenced by others in food choices, more fads, and junk food
4. Obesity often becomes apparent

C. Rest/Activity Needs

1. At 6 years, about 11 hours sleep needed; at 11 years, about 9 hours needed
2. Exercise essential for growth and muscle development

D. Safety Needs

1. Major concern for this group with its increased independence and abilities
2. Boys more accident-prone than girls
3. Must be taught safety precautions because accidents are leading cause of death in this age group

E. Psychosocial/Cognitive Development

1. Erikson's stage of industry versus inferiority
     a. sense of accomplishment at school and play
     b. fear of failure may develop
     c. much more competitive
2. Piaget's stage of concrete operations
     a. systematic reasoning about tangible or familiar situations
     b. decenters: considers more than one characteristic at a time
     c. reverses: images process in reverse

TABLE 8-6 Developmental Needs and Nursing Strategies: School-Age Children

Physical Needs

To complete control of body functions and self-care
Assess and maintain usual routines related to body function and self-care.
Allow independent self-care to extent feasible by treatment restrictions and child's tolerance.
Praise whatever self-care child does perform.

To develop fine motor skills
Provide materials for fine motor activities (pencils and crayons, scissors, Lego, computer games, hospital equipment safe for play that requires finger manipulation).
Encourage drawing pictures of body and body parts during discussions of disease and treatment. This gives nurse feedback on the accuracy of the child's interpretation of information.
Encourage child to "take notes" during patient education sessions—gives practice in fine motor dexterity for printing or writing.
Teach child to participate in treatments that give practice in fine motor skills.

Intellectual Needs

To develop rational thinking, reality orientation
Provide scientific descriptions of the child's disease and body responses during educational sessions or in reply to questions.
Offer a rationale for each procedure before doing it to help the child to maintain self-control during procedures and to participate when feasible.
Provide children with rules about what they may and may not do during hospitalization, because of the disease or during a treatment. Suggest writing out a list of rules to post at bedside.
Assess whether child perceives hospitalization as a punishment; intervene as for preschooler if so.
Provide opportunities for child to make decisions about routine, treatments, and daily care whenever choices actually exist. Encourage middle school-aged child to help devise a care plan.

To master concepts of conservation, constancy, and reversibility and to develop skills in classification and categorization
Allow child to participate in care by helping keep track on intake and output, writing down vital signs, counting the seconds or adding up the minutes it takes to complete a procedure.
Encourage the child who can tell time to inform the nurse when it is time for a procedure or when it is time to stop the procedure (when to take out thermometer, when to take off soaks, etc.).
Encourage scrapbook making, collection, diary keeping (according to child's interests) during hospital stay.

Use these concepts in teaching sessions.
Provide games that require use of these concepts (card games, board games).
Provide hospital school or tutor schoolwork.

To vocalize feelings during stress
Encourage verbalization of feelings associated with hospitalization, disease, procedures by asking questions ("How does it make you feel to have to miss school and be away from your friends?" or "Tell me what it is like to have to lie still for 30 minutes while those compresses are on.").
Schedule time to talk with child, time not associated with any specific care or procedure. Let child know this is a time she or he can talk about anything or ask any questions. Encourage parents to do the same.

Emotional-Social Needs

To have the opportunity to channel drives into socially acceptable behaviors
Do not place girls and boys in the same room.
Provide opportunities to interact with other hospitalized school-aged children.
Assess for preschool residual concerns about genitalia; manage as for preschooler.
Help maintain peer group contact via phone calls, letter writing, tape recordings, peer visitation, photo exchanges. (Teachers and parents are usually willing to help arrange these things.)
Arrange group education sessions for children with similar problems. Include discussions of how problems are similar and how they differ. Involve children in teaching each other about anatomy and physiology, disease process, and treatment, under nurse supervision.
Treat any separation anxiety as for preschooler.
Encourage parents to express affection toward their hospitalized school-aged children and to continue setting limits as before hospitalization.

To achieve industry and associated developing, self-concept
Praise cooperation efforts, self-care accomplishments, participation in treatments, and any other achievements. Praise honestly and often.
Provide opportunities for built-in successes several times daily. (Assign tasks the child is known to be able to accomplish.)
Provide opportunities for peer cooperation (solicit roommate's help in entertaining an immobilized child).
Actively involve child in care and treatments.
Balance quiet and solitary activity with action and peer interaction as tolerated.

Data adapted and compiled from Foster, R.L., Hunsberger, M.M., & Anderson, J.J. (1989). *Family-centered nursing care of children.* Philadelphia: W.B. Saunders Co.

---

 d. conserves: sees consistency in patterns
 e. reasons logically: thinks through situations and anticipates outcomes

F. Communication

1. At 6 years, uses language more as tool; swears and uses slang to test others' reactions
2. At 7 years, can print
3. At 8 years, writes cursive
4. By 9 years, participates in discussions
5. Preadolescent seems less communicative, often finding one close friend with whom to share feelings

G. Social Development

1. Friends more important than family; usually one special friend
2. Begins to develop relationships with adults other than parents
3. Increased social skills
4. More cooperative, but still may be highly competitive

V. THE ADOLESCENT (12 TO 19 YEARS)
(Table 8–7)

A. Normal Physical Development

TABLE 8-7 Developmental Needs and Nursing Strategies: Adolescents

Physical Needs	Involve school teachers in health care planning.
	Reinforce realistic career goals.
Support of rapid skeletal growth	
Provide nutritional information on diet, snacks, and weight control.	**Emotional-Social Needs**
Refer to dietitian for special dietary needs.	*To develop healthy attitudes about body image and sexuality*
Encourage consumption of nutritional snacks, rather than "empty calories."	Encourage verbalization of fears and concerns.
	Provide privacy.
To perform self-care skills associated with onset of puberty	Let youth have own belongings and wear own clothes.
Provide information on hygiene measures; means of independent bathing.	Assist with grooming needs (e.g., hair washing, nails).
Answer questions and provide counseling on reproductive system and function.	*To achieve independence*
Provide anticipatory guidance on preventive health maintenance, breast examinations, birth control.	Compliment the adolescent's strengths.
	Encourage self-care.
Physical exercise and mobility	Provide flexible limits.
Assist to move out of bed and around the unit.	Provide opportunities to participate in setting goals, planning care, and choosing options.
Recreation activities suitable to age and size.	Provide opportunities for appropriate decisions and control.
Acknowledge need for physical expression of frustration and provide innovative means.	*To have peer contact and approval*
Encourage physical and occupational therapy to increase independence, muscle strength, and mobility.	Provide opportunities for friends to visit and call.
	Suggest recreation activities that stimulate adolescents to gather.
Intellectual Needs	Arrange for unit meeting for adolescents.
	Suggest passes to go home or to school or social functions.
To receive scientific explanations	Opportunities for appropriate calls to friends.
Thorough explanation and preparation for procedures and instructions.	*To receive family suppport*
Use scientific terminology to explain illness.	Encourage parents to visit and stay when adolescent needs or wants them.
To participate in health care management decisions	Provide opportunities for meetings in which parents can discuss issues and get support.
Include client in planning guide.	Encourage sibling visits.
Give all instructions to client as well as parent. Orient to environment, routines, and expectations.	Give support to maintain the family unit.
	Encourage chaplain visits.
To achieve in academics and strive toward career goals	Encourage use of appropriate community resources.
Provide opportunity to complete schoolwork while hospitalized.	Provide community agency referrals.

Data adapted and compiled from Foster, R.L., Hunsberger, M.M., & Anderson, J.J. (1989). *Family-centered nursing care of children.* Philadelphia: W.B. Saunders Co.

1. Appearance
   a. second major period of rapid growth
   b. girls average 2.5 to 5 inches; boys average 3 to 6 inches
   c. developmental spurt also with puberty and development of adult reproductive status
   d. more clumsy because bones outgrow muscles
2. Other systems
   a. heart grows more slowly than rest of body, causing fatigue
   b. blood pressure, 100–120/50–70; pulse, 60–68; respirations, 16–20; girls have slightly higher basal temperature
   c. all teeth by 20 to 21 years
   d. auditory acuity peaks at 13 years and decreases thereafter

B. Nutritional Needs

1. Increased appetite
2. Females, 2100 to 2400 calories/day; males, 2800 to 3000 calories/day
3. Iron, calcium, and protein needs increased

4. Eating greatly influenced by peer group, fad diets, and eating disorders

C. Rest/Activity Needs

1. Activities consistent with peer group
2. Many competitive activities
3. More rest and sleep necessary

D. Psychosocial/Cognitive Development

1. Erikson's stage of identity formation versus identity diffusion
   a. asks, "Who am I? What am I going to do with my life?"
   b. works to become independent of parents and find one's own place in the world
   c. develops sexual identity
   d. needs successful experiences in youth to avoid becoming alienated and disillusioned
2. Piaget's stage of formal operations
   a. abstract and analytic thinking
   b. becomes philosophical

E. Social Development

1. May have difficulty with adults, authority figures
2. Still needs parental figures
3. Becomes sexually attracted and may be sexually active
4. Needs peer group with whom to identify
5. Has close friends of same sex

❓QUESTIONS

1. An appropriate response to a mother concerned about her 2-year-old's possessiveness and inability to play with others would be:

   ① "It is never too early to begin counseling."
   ② "Maria is demonstrating normal behavior for a child of her age."
   ③ "Maria has probably inherited her daddy's personality."
   ④ "You should strongly encourage Maria to interact with others and share her toys so that future problems can be prevented."

2. A 2-year-old is beginning to use the word "no" in response to almost all requests and insists on doing things by herself. According to Erikson, the developmental stage that must be achieved by this child at this age is:

   ① Autonomy
   ② Initiative
   ③ Industry
   ④ Identity

3. Freud referred to late childhood as the period of:

   ① The oral stage
   ② The anal stage
   ③ The Oedipal stage
   ④ The latent stage

4. The resting time between early childhood and adolescence when the sex drives are repressed is termed:

   ① The anal stage
   ② The Oedipal stage
   ③ Latency
   ④ Puberty

5. Generally, the sexual development of girls compared with boys is:

   ① Earlier
   ② Later
   ③ The same
   ④ Individualized

6. Erikson designates late childhood as a time of:

   ① Trust
   ② Autonomy
   ③ Initiative
   ④ Industry

7. The school-aged child's loyalty is placed on which of the following?

   ① The individual
   ② The family
   ③ The peers
   ④ The church

8. Intellectual development of a school-aged child becomes more flexible and systematic. Piaget termed this operation as:

   ① Sensorimotor
   ② Preoperational
   ③ Concrete
   ④ Formal

9. Knowing that there is as much water in a low quart container as in a tall quart container is an example of which of Piaget's stages?

   ① Preoperational
   ② Concrete
   ③ Formal
   ④ Generativity

10. Physical growth is slowest during the period of:

    ① Infancy
    ② Preschool
    ③ School age
    ④ Adolescence

11. The ability of a child to know that a ball of clay flattened out into a pancake or a long string is not really bigger is called:

    ① Reversibility
    ② Conservation
    ③ Configuration
    ④ Seriation

12. The ability to arrange articles according to size is called:

    ① Preconstruction
    ② Seriation
    ③ Configuration
    ④ Reversibility

13. The ability to understand that shapes can be reversed or that sequences have a beginning and an end and can be rerun is termed:

    ① Reversibility
    ② Conservation
    ③ Transposition
    ④ Seriation

14. Shyness in a school-aged child may be produced by:

① Shaming
② Encouraging
③ Lying
④ Ignoring

15. One remedy for decreasing shyness in children is:

① Finding ways to increase self-esteem
② Giving them adult responsibilities
③ Forcing them to meet strangers
④ Doing all their tasks for them

16. A parent who says to a child, "Do as you are told because I said so," is an example of a person who is:

① Disciplinarian
② Permissive
③ Authoritarian
④ Submissive

17. A parent who offers no guidelines, thus allowing the child to make his or her own decisions, is an example of:

① Authoritarian
② Disciplinarian
③ Submissive
④ Permissive

18. Which age group has the most difficulty coping with divorce in the family?

① Infant
② Young child
③ School-aged child
④ Adolescent

19. Motor coordination in the school-aged child:

① Increases

② Decreases
③ Stagnates
④ Fluctuates

20. Gross motor coordination is demonstrated by:

① Running
② Tying
③ Writing
④ Sewing

21. Emotionally, the 7- to 12-year span is one of relationships of:

① Groups with the same sex
② Opposite sex and intimacy
③ Oedipus complex
④ Electra complex

22. The girl's first menstrual period is termed:

① Prepubescence
② Socialization
③ Menarche
④ Maturation

23. You are caring for a 26-month-old boy who was admitted for severe diarrhea. The child is doing well and will be discharged tomorrow. His mother states that he does not usually nap at home. The most appropriate action during nap time would be to:

① Insist that he take a nap with all the children
② Put him down for a nap and turn out the lights
③ Hold him and rock him until he sleeps
④ Allow him simply to play quietly in his crib

24. Your client is a preschool child who is admitted for surgery. You should tell the client that:

① Surgery will be painless
② The child should not be afraid
③ Everyone is afraid at times
④ Crying is a sign of "babyishness"

ANSWERS AND RATIONALES

Guide to item identification (see pp. 4–5 for further details about each category):
  I, II, III, or IV for the phase of the nursing process
  1, 2, 3, or 4 for the category of client needs
  A, B, C, D, E, F, or G for the category of human functioning
  Specific content category by name; i.e., cholecystectomy

1. ② The toddler requires instant gratification of desires and at this age has no comprehension of sharing or desire to share. She also prefers to play next to, rather than with, other children—"parallel play."
III & IV, 4, A, Pediatrics growth and development

2. ① The toddler begins to realize she has some measure of control over her surroundings and begins to test the extent of her power by use of the word "no."
I, 4, A, Pediatrics growth and development

3. ④ Latency means quiet time or time without obvious changes.
I, 4, A, Pediatrics growth and development

4. ③ The hormone balance is similar in both sexes.
I, 4, A, Pediatrics growth and development

5. ① The pituitary gland activates the female hormones in preparation for menarche.
I & IV, 4, A, Pediatrics growth and development

6. ④ Energy is channeled into learning.
I & IV, 4, A, Pediatrics growth and development

7. ② Family continues to serve as a guide and security factor.
I & IV, 4, A, Pediatrics growth and development

8. ③ The ability to see an organized "whole" and its parts for application is developing.
I, 4, A, Pediatrics growth and development

9. ② The ability to transfer and conserve a volume is developed.
I, 4, A, Pediatrics growth and development

10. ③ This time is used to prepare the body for sexual development.
I, 4, A, Pediatrics growth and development

11. ② Transfer of volume and its application to change are developed.
I, 4, A, Pediatrics growth and development

12. ② The ability to relate small to large is developing.
I, 4, A, Pediatrics growth and development

13. ① Control of a physical world is present.
I, 4, D, Pediatrics growth and development

14. ① The school-age child listens to the significant "other's" negative remarks and internalizes them to be true, preventing a positive self-image.
I, 4, A, Pediatrics growth and development

15. ① Shyness results from derogatory remarks being internalized. To decrease shyness, a child needs to develop a positive sense of self.
I, 4, A, Pediatrics growth and development

16. ③ An authoritarian figure does not consider the child or the situation and needs control over both rather than teaching self-control.
I, 4, A, Pediatrics growth and development

17. ④ The parent has a low self-esteem, and giving the responsibility and control to the child assures the parent of being accepted by the child.
IV, 4, A, Pediatrics growth and development

18. ③ The school-aged child questions the reason for the divorce and sees self as a possible cause.
IV, 4, A, Pediatrics growth and development

19. ① The development of muscles and bones coincides with neurologic development; therefore, physical control is observed.
I, 4, A & F, Pediatrics growth and development

20. ① Large muscle groups of the legs are demonstrated in running. Small muscle groups are used for the other activities.
I, 4, F, Pediatrics growth and development

21. ① Resolution of the Electra and Oedipus complex permits an acceptance of one's own sexual orientation.
IV, 4, A, Pediatrics growth and development

22. ③ *Mena* means monthly and *arche* means first—subsequently "first monthly."
I, 4, D, Pediatrics growth and development

23. ④ Trying to force a toddler to take a nap is futile. Allowing quiet play in the crib allows for rest without unduly upsetting the child's routine.
III, 3, A, Pediatrics growth and development

24. ③ The child needs reassurance that what he or she is feeling is perfectly normal and that it is all right to be afraid.
III, 4, A, Pediatrics growth and development

OXYGENATION

Cardiovascular Disorders

I. CONGENITAL: ACYANOTIC HEART DEFECTS

A. Ventral Septal Defects (Fig. 8–1)

1. Assessment
   a. definitions
      (1) ventricular septal defect: abnormal opening between right and left ventricles; causes left-to-right shunting of blood; can vary in size from tiny to complete absence of septum; most common cardiac anomaly; small lesions may close spontaneously
      (2) atrial septal defect: abnormal opening between two atria; may also be patent foramen ovale; causes left-to-right shunting of blood; rarely symptomatic in childhood, although may eventually lead to pulmonary hypertension; repair of severe defects usually done between ages 2 and 4
   b. untreated leads to increased pulmonary pressures and congestive heart failure
   c. history of frequent upper respiratory infections
   d. loud murmur heard on auscultation at fifth intercostal space
   e. congestive heart failure frequent complaint with severe defects
   f. may exhibit failure to thrive
   g. small defects and about 10% of large defects close spontaneously within first 2 years of life
   h. surgical repair done on children between ages 1 and 2 if shunting of blood is severe; done before permanent damage occurs in the pulmonary vasculature
2. Planning, goals, expected outcomes
   a. family and infant are prepared for surgery
   b. family and infant are supported emotionally, and family is included in infant care
   c. family copes with infant's problem
3. Implementation
   a. prepare infant and parents for surgery to close defect
   b. provide emotional support to infant and family
   c. teach family to cope with reality of defect; surgical closure may be delayed to maximize child's growth before intervention
   d. prevent infection
   e. provide age-appropriate play therapy
   f. administer medications as ordered
   g. allow parents to remain with child and provide care as appropriate
4. Evaluation
   a. family and infant were prepared for surgery
   b. family and infant were supported emotionally
   c. family coped with infant's problem
   d. no congestive heart failure developed

B. Patent Ductus Arteriosus

1. Assessment
   a. definition: a normal fetal circulatory pathway that flows to the placenta that usually closes spontaneously within 10 to 15 hours after birth; failure of fetal ductus arteriosus to close after birth causes murmur and overload of left ventricle (see Fig. 8–1)
   b. signs and symptoms
      (1) preterm infants with patent ductus arteriosus usually symptomatic, whereas term infants with a small patent ductus arteriosus may be asymptomatic
      (2) widened pulse pressure
      (3) loud murmur on auscultation over second intercostal space
      (4) dyspnea on exertion
      (5) growth below expected norm
      (6) with severe defects may show signs of congestive heart failure
      (7) if untreated, may lead to endocarditis later in life
   c. usual treatment
      (1) may not be discovered until child older
      (2) preterm infants may have closure with indomethacin
         (a) indomethacin a prostaglandin inhibitor
         (b) inhibits prostaglandin and allows patent ductus arteriosus to heal spontaneously
         (c) given before infant 10 days old
         (d) oral or intravenous doses administered up to three times
      (3) if medication fails or for term infants, surgery used to close defect
2. Planning, goals, expected outcomes
   a. child and parents are adequately prepared for surgery
   b. symptoms are controlled until surgery
   c. family copes with child's problem
3. Implementation
   a. surgery to close defect performed when symptoms indicate, usually after 1 year of age
   b. provide emotional support to child and family
   c. teach family to cope with symptoms

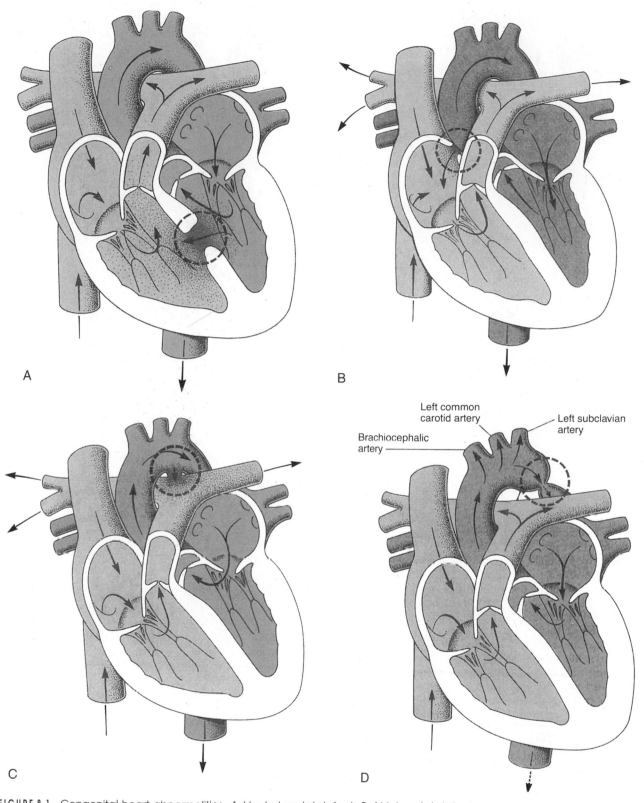

FIGURE 8-1 Congenital heart abnormalities. *A,* Ventral septal defect. *B,* Atrial septal defect. *C,* Patent ductus arteriosus. *D,* Coarctation of the aorta.

Illustration continued on following page

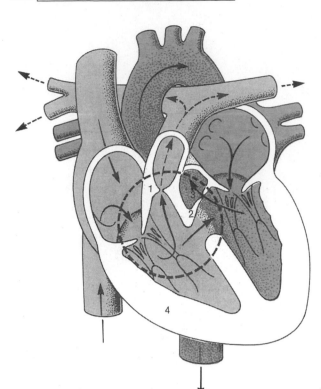

E

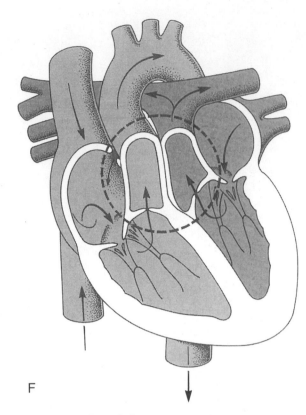

F

FIGURE 8-1 *Continued E,* Tetralogy of Fallot. *F,* Transposition of the great vessels. (From Betz, C.L., Hunsberger, M., & Wright, S. (1994). *Family-centered nursing care of children,* 2nd ed. Philadelphia: W.B. Saunders Co., pp. 1327, 1329, 1331, 1335, 1342.)

d. preoperative preparation and postoperative care as appropriate

e. mortality rate for elective closure low

f. prevent infection

g. administer medications as ordered

h. provide play therapy appropriate for developmental age

i. allow parents to stay in room and care for child as appropriate

4. Evaluation

a. child and parents were adequately prepared for surgery

b. symptoms were controlled until surgery

c. family coped with child's problem

d. child recovered from surgery without complications

C. Coarctation of Aorta

1. Assessment

a. definition: narrowing of aorta; usually causes hypertension in upper body and hypotension in lower body (see Fig. 8–1)

b. signs and symptoms

(1) hypertension in arms and hypotension in legs with absent femoral and pedal pulses

(2) history of cephalgia and epistaxis

(3) auscultation may not reveal any murmurs

(4) some infants symptomatic with congestive heart failure, failure to thrive, respiratory distress, poor weight gain, feeding problems, irritability, and tachycardia

(5) some children may be asymptomatic until later in childhood, when they complain of pain and weakness in their legs with exercise

c. usual treatment

(1) for symptomatic infants, defect is surgically corrected as soon as infant is medically stable

(2) for asymptomatic children, surgical repair is between ages 2 and 4

(3) repair may be surgical angioplasty or balloon angioplasty

(4) antibiotic prophylaxis is used to prevent endocarditis throughout the child's life

2. Planning, goals, expected outcomes
   a. surgery is delayed to allow child to grow
   b. child and parents are adequately prepared for surgery
   c. child recovers from surgery without complications
3. Implementation
   a. surgery resects aorta, insert graft, or dilate with balloon angioplasty treatments of choice
   b. teach parents care of child and include parents in daily routine
   c. provide preoperative and postoperative care as appropriate
   d. prevent infection and teach parents about need for antibiotic prophylaxis before any dental or surgical procedure
   e. provide age-appropriate play diversion for child
4. Evaluation
   a. surgery was delayed to allow child to grow
   b. child and parents were adequately prepared for surgery
   c. child recovered from surgery without complications

II. CONGENITAL: CYANOTIC HEART DEFECTS

A. Tetralogy of Fallot

1. Assessment
   a. definition: consists of four defects; right-to-left shunting of blood occurs with associated cyanosis
      (1) ventricular septal defect
      (2) right ventricular hypertrophy
      (3) pulmonary stenosis
      (4) overriding of aorta (see Fig. 8–1)
   b. signs and symptoms
      (1) cyanosis, periodic loss of consciousness, convulsions
      (2) older child with uncorrected defect assumes characteristic squatting position to facilitate breathing; preference for squatting position as child's activity increases
      (3) tetralogy of Fallot spells
         (a) characterized by periods of increased cyanosis, irritability, pallor, and tachypnea
         (b) may progress to flaccidity and loss of consciousness
         (c) usually occur first thing in morning
         (d) precipitated by crying, defecation, or feeding
         (e) if untreated, can progress to sei-

zures, cerebrovascular accidents, and death
      (4) clubbing of fingers
      (5) growth and development below expected norm
      (6) usually in poor eaters
   c. usual treatment
      (1) total surgical repair usually not performed in neonatal period; exact age when best done differs among institutions
      (2) palliative procedures, such as pulmonary shunts, may be done until corrective surgery can be done
      (3) complete surgical repair extensive with higher surgical risk
      (4) treatment of tetralogy of Fallot spells
         (a) place infant or child in knee-chest position
         (b) medications used include morphine or propranolol
         (c) oxygen may be used with medications
         (d) propranolol may be used routinely to prevent spells in children who are not surgical candidates
2. Planning, goals, expected outcomes
   a. preoperative cyanosis is minimized
   b. child and parents are adequately prepared for surgery
   c. child recovers from surgery without complications
3. Implementation
   a. assist with best position for breathing
   b. provide emotional support to child and family
   c. teach child and parent to cope with symptoms
   d. weigh child frequently and assess for symptoms of failure to thrive
   e. monitor cardiac and respiratory activity
   f. provide oxygen and maintain a pulse oximetry of at least 88 mm Hg
   g. meet infant or child's physical needs to prevent tetralogy of Fallot spells
   h. administer medication as ordered
   i. allow parents to remain in room and assist with child's care as appropriate
   j. preoperative preparation and postoperative care as appropriate
   k. prevent infection and teach parents about long-term problems
   l. surgery delayed to permit child to grow
4. Evaluation
   a. preoperative cyanosis was minimized
   b. child and parents were adequately prepared for surgery
   c. child recovered from surgery without complications

B. Transposition of Great Vessels

1. Assessment
   a. definition: pulmonary artery leaves left ventricle, and aorta leaves right ventricle (see Fig. 8–1); leads to severe hypoxia because unoxygenated blood is delivered to tissues; more common in males than females and occurs usually by birth
   b. signs and symptoms
      (1) dyspnea and cyanosis
      (2) tachycardia and tachypnea
      (3) clubbing of fingers in older children
      (4) infants may exhibit symptoms of congestive heart failure
2. Planning, goals, expected outcomes
   a. preoperative cyanosis is minimized
   b. child and parents are adequately prepared for surgery
   c. child recovers from surgery without complications
3. Implementation
   a. monitor cardiac and respiratory activity
   b. provide oxygen to maintain pulse oximetry above 75 mm Hg
   c. assess and weigh daily
   d. prevent infection
   e. monitor vital signs
   f. administer medications as ordered
   g. provide preoperative and postoperative care, as appropriate
   h. provide emotional support for child and family
   i. temporary shunt for oxygenated blood into general circulation may be done in infancy with surgical repair scheduled later
   j. include parents in daily care of child as appropriate
   k. allow rooming in as permitted by institution
   l. provide age-appropriate play and diversion
4. Evaluation
   a. preoperative cyanosis was minimized
   b. child and parents were adequately prepared for surgery
   c. child recovered from surgery without complications

III. CARDIAC SURGERY

A. Assessment

1. Preoperative observations
   a. vital signs to detect infection or congestive heart failure
   b. sleep/activity schedule to lessen stress in postoperative period
   c. bowel and bladder elimination, especially renal function
   d. fluid and food intake patterns to identify preferences and pattern of consumption
   e. monitor cardiac and respiratory function
   f. assess weight daily
2. Cardiac surgery most common in infants and toddlers with congenital heart abnormality

B. Planning, Goals, Expected Outcomes

1. Child and family are adequately prepared for surgery
2. Child recovers from surgery without complications

C. Implementation

1. Preoperatively
   a. familiarize child and family with environment, equipment, nursing personnel, and procedures
   b. use appropriate therapeutic play to practice postoperative procedures
   c. maintain preoperative schedule for least disruption
2. Postoperatively
   a. monitor vital signs continuously to detect pneumothorax, dehydration, and infection
   b. monitor pulse oximetry to reach level of greater than 92 mm Hg
   c. maintain patent airway
   d. monitor dressings for bleeding
   e. care for special apparatus, such as water-seal drainage (see Fig. 7–1)
   f. weigh daily
   g. administer medications as ordered
   h. monitor hydration, intravenous and oral fluids
   i. allow parents to remain with child and to provide care as appropriate
   j. increase activity as tolerated and appropriate for age
   k. provide emotional support for child and family
   l. discharge planning: foster independence; provide discharge teaching; prepare family for need for follow-up, prophylactic antibiotics, and other appropriate needs
   m. refer to follow-up agency

D. Evaluation

1. Child and family were adequately prepared for surgery

2. Child recovered from surgery without complications

IV. CHRONIC CONDITIONS

A. Congestive Heart Failure

1. Assessment
   a. definition: failure of myocardium resulting in engorgement of heart and blood vessels; eventually increased pressure in pulmonary or venous systems; most common in infant with a congenital abnormality, such as large septal defects or cyanotic defects
   b. signs and symptoms
      (1) cardiac enlargement shown on chest film
      (2) tachycardia with gallup rhythm
      (3) tachypnea
      (4) decreased urine output and edema
      (5) decreased peripheral pulses and mottling of the extremities
      (6) sweating and increased metabolic rate
      (7) hepatomegaly
      (8) failure to thrive
      (9) decreased exercise tolerance
   c. usual treatment
      (1) cardiac glycosides to improve cardiac function
      (2) medications to control symptoms, such as diuretics
2. Planning, goals, expected outcomes
   a. child's heart is maintained in compensated state
   b. child's condition does not deteriorate
   c. child and parents understand and comply with therapeutic regimen
3. Implementation
   a. assess vital signs as indicated by condition; changes in pulse and respiration can mean decompensation
   b. assess edema by checking weight gain and visible edema in dependent tissues and periorbital area of infants
   c. decrease cardiac demands by controlling activity, providing rest, and conserving energy; anticipate child's needs to avoid crying; decrease anxiety by teaching; maintain quiet environment
   d. reduce respiratory distress by using semi-Fowler's or Fowler's position; oxygen and humidity as ordered
   e. maintain nutritional status with small, frequent feedings and selection of nutritious, easily consumed, and easily digested foods with additional rest periods while feeding

   f. administer digitalis (see Table 7–5): count apical pulse for 1 full minute before administration; assess for toxicity and report vomiting, bradycardia, arrhythmias, or pulse deficit; monitor potassium levels
   g. administer diuretics (see Table 7–3): accurate intake and output; daily weights; encourage intake of potassium-rich foods, such as orange juice and bananas (see Table 5–4)
   h. restrict fluids; record child's usual pattern of intake and schedule restricted fluids in accordance with usual drinking habits; administer fluids in small container; educate child and parents
   i. restrict salt; monitor diet selection; educate parents and child (see Table 5–3)
   j. provide emotional support: keep parents informed of child's condition and scheduled therapies; allow parents rooming in as appropriate; encourage parental participation in child's care
   k. may be terminal condition: support parents' grief and remain with them; make child as comfortable as possible through providing comfort measures
4. Evaluation
   a. child's heart returned to compensated state
   b. child's condition did not deteriorate
   c. child and parents understood and complied with therapeutic regimen

B. Rheumatic Fever

1. Assessment
   a. definition: general systemic and chronic disease affecting connective tissues of heart, lungs, brain, and joints caused by antigen-antibody reaction to beta-hemolytic streptococci; usually follows streptococcal infection that occurred elsewhere in body
   b. between 1 and 5 weeks following initial infection (usually a sore throat), symptoms begin
      (1) lethargy
      (2) low-grade fever
      (3) anorexia
      (4) muscle and joint pain
      (5) carditis
      (6) chorea
      (7) polyarthritis
      (8) erythema marginatum
      (9) subcutaneous nodules
   c. laboratory studies confirm diagnosis
      (1) C-reactive blood protein

(2) positive throat culture for group A streptococci

(3) increased titer of antistreptococcal antibodies

(4) increased erythrocyte sedimentation rate

d. most common in school-aged child

e. usual treatment

(1) antibiotics, usually penicillin for streptococcal infection

(2) salicylates for joint pain

(3) steroids for inflammation

2. Planning, goals, expected outcomes

a. infection is detected early

b. child recovers from infection without complications

c. child and parents understand and follow therapeutic regimen

3. Implementation

a. maintain bed rest with continuous cardiac monitoring depending on presence of carditis and severity of cardiac symptoms

b. position comfortably with good body alignment and support for aching joints

c. provide age-appropriate and nonstressful diversional activities

d. continue observation of vital signs

e. select nutritious, appetizing meals and low-sodium diet to prevent edema

f. support child during frequent laboratory tests

g. provide emotional support for child and parents, and prepare for discharge that emphasizes balance of rest and activity periods

h. administer medications, especially salicylates for joint pain, steroids for inflammation (see Chapter 5 for side effects of steroids), and antibiotics for infection; educate parents and child concerning medications

i. monitor for gastrointestinal bleeding secondary to salicylates and steroids; monitor stools for occult blood

4. Evaluation

a. infection was detected early

b. child recovered from infection without complications

c. child and parents understood and followed therapeutic regimen

V. CARDIOPULMONARY RESUSCITATION (CPR)

A. Assessment/Implementation

Tell family to call 911 if outside the hospital

1. *Airway*

a. assess patency

b. if occluded, clean out child's mouth and open airway using head-tilt/chin-thrust maneuver

2. *Breathing*

a. determine whether child is breathing

b. if not, ventilate twice using mouth-to-mouth respiration

3. Circulation

a. after two breaths, check for carotid pulse (brachial pulse in infant)

b. if no pulse, using 5:1 ratio, compress chest five times, then ventilate

c. for infants, compress at 100 times/minute; for children age 1 to 8 years, rate 80 to 100 times/minute

Diseases of the Blood

I. SICKLE CELL ANEMIA

A. Assessment (Fig. 8–2)

1. Definition: hereditary trait causing breakdown of red blood cells carrying abnormal hemoglobin S; cells become crescent-shaped, carry less oxygen, and form thrombi easily

2. Defect leads to severe hemolytic anemia

3. Cells tend to be crescent-shaped when under low oxygen tension

4. Transmitted as autosomal recessive trait, particularly among African-Americans and Mediterraneans

5. Noncrisis state: symptoms of severe chronic anemia, enlarged spleen, jaundice from excessive red blood cell destruction, child tired and lethargic, may have gallstones, increased bone marrow spaces on x-ray

6. Crisis state: symptoms of thrombocytic crisis with occlusion of small blood vessels producing swelling of hands, feet, large joints, and surrounding tissues with severe pain, severely distended abdomen, and fever, followed with yellow sclera

B. Planning, Goals, Expected Outcomes

1. Early detection of children with sickle cell disease

2. Long-term complications minimized

C. Implementation

1. Prepare for laboratory studies, including sickle

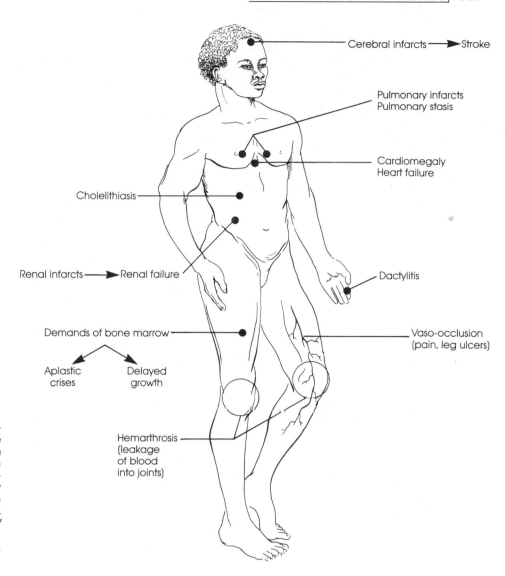

Cerebral infarts ➝ Stroke

Pulmonary infarts
Pulmonary stasis

Cardiomegaly
Heart failure

Cholelithiasis

Renal infarts ➝ Renal failure

Dactylitis

Demands of bone marrow

Vaso-occlusion
(pain, leg ulcers)

Aplastic
crises

Delayed
growth

Hemarthrosis
(leakage
of blood
into joints)

FIGURE 8-2 Potential effects of episodes of sickling. The fragility of the abnormal red blood cells results in their destruction and the formation of emboli and infarcts and the leakage of blood into the joints. Virtually every system of the body can be adversely affected. (From de Wit, S.C. (1992). *Keane's essentials of medical-surgical nursing,* 3rd ed. Philadelphia: W.B. Saunders Co., p. 447.)

cell slide test, sickle cell turbidity test, and hemoglobin electrophoresis
2. Provide supportive care with intravenous and oral fluids—increase fluid intake to 2 to 3 L/day
3. Monitor blood transfusions as ordered
4. Administer analgesics as ordered; pain can be extremely severe
5. Administer oxygen and monitor pulse oximetry
6. Teach child and parents concerning disease and therapy
7. Teach parents about availability of genetic counseling
8. Allow parents to room in and assist with care as appropriate

D. Evaluation

1. Sickle cell disease was detected early
2. Long-term complications were minimized

II. LEUKEMIA

A. Assessment

1. Definition: malignant blood disorder in which immature white blood cells increase in number, causing decrease in red blood cells and platelets in bone marrow; most common cancer in children, with acute lymphocytic leukemia the most common type; cure rate increasing with the use of chemotherapy and bone marrow transplantation
2. Signs and symptom
   a. anorexia
   b. nausea and vomitin
   c. weight loss
   d. fatigue
   e. pallor
   f. fever
   g. bone and joint pain
   h. abdominal pain

i. petechiae and bruises
j. enlarged spleen and liver
3. Diagnosed by presence of immature white blood cells, called blast cells, in blood and bone marrow
4. Most common in preschool children

B. Planning, Goals, Expected Outcomes

1. Leukemia is diagnosed early
2. Child and parents are adequately prepared for treatment regimen
3. *Child and parents are adequately prepared and cope with prognosis

C. Implementation

1. Prepare for diagnostic tests
2. Provide support during bone marrow biopsy
3. Provide supportive and symptomatic care
4. Provide emotional support to child and parents to handle chronic, sometimes fatal, disease
5. Support during administration of antineoplastic drugs (see Tables 7–22 and 7–23)
6. Observe meticulous medical asepsis to prevent infection
7. Maintain good nutrition
8. Provide careful skin and mouth care and care for all mucous membranes, especially of anus and rectal area
9. Allow parents to room in and participate in care as appropriate
10. Encourage age-appropriate toys and diversional activity
11. Prepare child and family for long-term survival with potential difficulties secondary to hospitalization and treatments for the disease
12. Provide for long-term follow-up of child
13. Encourage the use of support groups and resources from American Cancer Society
14. Provide referral for clergy and social service for child with terminal prognosis

D. Evaluation

1. Leukemia was diagnosed early
2. Child and parents were adequately prepared for treatment regimen
3. Child and parents were adequately prepared and coped with terminal prognosis

III. HODGKIN'S DISEASE

A. Assessment

1. Definition: malignancy of lymph system characterized by presence of large, primitive, malignant cells; most common in adolescents and young adults, rare before age 5 years; curable cancer with early diagnosis and treatment
2. Signs and symptoms
   a. history of frequent infections
   b. late afternoon fever with night sweats
   c. physical examination reveals enlarged, painless lymph nodes, especially in cervical or groin region
3. Usual treatment
   a. lymph node biopsy
   b. lymphangiogram
   c. staging laparotomy
   d. chemotherapy
   e. radiation therapy

B. Planning, Goals, Expected Outcomes

1. Client's condition is diagnosed early
2. Client is prepared for treatment regimen, including surgery, radiation therapy, and chemotherapy

C. Implementation

1. Prepare child for diagnostic tests, such as radiographs, lymph node biopsy, and lymphangiogram
2. Prevent infection
3. Provide emotional support to child and family to cope with diagnosis and treatment
4. Provide care for child receiving chemotherapy and radiation therapy
5. Prepare child and parents for long-term survival and need for continued follow-up
6. Provide discharge teaching for child and family

D. Evaluation

1. Client's condition was diagnosed early
2. Child and parents complied with therapeutic regimen

IV. HEMOPHILIA

A. Assessment

1. Definition: sex-linked autosomal recessive hereditary disorder of delayed blood coagulation caused by absence of clotting factor; disease occurs in males, whereas females are carriers
2. Easy bruising and bleeding into tissues

3. Injured areas show marked swelling and bruising
4. Symptoms dependent on area affected by bleeding, such as central nervous system symptoms if intracranial bleed
5. Diagnostic tests
   a. family history
   b. bleeding time and clotting time show prolonged intervals
   c. clotting factor analysis shows missing factor VIII or factor IX
6. Usual treatment
   a. replacement of deficient clotting factor and administration of cryoprecipitate
   b. local treatment, such as ice packs, Ace bandage wraps, and immobilization
   c. after bleeding stops, gentle massage to prevent contracture of joint
7. Complications
   a. formation of inhibitors (antibodies) that destroy factors
   b. human immunodeficiency virus (HIV) infection through administration of contaminated cryoprecipitate
      (1) rates of infection estimated at 80% to 90% of hemophilia A and 50% of hemophilia B clients who received cryoprecipitate before 1985
      (2) since 1985, better collection of donor serum
      (3) acquired immunodeficiency syndrome (AIDS) has replaced hemorrhage for this group as most common cause of death

B. Planning, Goals, Expected Outcomes

1. Child's condition is diagnosed early
2. Child experiences minimal complications
3. Child and parents understand and follow therapeutic regimen
4. Child and parents cope with chronic, usually fatal illness

C. Implementation

1. Provide support during frequent laboratory tests
2. Provide safe environment to prevent injury
3. Teach child and parents to understand nature of disease and factors to control
4. Assist child and parents in learning proper technique for cryoprecipitate administration
5. Provide support during blood transfusions
6. Refer to community agencies or support groups
7. Prepare child and family for outcome of HIV infection

D. Evaluation

1. Child's condition was diagnosed early
2. Child experienced minimal complications
3. Child and parents understood and complied with therapeutic regimen
4. Child and parents coped with chronic, usually fatal illness

V. INFECTIOUS MONONUCLEOSIS

A. Assessment

1. Definition: infectious disease, caused by the Epstein-Barr virus, results in increase in mononuclear white blood cells and signs of a general infection; thought to be only mildly contagious and spread by oral contact (sometimes called "kissing disease"); most common in adolescents
2. Signs and symptoms
   a. malaise; sore throat with pharyngitis; fever; enlarged liver, spleen, and lymph glands; lack of energy
   b. history of exposure; incubation period around 10 to 14 days
   c. macular type of skin rash on trunk
   d. positive Monospot test
3. Usual treatment
   a. no effective medication except acyclovir, which works in only high doses and is reserved for immunosuppressed clients
   b. rest and symptomatic treatment

B. Planning, Goals, Expected Outcomes

1. Transmission of virus is minimized
2. Child recovers from disease without complications

C. Implementation

1. Maintain bed rest as necessary and gradually increase activity as symptoms decrease
2. Administer antivirals as ordered
3. Administer nonsalicylate antipyretics as ordered
4. Maintain hydration with oral or intravenous fluids
5. Maintain good nutrition and provide diet as tolerated
6. Teach child and parents regarding need for rest and sleep
7. Maintain medical asepsis; isolation usually not necessary

8. Provide activities and diversions appropriate for age and activity level

D. Evaluation

1. Transmission of virus was minimized
2. Child recovered from disease without complications

Pulmonary Disorders

I. ACUTE DISORDERS

A. Upper Respiratory Infection

1. Assessment
   a. definition: viral or bacterial infection affecting upper respiratory tract; also called nasopharyngitis or "common cold"
   b. common in children of all ages
   c. signs and symptoms
      (1) fever
      (2) nasal congestion
      (3) sore throat
      (4) sneezing
      (5) rhinitis
      (6) cough
      (7) anorexia
      (8) irritability
   d. laboratory tests, such as throat culture, rarely done (mainly to rule out streptococcal infections)
2. Planning, goal, expected outcome: child recovers without complications
3. Implementation
   a. maintain bed rest or quiet environment until fever subsides
   b. maintain hydration with oral fluids
   c. administer antipyretics and decongestants as ordered (not aspirin because of risk of Reye's syndrome)
   d. humidify air to assist in decreasing congestion
   e. maintain adequate nutrition
4. Evaluation: child recovered without complications

B. Acute Otitis Media

1. Assessment
   a. definition: inflammation and infection of middle ear, frequently caused by infection-producing organism traveling through infant's shortened, widened eustachian tubes
   b. signs and symptoms
      (1) fever
      (2) pain in ears
      (3) irritability
      (4) restlessness
      (5) pulling or rubbing ears
      (6) rolling of the head
      (7) convulsions with high fever
   c. history of upper respiratory infection
   d. most common in infants
2. Planning, goals, expected outcomes
   a. child's condition is diagnosed and treatment begun early
   b. child and parents understand and follow therapeutic regimen
3. Implementation
   a. administer antibiotics and ear drops as ordered
   b. monitor vital signs
   c. encourage oral fluids to maintain hydration
   d. observe for ear drainage
   e. provide good skin care and cleanliness
   f. prepare for myringotomy as indicated
      (1) incision that opens tympanic membrane for drainage
      (2) may also include insertion of tubes to maintain patent incision for drainage
   g. teach child and family about cause and treatment of otitis media
4. Evaluation
   a. child's condition was diagnosed and treatment was begun early
   b. child and parents understood and complied with therapeutic regimen
   c. child experienced no hearing loss

C. Bronchiolitis

1. Assessment
   a. definition: inflammation of bronchioles usually caused by respiratory syncytial virus; results in thick mucus plugging bronchioles and trapping air in alveoli, leading to poor air exchange and difficulty in expelling air from lungs
   b. signs and symptoms
      (1) dry, nonproductive cough
      (2) shallow respirations
      3) air hunger and cyanosis (very late)
      (4) pale mucous membranes
      (5) dyspnea
      (6) irritability
      (7) retractions
      (8) rapid respirations
   c. slight fever
   d. most common in infants under age 18 months
2. Planning, goals, expected outcomes
   a. child recovers without complications
   b. child does not have recurrence of disease

3. Implementations
   a. maintain patent airway
   b. position for comfort and to ease respirations (Fowler's position or raise head of crib)
   c. humidify air and give oxygen as ordered
   d. monitor vital signs frequently, including oxygen perfusion and breath sounds
   e. maintain hydration with intravenous or oral fluids and feedings as indicated by dyspnea or tachycardia
   f. conserve energy: provide rest and activity as tolerated
4. Evaluation
   a. child recovered without complications
   b. child did not have recurrence of disease

D. Bronchitis

1. Assessmen
   a. definition: inflammation of mucous membrane of bronchial tubes *without* obstruction
   b. history of upper respiratory infection
   c. signs and symptoms
      (1) dry, nonproductive cough
      (2) irritability
      (3) fever
   d. most common in infants
2. Planning, goals, expected outcomes
   a. child recovers without complications
   b. child does not have recurrence of disease
3. Implementation
   a. humidify air
   b. maintain hydration by encouraging oral fluids
   c. monitor vital signs and oxygenation
   d. perform postural drainage as ordered
4. Evaluation
   a. child recovered without complications
   b. child did not have recurrence of disease

E. Pneumonia

1. Assessment
   a. definition: localized inflammation of lung tissues caused by primarily bacteria or viruses; may also be from aspiration
   b. signs and symptoms
      (1) nonproductive cough
      (2) fever
      (3) vomiting
      (4) diarrhea
      (5) convulsions with high fever
      (6) increased pulse and respirations
   c. laboratory tests showing increased white blood cell count

   d. chest radiograph positive for infiltrates
   e. most common in infants and toddlers
2. Planning, goals, expected outcomes
   a. child recovers without complications
   b. child and parents understand and follow therapeutic regimen
3. Implementation
   a. bed rest until fever diminishes
   b. maintain Fowler's position or elevate head of crib for comfort
   c. monitor vital signs frequently and oxygen perfusion and breath sounds
   d. maintain hydration by encouraging oral fluids, especially in children with tachycardia
   e. administer antipyretics and antibiotics (see Table 7–10) as ordered (not aspirin, which might lead to Reye's syndrome)
   f. control fever with sponge baths
   g. humidify air
   h. permit activity as tolerated, but prevent dyspnea and tachycardia
4. Evaluation
   a. child recovered without complications
   b. child and parents understood and complied with therapeutic regimen

F. Croup

1. Assessment
   a. definition: sudden attack of group of symptoms resulting from laryngospasm or obstruction of larynx; also called spastic laryngitis or laryngotracheobronchitis
   b. history of runny nose (rhinitis) or hoarseness
   c. signs and symptoms
      (1) barking cough
      (2) inspiratory stridor
      (3) retractions
      (4) restlessness
      (5) rapid respirations
   d. sudden onset of symptoms
   e. assess for symptoms of asphyxia
   f. fever may or may not be present
   g. usually occurs in children under age 5 years
   h. may have more than one attack
   i. attacks frequently occur at night
2. Planning, goals, expected outcomes
   a. child recovers without complications
   b. child and parents understand and follow therapeutic regimen
3. Implementation
   a. monitor vital signs frequently, including oxygen perfusion and breath sounds
   b. provide croup tent or mist tent for humidified oxygen

c. maintain calm manner and environment to avoid upsetting child

d. have tracheostomy tray at bedside for emergencies

e. provide emotional support to child and family

f. teach parents about emergency care at home; inhaling humidified air from steamy bathroom shower may relieve acute symptoms

4. Evaluation

a. child recovered without complications

b. child and parents understood and complied with therapeutic regimen

G. Tonsillitis and Adenoiditis

1. Assessment

a. definition: inflammation of tonsils and adenoids, caused by either bacteria or viruses and often accompanied by frequent upper respiratory infections

b. signs and symptoms

(1) sore throat, especially frequent bouts of strep throat

(2) difficulty in swallowing

(3) hoarseness

(4) nonproductive cough

c. noisy breathing or difficulty in breathing, "mouth breathers"

d. direct visualization of throat shows presence of redness and swelling of tonsils and adenoids

e. most common in preschoolers

2. Planning, goals, expected outcomes

a. child is adequately prepared for surgery

b. child and parents understand and follow therapeutic regimen

c. child recovers without complications

3. Implementation

a. administer antibiotics as ordered

b. provide supportive care of warm, salt-water gargles as age of child permits

c. maintain hydration by encouraging oral fluids as tolerated

d. prepare child and parents for surgery if chronic infections present

e. postoperative care

(1) monitor vital signs

(2) check throat and nares for bleeding

(3) observe for frequent swallowing that may indicate bleeding

(4) position client prone or flat with head to side initially

f. encourage cool nondairy product liquids when client is fully awake postoperatively

g. discharge instructions following surgery to include teaching child and parents concerning diet, fluids, activity, prevention of infections, and delayed hemorrhage due to tissue sloughing

4. Evaluation

a. child was adequately prepared for surgery

b. child and parents understood and complied with therapeutic regimen

c. child recovered without complications

H. Sudden Infant Death Syndrome (SIDS)

1. Assessment

a. definition: sudden, unexplained death of infant who was apparently healthy immediately before death; also known as "crib death"

b. often parent puts infant to bed and infant later discovered dead or infantile apnea noted (near-miss baby)

c. assess for any physical cause; autopsy usually rules out any preventable cause

d. research has not yet discovered cause of this syndrome

e. evaluate apnea in near-miss baby

2. Planning, goals, expected outcomes

a. parents cope with loss

b. parents learn care for near-miss SIDS baby

3. Implementation

a. emotional support crucial to family; parents often feel tremendous guilt

b. encourage psychologic counseling for parents, siblings, other family members, and caregivers

c. monitor for apnea/bradycardia continuously

d. teach parents continuous monitoring of near-miss SIDS baby

e. teach parents CPR

f. emotional support to parents of near-miss SIDS baby

4. Evaluation

a. parents coped with loss

b. parents verbalized and demonstrated care of near-miss SIDS baby

II. CHRONIC DISORDERS

A. Cystic Fibrosis

1. Assessment

a. definition: autosomal recessive hereditary disease caused by error in metabolism; generalized dysfunction of exocrine glands of lungs, pancreas, and liver; excessive amounts of mucus and sweat are produced, and these organs become obstructed

b. pancreatic involvement results in copious, bulky, greasy, foul-smelling stools containing large amounts of fat but no trypsin; infants eat well but do not gain weight

c. lung involvement consists of chronic cough and frequent upper respiratory infections

d. sweat gland involvement results in increased sweat chloride test over 60 mEq/L; salty "taste" to skin

e. poor absorption of fat-soluble vitamin D can lead to osteoporosis

f. pancreatic damage can lead to diabetes mellitus

g. prognosis: chronic disease that may shorten life span, but many children now survive to adulthood

h. family history of disease

2. Planning, goals, expected outcomes
   a. child's condition is diagnosed early
   b. child and parents understand and follow therapeutic regimen
   c. child and family are prepared for possible shortened life span

3. Implementation
   a. provide special nutrients and foods (especially pancreatic enzymes with food intake, vitamins, low-fat and high-protein diet, and additional salt during hot weather)
   b. prevent respiratory infection
   c. provide inhalation therapy, humidified air, percussion and postural drainage, breathing exercises, and mucolytic drugs as ordered to help break up mucus and keep lungs clear
   d. provide meticulous skin care to prevent irritation
   e. teach family concerning special care procedures, diet, and medications
   f. provide emotional support to family and child to accept and cope with this condition
   g. refer to Cystic Fibrosis Foundation and other community agencies

4. Evaluation
   a. child's condition was diagnosed early
   b. child and parents understood and complied with therapeutic regimen
   c. child and family prepared for possible shortened life span

B. Asthma

1. Assessment
   a. definition: obstructive airway disease caused by spasms of bronchioles owing to hypersensitivity of airways
   b. often caused by allergic response to pollen, food, or animal fur; can also be triggered by emotional upset
   c. history of respiratory problems in family
   d. chest radiograph rules out other causes
   e. most common in school-aged children

2. Planning, goals, expected outcomes
   a. child's asthma is controlled
   b. child and parents understand and follow therapeutic regimen

3. Implementation
   a. perform environmental study to remove allergens as much as possible
   b. monitor oxygen perfusion and breath sounds; wheezing often noted with some hypoxia
   c. administer bronchodilators as ordered (see Table 7–13)
   d. give steroids briefly to reduce inflammation, with care
   e. maintain hydration by encouraging fluids
   f. administer inhalation therapy and breathing exercises to maintain patency of bronchial tubes
   g. monitor theophylline levels
   h. teach child and parents to cope with condition

4. Evaluation
   a. child's asthma was controlled
   b. child and parents understood and complied with therapeutic regimen

C. Allergic Rhinitis (Hay Fever)

1. Assessment
   a. definition: allergic response to allergen, such as pollen, dust, fur, or food
   b. signs and symptoms
      (1) sneezing
      (2) watery and itchy eyes
      (3) runny nose
      (4) postnasal drip
   c. history of previous response to allergen
   d. allergy testing may be done
   e. most common in school-aged children and adolescents

2. Planning, goals, expected outcomes
   a. child's symptoms are controlled
   b. child and parents understand and follow therapeutic regimen

3. Implementation
   a. perform environmental study to remove allergens, if possible
   b. provide supportive therapy of decongestants and antihistamines as ordered

4. Evaluation
   a. child's symptoms were controlled

b. child and parents understood and complied with therapeutic regimen

Fluid and Electrolyte Balance

(See Chapter 7 for further, more specific information)

I. NORMAL FLUID AND ELECTROLYTE BALANCE

A. Assessment

1. Observe hydration of child; 73% of infant's weight is water
2. Laboratory tests for fluid and electrolyte levels

B. Planning, Goal, Expected Outcome

Child's fluid and electrolyte balance is maintained in homeostatic state

C. Implementation

1. Provide proper balance of electrolytes for homeostasis
2. Provide adequate hydration for proper body functioning
3. Take daily weight on same scale, at same time, in same clothes

D. Evaluation

Child remained in healthy homeostasis with correct fluid and electrolyte balance

II. FAILURE TO THRIVE

A. Assessment

1. Definition: failure to grow and develop within normal range; no apparent cause
2. Below 5th percentile for height and weight
3. Malaise, listlessness
4. Poor appetite, poor eating habits
5. Unresponsive to being held and cuddled
6. Laboratory tests rule out any specific disease entity
7. Evident in first few months of life
8. Assess parenting skills and assess for possible abuse or neglect

B. Planning, Goals, Expected Outcomes

1. Parents learn effective parenting skills
2. Infant's condition is diagnosed early
3. Infant begins to grow at normal rate

C. Implementation

1. Provide tender, loving care
2. Provide sensory stimulation: visual, auditory, and tactile stimulation needed
3. Give small, frequent feedings for weight gain; intravenous or nasogastric feedings may also have to be given
4. Provide emotional support to family
5. Encourage parents to assist in care; teach parents effective care of infant
6. Obtain extensive history and investigation of parenting and home situation

D. Evaluation

1. Parents learned effective parenting skills
2. Infant's condition was diagnosed early
3. Infant began to grow at normal rate

❓QUESTIONS

1. Sam is a 6-year-old admitted to the hospital for a diagnostic workup. He has been experiencing a low-grade fever, weight loss, and pain in his arms and legs. His admitting diagnosis is rheumatic fever. The pain most often associated with rheumatic fever:

   ① Results from involuntary muscle spasms
   ② Is located in the joints and migrates from one to the other
   ③ Is never associated with swelling or any other obvious symptom of the disease
   ④ May cause paralysis of the lower extremities

2. Rheumatic fever usually follows:

   ① Infections caused by beta-hemolytic streptococci
   ② Violent trauma to the body
   ③ Viral upper respiratory infections
   ④ Osteomyelitis

3. A child with rheumatic fever is placed on complete bed rest after the diagnosis has been confirmed. The nurse can best explain this to the client by telling him that:

   ① He must stay in bed or he will damage his heart and might die
   ② The doctor wants him in bed even if we have to restrain him
   ③ He must rest in bed while we will bring him everything he needs so that he can get well
   ④ He can play quietly in his room as long as he rests whenever he is even slightly tired

4. The physician orders aspirin every 4 hours for the child with rheumatic fever. Salicylates are given to treat rheumatic fever because they:

   ① Help destroy the bacteria causing it
   ② Keep the body temperature subnormal
   ③ Prevent cardiac involvement
   ④ Relieve the joint pain

5. The most potentially serious complication from rheumatic fever is:

   ① Cardiac involvement
   ② Disintegration of the joints
   ③ Rheumatoid arthritis
   ④ Cerebral involvement

6. Maternal factors that may possibly predispose to the birth of a child with a heart defect include:

   ① Early maternal age
   ② Tuberculosis in remission
   ③ Excessive weight gain
   ④ Rubella during the first trimester of pregnancy

7. A symptom *not* associated with prolonged vomiting in infants is:

   ① Decreased skin turgor
   ② Increased urine output
   ③ Metabolic alkalosis
   ④ Decreased blood volume

8. Mary has returned to her room following a tonsillectomy. A symptom that does *not* indicate hemorrhage is:

   ① Increased pulse and respiration
   ② Frequent swallowing
   ③ Complaint of sore throat
   ④ Vomiting bright red blood

9. Tony, age 5 months, is diagnosed with asthma and placed on bronchodilators and steroids. Because Tony is receiving steroids, the nurse should assess for:

   ① Increased respirations
   ② Decreased respirations
   ③ Fluid retention
   ④ Increased fluid output

10. Infants under evaluation for prolonged periods of coughing and episodes of large bulky stools may undergo which of the following diagnostic studies?

    ① Sweat electrolytes for cystic fibrosis
    ② Gastric pH for gastroesophageal reflux
    ③ Barium enema for intussusception
    ④ Arterial blood gases to determine oxygenation

11. Alecia, age 2 years, is brought to the emergency department after waking up with a barky cough and stridor. On arrival at the emergency department, she is in no respiratory distress and afebrile. The diagnosis is spasmodic croup. The nurse instructs the parents to:

    ① Perform percussion and postural drainage before putting Alecia to bed
    ② Encourage frequent coughing and deep breathing
    ③ Run a cool mist vaporizer in her room at night
    ④ Follow the schedule of antibiotic therapy

12. Tara, age 3 years, is admitted to the pediatric unit with a left lower lobe pneumonia. She has a temperature of 39.5° C and is complaining of chest pain. Respirations are shallow with a rate of 60. Nursing interventions for Tara would include:

    ① Forcing oral fluids
    ② Positioning Tara on her left side with head elevated
    ③ Administering intravenous morphine for pain
    ④ Provision of a high-calorie diet

13. What is the primary factor that causes the observable clinical signs in cystic fibrosis?

    ① Abnormal secretion of most of the exocrine glands
    ② Hyperactivity of the parasympathetic nervous system
    ③ Mechanical obstruction of gland secretion
    ④ Hypoactivity of the sweat glands

14. Which of the following best describes why cystic fibrosis can predispose a child to bronchitis?

    ① Elevated sodium in saliva can irritate the mucous membranes in the nasopharynx·

    ② Related cardiac defects and congestive heart failure can cause increased respiratory distress
    ③ Neuromuscular irritability can cause constriction of the bronchioles
    ④ Thick secretions block the respiratory tract, causing impaired drainage from the bronchi

15. The preschooler with allergic rhinitis would most likely *not* experience symptoms when:

    ① Eating eggs
    ② Playing with the dog
    ③ Rolling in the grass
    ④ Lying on the rug watching television

16. During an asthmatic attack, proper positioning can facilitate respirations. Respiratory effort is assisted if the child:

    ① Lies flat and is turned side to side frequently
    ② Sits upright and leans over a table
    ③ Lies on his or her side with head up 30 degrees
    ④ Lies flat with legs raised to promote venous return

ANSWERS AND RATIONALES

Guide to item identification (see pp. 4–5 for further details about each category):

I, II, III, or IV for the phase of the nursing process
1, 2, 3, or 4 for the category of client needs
A, B, C, D, E, F, or G for the category of human functioning
Specific content category by name; i.e., cholecystectomy

1. Migratory polyarthritis is a common symptom
② that does not cause permanent joint destruction.
IV, 2, B & E, Rheumatic fever

2. The causative agent for rheumatic fever is the
② beta-hemolytic streptococcus.
IV, 2, B & E, Rheumatic fever

3. A child cooperates better if he knows the reason
③ for the restrictions and also knows that all of his needs will be met.
III, 2, B & E, Rheumatic fever

4. Aspirin is a nonsteroidal anti-inflammatory
④ agent that helps relieve the joint pain.
IV, 2, B & E, Rheumatic fever

5. Valvular heart damage is common following
① rheumatic fever, especially mitral valve disease.
IV, 2, B & E, Rheumatic fever

6. Rubella or measles during the first trimester in
④ the mother can lead to serious heart defects in the fetus.
IV, 4, B, Rubella

7. The fluid and electrolyte imbalance from pro-
② longed vomiting in an infant would lead to a decrease in the urine output.
I, 4, B, Fluid & electrolytes

8. A complaint of a sore throat, although a normal
③ postoperative complaint, does not signify hemorrhage.
I, 2, B, Tonsillitis

9. Steroids often cause the child to retain sodium
③ and fluid.
IV, 2, B, Asthma

10. Sweat electrolytes are elevated in children with
① cystic fibrosis. These children demonstrate coughing as well as unusual stooling as the first signs and symptoms of the disease.
I, 1, B, Cystic fibrosis

11. Laryngeal spasm is relieved by provision of a
③ high-humidity atmosphere, especially at night.
III, 2, B, Croup

12. Children are generally more comfortable semi-
② erect, lying on the affected side to splint the chest wall and to reduce painful pleural rubbing. Children who are dyspneic are given nothing by mouth because of the danger of aspiration.
III, 2, B, Pneumonia

13. The primary abnormality in cystic fibrosis is an
① abnormality in the secretions of the exocrine glands, resulting in production of thick mucus.
I, 2, B, Cystic fibrosis

14. Thick secretions cause impaired drainage from
④ the bronchi, leading to chronic cough, bronchitis, and bronchopneumonia.
I, 2, B, Cystic fibrosis

15. Allergic rhinitis results from inhalation of cer-
① tain airborne particles.
I, 1, B, Allergic rhinitis

16. The child in respiratory distress is better able to
② breathe in a sitting position.
III, 2, B, Asthma

SENSORY/PERCEPTUAL ALTERATIONS

Disorders of the Cerebral or Central Nervous System

I. SEIZURE DISORDERS

A. Epilepsy

1. Assessment
    a. definition: recurrent, transient attacks of disturbed brain function resulting in convulsive symptoms of a general or localized nature
    b. idiopathic epilepsy: no identifiable cause; may be related to genetic defect in metabolism in brain
    c. organic epilepsy: history of phenylketonuria, hypoglycemia; prenatal, birth, or postnatal injury; central nervous system infection; trauma; genetic influences; toxic effects; brain tumors
    d. careful assessment and recording of seizure activity help to specify type of disorder and appropriate treatment
    e. classification of seizures
        (1) generalized seizures
            (a) *absence seizure (petit mal):* brief loss of consciousness; "staring" expression with immediate return to alert state
            (b) *tonic-clonic seizure (grand mal):* tonic (stiffening) and clonic (twitching) phases; may be accompanied by aura; loss of consciousness; incontinence; may be apneic with cyanosis; can progress to status epilepticus, a prolonged seizure and medical emergency
            (c) *myoclonic seizure:* single or repetitive muscle flexion spasms
            (d) *atonic seizure:* brief loss of posture or muscle tone
            (e) *infantile spasms:* massive myoclonus; occurs in infants 3 to 8 months of age
        (2) *partial seizures:* involve a localized area of cerebral cortex
            (a) *simple partial:* localized motor or sensory disturbance, usually without loss of consciousness
            (b) *complex partial:* psychomotor, temporal lobe seizures; often accompanied by tongue, hand, feet, or trunk; may or may not involve loss of consciousness
    f. preparation and support during electroencephalogram
    g. assessment of neurologic signs
2. Planning, goals, expected outcomes
    a. child's condition is diagnosed before problems occur
    b. child and parents understand and follow therapeutic regimen
    c. child does not suffer injuries from seizures
    d. child and family cope with chronic illness
3. Implementation
    a. assess children for presence of epilepsy if seizure activity occurs
    b. provide safe environment for child: safe toys; quiet surroundings; protect during seizure
    c. teach parent and child concerning nature of disorder, self-help activities, safety, proper medication administration and side effects, emergency procedures
    d. provide emotional support to understand disorder and cope with long-term care
    e. administer anticonvulsant medications (Table 8–8)
    f. have emergency equipment available for resuscitation, suction, CPR
    g. refer to national foundations and community support groups

TABLE 8-8 Properties of Some Commonly Used Anticonvulsant Drugs

Drug	Side Effects	Comments
Luminal (phenobarbital)	Drowsiness, irritability, hyperactivity	Safest overall medication; bitter, often combined with other drugs
Dilantin (phenytoin)	Ataxia, insomnia, motor twitching, gum overgrowth, hirsutism (hairiness), rash, nausea, vitamin D and folic acid deficiencies	Generally effective and safe; regular massaging of gums decreases hyperplasia; used in combination with phenobarbital or primidone
Depakene (valproic acid)	Gastrointestinal disturbance, altered bleeding time, liver toxicity	Monitor blood counts; take with food or use enteric-coated preparations; potentiates action of phenobarbital and other drugs
Mysoline (primidone)	Ataxia, vertigo, anorexia, fatigue, hyperirritability, dermatitis	May be used alone or in combination; side effects minimized by starting with small amounts
Valium (diazepam)	Headache, tremor, fatigue, depression	Used in combination or alone
Clonopin (clonazepam)	Behavior changes, ataxia, anorexia, nystagmus	Effective for most minor motor seizures

Modified from Thompson, E.D. (1990). *Introduction to maternity and pediatric nursing,* 2nd ed. Philadelphia: W.B. Saunders Co. (p. 641).
Note: The physician determines the child's medication by the type of seizure and other factors. The goal is to achieve the best control with the minimum dosage and the least number of side effects. An important aspect of nursing intervention includes reinforcing the need for drug supervision and compliance.

4. Evaluation
  a. child's condition was diagnosed early before complications occurred
  b. child and parents complied with therapeutic regimen
  c. child did not suffer injuries from seizures
  d. child developed normally and coped with chronic disease

B. Febrile Seizures

1. Assessment
  a. definition: seizures caused by high temperature (above 102° F or 38.8° C)
  b. generalized seizure characterized by tonic and clonic movements and loss of consciousness
  c. significantly elevated temperature
  d. history of recent infection or illness or fever
2. Planning, goals, expected outcomes
  a. child and parents understand and follow therapeutic regimen
  b. child recovers from disease without complications
3. Implementation
  a. prevent injury and ensure safety during seizure
  b. monitor vital signs continuously
  c. medicate as ordered, antipyretics (acetaminophen [Tylenol])
  d. use nursing measures to lower temperature; e.g., tepid sponge baths
  e. have emergency equipment for suctioning and resuscitation at bedside
  f. provide emotional support to child and family
  g. teach parent care during seizure and prevention of injury
  h. teach parents safe measures (i.e., fever reduction) to minimize episodes of seizure activity
4. Evaluation
  a. child and parents complied with therapeutic regimen
  b. child recovered without complications

II. CONGENITAL DISORDERS

A. Cerebral Palsy

1. Assessment
  a. definition: group of disorders caused by disruption of motor centers in the brain; cause usually interruption of oxygen supply to brain occurring prenatally, during birth, or from accident or disease
  b. motor development, difficulty with voluntary motor movements, developmental delays
  c. involuntary, random movements may be present
  d. histories of pregnancy and labor and delivery
  e. history of childhood accident or serious illness
  f. observation of weakness and spasticity of the extremities
  g. vision, speech, and hearing disabilities may also be present
  h. cerebral palsy from disease or accident can be manifested at any age
2. Planning, goals, expected outcomes
  a. child's diagnosis is made early
  b. child and parents understand and follow therapeutic regimen
  c. child and family cope with chronic disease
3. Implementation
  a. individualize care to specific needs of child
  b. provide early infant stimulation and early educational intervention
  c. maintain good body alignment, prevention of contractures, reinforcement of physical therapy or other ordered exercises
  d. maintain good nutrition; feeding and oral control should be considered
  e. prevent infection
  f. provide emotional support to child and family to accept long-term care; no cure
  g. teach parents and child concerning supportive appliances (e.g., braces), activities of daily living, expected growth and development; use team approach with child, family, nurse, physician, speech therapist, and so on
  h. refer to national organizations and local support groups for assistance
4. Evaluation
  a. prenatal or birth injury was diagnosed in infancy
  b. child and parents complied with therapeutic regimen
  c. child coped with disorder and altered lifestyle

B. Hydrocephalus

1. Assessment
  a. definition: increased intracranial pressure caused by overabundance of cerebrospinal fluid within brain; this accumulation may be due to blockage of flow of cerebrospinal fluid or to inadequate absorption, resulting in enlarged head and possible brain damage and retardation
  b. increased head circumference and change in shape, engorged scalp veins
  c. separating suture lines and bulging fontanels in infant

d. eye abnormalities may be present: strabismus, nystagmus, and "sunset sign" (sclera visible above iris)

e. malaise, lethargy may be present

f. poor neck control; inability to support head in upright position

g. feeding problems, anorexia, projectile vomiting, high-pitched cry

h. diagnostic tests, may include computed tomography (CT) scan

i. treated with insertion of shunt to drain fluid from brain

2. Planning, goals, expected outcomes

a. child and parents are adequately prepared for surgery

b. child suffers minimal complications from disease

3. Implementation

a. if surgery to implant ventriculoperitoneal shunt planned, preoperative care intended to prevent infection, maintain good nutrition, provide for emotional support of child and family, and make the child as comfortable as possible

b. postoperative care includes maintaining patent airway, observing neurologic and vital signs closely, supporting head and neck during any movement, preventing infection, assessing for shunt malfunction, and providing emotional support to child and family

   (1) signs of infection include fever, irritability, vomiting, altered level of consciousness, signs of increased intracranial pressure

   (2) signs of shunt malfunction include increasing head size and signs of increased intracranial pressure

c. prevention of complications such as infection or obstruction of shunt important during all phases of care

d. teach family care of child and strategies to prevent or decrease long-term complications

e. be sure family understands need for long-term follow-up

f. assess family's understanding of problems and ability to care for child at home; arrange visiting nurse if needed

4. Evaluation

a. child recovered from surgery without complications

b. child experienced minimal complications from disorder

C. Down Syndrome

1. Assessment

a. definition: chromosomal defect (trisomy 21, or extra chromosome), resulting in characteristic physical changes and mental retardation

b. history of mother: Down syndrome often associated with advanced maternal age

c. presence of particular physical characteristics

   (1) round face

   (2) thick, protruding tongue

   (3) almond-shaped eyes (origin of "mongoloid" description)

   (4) small, flat nose

   (5) poor muscle tone

d. developmental tests show slow motor development and varying degrees of mental retardation

e. hands show transverse palmar crease (simian crease)

f. integumentary system usually shows dry, cracked skin

g. child usually happy and smiling

h. usually diagnosed at birth or shortly after

2. Planning, goals, expected outcomes

a. child and family cope with diagnosis

b. child develops to maximal potential

3. Implementation

a. individualize all care according to the needs of the child

b. emotionally support parents, who expected "perfect baby"

c. teach parents and family about syndrome and reasonable expectations and goals for child

d. teach about normal growth and development and expectations for child

e. prevent infection; parent teaching to prevent infection

f. provide stimulation for child

g. teach parents care of child at home

h. genetic counseling for future pregnancies

i. refer to local agencies and support groups

j. include any siblings in teaching and emotional support

4. Evaluation

a. child and family coped with diagnosis

b. child developed to maximal potential

D. Mentally Handicapped Child

1. Assessment

a. definition: impairment of intelligence from unknown cause or injury or disease.

b. developmental testing results in classification according to intelligence quotient (IQ)

   (1) *educable mentally handicapped:* IQ between 50 and 75; capable of simple basic learning, social and sensorimotor skills can be developed; can learn activities of daily living

(2) *trainable mentally handicapped:* IQ between 35 and 50, can usually learn to communicate and interact on basic level; can learn independence with supervision

(3) *severely retarded:* IQ between 20 and 35, constant supervision necessary; learning ability poor

(4) *profoundly retarded:* IQ below 20, minimal capacity to function at most basic level; requires custodial care

c. history of child and family for disease or injury

d. usually evident in infancy; may be diagnosed anytime during childhood, depending on cause

2. Planning, goals, expected outcomes
   a. family and child cope with diagnosis
   b. child develops to maximal potential

3. Implementation
   a. nursing care must be provided for child's developmental age, not chronologic age
   b. provide stimulation
   c. prevent infection
   d. techniques of behavior modification often useful
   e. provide emotional support to child and family
   f. teach family to cope with child's permanent condition and maximize his or her potential
   g. refer to local support agencies

4. Evaluation
   a. family and child coped with diagnosis
   b. child developed to maximal potential

E. Spina Bifida

1. Assessment
   a. definition: spinal defect caused by failure of laminae to fuse or by absence of laminae; usually occurs in lumbosacral area; complications from involvement of spinal cord may occur
   b. visualization of defect and resulting spinal cord involvement
      (1) *spina bifida occulta:* bony defect of laminae with visible dimple or indentation
      (2) *meningocele:* bony defect of laminae with protrusion of meninges and cerebrospinal fluid into membranous sac
      (3) *myelomeningocele:* bony defect with protrusion of meninges, cerebrospinal fluid, spinal cord, and spinal nerves into membranous sac; paralysis below level of defect usually occurs
   c. assess for involvement of lower extremities, impairment of bowel and bladder function

2. Planning, goals, expected outcomes
   a. child and parents are prepared for surgery
   b. child and family cope with permanent deficits

3. Implementation
   a. if sac is intact, priority is to maintain that sac to prevent infection and further damage to cord
   b. if surgical closure of defect planned, preoperative care includes optimum skin care, nutrition, hydration, prevention of infection, and position of comfort to prevent pressure on sac
   c. postoperative care includes prevention of infection, optimum skin care, nutrition, hydration, and position of comfort with good body alignment
   d. perform range-of-motion exercises to lower extremities
   e. provide bladder care, including Credé method of expelling urine as appropriate or teach family and, if appropriate, child intermittent catheterization procedures
   f. provide emotional support to child and family to accept condition and resultant lengthy treatment

4. Evaluation
   a. child recovered from surgery without complications
   b. child and family coped with permanent deficits

III. INFECTIOUS DISORDERS

A. Meningitis

1. Assessment
   a. definition: viral or bacterial infection of meninges and cerebrospinal fluid
   b. fever
   c. high-pitched cry, irritability
   d. physical examination reveals nuchal rigidity
   e. seizures likely
   f. in infant, bulging fontanels

2. Planning, goals, expected outcomes
   a. child and family understand and follow therapeutic regimen
   b. child recovers from disease without complications

3. Implementation
   a. prepare for and assist with lumbar puncture
      (1) in bacterial, fluid cloudy with white blood cells, low glucose, and bacteria may be present
      (2) in viral, fluid may appear clear
   b. administer antibiotics as ordered for bacterial or antivirals for viral; initially intravenous route may be used to ensure optimum immediate dosage; intramuscular and oral doses follow as child's condition improves
   c. monitor vital signs

d. monitor neurologic signs and level of consciousness; institute seizure precautions
e. intravenous line may be used to give fluids and as vehicle for drug administration
f. fluids restricted to prevent increased intracranial pressure
g. administer sponge baths and acetaminophen to reduce high fever
h. maintain quiet environment when irritable
i. provide emotional support for child and family
4. Evaluation
a. child and parents complied with therapeutic regimen
b. child recovered without complications

B. Reye's Syndrome

1. Assessment
a. definition: acute encephalopathy following a viral infection
b. history of severe and persistent vomiting 1 to 7 days after onset of viral illness, such as influenza or chickenpox
c. progression of symptoms to alteration in mental functioning, such as extreme sleepiness, disorientation, hostility or combativeness, loss of consciousness
d. history of aspirin use has been connected with cause of Reye's syndrome
e. most survivors recover completely, but some suffer from minor to severe brain damage and resultant disability
2. Planning, goals, expected outcomes
a. parents understand nature of illness and institute preventive measures, such as not using aspirin during child's viral illness
b. child's diagnosis is made early
c. child and parents understand and follow therapeutic regimen
d. child and family cope with residual deficits
3. Implementation
a. quickly recognize symptoms and begin immediate supportive care, such as neurologic assessment and seizure precautions (extremely important); once mental changes have begun, progression may be rapid and may lead to death
b. maintain hydration with intravenous fluids as ordered
c. emergency equipment needed to assist respiration should be at the bedside
d. maintain seizure precautions
e. make accurate recording of signs, symptoms, and history; Reye's syndrome can be mistaken

for encephalitis, meningitis, diabetic acidosis, poisoning, or drug overdose
f. provide emotional support to the child and family; Reye's syndrome can lead to death in 3 to 5 days from the onset of vomiting
g. teach parents about signs and symptoms to be alert for and what to report to physician
h. provide preventive teaching about complications of viral illness for all parents; Reye's syndrome *not* communicable but occurs following viral infection; aspirin must not be used during a viral illness
i. reorient child gradually during recovery; provide toys and diversions appropriate for age and physical and mental condition
4. Evaluation
a. syndrome did not occur
b. diagnosis was made early
c. child and parents complied with therapeutic regimen
d. child and family coped with residual deficits

IV. BRAIN TUMORS

A. Assessment

1. Definition: abnormal growth within cranium; may be benign or malignant, but always treated to reduce size of tumor
2. Signs of increased intracranial pressure, including vomiting, headache, irritability, malaise, widening pulse pressure
3. Neuromuscular changes, including unsteady ambulation and incoordination
4. Sensory loss in sight, hearing, perception
5. Specific symptoms can assist in locating tumor site within brain
6. Most common in school-age years

B. Planning, Goals, Expected Outcomes

1. Child's increased intracranial pressure is diagnosed and treated early
2. Child and parents are adequately prepared for surgery and follow-up therapy
3. Child copes with any residual deficits

C. Implementation

1. With surgical removal, preoperative care involves maintenance of hydration, fluid restriction if indicated, good nutrition, safety, and specific care for individual symptoms

2. Postoperative care includes prevention of infection and continuation of preoperative care
3. Monitor vital signs and signs of increased intracranial pressure continually
4. Control fever with sponging, acetaminophen
5. Observe for seizures; institute seizure precautions
6. Prepare child for chemotherapy and support during course of medication administration
7. Prepare for radiation therapy and support during therapy
8. Provide emotional support for child and family; acceptance of condition and realistic future goals for child

D. Evaluation

1. Child's increased intracranial pressure was diagnosed and treated early
2. Child recovered without complications
3. Child coped with any residual deficits

V. DEGENERATIVE DISORDERS

A. Lead Poisoning

1. Assessment
   a. definition: poisoning from ingestion of lead from lead-based paints, plaster, exhaust accumulation, water and water fountains, lead solder in copper pipes; can be absorbed through skin, lungs, and gastrointestinal tract
   b. central nervous system symptoms appear gradually
      1) irritability
      (2) drowsiness
      (3) convulsions
      (4) weakness
      (5) vomiting
      (6) abdominal pain
      (7) constipation
   c. symptoms of encephalitis
   d. history reveals pica, or eating of nonfood substances
   e. death may occur; residual mental retardation possible
2. Planning, goals, expected outcomes
   a. child does not continue to ingest lead
   b. child recovers without permanent damage
3. Implementation
   a. collect urine and blood specimens for tests to determine amount of lead in child's body
   b. tell parents to study environment and remove sources of ingested lead
   c. administer anti–lead-absorbing medications

(chelation therapy); British antilewisite (BAL) (dimercaprol) or calcium disodium edetate (CaEDTA)
   d. teach child and family concerning sources of lead and substitute safe chew toys and objects
   e. refer to community agencies for ongoing follow-up
4. Evaluation
   a. child's environment was modified so that lead ingestion does not continue
   b. child recovered without permanent damage

Vision/Hearing/Speech

I. AMBLYOPIA

A. Assessment

1. Definition: "lazy eye," reduced visual acuity in one eye caused by inability of eyes to focus and work together for binocular vision; without treatment, blindness may occur in affected eye
2. History of blurred vision, double vision, problems with "blind spot"
3. Examination with Snellen eye chart pinpoints problem eye if child old enough to cooperate

B. Planning, Goals, Expected Outcomes

1. Child and parents understand and follow therapeutic regimen
2. Child recovers without complications

C. Implementation

1. Treatment usually application of patch to good eye so that child must use weak eye; this use focuses and strengthens weaker eye; length of treatment depends on severity and response to treatment
2. Provide emotional support to child and family; assist with coping mechanisms
3. Teach child and family importance of following treatment regimen faithfully
4. Response to treatment best during preschool years

D. Evaluation

1. Child and parents complied with therapeutic regimen
2. Vision returned to normal

II. STRABISMUS

A. Assessment

1. Definition: "cross-eye," failure of eyes to work to-

gether and focus on same object at same time for binocular vision; may be unilateral or bilateral
2. Assess for eye deviations
3. History of problems with vision
4. Defect responds best to treatment during the pre-school years

B. Planning, Goals, Expected Outcomes

1. Child and parents understand and follow therapeutic regimen
2. Child's vision becomes normal

C. Implementation

1. Apply patch to stronger eye to force weaker eye to focus

2. Corrective lenses and exercises may be prescribed
3. If conservative therapy does not correct problem, surgical intervention to correct muscle defects may be indicated
4. Provide emotional support to child and family to follow treatment regimen exactly
5. Teach child and family to understand the defect and methods to correct it for normal binocular vision

D. Evaluation

1. Child and parents complied with therapeutic regimen
2. Vision returned to normal level

❓QUESTIONS

1. When a congenital defect results in an increase in the intracranial pressure and size of the child's head, the child is said to have:

   ① Hydrocephalus
   ② Microcephalus
   ③ Anencephaly
   ④ A hydrocele

2. A symptom exhibited by infants with a cold that is rare in adults is:

   ① Nasal congestion
   ② Nasal discharge
   ③ A sore throat
   ④ A high fever

3. Sally Ponds, 4 days old, is admitted to the pediatric unit from the nursery with a diagnosis of Down syndrome. Which of the following are problems expected to develop in Sally?

   ① Slowed development once she reaches 1 or 2 years of age
   ② Profound mental retardation
   ③ More respiratory tract infections
   ④ Hearing problems

4. The symptom of Down syndrome most evident during the initial newborn assessment would be:

   ① Asymmetry of the gluteal folds
   ② Hypertonicity of the skeletal muscles
   ③ A rounded occiput
   ④ Simian creases on the palms and soles

5. Which of the following would an infant with Down syndrome need more than most babies?

   ① Frequent handling and rocking to keep her from crying
   ② Helping her parents learn to care for and about her
   ③ Teaching her parents to nipple-feed her
   ④ Preventing aspiration of formula by frequent burping

6. A common defect associated with Down syndrome is:

   ① Deafness
   ② Congenital heart defects
   ③ Hydrocephaly
   ④ Muscular hypertonicity

7. As Sally, an infant with Down syndrome, grows, her development lags and it is found that she is moderately retarded. Which of the following activities is best for her?

   ① Challenging, competitive situations
   ② Simple, repetitive tasks
   ③ Detailed tasks
   ④ Tasks that can be accomplished in less than 1 hour

8. Mary Spring, 7 years old, has spastic cerebral palsy involving all extremities and a history of grand mal seizures. She is admitted to the pediatric unit, accompanied by her parents, with a diagnosis of bronchopneumonia. Which of the following information is most essential to plan her nursing care?

   ① Ability to perform activities of daily living
   ② Immunizations received
   ③ Family history of illnesses
   ④ Reactions to previous hospitalizations

9. Mary is a 7-year-old with spastic cerebral palsy admitted for bronchopneumonia. Mary's rectal temperature is 103.6° F. To decrease her temperature, the PN should:

   ① Put her in a cool mist croupette with compressed air
   ② Sponge her trunk and extremities with tepid water
   ③ Encourage her to take clear liquids such as apple juice
   ④ Sponge her with a half water and half alcohol solution

10. Mary is a 7-year-old with spastic cerebral palsy admitted for bronchopneumonia. Mary had a tonic-clonic seizure (grand mal seizure). Which of the following interventions would be done first:

   ① Loosen her clothing and protect her from injury by padding the crib
   ② Maintain a patent airway by turning her head to the side and suction her if necessary
   ③ Remain with her and administer anticonvulsant medications as ordered by the physician
   ④ Describe and record events before the onset of the seizure, during the seizure, and after the seizure

11. Mary is a 7-year-old with spastic cerebral palsy admitted for bronchopneumonia. Mary is on a pureed diet. While feeding her, the PN sees that she has trouble eating because of a:

① Weakness of the muscles used in sucking and swallowing
② Delayed eruption of the lateral and central incisors
③ Inability to relax completely during meal time
④ Loss of appetite because of bronchopneumonia

12. Mary is a 7-year-old with spastic cerebral palsy admitted for bronchopneumonia. Which of the following interventions should the PN plan to implement each day before Mary's physical therapy?

① Decrease the tension in her muscles by placing her in a warm bath
② Administer a muscle relaxant as prescribed by the pediatrician
③ Provide a rest period in a quiet room with decreased stimulation
④ Decrease the tension in her muscles by massaging her extremities

13. Mary is a 7-year-old with spastic cerebral palsy admitted for bronchopneumonia. Mary's mother states, "Mary is not progressing. I'm going to take her to another doctor who will take better care of her and help her get well." This comment probably reflects her mother's:

① Anger at the health care team
② Denial of Mary's condition
③ Guilt feelings about Mary
④ A lack of understanding of cerebral palsy

14. Rapid diagnosis of Reye's syndrome is essential. To help parents prevent this life-threatening disorder, the nurse should teach which of the following?

① It is associated with all viral infections and occurs primarily during the warmer months
② Children recovering from a viral infection who suddenly begin to vomit should see the physician immediately
③ It is a self-limiting disorder but may precipitate liver failure if it is not treated immediately
④ Aspirin administration during the febrile period seems to decrease long-term complications

15. Children receiving phenytoin (Dilantin) to control seizures are instructed to:

① Take it with Maalox to reduce gastric upset
② Brush teeth frequently and see dentist regularly
③ Eat a high-fiber diet to reduce constipation
④ Stay away from known sources of infection

ANSWERS AND RATIONALES

Guide to item identification (see pp. 4–5 for further details about each category):
   I, II, III, or IV for the phase of the nursing process
   1, 2, 3, or 4 for the category of client needs
   A, B, C, D, E, F, or G for the category of human functioning
   Specific content category by name; i.e., cholecystectomy

1. ① The condition resulting when fluid causes an increase in the size of the skull and increased intracranial pressure is called hydrocephalus.
I, 4, C, Hydrocephalus

2. ④ Infants are much more likely to develop high fevers from a trivial cold than are adults.
I, 4, C, Febrile seizures

3. ③ Babies with Down syndrome have decreased muscle tone, which compromises breathing and coughing, leading to a likelihood of upper respiratory tract infections.
I, 2, B & C, Down syndrome

4. ④ Simian creases are the only symptom always observable. Other physical characteristics may suggest Down syndrome.
I, 4, B & E, Down syndrome

5. ② Parents' response to the child may greatly influence their ability to care for the child. Learning about the child and Down syndrome may help them give better care.
III, 3, C, Down syndrome

6. ② Babies with Down syndrome have a high incidence of congenital heart disease, especially atrial defects.
I, 2, B & C, Down syndrome

7. ② A child who is moderately retarded is unable to follow complicated procedures or remember detailed directions. Simple repetitive tasks provide all the challenge needed.
III, 4, A & C, Down syndrome

8. ① When a child with cerebral palsy is hospitalized, routines used at home should be followed, so it is important to know her abilities.
II, 1, C, Cerebral palsy

9. ② Tepid sponge baths reduce temperature by promoting evaporation. Alcohol baths may reduce temperature too rapidly, leading to vascular collapse/vasoconstriction, which defeats the purpose of the cool applications.
II, 1, D & C, Cerebral palsy

10. ② The most important action during a grand mal seizure is to maintain a patent airway. Accumulated secretions must be removed from the nasopharynx.
II, 1, B & C, Seizures

11. ① Children with cerebral palsy often have feeding difficulties because of poor sucking ability and persistent tongue thrust. She needs to sit up to promote swallowing.
I, 1, C & F, Cerebral palsy

12. ③ Children with cerebral palsy tire easily but find it difficult to relax. A period of rest should be provided before physical therapy.
III, 1, C, Cerebral palsy

13. ② Parents of handicapped children experience a period of mourning for the normal child they were expecting. Denial of the child's condition is expressed by consulting a variety of physicians, one of whom, it is hoped, will change the child's diagnosis.
IV, 3, G, Cerebral palsy

14. ② Reye's syndrome appears to follow a mild viral infection from which the child is recovering. The child then begins to vomit suddenly. It is important that parents recognize the potential severity of this symptom and seek immediate medical attention.
III, 1, C, Reye's syndrome

15. ② A common side effect of prolonged Dilantin administration is gum hyperplasia.
III, 2, C, Seizures/medications

PROTECTIVE FUNCTIONS

Immunization (Table 8–9)
Trauma/Accidents (Table 8–10)

I. ACCIDENTS

A. Assessment

1. Major cause of death of children; as independence increases during toddler and preschool years, risk of accidents increases; as environment broadens during school-age years and adolescence, accidents continue to be major threat
2. Determination of risk of environment
3. Determination of risk due to age and growth and developmental level of child

B. Planning, Goals, Expected Outcomes

1. Parents understand risk of accidents and help prevent them
2. Child does not suffer injury

C. Implementation

1. Teach parents concerning accident prevention and supervision

TABLE 8-9 Immunization Guide

Age	Immunization
2 months	Diphtheria Pertussis } DPT Tetanus Oral poliovirus vaccine (trivalent)
4 months	Diphtheria Pertussis } DPT Tetanus Oral poliovirus vaccine (trivalent)
6 months	Diphtheria Pertussis } DPT Tetanus Oral poliovirus vaccine (trivalent) (given in high-risk areas)
15 months	Tuberculin test (at or preceding measles vaccine) Measles } MMR Mumps } Singly or combined Rubella
18 months	Diphtheria Pertussis } DPT Tetanus Oral poliovirus vaccine (trivalent)
24 months	*Haemophilus* b polysaccharide vaccine (HBPV)
4–6 years	Diphtheria Pertussis } DPT Tetanus Oral poliovirus vaccine (trivalent)
14–16 years	Tetanus Diphtheria } TD (every 10 years) (adult form)

2. Provide specific teaching concerning vehicle safety, home safety, and water safety
3. Teach emergency first aid, poison control information, and rescue squad information
4. Guide parents to teach children safety

D. Evaluation

1. Parents decreased risk of accidents
2. Child was not injured

Communicable Diseases (Table 8–11)

I. VIRAL DISEASES

A. Measles (Rubeola)

1. Assessment
   a. spread by direct contact with droplets; incubation period of 10 to 14 days
   b. prodromal symptoms of fever, malaise, cough, coryza, Koplik's spots
   c. conjunctivitis, photosensitivity
   d. preventable by immunization
   e. rash, maculopapular
2. Planning, goals, expected outcomes
   a. child is immunized
   b. child recovers without complications
3. Implementation
   a. assess for signs and symptoms
   b. provide supportive care during fever; administer antipyretics and sponge to lower temperature but *never* aspirin
   c. provide quiet environment; dim room if photophobia present
   d. humidify air to ease coryza and cough
   e. provide gentle skin care; keep skin clean; apply topical lotions or medicated baths for itching
   f. maintain respiratory isolation to prevent spread of virus
   g. observe for complications of otitis media, pneumonia, croup, encephalitis
4. Evaluation
   a. child was immunized
   b. child recovered without complications

B. Rubella (German Measles)

1. Assessment
   a. low-grade fever, malaise, conjunctivitis, coryza, sore throat, cough, swollen lymph glands; rash pinkish red and maculopapular
   b. preventable by immunization
2. Planning, goals, expected outcomes
   a. child is immunized
   b. child recovers without complications

TABLE 8-10 Typical Accidents According to Developmental Age and Prevention Strategies

Prevention Strategies Requiring Repeated Monitoring Across Various Ages

Automobile:	Use of child-restraint device in automobile (check at *each* visit)
	Never leave child alone in car
Burns:	Reduce hot water temperature
	Purchase and install smoke alarm
	Use nonflammable clothing and toys
Poisonings:	Safe storage of drugs, corrosives, and chemicals
	Use child-resistant caps on drugs
	Syrup of ipecac in the home
	Poison control number placed at telephone
Play:	Monitor safety of toys, activities, and sports appropriate to age
Drowning:	Supervise children around water
	Encourage swimming lessons

Developmental Landmarks	Event and Preventive Strategies
Infant (0 to 4 months)	
Can roll, reach, grasp, and mouth objects	Motor vehicle accidents
	Child-restraint device
	Falls
	Protect from falls during dressing, etc.
	Keep one hand on baby
	Suffocation/aspiration
	Avoid use of plastic bags in and near crib and changing area
	Avoid bottle propping
	Check crib safety
	Do not tie pacifier around neck
	Keep small objects and toys with removable parts out of crib
	Do not use pillows or excess blankets
	Burns
	Water temperature of bath should be checked with wrist or back of hand
	Avoid handling hot foods or liquids near baby
	Drowning
	Nonskid bottom in tub
	Keep hand on baby in tub at all times
Infant (4 to 6 months)	
Is mobile and is developing some fine motor skills	Motor vehicle accidents
Can roll over	Continue use of child-restraint device
Touches, reaches, and grasps to learn about environment	Falls
Begins to understand off-limit areas (e.g., stove)	Discourage use of walkers
	Use gates at stairs
	Highchair safety
	Suffocation, aspiration, strangulation
	Keep drapery cords and mobiles out of reach
	Avoid hard foods, such as raw vegetables, peanuts, popcorn
	Avoid use of toys with small parts
	Ingestions, poisonings
	Place all harmful products out of reach
	Remove poisonous plants from child's reach
	Burns
	Begin to teach meaning of "hot" and off-limit areas
	Drowning
	Never leave child alone in tub
Infant (6 to 12 months)	
Creeps, crawls, is inquisitive	Motor vehicle accidents
Pincer grasp has developed by 8 months	Continue use of child-restraint device
Pulls self up and other things down	Falls (from windows, down stairs, and from outdoor play equipment)
May begin table foods around 8–9 months	Keep crib away from window
Holds own bottle and begins to drink from cup	Constant supervision is required to prevent falls
Teeth are developing	Suffocation, aspiration, strangulation
Has the capability to chew a teething biscuit and soft cooked foods	Child should sit when eating to prevent aspiration
	Continue to avoid hard foods
	Cut foods into small pieces
	Burns
	Keep vaporizer beyond child's reach
	Supervise constantly, especially in kitchen and bathroom
	Drowning
	Same as for 0–6 months

Table continued on following page

TABLE 8-10 Typical Accidents According to Developmental Age and Prevention Strategies *Continued*

Developmental Landmarks	Event and Preventive Strategies

Toddler (1 to 3 years)
Walks, runs quickly, and often darts onto the street
Is more independent and developing autonomy (will stray farther from a parent)
Not aware of dangers but is intent on exploration
Has unsteady gait
By 3 years has full set of deciduous teeth
Can reach higher and open lids, can turn doorknobs
May be learning to swim but continues to need supervision
	Teaching of child should begin at this age
	Motor vehicle accidents (as a passenger, cyclist, and pedestrian)
	    Reaffirm importance of car seat even if toddler resists
	    Ride in center of back seat (restrained)
	    Teach to stay off streets with riding toys and tricycle
	    Cannot be trusted, therefore requires supervision
	    Provide a fenced-in play area if possible
	Falls
	    Open windows from the top
	    Remove objects from crib that child could stand on to climb out window
	Suffocation, aspiration
	    Table foods can be given but avoid nuts and other small, hard foods
	    Teach the danger of plastic bags and similar items
	    Teach the child not to run with popsicle sticks or lollipops in mouth
	Burns
	    Expand on teaching about hot things. Especially teach about hot water, the stove, and hot food on the stove
	Ingestions, poisonings, trauma
	    Reevaluate placement of poisons and medicines
	    Keep sharp objects out of reach
	    Use only child-resistant containers for poisons and medicines
	    Teach child about poisons
	Drowning
	    Close supervision around water
	    Teach not to run around pools or other bodies of water
	    Supervise in tub

Preschool (3 to 5 years)
Eager to learn and capable of understanding simple explanations
Has the motor and coordination skills to ride a tricycle and is learning to ride a bicycle
Curious and explorative, particularly outdoors
Active in playground and outdoor play
Motor abilities exceed cognitive skills, therefore, child engages in physical activities without foreseeing danger
Is more independent and may walk or ride bike in the neighborhood with less supervision than when a toddler
Engages in sex play
Engages in dramatic play
	All aspects of safety should be taught to child
	Motor vehicle, pedestrian, cycle accidents
	    Begin to teach how to cross street safely
	    Teach rules of the road
	    Teach purpose of car seats and seat belts
	Falls, trauma
	    Caution against climbing into unsafe areas, marshy lands, drainage pipes, unsafe buildings
	    Teach child how to handle scissors
	Suffocation, aspiration
	    Teach child not to run while eating
	    Teach child not to crawl into areas where he or she could be entrapped (refrigerators, drainage pipes, excavation areas)
	Burns
	    Teach fire escape rules
	    Caution child against playing with matches
	    Keep matches out of reach
	Drowning
	    Begin organized swimming lessons
	    Never leave alone in bath or while swimming
	Street safety
	    Teach child not to accept rides or foods without permission of parents
	Bodily injury
	    Teach child not to insert objects into body orifices
	Ingestion/inhalation
	    Expand on teaching about poisons and medicines
	    Include teaching about cosmetics and sprays, which child may use in playing house

3. Implementation
    a. administer antipyretics for fever, but do not use aspirin
    b. provide supportive care for comfort
    c. use topical lotions or medicated baths to decrease itching
    d. teach child and family to avoid contact with pregnant women

4. Evaluation
    a. child was immunized
    b. child recovered without complications

C. Roseola (Exanthema Subitum)

1. Assessment

TABLE 8-10 Typical Accidents According to Developmental Age and Prevention Strategies *Continued*

Developmental Landmarks	Event and Preventive Strategies
School-age (6 to 12 years)	
More coordination in motor skills	All aspects of safety should be taught to child
Runs, skips, jumps, climbs, constantly on the move	Motor vehicle accidents
Active in sports	Pedestrian safety needs to be repeated
Increasing independence and need for peer acceptance	Bicycle safety must be emphasized
Curiosity about sexuality	Bodily injury, fractures
	Teach how to prevent injury from cold
	Teach safety related to hobbies, handicrafts, sports, mechanical equipment
	Drowning
	Water safety
	Supervise water sports
	Burns
	Teach child appropriate use of matches and campfires
	Firearms
	Teach respect of firearms
	Avoid keeping a loaded weapon in house
	Bodily harm and trauma
	Reinforce to avoid taking things or getting into a car of anyone without parents' knowledge
	Teach child about harmful use of drugs, alcohol, and cigarettes
	Sex education to make child aware of "good touching" and "bad touching" to prevent sexual abuse
Adolescent (13 to 18 years)	
Drive motor vehicles (cars, motorcycles)	All aspects of safety should be taught to adolescent
Peer pressure and peer acceptance predominates	Motor vehicle accidents
Risk taking to establish self with peers is common	Reemphasize use of seat belts
Activities in work and sports involve dangerous equipment	Emphasize the danger of alcohol and drug use (especially related to motor vehicle accidents)
Independence in all activities	Bodily injury and trauma
	Teach proper use of equipment and maintenance of equipment
	Drowning
	Teach water safety
	Instruct in the use of emergency care equipment
	Teach CPR
	Firearms
	Close supervision regarding firearms is required
	No loaded weapon in house

From Foster, R.L., Hunsberger, M.M., & Anderson, J.J. (1989). *Family-centered nursing care of children.* Philadelphia: W.B. Saunders Co.

a. observation for persistent high fever; maculopapular rash appears as fever subsides

b. most common in infant under 1 year; no immunization available

2. Planning, goal, expected outcome: child recovers without complications

3. Implementation

  a. observe for febrile seizures; take seizure precautions

  b. administer antipyretics; anticonvulsants may also be given *(avoid aspirin)*

  c. teach family to lower fever with tepid sponge bath

4. Evaluation: child recovered without complications

D. Varicella Zoster (Chickenpox)

1. Assessment

  a. prodromal symptoms of malaise, anorexia, fever

  b. rash appears first as macule, then papule, then vesicle; itching intense

  c. immunization now available

2. Planning, goal, expected outcome: child recovers without complications

3. Implementation

  a. skin care important to prevent secondary bacterial infection

  b. do not ever use aspirin to treat fever because of risk of Reye's syndrome

  c. administer diphenhydramine hydrochloride (Benadryl) or antihistamines to ease itching; apply topical lotions or medicated baths

  d. teach child and family concerning scratching; pressure, calamine lotion, baths, and fresh linen help

  e. acyclovir (Zovirax) may be given to decrease severe symptoms

  f. observe for complications of encephalitis, pneumonia, sepsis

  g. isolate to prevent spread until vesicles dried

TABLE 8-11 Clinical Presentation of Infection

System Involved	Signs and Symptoms
Central nervous system	Lethargy or irritability
	Jitteriness or hyporeflexia
	Tremors or seizures
	Coma
	Full fontanel
	Abnormal eye movements
	Hypotonia or increased tone
Respiratory system	Cyanosis
	Grunting
	Irregular respirations
	Tachypnea or apnea
	Retractions
Gastrointestinal tract	Poor feeding
	Vomiting (may be bile stained)
	Diarrhea or decreased stools
	Abdominal distention
	Edema or erythema of abdominal wall
	Hepatomegaly
Skin	Rashes or erythema
	Purpura
	Pustules or paronychia
	Omphalitis
	Sclerema
Hematopoietic system	Jaundice
	Bleeding
	Purpura or ecchymosis
	Splenomegaly
Circulatory system	Pallor, cyanosis, or mottling
	Cold, clammy skin
	Tachycardia or arrhythmia
	Hypotension
	Edema
Whole body system	"Not doing well"
	Poor temperature control (fever or hypothermia)

Adapted from Gotoff, S., & Behrman, R. (1972). Neonatal septicemia. *J. Pediatr.*, 16:142. Reprinted from Klaus, M., & Fanaroff, A. (1979). *Care of the high risk neonate*, 2nd ed. Philadelphia: W.B. Saunders Co.

4. Evaluation: child recovered without complications

E. Mumps

1. Assessment
   a. prodromal symptoms: fever, headache, earache aggravated by chewing and talking
   b. enlarged, tender, and painful parotid glands
   c. preventable by immunization
2. Planning, goals, expected outcome
   a. child is immunized
   b. child recovers without complications
3. Implementation
   a. diet and fluids for bland, nonirritating, palatable foods
   b. administer analgesics and antipyretics as necessary; elixirs may be more easily tolerated than tablets (do not use aspirin)
   c. if orchitis develops, scrotal support may ease discomfort
   d. observe for complications of encephalitis, hepatitis, deafness, sterility (adult male)

4. Evaluation
   a. child was immunized
   b. child recovered without complications

F. Poliomyelitis

1. Assessment
   a. observe for symptoms of fever, sore throat, vomiting, anorexia, abdominal pain
   b. symptoms may disappear with apparent recovery, but then central nervous system paralysis appears
   c. preventable by immunization
   d. postpolio syndrome may occur 30 to 40 years later
2. Planning, goals, expected outcomes
   a. child is immunized
   b. child and parents understand and follow therapeutic regimen
   c. child recovers without complications
   d. child and family cope with resultant deficits
3. Implementation
   a. provide supportive care and bed rest as appropriate
   b. assist with ventilation as necessary
   c. assist with physical therapy as necessary
   d. position for good body alignment and support
   e. monitor for complications: respiratory arrest, permanent paralysis
4. Evaluation
   a. child was immunized
   b. child and parents complied with therapeutic regimen
   c. child recovered without complications
   d. child and family coped with resultant deficits

II. BACTERIAL DISEASES

A. Diphtheria

1. Assessment
   a. causative organism *Corynebacterium diphtheriae*
   b. signs and symptoms
      (1) coryza without generalized symptoms of common cold
      (2) epistaxis
      (3) sore throat
      (4) fever
   c. physical examination for whitish gray membrane on tonsils or larynx
   d. preventable by immunization
2. Planning, goals, expected outcomes
   a. child is immunized
   b. child recovers from illness without complications

3. Implementation
   a. maintain strict isolation
   b. maintain bed rest
   c. humidify air
   d. administer antibiotics: usually penicillin or erythromycin (see Table 7–10)
   e. monitor for respiratory obstruction: tracheostomy tray at bedside
4. Evaluation
   a. child was immunized
   b. child recovered without complications

B. Pertussis (Whooping Cough)

1. Assessment
   a. causative organism *Bordetella pertussis*
   b. symptoms similar to those of upper respiratory infection—rhinitis, fever, cough
   c. cough that becomes more severe and paroxysmal
   d. preventable by immunization
      (1) can be fatal in unimmunized child
      (2) vaccine is controversial
      (3) slight risk of neurologic damage with convulsions, encephalitis, and death
      (4) sometimes child simply given diphtheria and tetanus (DT) vaccine rather than DPT
      (5) after DPT, further pertussis should not be given to children who have hypotensive or neurologic side effects
      (6) risks and benefits should be carefully explained to parents so informed decision can be made
2. Planning, goals, expected outcomes
   a. child is immunized
   b. child recovers without complications
3. Implementation
   a. be sure that parents understand risk of not immunizing child
   b. maintain bed rest and quiet environment when fever present
   c. humidify air
   d. maintain adequate hydration and nutrition
   e. observe for signs of airway obstruction
   f. provide emotional support for child and family
4. Evaluation
   a. child was immunized
   b. child recovered without complications

C. Scarlet Fever

1. Assessment
   a. causative organism group A beta-hemolytic streptococci
   b. prodromal symptoms of high fever, tachycardia, headache, chills, vomiting, malaise
   c. physical examination for red, enlarged tonsils and strawberry-red tongue
   d. no immunization available
2. Planning, goals, expected outcomes
   a. child's condition is diagnosed early
   b. child and parents understand and follow therapeutic regimen
   c. child recovers from infection without complications
3. Implementation
   a. maintain bed rest during fever
   b. administer antibiotics; usually intramuscular penicillin, progressing to oral penicillin
   c. teach child and family emphasizing importance of antibiotic therapy
   d. administer analgesics as indicated; gargles and lozenges may also be used to ease sore throat
   e. maintain adequate hydration by encouraging nonirritating fluids and bland foods
   f. observe for and teach parents to observe for complications, such as otitis media, rheumatic fever, glomerulonephritis, peritonsillar abscess
   g. prophylactic antibiotic therapy may be indicated for contacts
4. Evaluation
   a. child's condition was diagnosed early
   b. child and parents complied with therapeutic regimen

Abuse

I. ABUSE OF CHILDREN

A. Assessment

1. Definition: physical, sexual, nutritional, or emotional maltreatment or negligence of children by parents or others in position of caregiver (see Chapter 10)
2. Risk factors
   a. unplanned pregnancy
   b. premature birth
   c. stepchildren
   d. high expectations of children
   e. chronic disease
   f. mental retardation
   g. poverty
   h. high social stresses, such as divorce, joblessness, and homelessness
   i. parents themselves often abused as children
3. Physical examination of child: unexplained scars, bruises, burns, and other injuries
4. Discrepancies in accounts from parents, child, and others as to how injury occurred

5. Emotional interaction with child difficult; child withdraws from contact; passive, noncommunicative
6. Incidence of child abuse epidemic proportions
    a. difficult to estimate actual levels
    b. only statistics are reported cases, which may be much lower than actual
    c. estimates of 50 per 1000 children or higher

B. Planning, Goals, Expected Outcomes

1. Abuse is prevented
2. Abuse is detected early
3. Child and family are supported

C. Implementation

1. Nurses have legal responsibility to report incidents of suspected abuse to proper authorities
2. Optimize bonding of infant and parent at every opportunity
3. Teach growth and development and reasonable expectations to parents
4. Be nonjudgmental but also fulfill legal obligations
5. Provide physical and emotional care for the child, including a safe environment and nonthreatening interaction
6. Teach parents alternative methods of coping

D. Evaluation

1. Abuse was prevented
2. Abuse was detected
3. Child and family were supported

Poisoning
I. POISONING IN CHILDREN (see Table 8–10)

A. Assessment

Unusual behavior or evidence of empty container near children

B. Planning, Goal, Expected Outcome

Poisoning is prevented

C. Implementation

1. Teach family to prevent poisonings by locking medicines and dangerous chemicals out of child's reach
2. Contact nearest poison control center for important information when poisoning suspected; current first aid standard to contact poison center for any directions

3. Teach child, beginning in infancy, to avoid dangers
4. Teach family to have poison control center phone number posted in home
5. Teach family to have syrup of ipecac and charcoal on hand to use per instructions from poison control center

D. Evaluation

Accidental poisoning was prevented

Skin Disorders
I. BURNS

A. Assessment

1. Destruction of body tissue caused by coagulation of cells; most frequent accidental injury to infants and young children
2. Definition/pathophysiology: burns are injuries to skin caused by agents such as heat, electricity, chemicals, or radiation
3. Classification
    a. amount of body surface
        (1) rule of nines, a way of expressing portions of body surface burned
            (a) head and neck: 9%
            (b) anterior trunk: 18%
            (c) posterior trunk: 18%
            (d) each arm: 9%
            (e) each leg: 18%
            (f) genitalia and perineum: 1%
    b. depth of burn, old method
        (1) first-degree: involves epidural layer only
        (2) second-degree: involves superficial to deep dermis
        (3) third-degree: involves all layers of dermis, extends into subcutaneous tissues
        (4) fourth-degree: includes muscle and bone
    c. depth of burn, new method
        (1) partial-thickness: epidermal appendages (sweat and oil glands and hair follicles) intact and wound heals itself if no further injury occurs
        (2) full-thickness: involves all layers of skin and destruction of epidermal appendages and requires grafting for healing to occur
4. Signs and symptoms
    a. first-degree: red, dry skin and pain
    b. second-degree: mottled white to cherry-red, skin, moist with or without blisters and extreme pain
    c. third-degree: white and leathery to charred skin, dry without elasticity and little or no pain
    d. fourth-degree: skin charred to dead white, without pain

e. pulmonary involvement: respiratory wheezing or distress, redness of face and neck, or cough and sooty sputum

5. Usual treatment
   a. depth of wound assessed
   b. intravenous Ringer's lactate to maintain fluid balance and prevent shock
   c. pain medication: often intravenous morphine for severe pain
   d. continuous replacement of lost fluids with care to prevent fluid overload
   e. monitor respiratory status if upper respiratory tract burned
   f. open method
      (1) wounds left open to air in sterile settings
      (2) wet compresses or soaks used to debride burn
   g. closed method
      (1) occlusive dressings with silver sulfadiazine antibiotic cream to control infection
      (2) debridement of wound
   h. skin grafting
      (1) split-thickness graft for less severe and shallow burns
      2) full-thickness graft for severe and deep burns

B. Planning, Goals, Expected Outcomes

1. Burns are prevented
2. Child recovers from burns without complications
3. Child regains maximal function

C. Implementation

1. Prevent infection
2. Maintain alignment and support to all extremities
3. Maintain adequate nutrition and hydration; intravenous fluids may be used initially
4. Choice of treatment depends on type, extent, and depth of burn; open method with reverse isolation, sterile wet dressings (silver nitrate or similar drug), cream, skin grafts may be used

D. Evaluation

1. Burns were prevented
2. Child recovered from burns without complications
3. Child regained maximal functioning

II. INFANTILE ECZEMA

A. Assessment

1. Inflammation of skin (atopic dermatitis) caused by allergic reaction to some allergen

2. Observe skin for redness, swelling, papules, vesicles
3. Rash accompanied by itching, oozing, crusting; can occur on any part of body
4. Usually before age 2 years

B. Planning, Goals, Expected Outcomes

1. Allergens are identified and attacks prevented
2. Family and child understand and follow therapeutic regimen
3. Child recovers without complications

C. Implementation

1. Provide meticulous skin care to keep affected area clean and dry
2. Apply local ointments, creams, corn starch for itching
3. Prevent scratching with adequate stimulation and cuddling; suggest "mittens" to cover hands and elbow restraints only as necessary
4. Coordinate environmental study to find allergen and control or eliminate it as possible
5. Provide emotional support to child and family

D. Evaluation

1. Further attacks were prevented
2. Family and child complied with therapeutic regimen
3. Child recovered without complications

III. IMPETIGO

A. Assessment

1. Skin infection caused by *Streptococcus* or *Staphylococcus* bacteria
2. Observe skin for red vesicles and pustules
3. Assist with collection of culture for positive diagnosis
4. Can occur as break in hand-washing technique in hospital nursery or pediatric unit

B. Planning, Goals, Expected Outcomes

1. Infection is prevented
2. Child recovers without complications of more severe infection or scarring

C. Implementation

1. Follow strict hand-washing technique
2. Institute contact isolation with use of gowns and gloves
3. Administer parenteral, oral, or local antibiotics as ordered
4. Provide meticulous skin care
5. Provide emotional support to child and family

D. Evaluation

1. Infection was prevented
2. Child recovered without complications

IV. RINGWORM

A. Assessment

1. Fungal infection spread by direct contact: *(scalp—tinea capitis; body—tinea corporis; feet—tinea pedis)*
2. Observe for papules, dry scales; itching
3. Commonly spread in close proximity of day care or classroom situations

B. Planning, Goals, Expected Outcomes

Child recovers without complications

C. Implementation

1. Provide meticulous skin care; remove crusts after washing
2. Apply antifungal ointments as ordered; antifungal medication may also be given orally

D. Evaluation

Child recovered without complications

V. PEDICULOSIS

A. Assessment

1. Presence of lice on scalp and other hairy areas of body
2. Observe for nits or mature lice on examination of scalp and hairlines
3. History of intense itching, known contact
4. Recurs without treatment of all infected family members and environment

B. Planning, Goals, Expected Outcomes

1. Lice infestation is prevented

2. Child recovers from infestation without complications

C. Implementation

1. Shampoo and wash with special solution, such as Kwell or Rid
2. Wash all clothing, hats, bed linens in hot wash to destroy nits and eggs
3. Teach child and family to prevent recurrence by identifying source of contamination, teaching children not to share combs, and so on
4. Provide emotional support to child and family, often embarrassed by problem

D. Evaluation

1. Lice infestation was prevented
2. Child recovered without complications

VI. HIVES (URTICARIA)

A. Assessment

1. Allergic reaction to food, drugs, or other allergen
2. Observe bright red, raised rash in patches; intense itching of affected areas
3. History of exposure to known allergen
4. Assist with allergy testing to identify specific allergen
5. Assess for progression of hives to anaphylactic shock (emergency situation)

B. Planning, Goals, Expected Outcomes

1. Allergens are identified
2. Child and family understand and follow therapeutic regimen
3. Child recovers without complications

C. Implementation

1. Assist with environmental study to isolate and remove allergen if possible
2. Administer antihistamines or diphenhydramine hydrochloride (Benadryl) to decrease inflammation and itching
3. Provide meticulous skin care to prevent infection; use topical lotions and medicated baths to decrease itching
4. Teach child and family measures to decrease itching and avoid infection

5. Provide emotional support to child and family
6. Desensitization may be useful to prevent recurrence

D. Evaluation

1. Allergens were identified
2. Child and family complied with therapeutic regimen

VII. ACNE VULGARIS

A. Assessment

1. Inflammation of sebaceous glands; overactive sebaceous glands become blocked with sebum
2. Observe face, chest, and back for comedones (noninflamed, impacted sebaceous glands) or papules and pustules (inflamed glands)
3. History of client's age and diet
4. Usually occurs during adolescence

B. Planning, Goal, Expected Outcome

Adolescent recovers without complications

C. Implementation

1. Provide meticulous skin care to keep affected areas clean and dry
2. Teach client concerning hygiene and avoidance of stress
3. Administer oral medications or local creams and ointments as ordered, such as tetracycline or tretinoin (Retin-A)
4. Teach that treatment does not produce immediate results
5. Provide emotional support to adolescent and family

D. Evaluation

Adolescent recovered without complications

Perioperative Period
I. PREOPERATIVE PREPARATION
(Table 8–12)

A. Assessment

1. Assess child's developmental level and choose activities and words appropriate to that level
2. Assess child's knowledge of what to expect
3. Postoperative period can be less stressful and uncomfortable if child has been prepared preoperatively

B. Planning, Goals, Expected Outcomes

1. Child and parents are adequately prepared for surgery
2. Child recovers from surgery without complications

C. Implementation

1. Because fear increases tension and pain, basic principle for preparation for hospitalization is to decrease fear of unknown
2. All hospital procedures should be explained in way geared to child's level of comprehension
3. Involve family members in child's care to lessen anxiety of both parents and child
4. As child's development permits, let child participate in decision making; give child choices to make; avoid yes-no answers
5. Be truthful in explanations; explain at level of child's understanding, but do not lie to child
6. Therapeutic plan can assist child to handle anxiety and fear
7. Maintain familiar routine with familiar objects and toys
8. Safety important at all times; appropriate restraints should be used as necessary for child's safety
9. Medication administration should be matter-of-fact and cheerful; allowing child, if appropriate for age, to choose if injection to be given "in this leg or your other leg" makes child feel able to exercise some control over stressful situation
10. Preoperative teaching for specific surgeries should be geared to developmental level of child; describing anesthesia as "sleepy air," and assuring children they will not feel any pain can lessen anxiety
    a. infant: separation anxiety threatening; provide sensory stimulation; provide tender, loving care and cuddling and encourage parents to participate in care
    b. toddler: developmental stages may be disrupted during hospitalization; maintain rituals and routines to give child sense of control over frightening situations; explain to family that regression is normal behavior
    c. preschool child: sense of independence may be disrupted during hospitalization; therapeutic play and puppets can help work through anxiety, frustration, and painful experiences; answer questions honestly and en-

TABLE 8-12 Summary of Preparation of the Child for Surgery

Procedure	Modification
Consent	Parent or legal guardian
Blood work	Age-appropriate restraint
Urinalysis	Age-appropriate collection (U-bag)
	Assist school-aged child
	Age-appropriate instructions
Evaluate for respiratory infection, nutritional status	Use more objective observations in infants and toddlers because of child's limited verbal skills
Allergies	Indicate clearly on chart
Nothing by mouth (NPO)	Increase fluids prior to NPO status
	Length of time may vary with age and surgery (6–12 hours)
	If surgery is late, place appropriate notice on child—"Do not feed me"
	Remove goodies from bedside stand—no gum
	Supervise hungry, ambulatory patients carefully
Vital signs	Approach child carefully, explain, demonstrate, allow more time
Void before surgery	Not always possible in infants and toddlers
Bath	Hospital gown—also may wear underwear or pajama bottoms, depending on age, type of surgery
Identification	Ident-a-band
Teeth	Check for loose teeth, orthodontic appliances
Skin preparation	May be done in operating room (OR)
Nails	Trim, remove nail polish
Enemas	Not routine
Transportation	Crib or stretcher—parents may accompany to OR door
Emotional preparation	Preoperative tour
	Group and individual puppet play
	Body drawings of parts involved
	Play selected by child as mode of expression
	Support parents during surgery
Sedation	Usually 20 minutes before surgery
Record all pertinent data	Essentially the same, with pediatric modifications as indicated by the above

courage parents to do same; child-size wheelchairs, stretchers, and carts help to avoid feeling of being overwhelmed; regression is normal behavior

d. school-aged child: honest explanations important; children of this age value privacy; absence from peer group increases anxiety; opportunities for choices help foster sense of control; as child's condition permits, tutor or schoolwork assignments help child keep pace with class; provide outlets for frustration through physical activity as appropriate

e. adolescent: absence from peer group and social activities threatening; body image fragile; privacy important; maintain independence as much as possible; access to telephone and privacy for conversations may lessen resentment at separation from peer group; answer all questions honestly; heterosexual relationships important at this age; depending on seriousness of adolescent's condition, concern for future may produce anxiety

11. Use play therapy with surgical garb and some equipment so child can play and express fears about procedures

12. Telling child all details specific to surgery, such as intravenous infusions, dressings, tubes, medications, casts, traction, limitations of movement after surgery, where pain will be felt, limitations in diet, and frequent vital sign checks, avoids surprise when the child awakens in recovery room

13. Answer all child's questions honestly at child's comprehension level

14. Provide emotional support to both child and family to lessen anxiety

D. Evaluation

1. Child was adequately prepared for surgery
2. A lower-than-expected rate of postoperative complications occurred

II. POSTOPERATIVE PERIOD (Tables 8–13 and 8–14)

A. Assessment

1. Determine how well the child has been prepared preoperatively and fill in the gaps in child's knowledge
2. Assess vital signs, wounds, intravenous lines, pain, and any postoperative complications

B. Planning, Goal, Expected Outcome

Child recovers from surgery without complications

TABLE 8-13 Summary of Postoperative Care of the Child

Procedure	Modification
Return from recovery room	Notify parents Smaller patients generally in crib Age-appropriate safety precautions
Note general condition, alertness	Infant and toddler cannot verbalize fear or pain
Vital signs	Every 15–30 minutes until stable Blood pressure is sometimes omitted in infant
Evaluate for shock	Essentially same
Assess operative site for bleeding, dressing intactness	Essentially same Elevate casted extremities Circle drainage
Restraints	May be necessary to protect IV Remove periodically for range of motion
Connect dependent drainage (urinary catheter, Levin tubes, oxygen)	Prepare child for sight and noises of equipment, draw pictures to clarify purpose
Position patient	Abdomen or side unless contraindicated; no pillow
IV line	Should have pediatric adapting device Monitor rate meticulously, as infants and small children respond quickly to fluid shifts Measure and record intake and output
Assess elimination	Bowel and bladder
Relief of pain	Hold, comfort small children unless contraindicated Be sensitive to behavioral changes, such as increase in irritability, crying, regression, nail biting, passivity, withdrawal Administer pain relievers Involve parents in care Provide transitional object such as blanket, favorite toy, pacifier Be aware of transcultural considerations that provide familiarity and comfort
Nothing by mouth (NPO)	Until fully awake, babies are started on clear fluids by bottle unless contraindicated Avoid brown- or red-colored liquids, which may be confused with old or fresh blood Monitor bowel sounds
Consider diet	Advance clear, full liquids, soft regular
Observe for complications	Turn, cough, deep breathe, dangle feet, early ambulation—less of a problem in children Splint operative site with hands when child coughs

C. Implementation

1. Continuity of nursing personnel lessens anxiety of children
2. Continue to explain all procedures to child; use words appropriate to child's vocabulary and provide demonstrations with puppets or dolls to increase understanding
3. Teach family how to participate in child's care and allow participation as appropriate
4. Honestly tell child when to expect pain; administer pain medication as needed
5. Provide basic postoperative care, such as vital sign checks, observation of dressings, intake and output, intravenous infusion, Foley catheters, nasogastric tubes, diet limitation, and assessment of level of consciousness
6. Maintain safety at all times
7. Provide emotional support to child and family
8. Referrals to community agencies and support groups should be made as appropriate to the child's surgical procedure
9. Provide care per developmental level

D. Evaluation

Child recovered from surgery without complications

Immune Disorders

I. HUMAN IMMUNODEFICIENCY VIRUS AND ACQUIRED IMMUNODEFICIENCY SYNDROME

(See Chapter 7 for detailed information on HIV/AIDS)

A. Assessment

1. Symptoms vague and nonspecific
2. Blood test reveals presence of HIV

TABLE 8-14 Hospital Play Nursing Intervention for Various Age Levels

Age	Play	Nursing Intervention
1–3 months	Rattle, music boxes, mobiles. Do not discourage finger-mouth activity. Allow free movements when possible.	Cuddle, rock, talk softly. Encourage liberal parent contact. Anticipate needs.
3–6 months	Play peek-a-boo, provide soft toys, squeaky toys, music boxes	Smile, talk softly. Provide same caregiver. Use pacifier if oral feedings are restricted.
6–18 months	If child has own toy or blanket, encourage keeping it with child. Use mirror reflectors for immobilized child. Play identifying parts of body. Provide toys that child can mouth safely. Supervised crawling and walking when possible. Use sterilized toys. Play give-and-take games. Toy telephone, cloth books, pots and pans.	Nurture growth and development by encouraging participation in care; e.g., holding own bottle, but do not insist. Provide finger foods. Allow as much movement and exploring as environment and therapy allow.
18–24 months	Books, building toys, pictures, magic slates, action toys, foam blocks, toy telephones. Play games that show understanding of positive and negative demands.	Nurse or volunteer can read to child at child's level. Have child mimic word meanings. Use potty chair when possible. Allow child to help with daily care.
2–3 years	Read books and stories concerning separation and returning of visiting family. Coloring books, active and passive exercises, dolls, cars, clay, cuddly toys.	Provide alternatives instead of criticism. Understand and accept ritualistic behavior needs. Provide choices when possible. Allow child to assist with care. Use familiar terms for urination, defecation, pacifier, and so on. Use potty chair when possible.
3–6 years	Tape recorders can be used to listen to familiar voices or songs. Dolls, cars, television, radio, cuddly toys, picture books, easily won games, simple puzzles, pop-up books. Encourage peer contact when possible. Use doctor-nurse dress-up clothes.	Encourage independence when possible. Allow child to participate in planning and carrying out routine care.
6–12 years	Provide school activities when possible to keep up with peers. Write cards to friends and classmates. Play show-and-tell to explain equipment and procedures. Provide visual and verbal contact with peers. Electronic games, books, checkers, card games, paint, drawing pad, baseball cards, television, radio, crafts, toys involving large muscle coordination, weaving.	Separate male and female when appropriate and possible. Provide for privacy needs. Have child participate in decision making when possible and in self-care. Use reason and logic with child. Encourage self-expression. Hang up pictures child drew or painted. Provide private nook for personal items.
12–18 years	Provide school activities to avoid school problems on discharge. Write cards to friends and teachers. Provide hairstyling, deodorant, and pretty bedjacket when possible to enhance body image. Electronic games, checkers, chess, card games, puzzles, television, radio, crafts, weaving.	Separate sexes when possible. Have child help with ward activities when possible to feel useful. Set realistic standards and rules that may be required by diagnoses and therapy prescribed. Treat as an adult, do not talk down or order child. Provide private nook for personal items. Allow snack foods to be brought in.

From Leifer, G. (1982). *Principles and techniques in pediatric nursing,* 4th ed. Philadelphia: W.B. Saunders Co.

3. Often transmitted in utero from mother
4. May be from transfusions

B. Planning, Goals, Expected Outcomes

1. Child is supported throughout disease
2. Child does not experience opportunistic infections
3. Child and family understand and cope with terminal nature of illness

C. Implementation

1. Provide emotional support for child and family

2. Educate about ways HIV is transmitted and how to prevent transmission
3. Provide supportive care for symptoms
4. Prevent secondary infections

D. Evaluation

1. Child was supported throughout disease
2. Child did not experience opportunistic infections
3. Child and family understood and coped with terminal nature of illness

QUESTIONS

1. Bradley Mustin, age 2 years, has been brought to the clinic by his mother for an unexplained swollen arm. While assessing Bradley, the nurse notes several bruises over Bradley's shoulders, arms, legs, and buttocks in various stages of healing. Bradley is very quiet and refuses to look at the nurse. He also turns away from his mother. The nurse suspects Bradley is a victim of child abuse. The nurse should report her findings to:

   ① The physician
   ② The visiting nursing service
   ③ The county prosecutor
   ④ The appropriate government children's services agency

2. The first step of treatment of the family suffering from child abuse is:

   ① Assessment of the situation
   ② Immediate removal of the child from the home
   ③ Beginning criminal prosecution
   ④ Encouraging parent to attend support groups

3. When child abuse is suspected, the nurse assesses the mother and child for a negative parent–child fit. Which of the following statements by the mother may indicate a negative fit?

   ① "He's such a quiet child. He never gives me any trouble."
   ② "He really knows his own mind."
   ③ "He never tells me when his diaper is wet until it's too late. You'd think he'd learn."
   ④ "He didn't inherit my blue eyes. His are a light brown."

4. The nurse knows toddlers are the most common age group in which child abuse occurs. Erikson's developmental theory places the toddler in a conflict between:

   ① Trust versus mistrust
   ② Autonomy versus shame and doubt
   ③ Dependence versus independence
   ④ Initiative versus guilt

5. Jimmy Rogers, 5 years old, has had numerous upper respiratory infections, complicated with middle ear infections. The pediatrician has recommended that he have his tonsils and adenoids removed. Which of the following should the PN tell the surgeon about preoperatively?

   ① Jimmy's pulse is 92, respiratory rate is 24.
   ② Jimmy sometimes has difficulty swallowing.
   ③ Jimmy's upper right lateral incisor is loose.
   ④ Jimmy had an upper respiratory infection 2 weeks ago.

6. Jimmy Rogers, 5 years old, has had numerous upper respiratory infections, complicated with middle ear infections. The pediatrician has recommended that he have his tonsils and adenoids removed. The PN plans to explain the experience to Jimmy. What should the PN do first?

   ① Explain to Jimmy the need for preoperative medications
   ② Tell Jimmy that his parents will be waiting in his room after surgery
   ③ Describe the appearance of the recovery room and the operating room
   ④ Ask Jimmy to tell you what he knows about the procedure

7. Jimmy Rogers, 5 years old, has had numerous upper respiratory infections, complicated with middle ear infections. The pediatrician has recommended that he have his tonsils and adenoids removed. The PN is going to give Jimmy his preoperative medication. Jimmy asks, "Is it going to hurt?" The PN should reply:

   ① "If you lie very still, it won't hurt."
   ② "Shots don't hurt brave little boys."
   ③ "Yes, it will, but I'll stay with you until it stops."
   ④ "Yes, but it will only hurt for a little while."

8. Jimmy arrives in the recovery room after surgery for removal of his tonsils and adenoids. The best position for him is:

   ① Semi-Fowler's, with his head turned to the side
   ② Prone, with the head of the bed slightly elevated
   ③ On his back, with his head turned to the right side
   ④ On his abdomen, with his head turned to the side

9. When Jimmy, who has just had his tonsils and adenoids removed, starts to take fluids, which is best given first?

   ① Cool water
   ② Cranberry juice
   ③ Milk
   ④ Orange juice

10. Jimmy is going home after having his tonsils and adenoids removed. Which of the following should the parents be told to report to the physician after Jimmy's discharge?

  ① If a heavy, dirty gray membrane develops over the tonsillar area
  ② If he complains of a sore throat on the sixth postoperative day
  ③ If he complains of an earache without fever
  ④ If bleeding develops in the throat on the sixth postoperative day

11. A priority intervention for the child who has ingested Lysol is:

  ① Maintenance of hydration
  ② Removal of gastric contents by lavage
  ③ Observation for seizure activity
  ④ Prevention of vomiting

12. The long-term effects of lead poisoning are primarily related to:

  ① Neurologic damage due to cortical atrophy
  ② Prolonged anemia producing congestive heart failure
  ③ Decalcification of bones causing fractures
  ④ Kidney failure related to nephron damage

13. Which of the following should the mother of a child with varicella be instructed *not* to do?

  ① Administer aspirin for temperature above 101° F
  ② Keep fingernails short
  ③ Apply calamine lotion for itching
  ④ Encourage child's favorite liquids

14. When caring for Mark, who has varicella, the nurse prevents spread of the disease to other children by:

  ① Keeping Mark confined to his bed
  ② Placing Mark in a single room with the door closed
  ③ Wearing a mask whenever caring for Mark
  ④ Instructing all children who play with Mark to wash their hands

15. The most common cause of adolescent accidental injury involves:

  ① Motor vehicles
  ② Handguns
  ③ Skateboards
  ④ Alcohol

16. Gary has recently developed acne on his face. He asks you what happens to cause it to appear.

  ① Acne results from overactive estrogen that is eliminated through the pores in the skin.
  ② Acne is an inherited disorder that is transmitted via an autosomal recessive trait.
  ③ Acne is related to the overproduction of sebum, which blocks the sebaceous glands.
  ④ Acne is related directly to the excessive amount of masturbation engaged in by the adolescent.

ANSWERS AND RATIONALES

Guide to item identification (see pp. 4–5 for further details about each category):

I, II, III, or IV for the phase of the nursing process
1, 2, 3, or 4 for the category of client needs
A, B, C, D, E, F, or G for the category of human functioning
Specific content category by name; i.e., cholecystectomy

1. The law requires all medical professionals to
④ report any suspected child abuse to the appropriate governmental children's services department. If it is after hours, they often may be contacted through the sheriff's department.
III, 3, D, Child abuse

2. Without knowing the details of the situation,
① the nurse will not be able to decide the next action adequately. Removal from the parents is traumatic to the child and is therefore reserved as a last resort. Criminal procedures have proven fairly ineffective in changing the parents' behavior. Instead, they often blame the child for their trouble with the law. Without knowing the cause, the nurse cannot direct the parent to the correct support group.
I, 3, D, Child abuse

3. This indicates a normal behavior on the part of
③ the child that the parent sees in a negative and even unrealistic way.
I, 3, D & G, Child abuse

4. Because the toddler is striving for autonomy, he
② often ignores adult directives. If the parents are unaware of this normal reaction, they may find it frustrating and intolerable.
I, 3, A & D, Child abuse

5. Loose teeth are potential hazards during the an-
③ esthetic procedure. They may become dislodged and aspirated by the child.
III, 1, D, Perioperative care

6. The first step in the teaching/learning process
④ is to determine the child's present knowledge. Further explanations are then planned accordingly.
I, IV, D, Perioperative care

7. Simple, truthful explanations of procedures pro-
③ vide a basis for establishing trust with the school-aged child. The nurse should remain with Jimmy after the shot to encourage him to verbalize his feelings.
III, 1, A, G, & E, Perioperative care

8. Before the child is fully awake, he should be
④ placed on his abdomen with his head turned to the side to promote the drainage of secretions and to prevent aspiration. When alert, he may sit up but should remain in bed for the rest of the day.
III, 1, D, Perioperative care

9. Cool water or synthetic fruit juices are offered
① first. Red juices are avoided so that fresh blood in the emesis can be distinguished from ingested fluid. Citrus juices are avoided because they are irritating. Milk coats the throat, causing the child to clear his throat often, which may lead to bleeding.
III, 2, D, Perioperative care

10. Bleeding from 5 to 10 days postoperatively is
④ a possible complication of a tonsillectomy and adenoidectomy. This is the time when there is tissue sloughing as healing occurs. The sign noted is frequent swallowing, and it requires immediate medical attention.
III, 2, B & D, Perioperative care

11. To prevent reexposing the mucous membranes,
④ corrosive chemicals should not be removed from the stomach by emesis or lavage.
II, 1, D, Poisoning

12. Late effects include learning problems, seizures,
① mental retardation, and cerebral palsy.
I, 1, D, Lead poisoning

13. Aspirin should not be given owing to high risk
① of Reye's syndrome.
III, 2, D, Varicella/Reye's syndrome

14. Varicella is spread via droplets by direct or indi-
② rect contact.
III, 1, D, Varicella

15. Motor vehicles continue to be the leading cause
① of death in the adolescent period.
I, 1, D, Trauma/accidents

16. Acne is an inflammatory condition that involves
③ overactive sebaceous glands that become blocked with sebum.
III, 2, D, Acne vulgaris

MOBILITY

I. CONGENITAL MUSCULOSKELETAL DISORDERS

A. Congenital Clubfoot (Talipes Equinovarus)

1. Assessment
   a. definition: congenital malformation in which foot twisted inward; may affect one or both feet (Fig. 8–3)
   b. physical examination shows obvious defect; foot turns inward and adducted
   c. disorder usually diagnosed at birth or in early infancy
2. Planning, goals, expected outcomes
   a. child's condition is diagnosed early
   b. child recovers without complications
3. Implementation
   a. teach family to explain the condition to others
   b. treatment should begin as soon as possible; if not treated, bones, muscles, and tendons continue to develop abnormally
   c. less severe defects treated with application of Denis Browne splint for rotation, eversion, and dorsiflexion
   d. casts and surgery also used
   e. teach family and child cast care
   f. preoperative and postoperative care as appropriate
   g. teach family to continue prescribed routine after discharge
4. Evaluation
   a. child's condition was diagnosed early
   b. child recovered without complications

B. Congenital Dislocation of Hip

1. Assessment
   a. definition: congenital defect caused by shallow acetabulum, resulting in partial or com-

plete displacement of head of femur; often bilateral
   b. observe asymmetry of gluteal and thigh folds on affected side
   c. observe limitation of movement and abduction on affected side
   d. usually diagnosed when child is a newborn or is 1 to 2 months of age
2. Planning, goal, expected outcome: child recovers without complications
3. Implementation
   a. double or triple diapering can be sufficient to maintain abduction in the newborn
   b. hip spica cast applied to maintain abduction in older infant; brace or splint may also be used
   c. teach family care of infant, important for successful treatment
      (1) monitor area around cast for skin breakdown
      (2) teach parents how to keep cast dry and free of urine
      (3) warn parents not to let child put anything down cast
   d. provide emotional support to infant and family
4. Evaluation: child recovered without complications

II. TRAUMA

A. Fractures

1. Assessment
   a. signs and symptoms of fracture: limitation of movement, displacement, pain, swelling, discoloration, bone fragment protruding through the skin (compound)
   b. history of fall or traumatic injury
   c. accidents leading cause of death in children of all ages
2. Planning, goals, expected outcomes
   a. fractures are prevented
   b. fractures are treated and heal without complications
3. Implementation
   a. provide emotional support to child and family
   b. maintain safety
   c. prepare for closed or open reduction as ordered
4. Evaluation
   a. fractures were prevented
   b. fractures were treated and healed without complications

B. Casts (Fig. 8–4)

1. Assessment

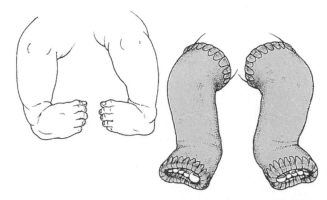

FIGURE 8-3 Bilateral talipes equinovarus (clubfoot) before and after application of plaster casts. Adhesive ``petals'' have been placed around the ends of the casts to prevent plaster from irritating the skin. (From Thompson, E.D. (1990). Introduction to maternity and pediatric nursing. Philadelphia: W.B. Saunders Co.)

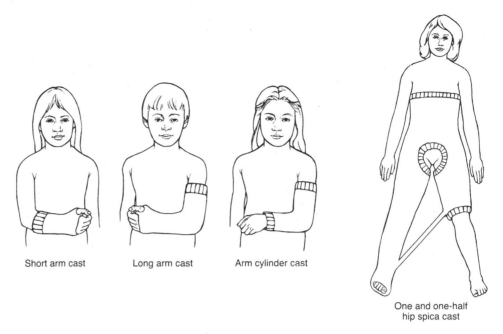

FIGURE 8-4 Types of casts used in children. (From Betz, C.L., Hunsberger, M., & Wright, S. (1994). *Family-centered nursing care of children,* 2nd ed. Philadelphia: W.B. Saunders Co., p. 1821.)

Short arm cast   Long arm cast   Arm cylinder cast   One and one-half hip spica cast   Short leg cast   Leg cylinder cast   Long leg cast

a. observe extremity distal to cast for color, motion, sensation, edema, and irritation
b. observe for unusual odor or bleeding
c. assess type of cast material used—either plaster or synthetic material (Table 8–15)
d. feel for warmth beneath cast
e. monitor top edge of cast for irritation

TABLE 8-15 Advantages and Disadvantages of Plaster Versus Synthetic Casting Materials

	Advantages	Disadvantages
Plaster	Readily conforms to body contours	Many layers required for adequate strength
	Inexpensive	Extended drying time
Synthetic/fiberglass	Lightweight	Delayed weight bearing
	Very strong for weight	Does not conform well to body contours
	Quick-drying	Dust may cause skin irritation
		Expensive

From Betz, C.L., Hunsberger, M., & Wright, S. (1994). *Family-centered nursing care of children,* 2nd ed. Philadelphia: W.B. Saunders Co.

f. assess for pain, which should decrease dramatically once cast applied
2. Planning, goals, expected outcomes
   a. circulation remains adequate
   b. fracture heals without complications
3. Implementation
   a. handle damp cast with palms to avoid finger tip indentations
   b. check pulse distal to cast; check capillary refill; check motion of phalanges; check sensation distal to cast
   c. protect cast from water, urine, and feces
   d. teach child and family concerning safety while fracture heals; how to cope with itching and irritation; importance of not putting or poking anything into cast
   e. tape top edge of cast (petal) to prevent crumbling
   f. encourage movement of uncasted extremities and any area distal to cast
   g. monitor for pain, hot spots, or odor

4. Evaluation
    a. circulation remained adequate
    b. fracture healed without complications

C. Traction

1. Types of traction (see Chapter 7)
    a. skeletal: pins, wires, or tongs for attachment
    b. skin: tape, moleskin, or bandages for attachment
    c. Bryant's: particular type of skin traction commonly used for infants and young children to treat fractured femur
2. Care of child in traction
    a. maintain traction alignment and constant pull
    b. maintain good body alignment and support
    c. teach child and family to allay anxiety
    d. provide meticulous skin care to avoid breakdown
    e. maintain hydration and good nutrition for healing and growth
    f. encourage exercises as ordered to prevent decalcification, contractures, and atrophy during immobilization
    g. observe affected extremity for color, motion, sensation, edema, and movement
    h. administer pain medications as necessary
    i. provide for age-appropriate diversional activities

III. OTHER DISORDERS

A. Juvenile Rheumatoid Arthritis

1. Assessment
    a. definition: systemic disease with chronic inflammation of one or more joints
    b. both infectious and autoimmune theories presented for etiology
    c. symptoms of edema, congestion, and visible swelling of joints and synovial tissues
    d. assess joint movement, limitation, and pain as disease progresses
    e. redness and warmth at involved joints
    f. intermittent rheumatoid rash (macules)
2. Planning, goals, expected outcomes
    a. child and parents understand and follow therapeutic regimen
    b. child maintains functional ability
    c. child adjusts to chronic disease and disability
3. Implementation
    a. observe involvement of individual joints, systemic symptoms, and progression of symptoms
    b. monitor fever

c. monitor affected joint warmth, redness, stiffness, and painful movement
    d. observe for involvement of eyes: photophobia, redness, discomfort, and vision problems; report them to physician
    e. provide exercise as ordered in nonacute states, with support to all joints
    f. provide emotional support to child and family
4. Evaluation
    a. child and parents understood and complied with therapeutic regimen
    b. child maintained functional ability
    c. child adjusted to chronic disease and disability

B. Scoliosis

1. Assessment
    a. definition: lateral "S"-shaped spinal curvature that occurs during growth spurt at puberty
    b. one shoulder or one hip higher than other, especially when child bends at waist
    c. one leg shorter than other
    d. complaints by child that clothes do not fit well or "look right"
    e. poor posture
    f. noticeable spinal curvature on examination of back
    g. more common in girls
2. Planning, goals, expected outcomes
    a. scoliosis is diagnosed early
    b. child recovers from therapy without complications
3. Implementation
    a. first treatment usually application of Milwaukee brace or splint
    b. spinal fusion with rod insertion necessary in more severe cases
        (1) monitor for postoperative complications
        (2) immobilize back as ordered
        (3) monitor neurovascular function in lower extremities
        (4) monitor bowel and bladder function
        (5) make sure brace fits and child and family know how to apply
    c. prepare emotionally and be sensitive to needs of adolescent; altered body image common
    d. if cast in place for several months, teach family care of adolescent and how to meet developmental needs
4. Evaluation
    a. child's scoliosis was diagnosed early

b. child's deformity was corrected without complications

C. Muscular Dystrophy

1. Assessment
   a. definition: hereditary, progressive degeneration of muscle; inherited as recessive trait
   b. muscle wasting and weakness
   c. increasing disability, with difficulty in walking, a "waddling gait," and difficulty in standing up
   d. muscle biopsy and electromyography may be done to assist in diagnosis
2. Planning, goals, expected outcomes
   a. diagnosis is made early
   b. maximal function is maintained
   c. child and family cope with altered lifestyle
3. Implementation
   a. prepare for and assist with diagnostic tests
   b. teach child and family to understand disease and accept fact that there is no cure; attempt to maximize child's potential
   c. assist with exercises as ordered to maintain function
   d. teach family to cope with assistive appliances, such as walkers, wheelchairs, crutches, braces, splints
   e. help with developmental testing to monitor child's progression; mild mental retardation frequently occurs
   f. refer to community agencies and support groups
   g. encourage genetic counseling for subsequent pregnancies
4. Evaluation
   a. child's diagnosis was made early
   b. maximal function was maintained
   c. child and family coped with altered lifestyle

D. Legg-Calvé-Perthes Disease (Osteochondritis Deformans Juvenilis)

1. Assessment
   a. definition: avascular necrosis of head of femur during rapid growth, followed by slow regeneration
   b. joint dysfunction with limp and limitation of motion
   c. history of child's complaining of pain; may or may not be preceded by trauma
   d. most common in white boys between 4 and 10 years of age
2. Planning, goals, expected outcomes
   a. child does dislocate femur
   b. child and parents understand and follow therapeutic regimen
   c. child recovers without complications
3. Implementation
   a. goal of nursing care to keep head of femur within acetabulum
   b. supportive devices, such as abduction brace, bed rest, traction, and casts, must be continued for 2 to 4 years; surgical correction usually permits child to return to normal activities within 3 to 6 months
   c. emotional support crucial to normally active child suddenly immobilized; family support extremely important
   d. activities need to be creatively used to maintain development of child; encourage child to begin new hobby or collection that can be done in bed
4. Evaluation
   a. child did not dislocate femur
   b. child and parents complied with therapeutic regimen
   c. child recovered function without complications

❓QUESTIONS

1. An example of a congenital anomaly in a new-born would be the presence of:

   ① Thrush
   ② Clubfoot
   ③ Purpura
   ④ Vernix

2. Brian, a 10-month-old, has a fractured femur. The most likely type of traction to be used would be:

   ① Buck's extension
   ② Bryant's traction
   ③ Balanced suspension traction
   ④ Skeletal traction

3. Which of the following best describes Legg-Calvé-Perthes disease?

   ① Dislocation of the head of the humerus
   ② Avascular necrosis of the femoral head
   ③ Evulsion of the tibial tuberosity
   ④ Pain around the brachial plexus

4. Acute pain is common for the child with Legg-Calvé-Perthes disease. Which of the following provides the most relief?

   ① Partial weight bearing on the affected side
   ② Bed rest and analgesics
   ③ Skeletal traction for 6 months
   ④ Repeated casting and muscle relaxants

5. Which of the following would be the best way for the PN to screen for scoliosis in school-aged children?

   ① Observe the students in the physical education class touching their toes
   ② Observe the physical education class for any students with a waddling gait
   ③ Advise students with knee pain to see a physician for radiographic follow-up
   ④ Observe the students in the physical education class for those with prominent buttocks

6. One of the students, Ellie, is found to have scoliosis. She is worried about how long the treatment for this is going to last. You should tell her that the treatment will last:

   ① For the rest of her life
   ② Until the curvature is less than 10 degrees
   ③ Until her body has reached bone maturity
   ④ About 2 to 3 years

7. It is recommended that Ellie, a student with scoliosis, have a Harrington rod insertion and spinal fusion. Which of the following is of greatest concern for the PN?

   ① Teenagers' need for privacy
   ② Presence of postoperative pain
   ③ Tolerance of the diet
   ④ Number of visitors each day

8. Sue is an infant with clubfoot and she is placed in a Denis Browne splint for discharge. Which of the following would be *inappropriate* in your discharge instructions?

   ① Prevent Sue from kicking or moving her legs
   ② Assess her feet regularly for signs of redness
   ③ Make sure that she always wears socks with her shoes
   ④ Maintain proper positioning within the splint

9. Harry, age 8 years, fell off his bike and broke his right tibia and fibula and had a cast applied. Which of the following is a priority nursing intervention in his immediate postoperative care?

   ① Have him cough and deep breathe every 2 hours
   ② Elevate the head of his bed 30 degrees
   ③ Elevate and support his right leg on pillows
   ④ Wash off any excessive plaster

10. One of the most important assessments for the nurse to make on Harry, who broke his right tibia and fibula, is neurovascular status. Which of the following findings would provide the least useful information on this?

    ① Finding that femoral pulses are strong and equal
    ② Absence of numbness or tingling beneath the cast
    ③ Presence of positive blanching
    ④ Complaints of pain and tightness around his right ankle

11. Which of the following best describes Bryant's traction?

   ① Fractured leg suspended under the knee and held in extension

   ② Bilateral lower extremities elevated with 90 degrees hip flexion

   ③ Fractured leg held in extension with a pin through the distal femur

   ④ Bilateral extension of the lower extremities

12. Alisha, age 14 years, fractured her femur and is placed in skeletal traction. Which of the following is *not* a part of Alisha's care?

   ① Clean pin sites daily with antibacterial ointment

   ② Elevate the head of the bed daily

   ③ Assess neurovascular status below the fracture every shift

   ④ Turn her from her back to unaffected side every 2 hours

ANSWERS AND RATIONALES

Guide to item identification (see pp. 4–5 for further details about each category):
I, II, III, or IV for the phase of the nursing process
1, 2, 3, or 4 for the category of client needs
A, B, C, D, E, F, or G for the category of human functioning
Specific content category by name; i.e., cholecystectomy

1. Clubfoot is a congenital anomaly occurring in
② newborns.
I, 4, E, Clubfoot

2. Bryant's traction is a type of skin traction used
② on young children, usually under 2 years of age,
to set fractures.
I, 1, E, Traction

3. This disease is characterized by avascular necro-
② sis of the head of the femur. It is not an infection
but is related to impairment of the blood supply.
I, 2, E, Legg-Calvé-Perthes disease

4. Bed rest and analgesics are used to help relieve
② the pain of this disease. The main goal besides
control of pain is the maintenance of function.
III, 1, E, Legg-Calvé-Perthes disease.

5. When children bend at the waist to touch their
① toes, a child with scoliosis has unlevel hips. The
PN should be able to screen easily for this problem by simply watching the students.
III, 4, E, Scoliosis

6. Scoliosis treatment must continue until the
③ bones have reached their maximum growth and
maturity is reached. As long as the bones are
growing, treatment must continue.
III, 2, E, Scoliosis

7. The presence of pain is an important assessment
② because of the extensive nature of the surgery
and the need for movement and exercise such as
coughing and deep breathing postoperatively.
Unless the pain is controlled, other postoperative complications are likely to occur.
I, 1, E, Scoliosis

8. The Denis Browne splint is designed so that as
① the infant kicks, the feet are automatically
moved into alignment. Limiting the child's kicking could delay development.
II, 4, E, Clubfoot

9. One of the major problems after fracture reduc-
③ tion and casting is edema and impairment of
circulation. For this reason, it is vital that the
affected limb be elevated to decrease the
swelling.
III, 2, E, Fracture, cast

10. It is important to check the neurovascular status
① distal not proximal to the cast. The other options
contain appropriate nursing interventions for
the child in a cast.
III, 2, E, Fracture, cast

11. Bryant's traction uses the child's body as count-
② ertraction. Bryant's traction is skin traction.
I, 2, E, Traction

12. When a child is in skeletal traction, it is impor-
④ tant to maintain the pull of traction without disruption. It is impossible to turn the child without
disrupting the skeletal traction.
III, 2, E, Skeletal traction

METABOLISM/ELIMINATION

Metabolic/Endocrine Disorders

I. CONGENITAL DISORDERS

A. Hypopituitary Dwarfism

1. Assessment
   a. definition: growth retardation caused by de-
      creased secretion of growth hormone
   b. delayed growth and development
   c. history of similar problem in family
   d. treatable if diagnosed early in development,
      before epiphyses close
2. Planning, goals, expected outcomes
   a. child's condition is diagnosed early
   b. child is treated and returns to normal
      growth pattern
3. Implementation
   a. provide emotional support to child and
      family
   b. administer growth hormone by injections as
      ordered
   c. teach child and family concerning importance
      of therapy and expected results

4. Evaluation
   a. child's condition was diagnosed early
   b. child returned to normal growth pattern with treatment

B. Congenital Hypothyroidism (Cretinism)

1. Assessment
   a. definition: severe deficiency of thyroid hormone caused by inborn errors of thyroid hormone synthesis, secretion, and use
   b. large, protruding tongue; dry, mottled skin; poor muscle tone; depressed reflexes; hoarse cry; coarse hair; and puffy eyes
   c. difficulty with feeding (slow, frequent choking)
   d. respiratory difficulties, including apnea, noisy respirations, and presence of nasal obstruction
   e. if not treated in infancy, dwarfed stature and mental retardation
   f. check developmental levels at well-child visits
   g. impaired development and mental retardation can be minimized if treated early in infancy
2. Planning, goals, expected outcomes
   a. child's diagnosis is made and treatment is begun early
   b. parents and child will understand and follow lifelong treatment regimen
3. Implementation
   a. prepare for and assist with diagnostic tests, such as thyroid function studies and protein bound iodine
   b. administer thyroid hormone replacement as ordered, such as levothyroxine sodium (Synthroid) (see Chapter 7)
   c. teach parent concerning importance of continued, lifelong replacement therapy
4. Evaluation
   a. child's diagnosis was made early
   b. child and parent followed lifelong therapeutic regimen

C. Phenylketonuria

1. Assessment
   a. definition: hereditary metabolic disorder resulting in failure of body to metabolize amino acid phenylalanine
   b. signs and symptoms of phenylalanine deficiency
      (1) failure to thrive
      (2) irritability due to failure to thrive
      (3) older children, bizarre behavior, resembles schizophrenia
      (4) anemia
      (5) anorexia
      (6) diarrhea
      (7) eczema
      (8) occasional seizures
   c. slow development noted by 3 to 6 months
   d. mental retardation preventable if detected and treated; usually diagnosed in infancy
   e. treatment is dietary in nature, so assessing parents' knowledge level important
2. Planning, goals, expected outcomes
   a. child's condition is diagnosed early
   b. child and parents understand and follow therapeutic dietary modifications
3. Implementation
   a. prepare for and assist with blood test for phenylketonuria; mandated by most state health departments after first feeding or by age 7 days by visiting nurse or at first clinic visit
   b. teach parents concerning importance of testing every child to detect this preventable cause of mental retardation
   c. teach parents about strict diet to eliminate phenylalanine from diet until child is 6 to 8 years old
   d. refer to and consult with dietitian for reinforcement of diet instruction with parents
   e. recommend genetic counseling for future pregnancies
4. Evaluation
   a. child's condition was diagnosed early
   b. child and parents understood and followed therapeutic dietary modifications

II. CHRONIC DISORDERS

A. Celiac Disease

1. Assessment
   a. definition: defect of metabolism characterized by malabsorption of gluten
   b. chronic diarrhea with greasy, bulky, foul-smelling stool
   c. history of anorexia, growth retardation, irritability, distended abdomen
   d. usually diagnosed between 6 and 18 months of age
2. Planning, goals, expected outcomes
   a. child's celiac disease is diagnosed early so that complications are prevented
   b. child and parents understand and follow therapeutic dietary modifications
3. Implementation
   a. collect stool specimens for determination of fat content; 72-hour stool collection, keep on ice

b. prepare for and assist with collection of blood specimens for determination of anemia

c. teach child and family special diet eliminating rye and wheat gluten (starch free and low fat); diet must be followed indefinitely, very difficult

d. provide emotional support to child and family, including referral to support groups

e. prevent respiratory tract infections, which may exacerbate celiac crisis (severe vomiting and diarrhea, dehydration, and acidosis)

4. Evaluation

a. child's condition was diagnosed early

b. complications were prevented

c. child and parents complied with therapeutic dietary modifications

B. Diabetes Mellitus

1. Assessment

a. definition: type I, insulin-dependent diabetes

b. Inadequate production of insulin by beta cells of pancreas or improper use of insulin results in glucose not being transported into cells leading to cellular starvation

c. rapid onset of symptoms in children
   (1) polydipsia (excessive thirst)
   (2) polyphagia (excessive hunger)
   (3) polyuria (excessive urine output)
   (4) weight loss
   (5) glycosuria (glucose in urine)
   (6) ketoacidosis

d. history of diabetes in family

2. Planning, goals, expected outcomes

a. diabetes is diagnosed early in its development

b. child and parents understand and follow therapeutic regimen

c. blood glucose is within normal limits so complications are minimized

3. Implementation

a. test blood for glucose; urine for ketones

b. assist with glucose tolerance test and other blood glucose tests for positive diagnosis

c. administer insulin as ordered (see Fig. 7–5)

d. provide emotional support for child and parents; difficult developmentally for many age groups
   (1) adolescent rebellion can lead to not following diet
   (2) adolescents often face peer pressure to conform with expected "norm"
   (3) diet of adolescent often less than nutritious

e. teach child and parents concerning importance of diet, exercise, urine testing and home blood glucose monitoring, skin care, and signs and symptoms of hyperglycemia and hypoglycemia (ketoacidosis and insulin reaction) (see Chart 7–6)

4. Evaluation

a. diabetes was diagnosed early in the course of disease

b. child and parents complied with therapeutic regimen

c. blood glucose remained within normal limits

d. child develops normally, with minimal complications

Upper Gastrointestinal Disorders

I. CONGENITAL DISORDERS

A. Cleft Lip and Cleft Palate

1. Assessment

a. definition: split or opening in upper lip that may extend through palate; developmental failure of bone and soft tissues of face to close properly

b. lip fissure; palate fissure visible on examination

c. may choke with feeding; milk may return through nostrils

d. more common in male infants

e. repair may be done in stages if defect severe, several surgeries over several years

2. Planning, goals, expected outcomes

a. parents and infant are adequately prepared for surgery

b. infant recovers from surgery without complications

c. infant receives adequate nutrition until surgery healed

3. Implementation

a. provide meticulous mouth care to prevent infection or skin breakdown or trauma
   (1) prevent trauma with Logan bar
   (2) provide mouth care to keep milk crusts from forming and interfering with healing

b. feed infant with Breck feeder; guard against aspiration, mother should breast-feed if possible

c. provide preoperative teaching for family as appropriate to prepare for closure of lip (as early as 2 to 4 weeks of age) or closure of palate (usually around 18 months of age)

d. teach family to feed infant and prevent infection preoperatively and postoperatively, proper positioning to prevent aspiration, frequent burping

e. postoperatively: side lying or supine position-

ing with elbow restraints to prevent rubbing on suture line, Logan Bar
f. teach family about developmental delays in speech as appropriate
g. provide emotional support for parents disappointed with a "less than perfect" child; encourage activities that promote bonding
h. provide for sucking needs for later speech development
i. provide comfort and help parents understand the need to decrease crying after repair because this puts stress on the suture line

4. Evaluation
a. parents and child were adequately prepared for surgery
b. child recovered from surgery without complications
c. adequate nutrition was maintained

B. Esophageal Atresia

1. Assessment
a. definition: developmental defect in which esophagus ends in blind pouch; if esophagus connected to trachea to form fistula, defect is called tracheoesophageal fistula
b. excessive amounts of saliva and drooling
c. choking, coughing, and respiratory distress during each feeding; regurgitation of all feedings; weight loss

2. Planning, goals, expected outcomes
a. infant and parents are adequately prepared for surgery
b. nutrition is maintained until surgical repair heals
c. infant recovers from surgery without complications
d. parents bond with infant

3. Implementations
a. prepare for passage of nasogastric tube or catheter to assess patency of esophagus; support infant during diagnostic testing
b. prepare for radiographic studies; teach family for all diagnostic testing, upper gastrointestinal series confirms diagnosis
c. suction nose and mouth as needed
d. maintain nutrition with gastrostomy tube or hyperalimentation preoperatively and until healing occurs
e. teach family and provide emotional support concerning surgical repair; not always successful
f. maintain patent airway, prevent aspiration

4. Evaluation
a. infant and parents were adequately prepared for surgery

b. nutrition was maintained until surgical repair healed
c. infant recovered from surgery without complications
d. successful parent-infant bonding occurs

C. Pyloric Stenosis

1. Assessment
a. definition: congenital hypertrophy of pyloric muscle fibers, resulting in narrowing of pylorus (Fig. 8–5)
b. projectile vomiting during or soon after feeding; formula appears undigested or mixed with mucus
c. weight loss and dehydration may occur
d. child very hungry and irritable, does not benefit from food eaten
e. presence of "olive pit" mass in stomach
f. more common in male infants

2. Planning, goals, expected outcomes
a. infant and parents are adequately prepared for surgery
b. infant recovers from surgery without complication
c. infant's nutrition is maintained until surgical repair heals

3. Implementation
a. prepare for surgical repair (pyloromyotomy) by Fredet-Ramstedt method
b. teach family and provide emotional support

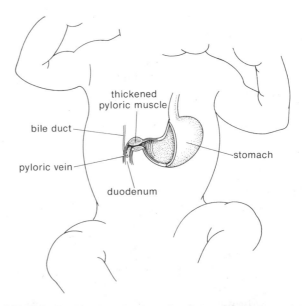

FIGURE 8-5 Pyloric stenosis. Hypertrophy, or thickening, of the pyloric sphincter blocks the stomach contents, causing the infant to regurgitate forcefully. Serious electrolyte imbalances ulitmately occur, and surgery is needed to correct the condition. (From Betz, C.L., Hunsberger, M., & Wright, S. (1994). *Family-centered nursing care of children*, 2nd ed. Philadelphia: W.B. Saunders Co., p. 1446.)

c. maintain hydration and nutrition preoperatively with intravenous fluids with adequate electrolytes, possible tube feedings or hyperalimentation

d. postoperatively: feedings begun slowly with small amounts of glucose water, progressing to formula

e. teach importance of feeding with head of bed elevated or in infant seat; turn to right side after feeding to aid in gastric emptying

4. Evaluation
   a. infant and parents were adequately prepared for surgery
   b. infant recovered from surgery without complication
   c. infant's nutrition was maintained until surgical repair healed

II. ACUTE DISORDERS

A. Gastroenteritis

1. Assessment
   a. definition: severe vomiting and diarrhea
   b. may be caused by viral or bacterial infection, allergies to food or drugs, laxatives, or other irritants
   c. frequent emesis or loose, watery stools expelled with force, explosive diarrhea
   d. symptoms of dehydration, including poor skin turgor, sunken fontanels, weight loss
   e. increased peristalsis and visible peristaltic waves
2. Planning, goal, expected outcome: child recovers without complications
3. Implementation
   a. maintain hydration; intravenous fluids as ordered, clear liquids with progression of diet as symptoms disappear, restore fluid and electrolytes
   b. record accurate intake and output, including diarrhea; daily weights
   c. establish isolation precautions (enteric) as appropriate for organism diagnosed; use care with stools
   d. record character, consistency, and number of emeses and stools
   e. provide meticulous skin care, especially to perineum and buttocks; apply medications locally as ordered such as petroleum jelly or A & D ointment
   f. provide emotional support to infant, including tender, loving care with cuddling
   g. teach family; encourage parents to participate in infant's care as desired
   h. be sure that parents know about diet at home

and good hygiene to prevent reinfection or spread to other family members

4. Evaluation: child recovered without complications

III. CHRONIC DISORDERS

A. Anorexia Nervosa and Bulimia

1. Assessment
   a. definition: eating disorders characterized by abnormal weight loss without physical reason caused by self-starvation (anorexia nervosa) or binge eating followed by self-induced purging with vomiting or laxative use (bulimia)
   b. history of psychologic disturbance concerning incorrect perception of body size (altered body image), compulsiveness, inability to perceive hunger, and poor self-esteem
   c. constipation, dry skin, anemia, weight loss, and amenorrhea
   d. most common in adolescent females
2. Planning, goals, expected outcomes
   a. client understands and follows therapeutic regimen
   b. client returns to normal eating pattern and returns to ideal body weight
   c. client develops realistic body image and shows improvement in self-esteem
3. Implementation
   a. provide adequate nutrition and hydration; often challenging to entire health team
   b. cooperate with behavior modification techniques and psychologic counseling
   c. client needs to get into stimulus-response conditioning program
   d. monitor vital signs and daily weight, watch water intake for artificial weight gain
   e. monitor daily intake of both food and fluids; record number of emeses or stools
4. Evaluation
   a. client understood and followed therapeutic regimen
   b. client returned to normal eating pattern and returned to ideal body weight
   c. client developed realistic body image and shows improvement in self-esteem

B. Obesity

1. Assessment
   a. definition: excessive weight over 20% of normal body weight for age, height, and body build
   b. assess eating habits and pattern
   c. most common during adolescence

2. Planning, goals, expected outcomes
   a. client understands and follows therapeutic dietary modifications and exercise
   b. client attains and maintains ideal body weight
3. Implementation
   a. provide emotional support and support psychologic counseling to discover cause of overeating
   b. prepare for diagnostic tests to rule out other causes
   c. teach client and parents concerning proper nutrition and choosing well-balanced meals
   d. provide dietary consultation as needed
   e. encourage behavior modification to change diet and exercise pattern
   f. encourage client to start exercise regimen
4. Evaluation
   a. client understood and followed therapeutic dietary modifications and exercise regimen
   b. client attained and maintained ideal body weight

Lower Intestinal Disorders

I. CONGENITAL DISORDERS

A. Megacolon (Hirschsprung's Disease)

1. Assessment
   a. definition: enlargement of portion of lower colon caused by lack of nerve cells in walls of colon
   b. lack of stools in newborn; progressive constipation as feeding and diet increase
   c. abdominal distention, anorexia
   d. colon thin, rubberlike
   e. vomiting bile-stained material
2. Planning, goals, expected outcomes
   a. child and parents are adequately prepared for surgery
   b. parents understand how to care for temporary colostomy
   c. child and parents adjust to temporary colostomy
   d. after closure of colostomy, bowel function returns to normal
3. Implementation
   a. prepare for barium enema and rectal biopsy to verify diagnosis
   b. monitor for signs and symptoms of obstruction
   c. administer daily enemas, irrigations, and stool softeners to evacuate colon for surgery
   d. provide emotional support to child and family
   e. maintain adequate nutrition; low-residue diet may be ordered
   f. if indicated, surgery done to resect nonfunctional portion of bowel, with temporary colostomy
   g. take temperature using axillary or tympanic route, avoid rectal
4. Evaluation
   a. child and parents were adequately prepared for surgery
   b. parents understood how to care for temporary colostomy
   c. child and parents adjusted to temporary colostomy
   d. after closure of colostomy, bowel function returned to normal

B. Imperforate Anus

1. Assessment
   a. definition: developmental abnormality in which anus ends in blind pouch; anal opening may be absent
   b. no stools within 24 hours of birth
   c. inability to insert rectal thermometer
2. Planning, goal, expected outcome: child recovers from surgery without complications
3. Implementation
   a. prepare for radiographs as ordered
   b. teach family about tests and surgery; provide emotional support
   c. teach parents about diet and postoperative care; anal dilations may continue to be needed
4. Evaluation: child recovered from surgery without complications

C. Omphalocele

1. Assessment
   a. definition: congenital defect of abdominal wall in which abdominal organs protrude into sac; abdomen covered with thin membrane
   b. presence of sac or membrane in place of abdominal wall
   c. outcome of surgery variable, depending on size of defect
2. Planning, goals, expected outcomes
   a. abdominal wall is closed as soon as possible
   b. child recovers without complications
3. Implementation
   a. maintain sterile environment to prevent infection
   b. cover omphalocele with sterile dressings moistened with sterile normal saline or with plastic wrap to avoid drying or cooling
   c. teach parents about surgical repair; provide emotional support
   d. record passage of any stools

4. Evaluation
    a. abdominal wall was closed as soon as possible
    b. child recovered without complications

D. Umbilical Hernia

1. Assessment
    a. definition: protrusion of portion of small intestine through weakness in umbilical ring
    b. presence of physical defect on examination
    c. more common in African-Americans
    d. classic symptom, crampy abdominal pain
    e. often reduces itself
2. Planning, goal, expected outcome: child recovers from surgery to reduce hernia without complication
3. Implementation
    a. teach family to avoid taping or binding hernia to reduce
    b. prepare for surgery; provide emotional support for child and family; surgery may be delayed unless symptoms persist
4. Evaluation: child recovered from surgery without complications

II. ACUTE DISORDERS

A. Intussusception

1. Assessment
    a. definition: telescoping (invagination) of one part of bowel into lower part (Fig. 8–6)
    b. sudden, severe colicky, paroxysmal abdominal pain; infant may draw legs up
    c. vomiting, presence of stools with blood and mucus, "currant-jelly" appearance

    d. signs of shock
    e. emergency situation; most common in male infants between 4 and 10 months of age
2. Planning, goals, expected outcomes
    a. infant and parents are adequately prepared for surgery
    b. infant recovers without complications
3. Implementation
    a. check vital signs frequently; monitor for shock
    b. prepare for barium enema to establish diagnosis; enema may also reduce invagination
    c. maintain hydration with intravenous fluids; infant usually NPO with nasogastric tube
    d. monitor for signs and symptoms of dehydration
    e. provide emotional support for infant and family
    f. surgery may be done if not reduced spontaneously or with enema; prepare infant and family
4. Evaluation
    a. infant and parents are adequately prepared for surgery
    b. infant recovered without complications

B. Appendicitis

1. Assessment
    a. definition: inflammation of appendix; sometimes follows obstruction or infection elsewhere in body, especially gastroenteritis
    b. pain in right lower quadrant with rebound tenderness (tenderness at withdrawal of palpating hand), abdominal rigidity
    c. classic symptom is positive McBurney's sign
    d. nausea and vomiting, elevated temperature, leukocytosis

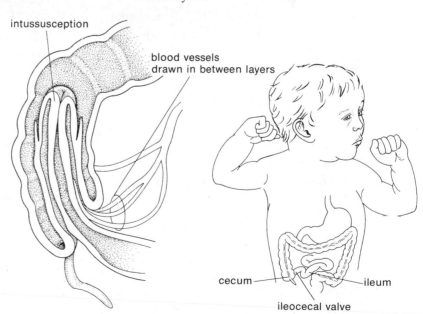

FIGURE 8-6 Intussusception. The most common type begins at or near the ileocecal valve, pushing into the cecum and onto the colon. At first, the obstruction is partial, but as the bowel becomes inflamed and edematous, complete obstruction occurs. (From Betz, C.L., Hunsberger, M., & Wright, S. (1994). *Family-centered nursing care of children*, 2nd ed. Philadelphia: W.B. Saunders Co., p. 1462.)

e. more common in school-aged children and adolescents

2. Planning, goals, expected outcomes
   a. child's diagnosis is made quickly before complications occur
   b. child recovers from surgery without complications

3. Implementation
   a. provide conservative care before definitive diagnosis; give client nothing by mouth (NPO); no laxatives, enemas, or pain medications; monitor vital signs
   b. maintain NPO status
   c. position client in low Fowler's position to help localize pain
   d. monitor for symptoms of ruptured appendix and peritonitis, such as sudden, severe abdominal pain and rigid, board-like abdomen
   e. teach child and parents and provide emotional support in preparation for surgery
   f. administer antibiotics; if appendix ruptured and peritonitis present, massive doses of antibiotics needed to control infection (see Table 7–10); maintain nasogastric tube
   g. administer pain medications as needed to keep child comfortable only after diagnosis made
   h. if incision is ruptured, provide care for open incision until infection clears up and incision is closed

4. Evaluation
   a. child's diagnosis was made quickly before complications occurred
   b. child recovered from surgery without complications

C. Pinworms

1. Assessment
   a. definition: parasitic worms that inhabit intestine, most common infestation in children
   b. spread easily by anal-oral contamination on hands, linens, or food; crowded conditions
   c. child scratches around anus in response to itching
   d. eggs or worms in the stool or on the anus seen on examination
   e. history of anorexia
   f. entire family should be treated to prevent infection
   g. classic symptom is poor sleep

2. Planning, goals, expected outcomes
   a. child's condition is diagnosed early
   b. child and parents understand and comply with therapeutic regimen
   c. child recovers without complications and reinfection does not occur

d. entire family is adequately treated and reinfection does not occur

3. Implementation
   a. collect laboratory specimen for examination with special collection blade or tongue blade covered with cellophane tape, sticky side out (tape test); should be collected in early morning before rising; deliver to laboratory while warm and fresh
   b. practice good hand-washing technique; teach child and family good hand-washing and hygiene habits; keep fingernails cut short to prevent transmission and reinfection
   c. isolate clothes and linens to prevent reinfection or contamination; wash at high temperature; dry 20 minutes in hot dryer; vacuum house well afterwards
   d. administer vermifuge medications: piperazine (Antepar) and pyrvinium pamoate (Povan) most commonly given
   e. teach child and parents that stools appear red from pyrvinium pamoate use so not frightened by change

4. Evaluation
   a. child's condition was diagnosed early
   b. child and parents understood and complied with therapeutic regimen
   c. child recovered without complications and reinfection did not occur
   d. entire family was adequately treated and reinfection did not occur

III. CHRONIC DISORDERS

A. Crohn's Disease (see also Chapter 7)

1. Assessment
   a. definition: chronic, recurrent inflammation of the small or large intestine; probably autoimmune in nature
   b. often affects portion of terminal ileum
   c. patchy, skipped inflammatory lesions
   d. also called regional enteritis or regional ileitis
   e. regional symptoms, such as acute, crampy, low abdominal pain, often described as colicky in nature, fever, abdominal distention, and tenderness
   f. chronic diarrhea, up to 20 or more stools a day with flatulence and steatorrhea
   g. may develop perianal fistulas and abscesses
   h. history of weight loss and anemia from diarrhea and malabsorption
   i. characteristic radiographic pattern of skipped lesions
   j. most common in late adolescence and young adulthood; more common in upper-class and middle-class individuals

2. Planning, goals, expected outcomes
   a. client's diarrhea is controlled
   b. client understands and follows therapeutic regimen
   c. disease remains in remission as long as possible
   d. client is adequately prepared for surgery if necessary
   e. client recovers from surgery without complications
3. Implementation
   a. encourage rest and relaxation
   b. maintain adequate nutrition and hydration; may need parenteral fluids and nutrition; small frequent feedings, bland diet
   c. teach dietary modification; usually soft, low-fiber diet recommended
   d. administer medications as ordered
      (1) steroids, to treat inflammation
      (2) antidiarrheals, such as diphenoxylate hydrochloride and atropine sulfate (Lomotil), to treat diarrhea
      (3) antispasmodics, such as propantheline bromide (Pro Banthine), to control intestinal spasms (Tables 7–31 and 7–32)
   e. encourage psychologic counseling for support and stress management
   f. prepare for surgery, both physically and mentally
4. Evaluation
   a. child's diarrhea was controlled
   b. client understood and complied with therapeutic regimen
   c. disease remained in remission as long as possible
   d. client adequately prepared for surgery
   e. client recovered from surgery without complications

B. Ulcerative Colitis (Granulomatous Colitis)

1. Assessment
   a. definition: chronic, recurrent, inflammatory, and ulcerative disease of colon
   b. differs from Crohn's disease by presence of patchy granulomas and ulcerations
   c. usually starts at rectum and extends upward
   d. may lead to perforation; increases risk of colon cancer
   e. history of chronic diarrhea, predefecation crampy, abdominal pain, and distention
   f. weight loss and anemia
   g. cardinal symptom—presence of blood and mucus in stools

   h. most common in older adolescents and young adults 15 to 40 years of age
2. Planning, goals, expected outcomes
   a. client's diarrhea and other symptoms are controlled
   b. client understands and follows therapeutic regimen
   c. disease remains in remission as long as possible
   d. client is adequately prepared for surgery if necessary
   e. client cares for and copes with possible permanent colostomy or ileostomy
   f. client recovers from surgery without complications
3. Implementation
   a. prepare client for radiographic and colonoscopic examinations to confirm disease
   b. maintain adequate hydration
   c. maintain adequate nutrition; soft, bland, low-fiber diet may be ordered, small frequent feedings; may require hyperalimentation for adequate nutrition
   d. provide emotional support to client and family, explain and teach to relieve stress level and help alleviate symptoms
   e. assess pain
   f. administer steroids to decrease inflammation as ordered
   g. administer antidiarrheals, antibiotics (sulfonamides), and antispasmodics as ordered
   h. teach client and family to cope with disease or with colostomy or ileostomy
   i. teach care of ileostomy (usual surgery)
      (1) drainage extremely irritating, so avoid getting any drainage on skin; fit pouch well
      (2) empty pouch three to four times per day
      (3) amount of drainage depends on child's weight
      (4) increased amounts of ileostomy drainage can lead to severe dehydration and electrolyte imbalance; teach parent to report this to physician immediately
4. Evaluation
   a. client's diarrhea and other symptoms were controlled
   b. client understood and complied with therapeutic regimen
   c. disease remained in remission as long as possible
   d. client was adequately prepared for surgery
   e. client was cared for and coped with possible permanent colostomy or ileostomy
   f. client recovered from surgery without complications

Renal/Urinary Disorders

I. CONGENITAL DISORDERS

A. Epispadias and Hypospadias

1. Assessment
   a. definition: congenital malformation of penis in which urethra opens on dorsal surface of penis (epispadias) or behind glans penis on the ventral surface (hypospadias)
   b. obvious physical defect; defect can be present in varying degrees and, if accompanied by undescended testicles or other anomalies, may leave sex of infant in doubt at birth; may need chromosomal studies
   c. may be noted during urination when stream malpositioned; nursery nurses usually pick this up
   d. normal return of function depends on degree of defect, how far off glans penis defect occurs
2. Planning, goals, expected outcomes
   a. child and parents understand and cope with process of surgical repair
   b. child recovers from surgery without complications and with maximal return of function
3. Implementation
   a. surgical correction necessary to improve physical appearance of penis for psychologic reasons and to improve physical function for urinary and reproductive reasons
   b. teach family concerning surgical correction and expected results
   c. provide emotional support to child and family; if repair done in stages, repeated surgeries and fear of castration and mutilation can lead to psychologic problems
   d. postoperative care to prevent infection and meet psychologic and emotional needs
4. Evaluation
   a. child and parents understood and coped with process of surgical repair
   b. child recovered from surgery without complications and with maximal return of function

B. Cryptorchidism

1. Assessment
   a. definition: failure of one or both testes to descend into scrotum before birth
   b. inability to palpate testes within scrotal sac, differs from retractable testicles that may be milked down into scrotum
   c. testes may descend normally shortly after birth
   d. undescended testes predispose to testicular cancer
   e. not painful
2. Planning, goals, expected outcomes
   a. child's testes descend normally
   b. child recovers from surgery without complications
3. Implementation
   a. treatment may not be begun in infancy; testes can descend spontaneously during early childhood, but usually treated before age 1 to 2 years
   b. provide emotional support to family concerning treatment and expected results; often concerned with future fertility issues, usually not a problem if testicles brought down shortly after birth
   c. administer hormones (human chorionic gonadotropin) as ordered to promote descent of testes
   d. prepare child and family for surgery (orchiopexy)
4. Evaluation
   a. child's testes descended normally
   b. child recovered from surgery without complications

II. ACUTE DISORDERS

A. Wilms's Tumor (Nephroblastoma)

1. Assessment
   a. definition: fast-growing malignant tumor of kidney
   b. palpation of mass on either side of abdomen or in costovertebral area, usually occurs on left side
   c. hematuria occasionally, fever, and hypertension
   d. prognosis good for early diagnosis and treatment of child under 1 to 2 years of age
2. Planning, goals, expected outcomes
   a. diagnosis is made early
   b. child and parents understand and comply with treatment regimen
   c. child recovers without complications
3. Implementation
   a. *Do not palpate abdomen or mass* to prevent spreading; have sign above bed stating this
   b. surgery usually scheduled as soon as possible; chemotherapy and radiation therapy may be used postoperatively; nephrectomy done if remaining kidney functioning normally
   c. monitor bowel sounds to detect signs of obstruction
   d. teach family and provide emotional support

concerning serious nature of tumor, expected treatment, and outcome
4. Evaluation
   a. child's diagnosis was made early
   b. child and parents understood and complied with treatment regimen
   c. child recovered without complications

B. Acute Glomerulonephritis

1. Assessment
   a. definition: inflammation of glomeruli; may occur as antigen-antibody reaction to infection, such as beta-hemolytic streptococcus
   b. high fever, vomiting, oliguria, hematuria (like tea), fatigue, anemia, edema (especially of face), pallor
   c. history of streptococcal infection 1 to 2 weeks previously
   d. more common in preschool children
2. Planning, goals, expected outcomes
   a. child's diagnosis is made early
   b. child recovers without urinary complications
3. Implementations
   a. maintain bed rest throughout fever and active symptoms
   b. administer antibiotics as ordered; if streptococcal infection, give penicillin
   c. administer antihypertensives as ordered (see Table 7–3) such as reserpine
   d. monitor vital signs, especially temperature and blood pressure, early signs of complications
   e. monitor intake and output and daily weights; observe for edema, especially facial; administer furosemide or diazide as ordered
   f. maintain adequate nutrition; diet may be restricted in salt and fluid as kidney function indicates
   g. test urine for protein and elevated specific gravity (assesses kidney's ability to concentrate urine)
   h. arrange for home visits for assistance with home management
4. Evaluation
   a. child's diagnosis was made early
   b. child recovered without urinary complications

III. CHRONIC DISORDERS

A. Nephrotic Syndrome (Nephrosis)

1. Assessment
   a. definition: degenerative and noninflammatory disease of glomeruli of kidneys, resulting in edema and large amounts of protein in urine (proteinuria)
   b. classic symptom: edema of face and generalized edema over whole body, weight gain, scrotal edema
   c. malnutrition, respiratory distress secondary to pleural effusion, and irritability; weight loss masked by edema
   d. history of frequent infections; increased susceptibility to infections
   e. laboratory tests reveal albuminuria, white blood cells in urine, lipids in urine, decreased blood proteins, increased sedimentation rate, increased blood lipids and cholesterol
   f. treatment may continue for 12 to 18 months or longer
   g. more common in preschool children
2. Planning, goals, expected outcomes
   a. infections are prevented
   b. child remains in remission as long as possible
   c. child and parents understand and follow therapeutic regimen
3. Implementation
   a. prevent infections
   b. provide meticulous skin care and position changes to avoid skin breakdown; use special beds or mattress and scrotal support
   c. monitor intake and output, daily weights
   d. test urine for protein and albumin
   e. administer diuretics as ordered (see Table 7–3)
   f. administer steroids as ordered to control inflammation (see Table 7–17)
   g. observe for drug side effects and toxicities
   h. maintain adequate nutrition; diet modifications may include high protein and low salt (see Tables 5–3 and 5–10)
   i. because this is a chronic disease, teach child and parents home care, medication administration, and prevention of infections; crucial to success of therapy
   j. provide emotional support to child and parents to accept conditions and to follow through in treatment regimen
4. Evaluation
   a. infections were prevented
   b. child remained in remission as long as possible
   c. child and parents understood and complied with therapeutic regimen

❓ QUESTIONS

1. Jeremy, 4 1/2 years old, has been admitted to the hospital with the diagnosis of nephrosis. The classic symptom seen in the child with nephrosis is:

   ① Hematuria
   ② Edema
   ③ Petechial rash
   ④ Dehydration

2. A urinalysis for a child with nephrosis would reveal:

   ① Gross albuminuria
   ② Gross hematuria
   ③ Glycosuria
   ④ No significant abnormalities

3. The diet ordered for a child with nephrosis would be most likely to contain:

   ① Decreased amounts of protein and possibly sodium
   ② Decreased amounts of sodium and limited fluids
   ③ Increase in fiber and vitamin content with increased fluid
   ④ Increased amounts of protein and possibly decreased amounts of sodium

4. Andy, age 2 years, suffers from nephrosis and has been on steroids for 6 months. As a result of steroid therapy, he would be *unlikely* to suffer from:

   ① Cushing's syndrome
   ② Depression
   ③ Delayed wound healing
   ④ Increased growth spurts

5. A severe emergency that may occur when a portion of the intestine becomes trapped in a passageway and the blood supply is impaired is known as a:

   ① Hernia
   ② Reducible hernia
   ③ Strangulated hernia
   ④ Irreducible hernia

6. Phenylketonuria is caused by:

   ① Faulty metabolism of phenylalanine
   ② Excessive ketone bodies in the urine
   ③ Faulty metabolism of trypsin, amylase, and lipase
   ④ Embryonic defect

7. A child is admitted with acute appendicitis. The most comfortable position for this child would be:

   ① Left lateral Sims's
   ② Prone
   ③ Supine
   ④ Semi-Fowler's

8. Pinworms may be transmitted by:

   ① Droplet infection
   ② Stepping on the worms or eggs
   ③ Improper hand washing after bowel movements
   ④ Using the same comb or brush

9. Adam is the third child born to Mr. and Mrs. Lewis; he is their first son and weighed 8 pounds at birth. They were shocked to learn that he had a complete cleft lip and palate. Mrs. Lewis was quite alarmed by the appearance of her baby and for some time she was unable to look at him without crying. Adam's lip will be repaired in 3 weeks, his palate later. Preoperatively, which of the following are necessary for Adam?

   ① Feed him in a flat position for ease of swallowing
   ② Feed him with a syringe
   ③ Offer small, frequent feedings so as not to tire him
   ④ Burp him frequently during feeding

10. In the recovery room after repair of a complete cleft lip and palate, Adam suddenly becomes cyanotic. Which of the following would you do first?

    ① Call for assistance
    ② Administer oxygen
    ③ Check for obstruction in the mouth
    ④ Insert an oral airway

11. The *best* position for Adam, who had a repair of a complete cleft lip and palate, while in the recovery room is:

    ① Prone with the head turned to one side
    ② Left lateral Sims's
    ③ Propped on his side
    ④ Flat on his back

12. Postoperatively, following repair of a complete cleft lip and palate, the nurse should feed 3-week-old Adam slowly by using a:

  ① Premature-type nipple
  ② Rubber-tipped Asepto syringe/Breck feeder
  ③ Newborn nipple
  ④ Nasogastric tube

13. It is important to prevent crying in the infant after repair of a complete cleft lip and palate because:

  ① Cyanosis is common postoperatively
  ② Adam could feel rejected if he is allowed to cry
  ③ He could injure a fresh suture line
  ④ Crying interferes with his feedings

14. Adam, an infant with a complete cleft lip and palate repair, will be discharged before the sutures have been removed. You should teach his mother to:

  ① Avoid contact with the suture line
  ② Carefully remove crusts that have formed on the suture line with soap and water
  ③ Apply zinc oxide ointment on the suture line before feeding
  ④ Gently cleanse the suture line with peroxide on a cotton swab

15. Carl, age 10 years, has a history of a strep throat 2 weeks ago. Now he has edema around his eyes, has decreased urine output, and complains of headache. He is admitted to the hospital with a diagnosis of acute poststreptococcal glomerulonephritis. The nurse would expect Carl's urine to:

  ① Be cloudy yellow
  ② Test +4 for protein

  ③ Have specific gravity of 1.005 or less
  ④ Be increased in quantity

16. The diet allowed Carl, suffering from acute poststreptococcal glomerulonephritis, should:

  ① Contain extra protein
  ② Consist of favorite foods
  ③ Be severely salt restricted
  ④ Provide a maximum of 120 mL of fluid

17. Carl was admitted with acute poststreptococcal glomerulonephritis. Carl's parents are concerned about his prognosis. The best response by the nurse is:

  ① Most children recover with no renal damage
  ② He may require medicine to control his blood pressure
  ③ There's a chance the disease could recur at any time
  ④ Permanent renal damage cannot be evaluated for a year

18. Preoperative care for the child suspected of having Wilms' tumor includes:

  ① Every shift takes abdominal circumferences
  ② Avoidance of palpating abdomen
  ③ Monitoring for intestinal obstruction
  ④ Assessing for signs of infection

19. Which of the following is *not* a classic sign of type I or insulin-dependent diabetes?

  ① Polyuria
  ② Weight gain
  ③ Polydipsia
  ④ Polyphagia

ANSWERS AND RATIONALES

Guide to item identification (see pp. 4–5 for further details about each category):

I, II, III, or IV for the phase of the nursing process
1, 2, 3, or 4 for the category of client needs
A, B, C, D, E, F, or G for the category of human functioning
Specific content category by name; i.e., cholecystectomy

1. Edema is the prime clinical symptom of nephrosis. It may become so severe that the child may gain to twice his normal weight.
② I, 2, F, Pediatrics nephrosis

2. Laboratory tests show "marked proteinuria," with blood not usually present.
① IV, 1, F, Pediatrics nephrosis

3. Increase in dietary proteins, although contrary to dietary treatment of most kidney disorders, is needed for replacement of urinary protein loss and for maintaining correct blood albumin levels.
④ III & IV, 4, F, Pediatrics nephrosis

4. Growth is retarded in children on long-term steroid therapy.
④ IV, 2, F, Pediatrics nephrosis

5. A hernia that is not reducible and has a compromised blood supply is called a strangulated hernia. If it is not treated immediately, it can result in gangrene of that portion of the bowel.
③ I, 2, F, Hernia

6. Improper metabolism of phenylalanine leads to a build-up of phenylketonuria.
① IV, 4, F, Phenylketonuria

7. Side lying with the right leg drawn up is the most comfortable position.
① III, 2, C, Appendicitis

8. Pinworms are transmitted through the rectal-to-hands-to-oral route. Good hand washing after bowel movements decreases their transmission.
③ I, 2, A, G–H, Pinworms

9. Frequent burping is necessary because he tends to swallow large amounts of air. He must be fed upright to make swallowing easier and decrease the chance of aspiration. Straws are not to be
④ used because he is not to form a vacuum seal that may injure his mouth.
III, 1, F, Cleft lip and palate

10. Making sure that the airway is free of mechanical obstruction is the priority.
③ III, 2, F, Cleft lip and palate

11. This is the best position for safety. The foot of the bed may also be elevated to prevent further aspiration of drainage.
③ III, 2, F, Cleft lip and palate

12. To prevent regurgitation through the nose and sucking during the postoperative period, use a rubber-tipped Asepto syringe (Breck feeder).
② III, 2, F, Cleft lip and palate

13. Prevent crying to minimize undue stress to the suture line. Cuddling, holding, and other comfort methods are effective.
③ III, 2, F, Cleft lip and palate

14. The best way to remove crusts is with peroxide. Arm/elbow restraints are used to prevent the infant from rubbing the suture line. If ordered, use A & D Ointment or mineral oil to keep the area lubricated because zinc oxide dries the area. It is important to protect and lubricate the incision so that the closure is more appealing. A poor scar is considered a failure.
④ III, 2, F, Cleft lip and palate

15. The urine is cola-colored, it contains albumin, output is low, and specific gravity is high.
② I, 2, E, Glomerulonephritis

16. The diet should be as unrestricted as possible because these children are anorexic. Sodium does not need to be restricted unless there are problems with the blood pressure.
② III, 2, E, Glomerulonephritis

17. Children with poststreptococcal glomerulonephritis usually recover without any residual effects.
① III, 2, E, Glomerulonephritis

18. Because the tumor tends to be fragile and can rupture and disseminate when palpated, the nurse should never palpate the abdomen.
② III, 2, E, Wilms's tumor

19. Classic signs and symptoms of type I insulin-dependent diabetes include weight loss despite polyphagia.
② I, 1, E, Diabetes

BIBLIOGRAPHY

Bates, B. (1994). *A guide to physical examination and history taking,* 6th ed. Philadelphia: J.B. Lippincott Co.

Behrman, R.E., & Vaughan, V.C. (1987). *Nelson textbook of pediatrics,* 13th ed. Philadelphia: W.B. Saunders Co.

Betz, C.L., Hunsberger, M., & Wright, S. (1994). *Family-centered nursing care of children,* 2nd ed. Philadelphia: W.B. Saunders Co.

Bolander, V.R. (1994). *Sorensen and Luckmann's basic nursing: A psychophysiologic approach,* 3rd ed. Philadelphia: W.B. Saunders Co.

Davis, J., & Sherer, K. (1994). *Applied nutrition and diet therapy for nurses,* 2nd ed. Philadelphia: W.B. Saunders Co.

Foster, R.L., Hunsberger, M.M., & Anderson, J.J. (1989). *Family-centered nursing care of children.* Philadelphia: W.B. Saunders Co.

Gorrie, T.M., McKinney, E.S., & Nurray, S.S. (1994). *Foundations of maternal newborn nursing.* Philadelphia: W.B. Saunders Co.

Govoni, L.E., & Hayes, J.E. (1992). *Drugs and nursing implications,* 7th ed. Norwalk, CT: Appleton & Lange.

Guyton, A.C. (1991). *Textbook of medical physiology,* 8th ed. Philadelphia: W.B. Saunders Co.

Hodgson, B.B., Kizior, R.J., & Kingdon, R.T. (1995). *Nurse's drug handbook, 1995.* Philadelphia: W.B. Saunders Co.

Ingalls, A.J., & Salerno, M.C. (1991). *Maternal and child nursing,* 7th ed. St. Louis: Mosby–Year Book.

Lehne, R.A., Moore, L., Crosby, L., & Hamilton, D. (1994). *Pharmacology for nursing care,* 2nd ed. Philadelphia: W.B. Saunders Co.

Linton, A.D., Matteson, M.A., & Maebius, N.K. (1995). *Introductory nursing care of adults.* Philadelphia: W.B. Saunders Co.

Matassarin-Jacobs, E. (1994). *Saunders review for NCLEX-RN,* 2nd ed. Philadelphia: W.B. Saunders Co.

Monohan, F.D., Drake, T., & Neighbors, M. (1994). *Nursing care of adults.* Philadelphia: W.B. Saunders Co.

Murray, R.B., & Zentner, J.P. (1993). *Nursing assessment and health promotion through the lifespan,* 5th ed. Englewood Cliffs, NJ: Prentice-Hall.

Thompson, E.D. (1987). *Pediatric nursing: An introductory text,* 5th ed. Philadelphia: W.B. Saunders Co.

Whaley, L.F., & Wong, D.L. (1994). *Nursing care of infants and children,* 4th ed. St. Louis: Mosby–Year Book.

9

The Childbearing Family

YOUNG ADULT DEVELOPMENT

I. PHYSIOLOGIC DEVELOPMENT

A. Females

1. Reproductive system
   a. maturation process begins during puberty
   b. influenced by hormones
   c. responsible for development of secondary sexual characteristics
2. Estrogen: secreted by maturing ovarian follicle and responsible for
   a. growth and development of ovaries, uterus, and vagina
   b. enlargement of breasts
   c. development of secondary sex characteristics
   d. aiding in growth of skeleton, resulting in cessation of bone growth
3. Progesterone: secreted by corpus luteum or, if pregnancy occurs, secreted by placenta
   a. prepares lining of uterus for implantation of embryo
   b. decreases rapidly with estrogen if fertilization does not occur
4. Menstrual cycle
   a. begins at puberty (menarche), ends at menopause
   b. usually on 28-day cycle
   c. consists of four phases
      (1) menstruation phase
         (a) lasts 4 to 6 days, shedding of endometrial lining
         (b) luteinizing hormone (LH), estrogen, and progesterone at lowest level
         (c) follicle-stimulating hormone (FSH) rises, which enables graafian follicle to begin to mature
      (2) proliferative phase
         (a) uterine lining grows and thickens, leveling off at ovulation
         (b) estrogen level increases
         (c) lasts about 9 days

(3) secretory or luteal phase
   (a) initiated by ovulation in response to surge of LH
   (b) corpus luteum produces large quantities of progesterone and estrogen
   (c) uterine lining prepared to receive and nourish fertilized ovum
   (d) implantation occurs 7 to 10 days after ovulation
   (e) fertilized ovum produces human chorionic gonadotropin (hCG), which stimulates continued estrogen and progesterone production; responsible for positive pregnancy test
(4) premenstrual or ischemic phase
   (a) occurs only if fertilization does not occur
   (b) progesterone and estrogen levels decrease as corpus luteum degenerates
   (c) arteries in endometrium constrict, causing uterine lining to shrink and die
   (d) lasts 3 to 5 days

B. Males

1. Reproductive system
   a. maturation begins at puberty
   b. influenced by hormones
   c. responsible for development of secondary sex characteristics
2. Testosterone: produced by interstitial cells in testes and responsible for
   a. producing sex drive and potency
   b. enlargement of scrotum and elongation of penis
   c. causing seminiferous tubules of testes to produce sperm
   d. developing secondary sexual characteristics

361

(1) affects height
(2) increases size and number of muscles
(3) promotes cessation of bone growth

3. Sperm
   a. develop in testes
   b. mature and remain in epididymis 2 to 10 days
   c. move into vas deferens after maturing

4. Reproduction
   a. sperm mixes with seminal fluid to form semen
   b. semen may be secreted during intercourse before ejaculation
   c. ejaculation helps to propel sperm toward uterus

II. PSYCHOLOGIC DEVELOPMENT

A. Females and Males

1. Similar for both sexes
2. Major developmental tasks: Erikson's stage of intimacy versus isolation
   a. achieve relative independence from parental figures and develop sense of responsibility for own life
   b. increased self-development and achievement of appropriate roles and positions in society
   c. begin to develop personal lifestyle away from home; begin work life
   d. adjust to marital relationships and intimacy with another person
   e. develop parenting behaviors for offspring or for society if childless
   f. integrate personal values with career development and socioeconomic constraints

PSYCHOLOGIC AND PHYSICAL CHANGES DURING PREGNANCY

I. MATERNAL DEVELOPMENTAL TASKS OF PREGNANCY

A. Tasks

1. Pregnancy validation: first trimester
   a. often shock and denial first
   b. introversion begins and lasts 7 to 8 months; encouraged by weight gain and other outward signs of pregnancy
2. Fetal embodiment: second trimester
   a. attempts to incorporate fetus into her body image as integral part of self
   b. readjusts to life roles
   c. develops feeling of inner strength
   d. appears to be time of maturation

3. Fetal distinction
   a. encouraged by quickening
   b. fetus becomes distinct and apart from herself
   c. daydreams about baby and herself as mother; dreams are often unrealistic
4. Role transition: third trimester
   a. separates fetus from herself and makes concrete plans
   b. becomes more anxious and wants pregnancy to end
   c. may express fear of unknown
   d. wish for healthy baby

II. EFFECTS ON BODILY SYSTEMS

A. Effects

1. Reproductive system
   a. amenorrhea occurs; ovulation inhibited by increased progesterone and estrogen levels
   b. softening of cervix (Goodell's sign) due to increased blood supply
   c. softening of lower segment of uterus (Hegar's sign)
   d. purplish hue to vaginal mucosa (Chadwick's sign)
   e. uterus enlarges
   f. secretions of vaginal cells increase: leukorrhea, acts as body's first line of defense against infection
2. Endocrine system
   a. fatigue result of increased hormonal levels, causing sodium and water retention and smooth muscle relaxation
   b. hCG produced by 14th day
      (1) secreted by trophoblastic tissue of conceptus
      (2) critical to corpus luteum
      (3) measured as part of pregnancy test
   c. melanocyte-stimulating hormone (MSH) causes increased pigmentation in localized areas
   d. estrogen produced by corpus luteum first 5 weeks, then by placenta, with levels rising throughout pregnancy; main functions of estrogen:
      (1) growth of uterine muscles and ability of uterine muscles to contract
      (2) aids in development of breast ducts and secretory system to prepare for lactation
   e. progesterone produced by corpus luteum for first 5 weeks, then by placenta; functions of progesterone include:
      (1) acting as regulatory mechanism to handle increased needs of woman and fetus

(2) causing slight increase in basal metabolic rate

(3) causing smooth muscle of uterus to relax

(4) sustaining pregnancy

(5) relaxing uterine muscle

(6) causing endocervical glands to secrete thick mucus, impedes sperm migration

   f. aldosterone increases

3. Cardiovascular system

   a. main functions:

     (1) deliver blood to uterine vessels at pressures adequate to fulfill requirements of placental circulation

     (2) bring about physical, chemical, and cellular changes in blood to provide adequate oxygen exchange between mother and fetus

   b. major changes include:

     (1) cardiac enlargement

     (2) cardiac output increased by 30% to 50%

     (3) increased cardiac rate and stroke volume

     (4) blood volume increased 30% to 50%

     (5) increased potential for varicose veins

     (6) pseudoanemia due to increased fluid volume

4. Respiratory system

   a. increased volume of air per minute

   b. increased alveolar ventilation

   c. improved exchange of CO_2 and O_2 at cellular level

   d. increased estrogen leads to nasal swelling and stuffiness

   e. enlarging uterus puts pressure on diaphragm, decreasing respiratory movement

5. Urinary system

   a. increased renal blood flow

   b. increased renal plasma flow

   c. increased glomerular filtration rate, increasing efficiency of clearance, resulting in polyuria

   d. increased susceptibility to infection from dilation of ureters and renal pelvis

   e. pressure from uterus and loss of bladder tone, leading to urinary frequency

6. Gastrointestinal system

   a. increased appetite and thirst

   b. increased food requirements

   c. decreased gastric acids and pepsin levels

   d. heartburn, caused by esophageal reflux

   e. increased time of contents in bowel, leading to increased absorption of water and to constipation

   f. delayed gastric emptying time, resulting in better absorption of nutrients, especially glucose and iron

III. SIGNS OF PREGNANCY

A. Presumptive, Probable, and Positive Signs

1. Presumptive signs: more subjective signs; cannot be used to diagnose pregnancy

   a. amenorrhea

     (1) other causes may be strenuous exercise, changes in nutrition, and endocrine problems

     (2) menses may not cease immediately with pregnancy

   b. nausea and vomiting

     (1) present in 50% of all pregnancies

     (2) referred to as "morning sickness," but can occur at any time

     (3) common food or odor distaste an early problem

     (4) hCG secretion a major cause

   c. breast changes

     (1) result of progesterone secretion

     (2) increase in size, tenderness, and darkening of the areola

   d. urinary frequency

     (1) extra pressure on bladder from enlarging uterus

     (2) blood supply to pelvis increased

     (3) frequency and urgency common in first trimester until uterus enlarges enough during second trimester to rise into abdomen

   e. fatigue

     (1) exact cause unknown

     (2) sometimes the most common early sign of pregnancy in healthy young women

   f. quickening

     (1) faint abdominal fluttering felt by mother at 18 to 20 weeks

     (2) sometimes used as reference point in determining gestational age

2. Probable signs: objective signs determined during physical examination; result of vascular congestion in pelvis

   a. uterine enlargement

     (1) occurs irregularly at beginning

     (2) uterus above pubic symphysis by 12th week

     (3) reaches umbilicus by 20 to 22 weeks

   b. Hegar's sign

     (1) softening of lower uterine segment

     (2) occurs in second and third months of pregnancy

   c. Goodell's sign

     (1) softening of cervix and vagina

     (2) caused by vascular congestion of pelvis

d. Chadwick's sign
   (1) one of earliest signs of pregnancy but may not be significant after first pregnancy
   (2) bluish or purplish discoloration of cervix, vagina, and vulva
   (3) caused by vascular congestion of pelvis
e. ballotment: rebounding of fetus against examiner's fingers on palpation
f. Braxton Hicks contractions: irregular, painless contractions throughout pregnancy
g. abdominal enlargement
   (1) gradual process
   (2) more rapid after 12th week, when uterus rises into abdominal cavity
h. abdominal striae
   (1) stretch marks
   (2) occur when elastic tissue stretched beyond its capacity
   (3) found on breasts, abdomen, thighs, and buttocks
i. skin pigmentation changes
   (1) results from hormonal changes
   (2) nipples may darken
   (3) linea nigra: brown or pink line from umbilicus to pubic symphysis
   (4) chloasma gravidarum: mask of pregnancy
j. positive pregnancy test
   (1) measures hCG
   (2) 90% to 98% reliable
3. Positive signs: absolute indicators of pregnancy
   a. fetal heart sounds
      (1) may be heard at 10 to 12 weeks by Doppler examination
      (2) may be heard through regular fetoscope by 18 to 20 weeks
      (3) normal rate 120 to 160 beats/minute
   b. fetal movements: felt by second trimester
   c. ultrasound study of fetus
      (1) at 6 to 8 weeks, fetal identification positive
      (2) earliest positive method of diagnosing pregnancy

PREGNANCY

I. PRENATAL DEVELOPMENT

A. Conception

1. Fertilization of egg by sperm
   a. human body cells normally contain 46 chromosomes; of these, 2 are sex chromosomes
   b. sperm and ovum each contain 22 chromosomes and 1 sex chromosome
   c. the sex chromosome is either an X or a Y chromosome
   d. a female develops if the sex chromosomes are X and X
   e. a male develops if the sex chromosomes are X and Y
   f. the sex chromosome of the sperm determines the sex of the fetus
2. Fertilized egg normally implants into upper portion of uterine wall 7 to 10 days after conception
3. Known as zygote until third week

B. Embryonic Stage: Third to Eighth Week

1. Embryo
   a. differentiates into three distinct layers
      (1) ectoderm
      (2) mesoderm
      (3) endoderm
   b. critical period of organ development, disruption can cause abnormal development, effect of teratogens most significant at this time
   c. size approximately
      (1) 2 mm at 3 weeks
      (2) 5 mm at 4 weeks
      (3) 12 mm at 6 weeks
      (4) 3 cm at 8 weeks and weighs 2 g
   d. fingers, toes, eyes, mouth, nose, and ears formed
   e. differentiation of sexes occurs
   f. heart function and fetal circulation established
2. Placenta
   a. developed by the first month of pregnancy
   b. provides fetal oxygenation, nutrition, and elimination
   c. produces progesterone, estrogen, hCG, and human placental lactogen (hPL)
3. Umbilical cord
   a. develops at same time as placenta
   b. connects fetal circulation to placentac.
   c. consists of two arteries and one vein
   d. attaches at center of placenta in normal development
   e. is about 55 cm long and 2 cm in diameter
4. Amniotic sac
   a. surrounds the fetus and fetal side of placenta
   b. is made up of two membranes, chorion and amnion
   c. contains amniotic fluid
      (1) between 500 and 1000 mL by end of pregnancy
      (2) protects the embryo
      (3) allows fetal movement
      (4) provides a constant temperature
      (5) is swallowed by the fetus
      (6) is primarily water but contains small

amount of protein, glucose, fetal hair, fetal urine, and vernix caseosa

vein and ascending vena cava, bypassing fetal liver

C. Fetal Period

1. Lasts from start of third month to delivery
2. General development
   a. by 12 weeks
      (1) eyes, ears, mouth, nose, heart and circulatory system, limbs, tail, spinal cord, and bones present
      (2) bile secreted into stomach
      (3) fetus weighs 45 g, moves body parts, and swallows
   b. refinement and completion of all systems occurs
   c. by 20 weeks
      (1) fetal hair grows, skeleton hardens, sex visible, and fetal heart audible
      (2) fetus able to suck and swallow
      (3) weight: about 450 g
   d. by 28 weeks
      (1) eyelids open
      (2) skin red and wrinkled, with vernix caseosa
      (3) surfactant production begins
      (4) some nervous system regulation begins
      (5) testes descend into scrotum
      (6) weight: about 1250 g
   e. by 36 weeks
      (1) increased fat deposits, nervous and breathing systems, and blood developed enough to support extrauterine life
      (2) lanugo decreases, with vernix caseosa
      (3) weight: 2600 to 2750 g
   f. major development of brain and nervous system during last 3 months
3. Fetal circulation (Fig. 9–1)
   a. placenta supplies oxygen and nutrients and removes wastes; responsible for:
      (1) metabolism, fetal digestive tract
      (2) oxygenation and waste removal, fetal lungs and kidneys
      (3) endocrine secretions, major endocrine gland
   b. umbilical cord contains two arteries and one vein
      (1) vein brings oxygen to fetus
      (2) arteries remove wastes from fetus
   c. major bypasses in fetal circulation
      (1) foramen ovale, opening between right and left atria of heart, bypassing lungs
      (2) ductus arteriosus, connects pulmonary artery to aorta, bypassing the lungs
      (3) ductus venosus, connecting umbilical

II. PRENATAL PERIOD

A. Prenatal Care

1. Initial assessment
   a. complete history and physical examination
   b. assess tolerance to pregnancy
      (1) past pregnancies and outcomes
      (2) family situation
      (3) expectant mother's educational needs
   c. presence of any health problems
   d. estimated date of delivery, Nägele's rule (take first day of last menstrual period, subtract 3 months and add 7 days)
   e. pelvic measurements
   f. vital signs, weight, and laboratory tests
   g. fetal heart rate and presentation
2. Nutritional status
   a. gain 25 to 30 pounds, if weight normal before conception
      (1) underweight women should be encouraged to gain to normal weight plus 25 to 30 pounds
      (2) overweight women must watch weight carefully
      (3) suggested weight gain with twins, approximately 44 pounds
   b. increased calories needed to meet requirements for mother and baby (see Chapter 5)
   c. increased protein, vitamins, and minerals, especially calcium and iron
   d. sodium not restricted unless specifically ordered
   e. diet based on four basic food groups
3. Prenatal visits
   a. initial visit for pregnancy test
   b. monthly visits for the first 7 months if pregnancy without problems
   c. during eighth month, visits usually every 2 weeks, and then weekly during last month until delivery

B. Environmental Risks to Pregnancy

1. German measles (rubella)
   a. can cause major defects in fetus between second and sixth weeks after conception
   b. measles titer should be done before pregnancy to determine risks
2. Sexually transmitted diseases
   a. chlamydial infection

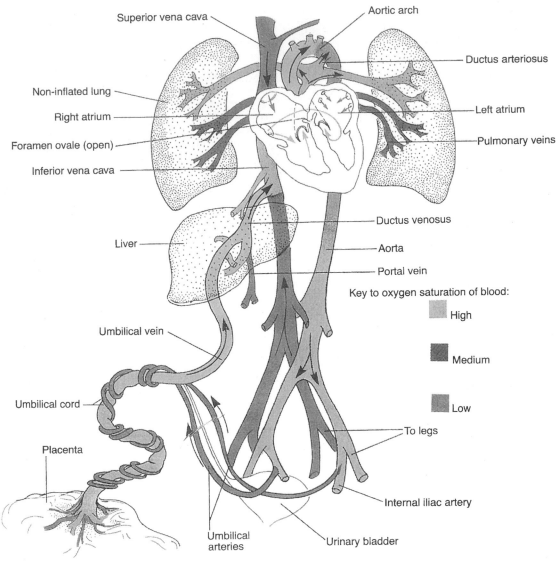

Superior vena cava

Aortic arch

Ductus arteriosus

Non-inflated lung

Right atrium

Foramen ovale (open)

Inferior vena cava

Left atrium

Pulmonary veins

Liver

Ductus venosus

Aorta

Portal vein

Key to oxygen saturation of blood:

High

Medium

Low

Umbilical vein

Umbilical cord

To legs

Placenta

Internal iliac artery

Umbilical arteries

Urinary bladder

FIGURE 9-1 Fetal circulation. (From Gorrie, T.M., McKinney, E.S., & Murray, S.S. (1994). *Foundations of maternal newborn nursing*. Philadelphia: W.B. Saunders Co., p. 112.)

(1) most common sexually transmitted disease, especially high in teenagers

(2) transmission to neonates of infected mothers during passage through birth canal

(3) must be careful with timing of treatment because doxycycline or tetracycline used

    (a) can interfere with tooth enamel formation and cause discoloration of teeth

    (b) best not to use during last trimester, but side effects of medication better than transmission of chlamydial infection to infant

b. syphilis

(1) passed to fetus; usually leads to spontaneous abortions

(2) treated with penicillin up to last trimester; important to prevent congenital syphilis

(3) increased incidence of mental subnormality and physical deformities

c. herpes

(1) contamination of fetus after membranes rupture or with vaginal delivery

(2) generalized herpes results in 100% mortality

(3) cesarean section indicated if labor occurs during an episode

d. gonorrhea

(1) fetus contaminated during vaginal delivery

(2) risks to neonate: ophthalmia neonatorum, pneumonia, sepsis

(3) problems avoided if treatment given before delivery

e. human immunodeficiency virus (HIV)

(1) risk of transmission to fetus estimated from 30% to as high as 75%

(2) newborn may be asymptomatic at birth, but signs and symptoms usually develop during first year of life

(3) no effective treatment or prevention if mother HIV positive

f. group B streptococcus infection

(1) most common cause of neonatal sepsis in United States

(2) treatment in last semester with ampicillin can prevent transmission to neonate during labor

(3) can lead to postpartal infections in mother

3. Drugs, alcohol, tobacco

a. drugs cross placenta

(1) no drugs unless prescribed by physician

(2) no over-the-counter medications

(3) no illegal drugs

b. alcohol during pregnancies may lead to fetal alcohol syndrome, physical abnormalities, congenital anomalies, growth deficits, or jitteriness

c. cigarette smoking

(1) leads to low birth weights and higher incidence of birth defects and stillbirths

(2) research indicates that even second-hand smoke is harmful

4. Radiation exposure

a. no level of radiation safe; women should always be asked about possibility of pregnancy before radiographs are taken

b. increased risk of spontaneous abortion

c. increased risk of physical deformities

5. Other risk factors

a. stress causes increased activity in fetus in response to increased epinephrine

b. women over age 35 years have greater risk of genetic abnormalities

c. girls under age 15 years have greater risk of stillbirths, spontaneous abortions, and premature births

C. Diagnostic Tests During Pregnancy

1. Pregnancy test

a. measures hCG in urine

b. accurate early in pregnancy

2. Ultrasound

a. identifies fetal and maternal structures

b. PN responsibilities

(1) explain test to client

(2) have client drink six to eight glasses of water, without voiding, before test

3. Amniocentesis: determines genetic disorders, sex, and fetal lung maturity (lecithin:singlemyelin [L:S])

4. Oxytocin challenge test or stress test: determines fetal well-being and ability of fetus to withstand stress of labor

5. Non–stress test: evaluates fetal heart rate in response to fetal movement

6. Maternal estriol levels: provides information about stability of fetal-placental/maternal unit

7. Chorionic villus sampling: aspiration of small sample of chorionic villus tissue at 8 to 12 weeks' gestation to detect genetic abnormalities

8. Maternal serum alpha-fetoprotein: assesses quantity of fetal serum proteins that, if elevated, are associated with neural tube defects

9. Biophysical profile: looks at fetal hypoxia and fetal compromise by measuring five parameters of fetal activity—fetal heart rate, fetal breathing movements, gross fetal movements, fetal tone, and amniotic fluid volume

D. Discomforts of Pregnancy

1. First trimester

a. nausea and vomiting due to elevated hCG levels and changes in carbohydrate metabolism

(1) small, frequent meals

(2) dry crackers often help

(3) drink liquids between meals

b. fatigue

(1) get plenty of rest

(2) usually disappears, then returns during late third trimester

c. urinary urgency and frequency because of pressure of fundus on bladder

(1) do not limit fluid intake

(2) burning and disagreeable odor abnormal

(3) decreases in second trimester

d. breast tenderness from increased levels of estrogen and progesterone

e. increased vaginal discharge from hyperplasia of mucosa and increased mucus production

(1) take shower daily

(2) do not use commercial vaginal cleansing products

f. nasal stuffiness and epistaxis from elevated estrogen levels

2. Second and third trimester

a. heartburn: from esophageal reflux

(1) avoid caffeine and spicy foods

(2) sit up after meals

b. ankle edema: from venous stasis

(1) elevate legs when sitting and do not cross legs

(2) avoid prolonged standing

(3) wear support stockings

c. varicose veins: from weakening walls of veins or faulty valves

(1) elevate legs when sitting and do not cross legs

(2) avoid prolonged standing

(3) wear support stockings

d. hemorrhoids: from increased venous pressure or constipation

(1) avoid constipation

(2) increase bulk and fluid in diet

e. constipation: from sluggish bowel from progesterone and steroid metabolism, displaced intestines, and iron supplements

(1) increase fluid and bulk in diet

(2) maintain regular exercise regimen

f. backache from exaggerated lumbosacral curve from enlarged uterus

(1) maintain good body mechanics and posture

(2) wear low-heeled shoes

(3) sit in chairs with proper back support

g. leg cramps: from pressure on nerves

(1) stretch and exercise legs

(2) maintain good posture and body mechanics

h. faintness: a result of orthostatic changes

(1) change position slowly

(2) sit up for several minutes before rising

i. shortness of breath: from pressure on diaphragm

(1) rest with head elevated

(2) sleep in reclining position rather than flat

E. Complications of Pregnancy

1. Pregnancy-induced hypertension (PIH)

a. also known as toxemia

b. leading cause of maternal mortality

c. incidence

(1) common in teenagers, low-income mothers, and women over age 35

(2) women with previous history of hypertension

(3) multiple pregnancy; e.g., twins

d. cause unknown; predisposing factors include

(1) diabetes mellitus

(2) hypertension

(3) kidney disease

(4) obesity

(5) protein malnutrition

(6) previous hydatidiform mole—gestational trophoblastic disease

(7) excessive amniotic fluid (hydramnios)

(8) family history of PIH

e. symptoms

(1) hypertension

(2) proteinuria

(3) generalized edema

f. classified as preeclampsia and eclampsia

(1) mild preeclampsia

(a) edema minimal

(b) blood pressure only about 30 mm Hg higher systolic and 15 mm Hg higher diastolic

(c) proteinuria of +1 or +2

(2) severe preeclampsia

(a) sudden, severe edema with rapid weight gain

(b) systolic blood pressure 40 mm Hg or more higher and diastolic 20 mm Hg or more higher

(c) proteinuria +3 or +4 with oliguria

(d) blurred vision and headaches

(e) hyperreflexia

(f) epigastric pain from engorgement of liver, usually precedes convulsions

(3) eclampsia

(a) fever

(b) convulsions

(c) severe hypertension

g. treatment

(1) mild

(a) close monitoring of blood pressure

(b) high-protein, moderate-sodium diet

(c) bed rest in left lateral recumbent position

(2) severe

(a) hospitalization

(b) monitor vital signs, fetal heart tones, urine output, and maternal daily weights

(c) maintain high-protein, moderate-sodium diet

(d) monitor closely for convulsions

(e) maintain quiet, nonstressful environment

(f) if continues and hypertension severe, intravenous magnesium sulfate administered carefully (Table 9–1)

(g) assess deep tendon reflexes and clonus

h. only real cure, termination of pregnancy

i. attempt to control hypertension long enough to deliver viable fetus

2. HELLP syndrome: *h*emolysis, *e*levated *l*iver enzymes, *l*ow *p*latelet

a. potentially life-threatening complication, variation of PIH

b. pathophysiology

(1) hemolysis from erythrocyte rupture during passage through small damaged blood vessels

TABLE 9-1 Drugs Affecting Reproduction

Uterine Smooth Muscle Stimulants

DESCRIPTION: Drugs that stimulate uterine smooth muscle, especially the gravid uterus; sensitivity of uterus increases during gestation and increases sharply before parturition

USES: For initiation and improvement of uterine contractions for term or preterm delivery in maternal or fetal distress situations; postpartum to control postpartum bleeding or hemorrhage; nasal oxytocin indicated for initial letdown of milk

SIDE EFFECTS: Fetal bradycardia; anaphylaxis; hemorrhage; nausea, vomiting; uterine hypertonicity; rupture of uterus; water intoxication

NURSING IMPLICATIONS: Obtain good obstetric history; do not administer IV without physician available; have magnesium sulfate ($MgSO_4$) on hand to treat tetany; use infusion pump with IV; monitor mother and fetus continually during administration; monitor for postpartum bleeding; monitor uterine contractions

EXAMPLE: oxytocin (Pitocin)

---

  (2) elevated liver enzymes secondary to obstructed hepatic blood flow from fibrin deposits

  (3) low platelets are due to vascular damage from vasospasms; platelets aggregate at sights of damage, leading to thrombocytopenia

 c. signs and symptoms

  (1) upper right quadrant pain and tenderness secondary to liver distention

  (2) nausea, vomiting, severe edema

  (3) hyperbilirubinemia and jaundice may occur

  (4) anemia, thrombocytopenia, elevated liver enzymes

 d. treatment

  (1) hospitalization with strict bed rest

  (2) volume expanders

  (3) antithrombotic medications

 e. poor maternal and perinatal outcomes, with up to 25% maternal and 60% fetal mortality

3. Hyperemesis gravidarum: persistent nausea and vomiting, after first trimester, causing dehydration and starvation

 a. cause unknown but related to psychologic factors

 b. treatment

  (1) correct electrolyte imbalance and dehydration

  (2) carefully monitor intake and output

  (3) provide good oral care before meals

  (4) try small meals, not highly seasoned or odorous

  (5) have someone other than the pregnant woman prepare food

  (6) provide emotional support

4. Hemorrhagic disorders

 a. abortion: termination of pregnancy before fetus is viable, 20 weeks or weight of 500 g

  (1) types

   (a) spontaneous: natural causes; sometimes termed miscarriage or complete abortion

   (b) induced: therapeutic or elective reasons

   (c) threatened: bleeding, cramping, and backache but cervix remains closed

   (d) imminent or inevitable: persistent cramping and bleeding with dilation of cervix and rupture of membranes

   (e) incomplete: portion of products of conceptions expelled, usually fetus, but placenta remains

   (f) missed: fetus dies in utero without being expelled; may expel after about 6 weeks or may need dilatation and curettage (D&C)

   (g) habitual: loss of three or more consecutive pregnancies, preterm

  (2) nursing interventions

   (a) maintain bed rest

   (b) monitor vital signs

   (c) monitor amount of bleeding and loss of tissue

   (d) provide emotional support to parents

 b. ectopic pregnancy: implantation of fertilized ovum in site other than endometrial lining of uterus

  (1) usually occurs in fallopian tubes

  (2) diagnostic tests

   (a) beta-hCG

   (b) endovaginal ultrasound

   (c) culdocentesis

  (3) causes

   (a) pelvic inflammatory disease

   (b) tubal adhesions

   (c) endometriosis

  (4) rupture of tube when fetal size increases, with severe pain and bleeding, may have referred shoulder pain

   (a) often requires blood transfusions and fluid replacement

   (b) untreated may lead to shock and death

  (5) surgical removal

   (a) if diagnosed before rupture, tube may be left intact

   (b) if after rupture, fetus and affected tube removed

 c. gestational trophoblastic disease (hydatidiform mole): rare condition of abnormal change

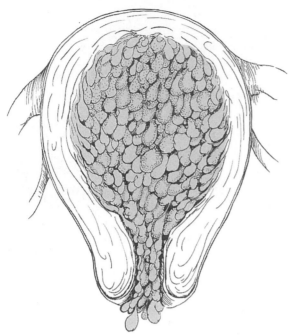

FIGURE 9-2 Drawing of a uterus containing a hydatidiform mole. (From Gorrie, T.M., McKinney, E.S., & Murray, S.S. (1994). *Foundations of maternal newborn nursing.* Philadelphia: W.B. Saunders Co., p. 636.)

of placental villi into grape-like cysts filled with viscid material (Fig. 9–2)

    (1) signs and symptoms
        (a) uterus larger than expected for gestational age
        (b) higher-than-normal level of hCG
        (c) prolonged, severe nausea and vomiting
        (d) ultrasound shows no sign of fetus
        (e) signs of PIH
    (2) embryo dies and mole grows rapidly
    (3) often brown vaginal discharge
    (4) treated by D&C; avoid pregnancy for 1 year
    (5) hCG levels once weekly until negative titer
    (6) chest x-ray every 2 months for 1 year
    (7) increases incidence of choriocarcinoma

d. placenta previa: improperly implanted placenta in lower uterine segment or over internal os (Fig. 9–3)
    (1) types
        (a) low or marginal: placenta attached close to internal cervical os
        (b) partial: small part of placenta over internal cervical os
        (c) complete: placenta completely over internal cervical os
    (2) as lower uterine segment dilates and effaces, placental villi torn from uterine wall

    (3) classic symptom painless vaginal bleeding after 7 months
    (4) treatment for incomplete placenta previa is attempt to continue pregnancy until fetus viable
    (5) may require cesarean section for delivery

e. abruptio placentae: premature separation of placenta from uterine wall (Fig. 9–4)
    (1) medical emergency
    (2) classic symptom: painful vaginal bleeding
    (3) abdomen is board-like and symptoms of shock
    (4) hasten labor if bleeding not severe
    (5) cesarean section for severe bleeding

5. Infectious diseases
  a. cystitis
    (1) causative organism is usually *Escherichia coli*

Marginal

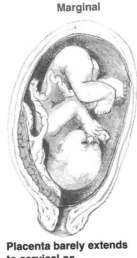

Placenta barely extends to cervical os

Partial

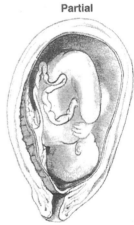

Placenta partially covers cervical os

Total

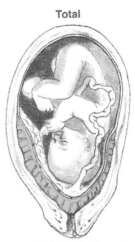

Placenta completely covers cervical os

FIGURE 9-3 Three types of placenta previa. (From Gorrie, T.M., McKinney, E.S., & Murray, S.S. (1994). *Foundations of maternal newborn nursing.* Philadelphia: W.B. Saunders Co., p. 669.)

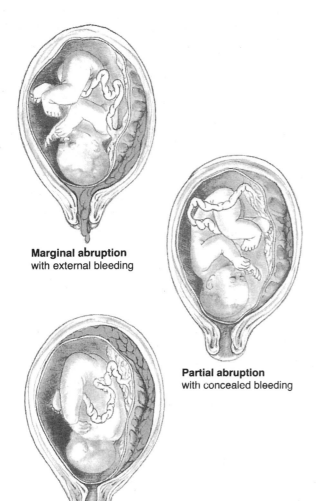

Marginal abruption
with external bleeding

Partial abruption
with concealed bleeding

Complete abruption
with concealed bleeding

FIGURE 9-4 Three types of abruptio placentae. (From Gorrie, T.M., McKinney, E.S., & Murray, S.S. (1994). *Foundations of maternal newborn nursing.* Philadelphia: W.B. Saunders Co., p. 671.)

    (2) antibiotics usually control
    (3) tetracycline contraindicated because of effect on fetus
    (4) instruct woman on proper perineal cleansing
  b. pyelonephritis
    (1) intravenous antibiotics required
    (2) increase fluid intake to help wash out bacteria
    (3) maintain acid urine with fluids such as cranberry juice
  c. *TO*xoplasmosis, *R*ubella, *C*ytomegalovirus, *H*erpes (TORCH)
    (1) toxoplasmosis
      (a) organism transmitted through feces of infected animals
      (b) avoid changing cat litter box

      (c) although mother recovers, fetus affected
      (d) fetal damage greatest if infection in first 20 weeks
    (2) rubella or German measles
      (a) causes chronic infection in fetus
      (b) exposure in first trimester often results in fetal death
      (c) in second trimester leads to hearing loss and other abnormalities, including growth retardation
      (d) draw rubella titer in all women at first prenatal visit; if low, must avoid exposure
      (e) vaccinate, if possible, at least 3 months before pregnancy occurs, if woman's titer low, or after pregnancy
    (3) cytomegalovirus
      (a) herpesvirus
      (b) may be present in adults without symptoms
      (c) presence of antibodies means mother has virus
      (d) no treatment currently
      (e) may cause severe damage to fetus or even fetal death
    (4) herpesvirus, type 2, herpes simplex
      (a) symptoms of herpes simplex in mother
      (b) may cause spontaneous abortion in first trimester
      (c) fetus may be infected during vaginal delivery, cesarean section indicated
      (d) if infected during vaginal delivery, high incidence of fetal death
6. Noninfectious diseases
  a. diabetes mellitus: inherited metabolic disorder caused by insulin deficiency
    (1) gestational diabetes: diabetes that is first diagnosed during pregnancy
    (2) pregnancy increases mother's need for insulin
    (3) fetus compensates by oversecreting insulin, resulting in excessively large fetus
    (4) increased incidence of stillbirth; congenital abnormalities; fetal, maternal, and neonatal complications
  b. cardiac disease
    (1) unable to cope with added volume and increased cardiac output
    (2) symptoms of fatigue and shortness of breath, palpitations, tachycardia, murmurs, rales, and hemoptysis
    (3) classified and treated based on the severity of symptoms

c. Rh incompatibility
  (1) Rh-negative mother and Rh-positive fetus
  (2) mother produces antibodies against Rh antigens
  (3) first pregnancy fetus not usually affected because this occurs near time of delivery, but subsequent fetuses affected
  (4) Rh_o (D) immune globulin, RhoGAM, given to destroy antibodies in mother's blood stream; given at 28 weeks' gestation and within 72 hours after termination of pregnancy
  (5) once sensitized, effect is permanent and no treatment available

QUESTIONS

1. In which of the following situations is the fetus at highest risk if born to an Rh-negative mother?

   ① First pregnancy, Rh-positive fetus
   ② First pregnancy, Rh-negative fetus
   ③ Second pregnancy, Rh-positive fetus, mother received RhoGAM right after first delivery
   ④ Second pregnancy, Rh-positive fetus, mother received RhoGAM before second pregnancy

2. Which of the following statements is not true concerning a hydatidiform mole (gestational trophoblastic disease)?

   ① It is a malignant neoplasm
   ② Bleeding is associated with its presence
   ③ The uterus enlarges out of proportion to gestational age
   ④ Transparent vesicles resembling grapes develop from the chorion

3. Judy is a 16-year-old single primigravida whose membranes ruptured spontaneously. She has a slight bloody show and contractions 10 to 12 minutes apart that last about 20 seconds. Her chart indicates that she was seen by a physician for the first time 2 weeks ago. Judy's pregnancy is considered high risk because of:

   ① Lack of prenatal care
   ② Her age
   ③ Her marital status
   ④ All of the above

4. You plan to do as much teaching as possible to assist Judy, a 16-year-old primigravida with no prenatal care. The best time to do this would be:

   ① During the latent phase of labor, giving simple, short instructions
   ② During the active phase of labor, so that Judy will know what you are talking about
   ③ During transition, because now Judy knows that delivery is near
   ④ After delivery, when Judy is less anxious and more comfortable

5. Judy is a 16-year-old primigravida who received no prenatal care. She is now in labor with contractions 10 to 12 minutes apart. While taking Judy's vital signs, you discover that her blood pressure is 148/98, her face is edematous, and her urine shows 2+ protein. These are signs of:

   ① Normal progression of labor
   ② Preeclampsia
   ③ Gestational diabetes
   ④ Impending delivery

6. Judy is a 16-year-old primigravida who received no prenatal care. She is now in labor with contractions 10 to 12 minutes apart. While taking Judy's vital signs, you discover that her blood pressure is 148/98, her face is edematous, and her urine shows 2+ protein. The physician examines Judy and orders an infusion of $MgSO_4$ (magnesium sulfate). This drug is administered to:

   ① Stimulate labor
   ② Relieve discomfort
   ③ Prevent hemorrhage
   ④ Prevent convulsions

7. Which of the following occurs first in fetal development?

   ① Appearance of vernix caseosa
   ② Muscle contraction
   ③ Increased subcutaneous fat deposits
   ④ Secretion of urine by the kidneys

8. The fetus receives oxygen and excretes its wastes through:

   ① The amniotic fluid
   ② Two umbilical arteries and one umbilical vein
   ③ One umbilical artery and two umbilical veins
   ④ The lungs and kidneys

9. The first movements of the fetus in utero are referred to as:

   ① Lightening
   ② Quickening
   ③ Involution
   ④ Expulsion

10. The first movements of the fetus in utero are usually felt:

    ① 2 weeks before delivery
    ② At about 8 weeks
    ③ Within the first week after conception
    ④ Between 16 and 20 weeks of gestation

11. Normal changes that occur during pregnancy include:

    ① Increased vaginal discharge
    ② Persistent vomiting
    ③ Headaches and dizziness
    ④ Swelling of fingers and ankles on rising

12. The hemoglobin and hematocrit values change during pregnancy. The normal changes experienced include:

    ① A decrease in both because of the increased blood volume

    ② An increase in both because of the decreased blood volume

    ③ An increase in the hemoglobin and a decrease in the hematocrit

    ④ Neither actually changes significantly during pregnancy

13. Signs and symptoms of placenta previa include:
    ① Bleeding in the early months of pregnancy
    ② Painless bleeding in the last months of pregnancy
    ③ Sharp pains with the absence of bleeding
    ④ Separation of a normally implanted placenta

14. Your client is admitted with hyperemesis gravidarum. Your nursing interventions should include:
    ① Placing a padded tongue blade at the head of the bed
    ② Accurately measuring intake and output
    ③ Identification of foods especially nauseating to her
    ④ Limiting visitors

15. Your client is admitted with preeclampsia in week 32 of pregnancy. Her blood pressure is 160/110, she has 3+ albumin in her urine, and she is complaining of severe headaches. Which of the following should be included in your nursing care of this client?

    ① Complete bed rest
    ② Rest on the right side
    ③ Blood pressure measurement every shift
    ④ Limit fluids

16. Your client begins to experience convulsions. Your priority nursing intervention would be to:
    ① Run for help immediately
    ② Put on the call light and ask for help
    ③ Yell for help
    ④ Ask her roommate to get help

17. Which of the following nursing interventions would be appropriate for the pregnant client during a convulsion?
    ① Place a padded tongue blade between her teeth
    ② Put a blanket over the side rails to protect her
    ③ Monitor the fetal heart tones
    ④ Restrain her movements

18. The expectant mother at the greatest risk for pregnancy-induced hypertension would be a:
    ① 22-year-old Rh-negative multigravida
    ② 17-year-old primigravida with a positive roll-over test
    ③ 25-year-old anemic primigravida
    ④ 28-year-old slightly obese primigravida

19. Which of the following is *not* a cause of ectopic pregnancies?
    ① Adhesions of the fallopian tubes
    ② Congenital abnormalities of the fallopian tubes
    ③ Tumors outside the fallopian tube, pressing on it
    ④ Complete obstruction of the fallopian tubes

ANSWERS AND RATIONALES

Guide to item identification (see p. 4–5 for further details about each category):
 I, II, III, or IV for the phase of the nursing process
 1, 2, 3, or 4 for the category of client needs
 A, B, C, D, E, F, or G for the category of human functioning
 Specific content category by name; i.e., cholecystectomy

1. RhoGAM must be given within 72 hours after
④ delivery in Rh-incompatible births so that the mother does not form antibodies.
 I & IV, 4, A, Complications of pregnancy

2. A hydatidiform mole or gestational trophoblas-
① tic disease is considered a benign tumor, but follow-up for a malignancy is always recommended.
 I & IV, 2, A, Complications of pregnancy

3. All of these factors increase the risk of preg-
④ nancy.
 I, 4, C, Prenatal care

4. During the latent phase of labor, the client is
① fairly comfortable, and instructions regarding what to expect as labor progresses relieve anxiety and promote cooperation. A person under stress has limited ability to concentrate; thus, instructions should be short and simple.
 III, 4, C, Prenatal care

5. Classic signs and symptoms of preeclampsia
② are elevated blood pressure, proteinuria, and edema.
 I, 4, C, Prenatal care

6. Magnesium sulfate decreases nerve impulses
④ from the brain to the muscles.
 IV, 4, B, Prenatal care

7. The kidneys begin to secrete urine as early as
④ week 12 after conception.
 IV, 4, A, Fetal development

8. The normal umbilical cord contains two arteries
② and one vein.
 I, 4, A, Fetal development

9. The first fetal movement is quickening.
② IV, 4, A, Fetal development

10. Quickening usually occurs between weeks 16
④ and 20.
 I, 4, A, Fetal development

11. Increased vaginal discharge is normal and quite
③ common. All others require that the physician be notified.
 I, 4, A, Prenatal care

12. As the blood volume increases, the relative lev-
③ els of the hemoglobin and hematocrit are lowered.
 I, 4, A, Prenatal care

13. Because the placenta is located on or near the
② cervical os, as the cervix prepares for birth, painless bleeding occurs.
 I, 4, A & C, Prenatal care

14. Measurement of intake and output is important
② to make sure that the client is not developing a severe imbalance. Food should not be discussed because it often increases the nausea.
 III, 4, C, Prenatal/hyperemesis

15. Complete bed rest promotes diuresis. Client
① should rest on left side. Blood pressure is monitored frequently; fluids are not limited.
 III, 4, C, Prenatal/hyperemesis

16. The nurse must remain with the client experi-
② encing convulsions, protecting her from injury. Yelling may needlessly upset many other clients and family, and the call light should be answered immediately.
 III, 1 & 4, F, Preeclampsia

17. During the convulsion, the mother's protection
② must be the priority. The fetal heart tone can be monitored as soon as the convulsion is over. Padded tongue blades are rarely used. Do not restrain.
 III, 1 & 4, F, Preeclampsia

18. Younger clients are always at higher risk, and
② the roll-over test is usually accurate in detecting women at risk for pregnancy-induced hypertension.
 IV, 4, A, C, & E, Preeclampsia

19. If the fallopian tubes are completely obstructed,
④ fertilization cannot occur anywhere.
 IV, 4, A, Ectopic pregnancy

LABOR AND DELIVERY

I. NORMAL LABOR AND DELIVERY

A. Normal Labor Process

1. Onset: exact cause unknown
   a. contributing factors
      (1) enlarged uterus
      (2) aging placenta
      (3) hormonal changes
         (a) increased oxytocin
         (b) decreased estrogen
   b. lightening: fetal head settles into pelvis
   c. show: discharge of blood-tinged mucus from cervical canal
   d. cervical changes
      (1) cervix "ripens": becomes soft
      (2) effacement: thinning and shortening of cervix to 100%
      (3) dilation: opening of cervical os to 10 cm (complete dilation)
2. Spontaneous rupture of membranes
   a. verified by Nitrazine paper (pH), gives alkaline reaction (turns paper from yellow to dark blue)
   b. microscopic examination of fluid shows ferning pattern
   c. risk of infection increases in direct proportion to length of time membranes are ruptured before delivery
   d. risk of prolapsed cord
   e. if labor does not begin, may require induction
      (1) intravenous oxytocin (Pitocin) (see Table 9–1)
      (2) physician must be present
      (3) mother and fetus must be closely and continually monitored
   f. record time, color, and amount of fluid; presence of unusual odor; and fetal heart rate
   g. note presence of meconium-stained fluid if fetus is in vertex position; may indicate fetal distress
   h. observe for cord prolapse
3. Presentation and positions of fetus
   a. lie: relationship of long axis of fetus to long axis of mother
      (1) longitudinal
      (2) transverse
   b. attitude: degree of flexion of fetal head
   c. presentation: part of fetus coming through pelvis first
      (1) cephalic: head first
         (a) vertex: head well flexed onto chest
         (b) face: head hyperextended

TABLE 9-2 Fetal Presentations

Vertex	
ROA	Right occiput anterior
LAO	Left occiput anterior
ROP	Right occiput posterior
LOP	Left occiput posterior
ROT	Right occiput transverse
LOT	Left occiput transverse
Face	
RMA	Right mentoanterior
LMA	Left mentoanterior
RMP	Right mentoposterior
LMP	Left mentoposterior
RMT	Right mentotransverse
LMT	Left mentotransverse
Breech	
RSA	Right sacroanterior
LSA	Left sacroanterior
RSP	Right sacroposterior
LSP	Left sacroposterior
RST	Right sacrotransverse
LST	Left sacrotransverse
Shoulder	
RADA	Right acromiodorsoanterior
LADA	Left acromiodorsoanterior
RADP	Right acromiodorsoposterior
LADP	Left acromiodorsoposterior

      (2) breech: fetal buttocks or lower limbs first
      (3) shoulder: transverse lie with shoulder first
   d. position: relationship of presenting part to quadrants of maternal pelvis (Table 9–2)
4. Normal progression
   a. station: relationship of presenting part to ischial spine in maternal pelvis (Fig. 9–5)
      (1) presenting part above ischial spines measured as −1 cm, −2 cm, −3 cm, ballottable, or floating
      (2) presenting part even with ischial spines: 0 station, engagement

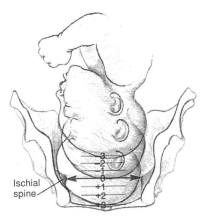

Ischial spine

FIGURE 9-5 Stations of the presenting part. (From Gorrie, T.M., McKinney, E.S., & Murray, S.S. (1994). *Foundations of maternal newborn nursing.* Philadelphia: W.B. Saunders Co., p. 281.)

      (3) presenting part below ischial spine progressing toward perineum, +1 cm, +2 cm, +3 cm, crowning

      (4) crowning: fetal head or presenting part seen on perineum during contraction

  b. cardinal movements: mechanisms of labor

      (1) descent, enlargement, flexion: may occur concurrently and continue during labor

      (2) internal rotation: fetal head reaches perineum

      (3) extension: head emerges from vaginal opening

      (4) external rotation (restitution): head re-aligns with shoulders

      (5) expulsion: delivery of fetus

  c. contractions: rhythmic, involuntary tightening of uterine muscles

      (1) frequency: time from beginning of one contraction to beginning of next

      (2) duration: time from beginning to end of one contraction

      (3) intensity

         (a) strength of contraction determined by palpation

         (b) described as mild, moderate, or strong

         (c) also can be measured by internal uterine monitor, which measures pressure of amniotic fluid; can be used only after membranes have ruptured

      (4) record and report to physician

         (a) change in pattern of contractions

         (b) tetanic contractions: those lasting more than 90 seconds

         (c) decreased relaxation between contractions

         (d) cessation of contractions

         (e) abrupt increase in pain

5. Factors influencing course of labor

  a. parity

      (1) primigravida: usual length of labor, 10 to 12 hours

      (2) multigravida: usual length of labor, 6 to 8 hours

  b. contractions

      (1) quality

      (2) frequency

  c. position, presentation, attitude, and lie of fetus

  d. maternal pelvic to fetal proportions

  e. maternal characteristics

      (1) physical status of mother

      (2) psychologic status of mother

      (3) prenatal education

      (4) attitude

      (5) support system

      (6) ability to relax and to cooperate with labor process

B. Assessment of Client in Labor

1. Impending labor

  a. nesting instinct

      (1) sudden burst of energy

      (2) want to clean house, rearrange furniture

      (3) make sure mother avoids overexertion

  b. weight loss

      (1) fluid loss

      (2) related to changes in estrogen and progesterone levels

  c. lightening

      (1) fetus moves into pelvic inlet

      (2) mother notices decreased pressure on diaphragm and urinary frequency

  d. increasing backache

      (1) hormone relaxin causes relaxation of pelvis

      (2) fetus moves lower into pelvis

  e. other

      (1) indigestion, nausea, and vomiting from changing hormone levels

      (2) increased pressure on bladder as fetus settles into pelvis

2. Active labor

  a. admission criteria

      (1) membranes leaking or ruptured

      (2) vaginal bleeding present

         (a) do not do rectal examination

         (b) do not do vaginal examination

         (c) do not give enema

      (3) contractions regular and effective with cervical changes

      (4) premature dilation and effacement present

      (5) abnormally high blood pressure, proteinuria, and edema present or known PIH

      (6) fetal heart rate and rhythm abnormal

      (7) mother in labor with history of multiparity with short labor

      (8) severe abdominal pain, not associated with contraction, present

  b. Leopold's maneuver

      (1) systematic palpation of abdomen

      (2) done to determine fetal position before delivery

  c. sterile vaginal examination

      (1) done to determine station, dilation, effacement, and presentation

      (2) done less frequently if membranes have been ruptured for a while

(3) *never do examination if active bleeding present*
d. maternal vital signs
  (1) on admission, establish baseline; also check prenatal record for baseline assessments
  (2) temperature: elevation may indicate dehydration or infection
  (3) pulse: elevation may indicate anxiety, bleeding, or maternal distress
  (4) blood pressure
    (a) hypotension: may indicate bleeding
    (b) hypertension: may indicate anxiety or preeclampsia (PIH)
e. rupture of membranes
  (1) spontaneous rupture of membranes
    (a) record and report time of rupture, color, amount, or unusual odor of fluid
    (b) assess fetal heart rate and for prolapsed cord
  (2) artificial rupture of membranes: amniotomy performed by physician
    (a) allows placement of fetal electrode
    (b) allows placement of internal uterine monitor
    (c) stimulates labor
    (d) induces labor
    (e) performed between contractions and not until fetal head engaged
    (f) record time of procedure, color, amount, and unusual odor of fluid
    (g) assess fetal heart rate and for prolapsed cord
  (3) premature rupture of membrane and at least 12 hours elapsed
    (a) if labor not started, intervention needed
    (b) oxytocin used to induce or to augment labor if some contractions occur
    (c) temperature should be taken every hour because of increased risk of infection
f. fetal assessment: cardiac activity
  (1) normal fetal heart rate, 120 to 160 beats/minute (bpm)
  (2) bradycardia: less than 120 bpm
  (3) tachycardia: greater than 160 bpm
  (4) classification of fetal decelerations
    (a) type I: early decelerations
      (i) start at onset of contraction
      (ii) most often due to head compression of infant
      (iii) pattern benign and requires no intervention
    (b) type II: late decelerations
      (i) slowdown of fetal cardiac activity, beginning after peak of contraction with slow return to baseline
      (ii) indicates uteroplacental insufficiency
      (iii) associated with high-risk pregnancies, uterine hyperactivity, and maternal hypotension
      (iv) requires intervention to decrease or eliminate fetal distress
        (*a*) decrease in uterine activity (stop oxytocin if applicable)
        (*b*) change maternal position to correct maternal hypotension
        (*c*) administer oxygen at 6 to 12 L/minute via mask
        (*d*) prepare for delivery
    (c) type III: variable deceleration
      (i) periodic and unpredictable
      (ii) most often due to cord compression
      (iii) most common pattern associated with fetal distress
      (iv) often alleviated by changing maternal position
      (v) if persistent and increasing, other intervention required
        (*a*) check for prolapsed cord
        (*b*) turn client or place in Trendelenburg position
        (*c*) administer oxygen at 6 to 12 L/minute via mask
        (*d*) prepare for delivery via cesarean section
  (5) fetal accelerations
    (a) usually benign and initiated by fetal activity
    (b) may precede late decelerations when associated with contractions
  (6) other signs of fetal distress
    (a) meconium-stained amniotic fluid with fetus in cephalic position
    (b) sudden, exaggerated fetal movement

C. Stages of Labor

1. First stage: period of time that elapses from beginning of regular contractions until cervix completely dilated and effaced
   a. latent phase

(1) dilation of cervix from 1 to 4 cm
(2) contractions
   (a) may be mild to moderate
   (b) occur every 4 to 5 minutes
   (c) last 30 to 40 seconds
(3) mother
   (a) may complain of backache; provide backrub, position on left side, and provide pillow for back
   (b) does not want to be left alone; stay with mother, encourage significant other to stay with mother
   (c) time to do any teaching such as breathing techniques, if needed

b. active phase
(1) dilation from 4 to 8 cm
(2) contractions
   (a) may be moderate to strong
   (b) occur every 2 to 4 minutes
   (c) last 45 to 60 seconds
(3) mother
   (a) may be more apprehensive; reassure her, provide support, and inform her of progress of labor and what to expect
   (b) does not want to be left alone; stay with mother, or have significant other stay with her
   (c) may be uncertain whether she can cope with contractions; encourage her, and use relaxation and breathing techniques

c. transition phase
(1) dilation from 8 to 10 cm
(2) contractions
   (a) may be moderate to moderately strong
   (b) occur every 2 to 4 minutes
   (c) last 45 to 90 seconds
(3) mother may
   (a) have increased bloody show; give frequent perineal care, change blue pads frequently, and assure mother this is normal
   (b) feel rectal pressure; encourage her not to push at this point and to use deep-breathing exercises
   (c) show marked restlessness; continue relaxation exercises and encourage mother
   (d) become nauseated; encourage deep breaths, provide frequent mouth care, ice chips, and whatever else allowed; clean mother up if vomiting occurs, and prevent aspiration

   (e) experience shaking of legs; provide blankets and gently massage legs
   (f) have perspiration on upper lids and forehead; change bed linens and gown as needed, and apply cold cloth to forehead; hydration important, give fluids or intravenous fluids, whatever allowed
   (g) display irritability and unwillingness to be touched; speak slowly and clearly, help mother focus attention on task, and be understanding
   (h) show frustration and inability to cope with contractions if left alone; do not leave mother alone, and encourage mother to focus on progress
   (i) be eager to be "put to sleep"; provide encouragement, advise mother of progress, and provide noninvasive pain relief through breathing and massage
   (j) be bewildered by intensity of contractions; tell her what to expect and encourage her about her progress

2. Second stage: lasts from time of complete dilation of cervix through delivery of baby
a. contractions
(1) may be moderate to moderately strong
(2) occur every 1 to 2 minutes
(3) last 60 to 90 seconds
b. mother may
(1) experience desire to move bowels
   (a) may have to move bowel if has not had a bowel movement today or if had a Fleet's enema that day; often does not actually have to move bowels, just feeling sensation of pressure
   (b) use pushing only when necessary
(2) panic when head reaches perineum
   (a) reassure mother
   (b) use breathing and relaxation techniques
(3) feel splitting sensation because of extreme vaginal stretching
   (a) assist with local anesthesia
   (b) assist with episiotomy
(4) be vague in communication
   (a) speak slowly and clearly to mother
   (b) avoid unnecessary distractions
(5) be amnesic between contractions
   (a) avoid unnecessary distractions
   (b) avoid explanations at this time
(6) have tremendous satisfaction or great pain with each push: praise progress

3. Third stage: lasts from after birth of baby until placenta expelled
   a. physical characteristics include
      (1) rise of fundus
      (2) uterus assumes globular shape
      (3) visible descent of cord, lengthening
      (4) trickle or gush of blood
   b. mother should be
      (1) alert
      (2) proud and happy
      (3) anxious to see baby
      (4) relieved
   c. nursing interventions
      (1) assess mother's vital signs
      (2) monitor for excessive bleeding
      (3) assist with episiotomy repair
      (4) lower mother's legs slowly and simultaneously
      (5) take mother to recovery room
4. Fourth stage: from after delivery of placenta to postpartum stabilization
   a. time, 2 to 4 hours
   b. assessments
      (1) fundus firm; in midline, at, or below umbilicus
      (2) lochia scant to moderate, rubra color
      (3) mother may be excited or exhausted; response individualized
   c. nursing interventions
      (1) palpate fundus every 15 minutes for first hour and massage fundus if boggy
      (2) check for bladder distention; offer bedpan
      (3) monitor vital signs for signs of shock
      (4) check vaginal drainage and report any fresh, heavy bleeding, especially if uterus is boggy
      (5) monitor mother on intravenous oxytocin to treat boggy uterus and hemorrhage
      (6) check perineum for signs of trauma
         (a) watch for swelling and hematoma formation
         (b) apply ice to perineum to treat pain and swelling

D. Anesthesia and Analgesia During Labor and Delivery

1. Analgesia: alters pain perception
   a. nonpharmacologic: relief of fear, tension, or pain syndrome
      (1) encourage mother and significant other to use Lamaze if prepared
      (2) relaxation
         (a) allows release of endorphins
         (b) good for tension and anxiety
         (c) can treat real physical pain

(3) education: information and understanding
(4) cognitive control: use of dissociation, imagery, and focusing
   b. pharmacologic
      (1) timing of depressant drug administration
         (a) respiratory depression of fetus may occur if given within 2 hours of delivery
         (b) progress of labor may be impeded if given during latent phase
         (c) should be administered during active phase of labor
      (2) classifications
         (a) sedatives/barbiturates: allow rest and sleep; can depress fetal respirations and heart rate
         (b) tranquilizers: promote relaxation and potentiate action of barbiturates and narcotics
         (c) narcotics: alter perception of pain
         (d) narcotic antagonist, naloxone (Narcan): administered to infant to reverse respiratory depression effects of narcotics; *note:* does not reverse effects of sedatives or tranquilizers
2. Anesthesia
   a. general
      (1) rarely used—emergency cesarean section only
      (2) produces unconsciousness
      (3) may cause severe respiratory depression of fetus or infant
   b. regional
      (1) subarachnoid block (saddle block)
         (a) dilation must be complete
         (b) may cause maternal hypotension, which causes fetal bradycardia
         (c) bearing-down reflex lost
      (2) epidural
         (a) given during first or second stage of labor
         (b) may prolong latent phase if given too early
         (c) loss of bearing-down reflex unless low-dose epidural, which allows for mother to feel "urge to push"
         (d) assess for maternal hypotension
      (3) pudendal block
         (a) infiltration of pudendal nerve
         (b) produces pain relief and relaxation of perineum
         (c) no fetal side effects if given properly
      (4) paracervical block
         (a) infiltration of tissues around cervix
         (b) given during first stage of labor

(c) lasts 1 to 2 hours
(d) rapid placental transmission, causing fetal bradycardia lasting up to 10 minutes; position mother on left side, increase fluid intake, monitor closely for maternal hypotension, and administer oxygen at 6 to 12 L/minute if maternal hypotension occurs
    (5) local
      (a) infiltration of perineal tissues
      (b) purpose: episiotomy
      (c) no fetal side effects

II. DEVIATIONS IN NORMAL LABOR PROCESS

A. Preterm Labor

1. Occurrence: before end of week 37 of gestation
2. Causes
   a. spontaneous rupture of membranes
   b. cervical incompetence
   c. uterine anomalies
   d. fetal anomalies
   e. multiple fetuses
   f. chronic maternal disease, such as diabetes or hypertension
3. Treatment
   a. bed rest
   b. medications to decrease or stop contractions (ritodrine, terbutaline sulfate [Brethine], isoxsuprine hydrochloride [Vasodilan], MgSO$_4$) (see Table 9–1)
   c. delivery, if fetus is viable
4. Contraindications for halting preterm labor
   a. rupture of membranes
   b. gross vaginal bleeding
   c. gross fetal anomalies
   d. severe maternal hypertension, eclampsia
   e. fetal demise

B. Precipitate Labor

1. Definition: labor lasting less than 3 hours
2. Nursing intervention: never attempt to hold back infant's head to slow or prevent delivery

C. Dystocia (Difficult Labor)

1. Hypotonic contractions
   a. contractions ineffective and irregular
   b. treatment
       (1) prostaglandin E$_2$ gel (Prepidil Endocervical Gel) to ripen cervix
       (2) oxytocin augmentation, if no complications present
   c. cesarean section for cephalopelvic disproportion, fetal distress, or maternal distress
   d. nursing interventions
       (1) provide rest for mother
       (2) offer emotional reassurance
       (3) monitor oxytocin infusion for effects on contractions and maternal response using fetal monitor with intrauterine pressure catheter
2. Hypertonic contractions
   a. decrease in resting tone between contractions, with uncoordinated activity between upper and lower uterine segments
   b. contractions painful but ineffective in producing cervical dilation
   c. treatment
       (1) sedation and analgesia
       (2) cesarean section for fetal distress
   d. nursing interventions
       (1) provide rest
       (2) offer emotional support
       (3) monitor for maternal exhaustion
       (4) administer medications as ordered
       (5) monitor fetal status
3. Rupture of uterus: may be partial or complete
   a. causes
       (1) prolonged labor with cephalopelvic disproportion
       (2) poorly managed induction of labor
       (3) unsupervised labor after previous cesarean section
   b. treatment: immediate laparotomy
   c. nursing interventions
       (1) report changes in contraction pattern, especially tetanic contraction with sudden cessation of contraction
       (2) monitor for signs of shock
       (3) be calm and supportive to mother
4. Prolapsed cord (Fig. 9–6)
   a. caused by rupture of membranes when presenting part not engaged in pelvis
   b. nursing interventions
       (1) relieve pressure on cord by placing mother in Trendelenburg or knee-chest position
       (2) notify physician immediately
       (3) do *not* attempt to replace cord into uterus
       (4) if cord protrudes outside vagina, cover with saline-moistened sterile towel
       (5) monitor fetal heart rate closely, may use internal fetal scalp electrode on presenting part
       (6) prepare for delivery by cesarean section

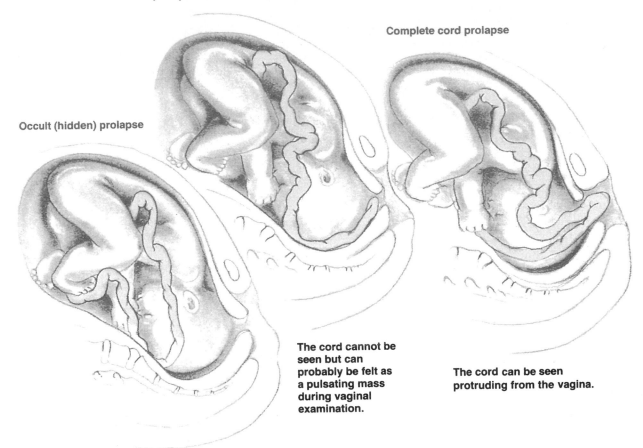

Cord prolapsed in front of the fetal head

Complete cord prolapse

Occult (hidden) prolapse

The cord cannot be seen but can probably be felt as a pulsating mass during vaginal examination.

The cord can be seen protruding from the vagina.

The cord is compressed between the fetal presenting part and pelvis but cannot be seen or felt during vaginal examination.

FIGURE 9-6   Variations of prolapsed umbilical cord. (From Gorrie, T.M., McKinney, E.S., & Murray, S.S. (1994). *Foundations of maternal newborn nursing.* Philadelphia: W.B. Saunders Co., p. 765.)

(7)   give client supplemental oxygen
(8)   increase intravenous fluid rate

D.   Complications with Amniotic Fluid

1.   Hydramnios
   a.   excessive amounts of amniotic fluid; over 2000 mL
   b.   cause unknown: associated with
      (1)   maternal diabetes mellitus
      (2)   Rh sensitivities
      (3)   fetal malformations of esophagus or neural tube anencephaly
   c.   problems associated with increased fluid amount
      (1)   2000 to 3000 mL causes some discomfort but no real problems
      (2)   greater than 3000 mL
         (a)   severe respiratory discomfort from pressure on diaphragm
         (b)   lower extremity edema from pressure on pelvic vessels
         (c)   abruptio placentae with rupture of membranes because of rapid change in uterine size
         (d)   postpartum hemorrhage from over-distended uterine muscles
         (e)   increased fetal mortality and increased risk of prolapsed cord with rupture of membranes
   d.   treatment
      (1)   identification of problem during prenatal period
      (2)   amniocentesis if maternal problems great
2.   Oligohydramnios
   a.   amniotic fluid less than 100 mL
   b.   associated with
      (1)   postmaturity
      (2)   intrauterine growth retardation
      (3)   fetal renal system abnormalities
   c.   labor may be dysfunctional

d. fetal hypoxia may occur from cord compression during labor

e. treatment: normal saline infusion via uterine catheter to prevent cord compression

III. OPERATIVE PROCEDURES

A. Episiotomy

1. Surgical incision into perineum
2. Rationale
   a. facilitate delivery
   b. prevent lacerations
      (1) first-degree laceration: tear in mucous membrane and skin only
      (2) second-degree laceration: includes above plus tear into perineal muscle
      (3) third-degree laceration: both of above plus tear into rectal sphincter
      (4) fourth-degree laceration: all of above plus tear into rectal mucosa
3. May be midline or mediolateral

B. Forceps

1. May be used to facilitate delivery, shortening the second stage of labor
2. High forceps: above 0 station—never recommended
3. Mid forceps: 0 station—only occasionally used
4. Low forceps (outlet forceps): baby's head on perineum—most common

C. Cesarean Delivery (Section)

1. Delivery of fetus through abdominal incision
2. Planned
   a. repeat of previous section
   b. prediagnosed placenta previa, herpes, or abnormal presentation
3. Emergency
   a. abruptio placentae: premature separation of placenta
   b. placenta previa: abnormal implantation of placenta, in which placenta partially or completely covers cervical os
   c. cephalopelvic disproportion
   d. abnormal presentation
   e. prolapsed cord
   f. fetal distress
   g. uterine dystocia
4. Types
   a. classic
      (1) midline section
      (2) performed when speed is important

b. transverse incision in lower uterus, "bikini cut"
   c. extraperitoneal
5. Nursing interventions
   a. remain calm
   b. insert Foley catheter
   c. be sure operative permit signed before administering any medications
   d. notify nursery
6. Postoperative care
   a. same as for every abdominal surgery client
   b. remember to monitor uterus as after any delivery
   c. attention to postpartum needs
   d. psychosocial support to facilitate mother–infant bonding

D. Vaginal Birth After Cesarean

1. Women should be offered opportunity for vaginal delivery even after cesarean section
2. Previous classic uterine incision contraindication for labor
3. Women who had a low uterine incision can have normal labor and delivery
4. If no labor associated with previous sections, labor proceeds similar to that of a primigravida
5. Should be prepared to have another section if labor does not progress or if problems develop

IV. SPECIAL CONCERNS

A. HIV Positive Mother During and After Delivery

1. Assessment
   a. knowledge of condition
   b. plans for discharge care of self and infant
   c. self-concept
   d. mother's knowledge of own prognosis and infant's prognosis
      (1) mother HIV-positive or with active AIDS
      (2) one third of infants born to HIV-positive mothers are HIV-positive
      (3) most of HIV-positive infants die within first 2 years
2. Nursing interventions
   a. use universal precautions guidelines from Centers for Disease Control and Prevention (CDC) (Table 9–3)
   b. provide routine postpartum care and support
   c. teach self-care
      (1) usual postpartum information
      (2) information needed to treat own disease
   d. teach infant care
      (1) HIV-positive infant, special needs

TABLE 9-3 Universal Precautions Guidelines from the Centers for Disease Control and Prevention

1. Precautions should be used in care of *all* patients
2. Barrier precautions to prevent skin and mucous membranes exposed
   a. Gloves for contact with blood and body fluids of mother and infant
   b. Masks, protective eye wear, and gowns for procedure that might involve droplet or splash exposure
3. Handwashing
   a. Immediately after exposure
   b. After removing gloves
4. Precautions to prevent needle-stick injuries
5. Health care workers with skin lesions should avoid direct patient contact until condition resolves

        (2) mother may be unable to care for infant
  e. encourage consultation with social services

3. Evaluation
   a. mother demonstrates feelings of self-worth
   b. mother verbalizes understanding of precaution
      (1) hand washing
      (2) breast-feeding discouraged; HIV can be transmitted in breast milk
      (3) interactions with family and friends
      (4) disposal of soiled materials from self and infant (if infant HIV-positive)
   c. mother verbalizes knowledge of support systems
   d. mother verbalizes knowledge of disease process and prognosis for self and infant (if infant HIV-positive)

? QUESTIONS

1. At 8 A.M. Susan, a 24-year-old gravida 3 para 1, arrives at the labor and delivery unit. She states that her "water broke" about 7:30 this morning and she has been having contractions 6 to 7 minutes apart lasting 30 seconds since that time. During the admission procedures, the LPN obtains Susan's temperature, pulse, and respiration, blood pressure, and fetal heart rate. Vital signs are taken on admission primarily because:

   ① It is hospital policy
   ② A baseline is necessary for further assessment
   ③ It is part of the admission record
   ④ The nursing care plan is based on this information

2. Susan is in active labor. Before taking the fetal heart rate, the nurse palpates Susan's abdomen to determine fetal position. This procedure is known as:

   ① Ritgen's maneuver
   ② Homans' sign
   ③ Leopold's maneuver
   ④ Chadwick's sign

3. Rupture of the membranes may be verified by testing:

   ① Fluid in the vagina with pH paper and obtaining an acid reaction
   ② Fluid in the vagina with pH paper and obtaining an alkaline reaction
   ③ Fluid in the vagina for glucose
   ④ Fluid in the vagina for meconium

4. Sterile vaginal examination reveals that Susan's cervix is dilated 2 to 3 cm and 50% effaced and the presenting part is at 0 station. Complete dilation of the cervix is considered to be:

   ① 10 cm
   ② 8 cm
   ③ 20 cm
   ④ 5 cm

5. Effacement refers to:

   ① The amount of show
   ② The size of the pelvis
   ③ The position of the infant's head
   ④ Thinning and shortening of the cervix

6. Station refers to:

   ① Position of the baby's head in relation to the ischial spines
   ② Degree of flexion of the baby's head
   ③ Relationship of the presenting part to the four quadrants of the maternal pelvis
   ④ Ballottement

7. Susan, who was admitted in active labor, is placed in bed, and the external fetal-maternal monitor is applied. The phonotransducer indicates fetal heart rate of 140 bpm. The normal fetal heart rate is:

   ① 60–90 bpm
   ② 90–120 bpm
   ③ 120–160 bpm
   ④ 160–190 bpm

8. To time the frequency of Susan's contractions, the nurse counts the time from:

   ① The beginning of one contraction to the beginning of the next contraction
   ② The end of one contraction to the beginning of the next contraction
   ③ The beginning of the contraction to the end of the contraction
   ④ The peak of one contraction to the peak of the next contraction

9. Susan's contractions are 2 to 3 minutes apart and lasting 60 seconds. She is 5 to 6 cm dilated and is using good breathing techniques. Susan requests some medication for discomfort. The nurse's best reply would be:

   ① "Sure, I'll get you something right away."
   ② "No, you're in transition, and if we give you anything, it will make your baby sleepy."
   ③ "You are in the active phase of labor now. I will check with the physician to see if you can have something."
   ④ "I thought you wanted to have natural childbirth."

10. Susan's contractions are 2 to 3 minutes apart and lasting 60 seconds. She is 5 to 6 cm dilated and is using good breathing techniques. Susan requests some medication for discomfort. The physician orders Demerol, 50 mg intramuscularly, to be given now. The nurse knows that:

    ① This is an incorrect dose
    ② Demerol can be given only by mouth
    ③ Demerol is a narcotic analgesic
    ④ The infant will require Narcan

11. Susan is taken to the delivery room. The physician does an episiotomy to facilitate the birth of the baby. An episiotomy is an incision into:

    ① The peritoneum
    ② The abdomen
    ③ The perineum
    ④ The cervix

12. As soon as possible after delivery, the baby is placed next to Susan and her husband is encouraged to stroke and talk to the baby. This helps to promote:

    ① Involution
    ② Bonding and attachment
    ③ Separation of the placenta
    ④ Breast-feeding

13. The placenta separates and is expelled during the:

    ① First stage of labor
    ② Second stage of labor
    ③ Third stage of labor
    ④ Fourth stage of labor

14. Doris is a primigravida at term who was scheduled for a cesarean section but was admitted in active labor with a breech presentation. Her membranes are intact, and she is 4 cm dilated and at −1 station. If her membranes rupture, she would be at risk for:

    ① A prolapsed cord
    ② A nuchal cord
    ③ Hemorrhage
    ④ Precipitate delivery

15. The LPN knows that a breech presentation means that the baby is in:

    ① A transverse position
    ② A vertex position
    ③ A buttocks presentation
    ④ Distress

16. Doris is a primigravida at term who was scheduled for a cesarean section but was admitted in active labor with a breech presentation. Her membranes are intact, and she is 4 cm dilated and at −1 station. The physician decides to do an immediate cesarean section and orders a Foley catheter inserted. The purpose of the catheter is to:

    ① Prevent rupture of the membranes
    ② Slow down labor
    ③ Prevent incontinence postoperatively

    ④ Prevent trauma to the bladder during surgery

17. To provide the best outcome for both the mother and the baby delivered by cesarean section, the anesthesia of choice would be a (an):

    ① Epidural
    ② General
    ③ Pudendal
    ④ Bier's block

18. Doris asks if she will be able to breast-feed her baby after a cesarean section. The nurse's best reply would be:

    ① "You will probably have a lot of pain, so perhaps you should consider bottle feeding."
    ② "Yes, and one of us will help you."
    ③ "You will have to ask the physician."
    ④ "Don't think about that now—you can decide later."

19. Karen is admitted to the labor floor in active labor. A diagnosis of PIH is made. An infusion of $MgSO_4$ is begun. While Karen is receiving the $MgSO_4$, you observe that her respirations are 8 and her patellar reflexes have decreased. This should be:

    ① Brought to the attention of the charge nurse immediately
    ② Considered to be the desired result
    ③ Recorded and monitored to see if it continues
    ④ Considered as an indication that a higher dose of medication is needed

20. As you care for Karen who has PIH and is receiving $MgSO_4$, you watch the fetal monitor for signs of fetal distress. Fetal distress may be indicated by:

    ① An increase in the frequency and duration of contractions
    ② Meconium-stained amniotic fluid when the baby is in a breech position
    ③ Decelerations in the fetal heart rate
    ④ Increased bloody show as Karen nears the end of transition

21. The most common type of fetal deceleration is:

    ① Early
    ② Late
    ③ Variable
    ④ Periodic

22. Early decelerations are most often due to:

① Cord compression
② Fetal head compression
③ Uteroplacental insufficiency
④ Prolapsed cord

23. When oxygen is administered via mask to relieve fetal distress, the correct rate is:

① 2–3 L/minute
② 4–6 L/minute
③ 8–10 L/minute
④ 15–20 L/minute

24. Labor progresses, and Karen delivers a healthy baby boy and is taken to the recovery room. The chart indicates a blood loss of approximately 350 mL. This is:

① Considered to be postpartum hemorrhage
② Normal
③ A sign of retained placenta
④ An indication that a transfusion will be needed

ANSWERS AND RATIONALES

Guide to item identification (see pp. 4–5 for further details about each category):

I, II, III, or IV for the phase of the nursing process
1, 2, 3, or 4 for the category of client needs
A, B, C, D, E, F, or G for the category of human functioning
Specific content category by name; i.e., cholecystectomy

1. While the other answers may be correct, it is
② most important to establish a baseline so that changes may be assessed.
I, 4, A, Labor and delivery

2. Ritgen's maneuver assists in delivery of the fetal
③ head. Homans' sign assesses for thrombophlebitis. Chadwick's sign is a bluish coloration of the vagina found early in pregnancy.
III, 4, A, Labor and delivery

3. The pH of amniotic fluid is 7.5, or alkaline. The
② pH of vaginal fluid is 5 to 6.5, or acidic.
III, 2 & 4, A, Labor and delivery

4. Complete dilation of the cervix is 10 cm.
① I, 1 & 4, A, Labor and delivery

5. Effacement is a thinning and shortening of the
④ cervix that occurs before or concurrent with dilation of the cervix.
I, 4, A, Labor and delivery

6. As the baby descends toward the perineum,
① progress is measured by the relationship of the presenting part to the ischial spines of the maternal pelvis.
I, 4, A, Labor and delivery

7. A fetal heart rate of less than 120 bpm is con-
③ sidered bradycardia, and an increase above 160 bpm is tachycardia. A 30-bpm deviation from the baseline may also be used to determine these conditions.
I, 4, A & B, Labor and delivery

8. Frequency is always timed from the beginning
① of one contraction to the beginning of the next contraction. Duration is the time period from the beginning of a contraction to the end of that contraction.
III, 4, A, Labor and delivery

9. During the active phase of labor is the optimum
③ time for the client to receive medication. An order must always be obtained from the physician, however, after complete assessment of the client's progress. Answer 2 is not a correct assessment of the client's progress, and answer 4 is judgmental.
III, 1 & 4, A & G, Labor and delivery

10. The dosage is within acceptable limits. The oral
③ route is the slowest acting. The infant will probably not require Narcan (naloxone) if the Demerol (meperidine) is given during the active phase of labor.
III, 1 & 4, A, Labor and delivery

11. An incision is made into the perineum to facili-
③ tate the delivery of the infant and to prevent lacerations.
I, 4, A, Labor and delivery

12. Early contact with the infant promotes a close
② relationship with both parents.
IV, 4, A & G, Labor and delivery

13. The first stage of labor is from the beginning of
③ contractions to complete dilation of the cervix. The second stage of labor is from complete dilation of the cervix through the delivery of the infant. The fourth stage of labor is the time from the delivery of the placenta to postpartum stability, about 2 hours.
I, 4, A, Labor and delivery

14. Rupture of the membranes when there is other
① than a cephalic presentation or when the presenting part is not engaged predisposes to a prolapsed cord. A nuchal cord is found around the back of the infant's neck. Precipitate delivery is a rapid delivery often without benefit of sterile preparations.
I, 4, A, Labor and delivery

15. In a transverse lie, the long axis of the infant is
③ crosswise to the long axis of the mother. A vertex is a head, or cephalic, presentation.
I, 4, A, Labor and delivery

16. During a cesarean section the bladder must re-
④ main empty to avoid trauma during surgery.
III, 4, A & D, Cesarean section.

17. General anesthesia predisposes the infant to res-
① piratory depression. A pudendal and a Bier's block are regional anesthetics that would have no effect on the abdomen.
IV, 4, A & D, Cesarean section.

18. A cesarean section is not a contraindication to
② breast-feeding. Encouragement and assistance
from the nursing staff decrease anxiety and promote successful breast-feeding.
III, 1 & 4, A & G, Cesarean section.

19. Respirations less than 14, absent patellar re-
① flexes, and urinary output of less than 24 mL/
hour are signs of magnesium toxicity, and the
physician should be notified immediately.
I & III, 1, 2, & 4, A, B, & C, Labor and delivery

20. Decelerations in the fetal heart rate indicate an
③ attempt by the fetus to compensate for stress.
I, 1, 2, & 4, A & B, Labor and delivery

21. Variable decelerations are the most common
③ type and are associated with cord compression
and are often relieved by a change in maternal
position.
I, 4, A & B, Labor and delivery

22. Early decelerations are most often due to fetal
② head compression as the head progresses through
the maternal pelvis. Late decelerations are considered ominous and are related to placental
insufficiency.
I, 4, A & B, Labor and delivery

23. The rate of oxygen administration must be great
③ enough to cross the placenta and reach the fetus.
III, 4, A & B, Labor and delivery

24. Normal blood loss during delivery is 300 to
② 450 mL. A blood loss of more than 450 to
500 mL is considered postpartum hemorrhage.
I, 2 & 4, A & B, Labor and delivery

POSTPARTUM PERIOD

INVOLUTION. Process occurring in time period
from delivery until reproductive organs return to pre-
pregnant state (usually about 6 weeks).

I. NORMAL POSTPARTUM PERIOD

A. Assessment

1. Fundus
   a. should be firm, 1 to 2 cm below umbilicus, in
      midline, and not palpable after day 10
   b. cramping sensation felt by mother as uterus
      contracts, called "afterpain"
      (1) more pronounced in multiparous clients
      (2) stimulated by breast-feeding
      (3) relieved by mild analgesic (acetamino-
          phen [Tylenol], ibuprofen [Motrin])
      (4) ergovine may be prescribed to hasten
          process
2. Lochia
   a. rubra: bright red; lasts 1 to 2 days
   b. serosa: pinkish to brown; lasts 2 to 10 days
   c. alba: whitish; usually appears after day 10
   d. amount: should be scant
   e. report: any foul odor or increase in bright
      red blood
3. Perineum and rectum
   a. check episiotomy suture line for intactness,
      bruising, edema, or hematoma
   b. check for hemorrhoids
   c. apply ice packs or anesthetic sprays as or-
      dered
   d. teach mother perineal care and proper applica-
      tion of perineal pads

   e. monitor for first bowel movement
      (1) usually within 3 days post partum
      (2) administer stool softener docusate so-
          dium (Colace) as ordered
   f. may use sitz bath or warm perineal pads for
      episiotomy discomfort
4. Vital signs
   a. temperature
      (1) elevation 2 to 3 days post partum and
          lasting less than 12 hours may be due to
          breast engorgement
      (2) elevation immediately after delivery may
          mean dehydration or beginning of in-
          fection
      (3) elevation greater than 100.2° F lasting or
          recurring for 24 hours or more may indi-
          cate endometritis, urinary tract infection,
          or other systemic infection
      (4) elevation accompanied by positive Ho-
          mans' sign may indicate thrombophle-
          bitis
   b. pulse
      (1) bradycardia (50 to 60 bpm) normal and
          may last 5 to 10 days
      (2) tachycardia may indicate pain, infection,
          anxiety, or excessive blood loss
   c. blood pressure
      (1) hypotension: blood loss
      (2) hypertension: ongoing disorder related to
          pregnancy, such as preeclampsia, PIH
5. Elimination
   a. urination
      (1) diuresis common first 24 hours and may
          last up to 5 days
      (2) be alert for signs of urinary tract infection
   b. defecation

(1) stool softeners, such as Colace, usually ordered
(2) monitor closely those patients with third-
degree or fourth-degree lacerations
c. diaphoresis (excessive sweating) is common
as body adjusts to eliminate excess fluid
6. Weight loss
a. 10 to 12 pounds lost immediately after delivery
from fetus, placenta, and fluid
b. 5 pounds lost in early postpartum period
through diuresis and diaphoresis
c. loss may be hastened by exercise and balanced diet
7. Lactation
a. controlled by secretion of hormones prolactin
and oxytocin
b. stimulated by sucking of infant
c. may be suppressed by medications, bromo-
criptine (Parlodel)
d. breast-feeding requires high-protein diet, with
500 additional calories and 2 to 3 quarts of
liquid daily
e. initial milk called colostrum, loaded with im-
munoglobulin A (IgA) antibodies
8. Other
a. Rh-negative mothers with Rh-positive fetus
(1) mother develops antibodies
(2) must be given RhoGAM within 72 hours
after delivery
b. mother who had low or no rubella titer
(1) rubella vaccine given
(2) may cause fever and symptoms of mild
case of measles
(3) mother should be told of dangers of becoming pregnant within 3 months after
vaccination, permit needs to be signed
that client understands the need not to
get pregnant for 3 months after vaccination and is willing to receive shot
9. Bonding and attachment
a. relationship formed between parents and infant that has lifelong effects
b. infants separated from parents at birth at risk
for difficulties in bonding
c. monitor for signs of bonding progression
d. create atmosphere on nursing unit to enhance bonding

II. POSTPARTUM COMPLICATIONS

A. Postpartum Hemorrhage

1. Blood loss greater than 500 mL
2. Causes
a. uterine atony
b. retained placenta
c. lacerations of reproductive tract

3. Control and correction of hemorrhage
a. massage fundus
b. additional oxytocin given
c. if bleeding continues and fundus boggy, client
may need to return to delivery room for sterile
examination to look for retained placenta fragments or other problem, such as cervical or
vaginal lacerations
d. blood loss may need to be replaced by transfusions

B. Puerperal Infections

1. Endometritis
a. predisposing factors
(1) prolonged labor
(2) postpartum hemorrhage
(3) premature rupture of membranes
(4) intrauterine manipulation
(5) anemia
(6) retention of placental fragments
b. assessment
(1) sustained fever 100.4° F or higher
(2) uterine tenderness
(3) profuse, foul-smelling lochia, sometimes
frothy
c. treatments and nursing interventions
(1) antibiotic therapy, usually intravenous
(2) Tylenol for temperature above 101° F
(3) sitz bath
(4) position to promote excretion of lochia
2. Mastitis (inflammation of breasts)
a. cause: usually due to *Staphylococcus aureus* derived from
(1) infant's nose or mouth
(2) mother herself because of poor hand
washing
(3) hospital personnel because of poor hand
washing
b. assessment
(1) usually appears third or fourth week of
puerperium
(2) marked by breast engorgement
(3) chills
(4) elevated temperature
(5) increased pulse rate
(6) hardness and redness of breasts
(7) pain in breast
c. treatment and nursing interventions
(1) antibiotic therapy
(2) administer pain medication as needed
(3) teach and maintain good hygiene
(4) breast-feeding may or may not be discontinued, since infection is not in the milk
ducts

C. Thrombophlebitis

1. Cause
   a. injury (bruise) to vein, thrombus, or clot forms at the site and attaches to vessel wall
   b. extension of infection from tissues surrounding vessel
   c. pregnancy, when women must be in bed for prolonged time
   d. overactivity in clients who have been on bed rest
2. Assessment
   a. soreness or stiffness in calf
   b. edema of leg
   c. redness over area affected
   d. pain in upper posterior calf on dorsiflexion of foot (Homans' sign)
   e. assumption of "frog-like" position (leg externally rotated, knee flexed)
   f. muscle ache, may be falsely assumed to result from wearing flat bedroom slippers postoperatively
   g. signs of circulatory obstruction (thrombus)
      (1) swelling
      (2) vasospasm followed by cyanosis
      (3) increasing coolness of area
      (4) loss of pulses distal to obstruction
   h. signs of pulmonary embolus
      (1) restlessness
      (2) severe shortness of breath
      (3) unrelieved chest pain
      (4) frothy blood-tinged sputum
      (5) respiratory arrest
3. Preventive measures
   a. initiate early ambulation as soon as possible in postpartum or postoperative period
   b. avoid keeping extremities in one position for long period of time
   c. avoid using knee gatch on bed
   d. do not sit with legs crossed
   e. use elastic stockings before thrombophlebitis occurs
4. Treatment and nursing interventions
   a. institute all preventive measures appropriate for this client
   b. avoid massaging or rubbing calf because of danger of breaking clot loose
   c. apply heat in form of warm, moist packs to area to promote circulation and provide comfort
   d. administer anticoagulants as ordered
      (1) intravenous heparin first
      (2) oral warfarin sodium (Coumadin) next and after discharge
   e. bed rest with affected leg elevated, without pressure behind knee
   f. apply support hose to unaffected leg only

   g. instruct client for discharge
      (1) wear support stockings (remove several times daily for short periods)
      (2) avoid prolonged sitting or standing
      (3) elevate extremity as much as possible
      (4) take precautions against injury to area
      (5) exercise extremity for 5 minutes every hour
      (6) take Coumadin as ordered
         (a) return per physician's orders for blood tests
         (b) do not stop taking Coumadin until told by physician
         (c) instruct on bleeding precautions

D. Urinary Tract Infections

1. Predisposing factors
   a. urinary stasis
   b. indwelling catheters
   c. renal disease
   d. lowered body resistance
2. Assessment
   a. some clients completely asymptomatic (diagnosis made by presence of bacteria in urine culture in more than 100,000 microorganisms/mL)
   b. dysuria
   c. urgency
   d. frequency
   e. burning sensation on voiding
   f. fever
   g. flank pain; costovertebral angle tenderness
3. Treatment and nursing interventions
   a. give antibiotics for 10 to 14 days
   b. encourage fluids, especially acid-ash fluids, such as cranberry juice
   c. obtain follow-up culture specimens after antibiotic therapy (disappearance of symptoms does not mean client has been adequately treated)

E. Wound Separations

1. Predisposing factors
   a. sutures or staples giving way
   b. obesity
   c. infections
   d. marked distention
   e. heavy coughing without splinting incision
   f. pulmonary or cardiovascular disease
   g. diabetes mellitus
   h. steroid therapy
2. Types of wound separations
   a. dehiscence: separation of wound edges down to peritoneum, without exposure of viscera

    b. evisceration: separation of wound edges, with protrusion of viscera through open incision

3. Assessment
   a. client complains feeling that something suddenly gave way in wound, complains of intense burning at operative site
   b. edges of wound separated, intestines may be exposed and gradually pushing out (observe for drainage of peritoneal fluid on dressing)
   c. pain, anxiety, and vomiting

4. Treatment and nursing interventions
   a. return client to bed in semi-Fowler's position with knees flexed to relieve tension on abdominal muscles
   b. notify surgeon immediately
   c. reassure client, keep client quiet and relaxed
   d. for eviscerations, prepare client for surgery and wound repair
   e. if intestines are exposed, cover with sterile dressing, wet with normal saline
   f. for smaller dehiscence, irrigations with saline or hydrogen peroxide may be ordered; wound eventually heals, by granulation, leaving wider scar

❓ QUESTIONS

1. Following a normal vaginal delivery, the client's vital signs, fundus, and lochia are checked every 15 minutes until stable. The fundus should be:

   ① Firm, below the umbilicus and in the midline
   ② Soft, below the umbilicus and in the midline
   ③ Firm, dextroverted and above the umbilicus
   ④ Soft, above the umbilicus and in the midline

2. A postpartum client is receiving an infusion of dextrose 5% in lactated Ringer's solution with oxytocin, 20 U, while in the recovery room. The purpose of the oxytocin is to:

   ① Decrease discomfort
   ② Prevent uterine tetany
   ③ Remove retained placental fragments
   ④ Prevent uterine atony

3. A nursing mother often does not menstruate for several months after delivery or until she discontinues breast-feeding. She should be taught that:

   ① Ovulation is suppressed and pregnancy is impossible while she is breast-feeding
   ② Ovulation is not suppressed and pregnancy is possible even though she is breast-feeding
   ③ The uterus will not return to a normal size while she is breast-feeding
   ④ If she does not begin to menstruate in 3 months, she should stop breast-feeding

4. The nurse notes that the lochia has a foul smell. The most appropriate nursing intervention is:

   ① Report immediately that the client may have an infection
   ② Nothing, as this is normal during the first few days after delivery
   ③ Begin vaginal irrigations to decrease the odor and increase client comfort
   ④ Stop the use of perineal pads for the next few days

5. When administering an enema to a postpartum client, it is important that the nurse:

   ① Use a small-caliber tube
   ② Administer no more than 100 mL of solution
   ③ Be careful not to irritate the perineum while inserting the rectal tube
   ④ Encourage the client to administer her own so she will learn how for home care

6. The incidence of postpartum thrombophlebitis has been decreased owing to which of the following nursing interventions?

   ① Early ambulation
   ② Immobilization and elevation of the lower extremities
   ③ Administration of anticoagulants routinely after the birth
   ④ Breast-feeding the newborn

7. Mary is a single 17-year-old who delivers a healthy baby girl. Two hours after Mary's delivery, you notice that Mary's fundus is firm, rising, and displaced to the right. This indicates:

   ① Postpartum bleeding
   ② A normal position
   ③ Retained placental fragments
   ④ A full bladder

8. Mary, who has just delivered a healthy baby girl, had a laceration into the vaginal mucosa and the perineal muscle. This is a:

   ① First-degree laceration
   ② Second-degree laceration
   ③ Third-degree laceration
   ④ Fourth-degree laceration

9. Mary, who just delivered a healthy baby girl, plans to bottle-feed her infant, and the physician orders medication to suppress lactation. Which of the following drugs is used for this purpose?

   ① Parlodel
   ② Motrin
   ③ Pitocin
   ④ Colace

10. Mary is a single mother who just delivered a healthy baby girl. Even though Mary's family has been supportive, she expresses concern about how she will support herself and her baby. Your best response would be:

   ① "You should have thought of that before you got pregnant."
   ② "Getting on welfare is probably your best bet."
   ③ "The baby's father has a responsibility to help you out."
   ④ "Tell me some of the things you have considered, and we can find out more about them."

11. Mary is a single mother who just delivered a healthy baby girl. Because of Mary's educational level, socioeconomic status, and age:

   ① She has special need for information about maternal and infant nutrition
   ② Her baby is at risk for neglect and abuse
   ③ She is at risk for postpartum complications
   ④ All of the above

ANSWERS AND RATIONALES

Guide to item identification (see pp. 4–5 for further details about each category):
I, II, III, or IV for the phase of the nursing process
1, 2, 3, or 4 for the category of client needs
A, B, C, D, E, F, or G for the category of human functioning
Specific content category by name; i.e., cholecystectomy

1. A soft, boggy uterus is associated with postpartum bleeding. If the fundus is firm, rising, and displaced to the right or left side, the client probably has a full bladder.
① IV, 4, A, Postpartum

2. Pitocin (oxytocin) promotes contraction of the uterus.
④ IV, 4, A & D, Postpartum/medications

3. Although menstruation usually does not occur, ovulation may occur, so lactation is not a method of contraception.
② III, 4, A, Postpartum

4. Foul odor may indicate the presence of an infection and should be reported to the physician so antibiotics can be started.
① III, 4, A & D, Postpartum

5. It is important to be gentle because the area around the episiotomy is easily irritated and
③ hemorrhoids are quite common.
III, 4, A & F, Postpartum

6. Early ambulation is the most effective and safe way to prevent thrombophlebitis.
① III, 4, A, B, E, Postpartum

7. The fundus should be firm, below the umbilicus, and in the midline. A firm, rising fundus often displaced to the right is an indication of a full bladder.
④ I & IV, 4, A & F, Postpartum

8. Second-degree lacerations include the skin, mucous membrane, and the muscles of the perineal block.
② I & IV, 4, A & D, Postpartum

9. Parlodel is a lactation inhibitor.
① I & III, 4, A & D, Postpartum

10. It is important to discover what plans and ideas the person has and explore those possibilities. Giving advice is judgmental, serves no useful purpose, and only increases the person's feelings of insecurity and any guilt feelings.
④ III, 4, A & G, Postpartum

11. A single teenaged mother usually has limited resources and coping mechanisms. Support systems can assist the mother in gaining maturity and in learning parenting skills. Her health status may also be lowered.
④ II & IV, 4, A & G, Postpartum

NEONATE

First 4 weeks of life

I. PHYSIOLOGIC DEVELOPMENT

A. Appearance

1. Head often misshapen; one fourth of total body size
   a. caput succedaneum
   b. molding
   c. cephalhematoma
2. Skin discolored and puffy
3. Protruding umbilical stump for first 3 weeks
4. Soft fontanels
   a. posterior closes in about 2 to 3 months
   b. anterior closes in about 8 to 18 months

B. Head Circumference

1. Measurement taken over eyebrows, just above eyes, across posterior occipital protuberance
2. Normal size about 14 inches (or 35 cm)
3. Head may be molded from birthing process

C. Cardiovascular System

1. Foramen ovale functionally closes after 1 minute; anatomically after 2 weeks
2. Ductus arteriosus functionally closes after 15 to 24 hours; anatomically closes in 3 weeks
3. Unstable temperature regulation system
   a. dependent on ambient (room) temperature and amount of covering
   b. observe facial color to gauge warmth
      (1) flushed face, too warm
      (2) pale or bluish face, too cold

D. Skin

1. Lanugo: downy hair, lost after few months
2. Vernix caseosa: cheesy skin covering that rubs off in several days
3. Milia: small collections of sebaceous secretions that disappear within several weeks
4. Hemangiomas: pink spots that may or may not be permanent
5. Mongolian spots: slate-colored areas found in African-Americans, Asians, or Mediterraneans, which normally fade; usually over sacrum and gluteal areas
6. Jaundice: yellowish discoloration of skin
   a. physiologic: normal by about day 3 or 4 and disappears in 1 week
   b. abnormal: occurs in first 24 hours, usually due to Rh incompatibility, trauma, or infection
7. Acrocyanosis: normal blueness of hands and feet
8. Desquamation: peeling of skin; normal for about 2 to 4 weeks after birth
9. Umbilical cord
   a. dries and shrinks rapidly, dropping off in 6 to 14 days
   b. area should be cleaned daily with alcohol or triple dye and watched for presence of infection

E. Weight/Length

1. Weight at birth is about 7 to 8 pounds
2. Normal loss of 10% of birth weight right after birth
3. Steady weight gain begins at 1 to 2 weeks, 1 1/2 to 2 pounds/month
4. Average length about 19 to 21 inches

F. Vital Signs

1. Unstable in newborn
2. Respirations vary from 50 to 80 right after birth to 35 to 50 soon thereafter
3. Temperature ranges from 97° F to 100° F, with body heat lost rapidly
4. Heart rate at birth is 120 to 150 bpm and varies from 170 to 180 bpm when crying to 90 bpm when asleep, dropping throughout first years of life
5. Blood pressure is 40 to 70 systolic, reaching 80/40 by end of first month of life

G. Elimination

1. Gastrointestinal
   a. Meconium: first fecal material passed 8 to 24 hours after birth
      (1) mix of amniotic fluid and intestinal glandular secretions
      (2) dark green, thick, sticky stool
   b. transition stools with mucus for first week
   c. 2 to 4 stools/day normal at first, decreasing to 1 to 2 stools/day
   d. breast-fed baby: stools soft, yellow, and pasty; more frequent than bottle-fed baby
   e. bottle-fed baby: stools more solid and yellow to brown
   f. stools are darker if infant is receiving iron
   g. stools are greener if infant is under bilirubin lamp
2. Genitourinary
   a. decreased ability to concentrate urine
      (1) more prone to dehydration
      (2) limited ability to reabsorb important substances
   b. voids soon after birth
   c. voids frequently during early life

H. Reflex Activities

1. Consummatory: survival, such as rooting and sucking
2. Avoidant: elicited by potentially harmful stimuli, such as Moro's reflex and blinking
3. Postural: tonic neck reflex seen when baby asleep
4. Exploratory: when awake and upright
5. Social: such as smiling
6. Attentional: orienting and attending
7. Born with reflexes, such as gag, sneeze, blink, suck, and grasp
8. Absence of any reflexes should be noted

II. SENSORY DEVELOPMENT

A. Vision

1. Can see at birth
2. Able to fixate points of contrast
3. Shows preference for human face
4. Can follow moving objects
5. Likes bright or contrasting colors

B. Hearing

1. Responsive to verbal stimuli
2. Avoid auditory overload
3. Attends to auditory toys

C. Sleep

1. Usually sleeps 15 to 20 hours/day at first
2. May begin sleeping through night after 4 to 6 weeks

III. CARE OF NEONATE

A. Immediate Assessment

1. Airway
   a. first concern after delivery, clearing airway
   b. use soft rubber bulb syringe to aspirate mouth gently and then the nose
   c. spontaneous breathing usually occurs soon after birth
   d. if breathing does not occur
      (1) immediate resuscitation
      (2) tactile stimulation
      (3) ventilation
      (4) use of naloxone (Narcan) to reverse narcotics given to mother
   e. signs of respiratory distress
      (1) flaring of nares
      (2) grunting
      (3) sternal and substernal retractions
2. Apgar: system of immediate assessment of newborn to evaluate physical status
   a. assess
      (1) heart rate
      (2) respiratory effort: frequency and regularity
      (3) muscle tone
      (4) reflex irritability
      (5) color
   b. each scored as 0, 1, or 2, then added together, with 10 being highest score
      (1) 7–10: condition good
      (2) 4–6: condition fair
      (3) 0–3: poor condition and need for further evaluation and care
   c. first assessment at 1 minute after delivery
   d. second assessment at 5 minutes
3. Assess for gestational age
   a. Dubowitz evaluation
      (1) done within 24 hours after birth
      (2) scoring system including evaluation of physical characteristics and neuromuscular tone
   b. also figured by counting weeks of fetal development from first day of mother's last normal period until delivery
4. Meconium aspiration
   a. suggestive of fetal distress in utero
   b. common if fetus is a cephalic presentation, with meconium-stained amniotic fluid
   c. neonate needs immediate suctioning
   d. may exhibit respiratory distress
      (1) mild, usually disappears in 48 hours
      (2) severe, may lead to aspiration pneumonia and require intensive care

B. Immediate Nursing Care

1. Prevention of infection
   a. sterile technique for cutting cord
   b. use of erythromycin ophthalmic ointment in eyes to prevent ophthalmia neonatorum (blindness from maternal gonococcal infection)
2. Provision of warmth
   a. use of preheated tables, warming lamps, and warm blankets
   b. dry neonate well
   c. can be placed on mother's chest, with direct contact providing body warmth
   d. cap on neonate to prevent heat loss
   e. place in warm Isolette or under radiant warmer
3. Vitamin K given intramuscularly to aid in clotting and preventing bleeding
4. Neonate footprinted and identification bracelets applied to mother and neonate before removing neonate from delivery room
5. Hepatitis B vaccine

C. Continuing Care of Neonate

1. Bonding: psychosocial attachment of neonate to mother and father
   a. both parents allowed to hold and touch neonate
   b. need to assure themselves of neonate's sex and wholeness
   c. parents encouraged to point out family resemblances
   d. way to begin to establish parental role and love of neonate
2. Screening tests
   a. phenylketonuria
      (1) screening for inability to metabolize phenylalanine
      (2) done after neonate feeds for first time, within first 24 hours, or done by visiting nurse at home or clinic
   b. hypothyroidism
   c. galactosemia
   d. hypoglycemia
3. Teaching infant care

a. mother needs to learn to care for infant
   (1) bathing
   (2) diapering
   (3) safety
   (4) care of umbilical cord

(5) need for sleep
b. feeding
   (1) bottle
   (2) breast-feeding

? QUESTIONS

1. The jaundice associated with erythroblastosis fetalis is generally seen:

   ① During the first 24 hours after birth
   ② 72 to 96 hours after birth
   ③ 96 to 120 hours after birth
   ④ 1 week after birth

2. Baby Boy Harris, 6 pounds, 1 ounce, was just delivered after a long labor. His initial Apgar is 3. Which of the following is the priority nursing intervention for this baby?

   ① Suction him
   ② Dry him with a warm towel
   ③ Ventilate him with 100% oxygen at 40 to 60 breaths/minute
   ④ Place baby under warmer to maintain body temperature

3. Baby Boy Harris, 6 pounds, 1 ounce, was just delivered after a long labor and is in the newborn nursery. In assessing his eyes and vision, which of the following would be an abnormal finding?

   ① Crossed eyes
   ② Absent blink reflex
   ③ Positive red reflex
   ④ Edema of the eyelids

4. Which of the following would be an abnormality in the newborn's cardiovascular system?

   ① Heart rate of 154
   ② Irregular heart beats
   ③ Acrocyanosis of the extremities
   ④ Circumoral cyanosis

5. Baby Boy Harris, 6 pounds, 1 ounce, who was just delivered after a long labor, is breathing with 10- to 15-second periods of apnea. The PN knows that this is a sign of:

   ① Normal newborn breathing
   ② Impending respiratory distress
   ③ Prenatal asthma
   ④ Impending respiratory infection

6. When you assess the newborn's renal system, which of the following would be considered abnormal?

   ① Urine specific gravity of 1.008
   ② First void after the first 24 hours
   ③ Voiding up to 20 times a day
   ④ "Brick dust"–colored urine with the first void

7. Which of the following is *not* part of the care of a newborn with hyperbilirubinemia?

   ① Withhold fluids during treatment
   ② Maintain neutral temperature
   ③ Administer phototherapy
   ④ Assist with exchange transfusions if needed

8. Baby Fran, 6 pounds, 8 ounces, was born today. She is in the newborn nursery and you are caring for her. Which of the following is appropriate when caring for the umbilical cord?

   ① Apply a petroleum jelly gauze dressing over the site
   ② Apply a simple dry dressing over the site
   ③ Clean the site daily vigorously with soap and water
   ④ Apply topical triple dye or bacitracin ointment initially and apply alcohol daily

9. Gastric emptying time in the newborn is about:

   ① 1 to 1 1/2 hours
   ② 2 1/2 to 3 hours
   ③ 1 1/2 to 2 hours
   ④ 3 to 3 1/2 hours

10. About how many calories/day does the average newborn need?

    ① 50 cal/kg/day
    ② 75 cal/kg/day
    ③ 120 cal/kg/day
    ④ 150 cal/kg/day

11. The newborn infant exhibits a number of reflexes at birth. Which reflex is *not* present at birth?

    ① Parachute reflex
    ② Moro's reflex
    ③ Sucking reflex
    ④ Extrusion reflex

12. Which of the following is *not* a risk factor for respiratory distress syndrome?

    ① Prematurity
    ② Maternal diabetes
    ③ Birth trauma
    ④ Post-term birth

ANSWERS AND RATIONALES

Guide to item identification (see pp. 4–5 for further details about each category):

I, II, III, or IV for the phase of the nursing process
1, 2, 3, or 4 for the category of client needs
A, B, C, D, E, F, or G for the category of human functioning
Specific content category by name; i.e., cholecystectomy

1. Pathologic jaundice appears within the first 24 hours after birth.
⓵ I, 4, A & E, Newborn

2. An Apgar score of 3 indicates a very depressed infant. He will be intubated and ventilated at a rate of 40 to 60 breaths/minute with 100% oxygen.
③ III, 4, A & B, Newborn

3. The blink reflex is a protective reflex that is present at birth; absence is abnormal.
② III, 2, A & C, Newborn

4. Circumoral cyanosis is an ominous sign of severe hypoxia and is not a normal finding.
④ III, 1, A & B, Newborn

5. Short periods of apnea are normal in the newborn and no action is needed.
① III, 1, A & B, Newborn

6. It is normal for the first voiding to be within the first 24 hours, not after it.
② III, 1, A & F, Newborn

7. It is important that the newborn be adequately hydrated to help prevent further complications from hyperbilirubinemia.
① III, 4, A & F, Newborn

8. The cord needs to dry and should be open to the air. An antibiotic ointment is applied initially and the cord cleaned daily with alcohol. The baby should receive sponge baths until the cord drops off.
④ III, 4, A, Newborn

9. Normal gastric emptying in the newborn is about 2 1/2 to 3 hours.
② III, 1, A & F, Newborn

10. The normal newborn needs about 120 cal/kg/day to grow normally.
③ III, 1 & 4, A & E, Newborn

11. The parachute reflex appears at about 7 to 9 months and remains indefinitely.
① III, 1, A & C, Newborn

12. The post-term infant is not at special risk for respiratory distress syndrome. The other options listed are risk factors for respiratory distress syndrome.
④ III, 1, A & B, Newborn

BIBLIOGRAPHY

Betz, C.L., Hunsberger, M., & Wright, S. (1994). *Family-centered nursing care of children,* 2nd ed. Philadelphia: W.B. Saunders Co.

Bobak, I.M., Jensen, M., & Zalar, M. (1993). *Maternity and gynecological care, the nurse and the family,* 5th ed. St. Louis: Mosby–Year Book.

Bolander, V.R. (1994). *Sorensen and Luckmann's basic nursing: A psychophysiologic approach,* 3rd ed. Philadelphia: W.B. Saunders Co.

Davis, J., & Sherer, K. (1994). *Applied nutrition and diet therapy for nurses,* 2nd ed. Philadelphia: W.B. Saunders Co.

Gorrie, T.M., McKinney, E.S., & Murray, S.S. (1994). *Foundations of maternal newborn nursing.* Philadelphia: W.B. Saunders Co.

Hamilton, P.M. (1993). *Basic maternity nursing,* 7th ed. St. Louis: Mosby–Year Book.

Ingalls, A.J., & Salerno, M.C. (1991). *Maternal and child health nursing,* 7th ed. St. Louis; Mosby–Year Book.

Lehne, R.A., Moore, L., Crosby, L., & Hamilton, D (1994). *Pharmacology for nursing care,* 2nd ed. Philadelphia: W.B. Saunders Co.

Linton, A.D., Matteson, M.A., & Maebius, N.K. (1995). *Introductory nursing care of adults.* Philadelphia: W.B. Saunders Co.

Matassarin-Jacobs, E. (1994). *Saunders review for NCLEX-RN,* 2nd ed. Philadelphia: W.B. Saunders Co.

Monohan, F.D., Drake, T., & Neighbors, M. (1994). *Nursing care of adults.* Philadelphia: W.B. Saunders Co.

Thompson, E.D. (1990). *Introduction to maternity and pediatric nursing.* Philadelphia: W.B. Saunders Co.

10

The Mental Health Client

COMMUNICATION, INTERACTION, AND BEHAVIOR

Involves exchange of attitudes, feelings, and ideas; done through:

1. *Active listening:* allowing individual to own problem, using techniques of reflection and clarification
2. *"I" messages:* clear and honest statements of fact about individual, rather than "you" messages, which put receiver on defensive

Communication Process

I. PROCESS

A. Assessment

1. Assess client's level of functioning and ability to process information
2. Observe what is happening to client at present time
3. Assess overall behavior and appearance of client
4. Identify environmental conditions that may affect communication process
5. Assess relationship between persons communicating
    a. sender's purpose
    b. content of message
    c. nonverbal manner in which message is conveyed
    d. effect of message on receiver
    e. receiver's personal characteristics
    f. feedback
6. Verbal versus nonverbal communication
    a. verbal refers to what is actually said
    b. nonverbal refers to message conveyed by means other than speaking
        (1) body language
        (2) facial expressions
        (3) gestures
        (4) distancing
        (5) often "implied" message
        (6) client may be unaware of these messages
    c. verbal and nonverbal messages may or may not be same
    d. if verbal and nonverbal messages are different, nonverbal is more likely to be accurate
    e. nonverbal communication easily misunderstood
7. Blocks and barriers to communication
    a. blocks (verbal)
        (1) asking why
        (2) inappropriately changing subject
        (3) excessive questioning
        (4) making judgments
        (5) giving false reassurance
        (6) using highly emotional words
        (7) giving advice
        (8) focusing on oneself
        (9) agreeing or disagreeing
    b. barriers (physical)
        (1) language differences
        (2) deafness
        (3) stuttering
        (4) muteness
        (5) blindness

B. Planning, Goals, Expected Outcomes

1. Client knows purpose of interaction
2. Client is able to understand messages being sent
3. Client is able to convey needs, feelings, and thoughts
4. Client develops agreement between verbal and nonverbal communication
5. Client maintains control over own life

C. Implementation

1. Identify situations to be discussed with client
    a. define purpose of relationship
    b. identify expectations
    c. provide safe, comfortable, and protective environment
2. Use active listening techniques to encourage client to describe what is happening, communication enhancers

405

a. ask client to clarify message received

b. use "I" messages rather than "you" messages, such as "I do not like what you are doing," not "you shouldn't do that"

c. use restatement

d. use open-ended sentences

e. avoid selective listening

f. avoid insensitive listening

3. Assist client to identify own thoughts and feelings

a. tune into verbal and nonverbal cues from client

b. maintain accepting, nonjudgmental attitude

4. Focus on client's verbal and nonverbal communication

a. assist client to recognize inconsistencies between verbal and nonverbal communication

b. give honest, nonbiased feedback to client

5. Allow client to problem solve

a. assist client to use problem-solving process

b. help client to identify goals, to meet individual needs

c. focus on positive aspects of client's attempt to communicate effectively

D. Evaluation

1. Communication, client centered
2. Client's ability to understand messages received is increased
3. Client's ability to communicate needs, feelings, and thoughts improved
4. Client's verbal and nonverbal communications consistent with one another
5. Client's coping mechanisms appropriate to situation

Interpersonal Relationships

I. INTERACTIONS

A. Between Two or More Persons Over Period of Time

II. THERAPEUTIC INTERPERSONAL RELATIONSHIPS

A. Characterized by

1. Acceptance
2. Honesty
3. Understanding
4. Empathy
5. Goal directed
6. Client centered
7. Time limited
8. Content specific
9. Purposeful
10. Structured

B. Phases

1. Initial, introductory, or orientation phase

a. guidelines for relationship established mutually

b. mutual problems and expectations identified

2. Working, problem solving, or working-through phase

a. problem-solving techniques developed for identified problems

b. methods of working through problems implemented and evaluated

c. focus on increasing client's independence

3. Terminating phase

a. closing of relationship planned for early in development of relationship

b. problems of termination anticipated and discussed openly

C. Assessment

1. Self-assessment questions for PN

a. do you honestly want to help?

b. are you able to experience positive attitudes toward others: caring, warmth, acceptance, interest, and respect?

c. can you give, or must you always be on receiving end?

d. can you enter into client's world and view what's happening from client's perspective?

e. can you allow client to grow by encountering his or her independence and, eventually, separation?

2. Client assessment

a. determine purpose of relationship with client

b. observe what is happening with client in here and now and how client perceives your assistance

c. identify developmental level of client so that realistic expectations of relationship are developed

d. assess verbal and nonverbal communication patterns of client

e. examine expectations of client and self in terms of outcome of relationship

D. Planning, Goals, Expected Outcomes

1. Client develops sense of trust
2. Client is able to verbalize thoughts and feelings clearly

3. Client is able to set goals for self within relationship
4. Client uses problem-solving process with ineffective behaviors
5. Client becomes as independent as possible and is able to terminate relationship in positive way

E. Implementation

1. Help identify times that trust occurs in client's behavior; for example, when client makes positive decision about life, respond by saying, "That was a positive choice you made. See, you can trust your own decisions."
   a. accept client as is
   b. be open, honest, and consistent in relationship with client
   c. demonstrate to client that you can be trusted; only make promises you can keep
2. Encourage client to verbalize thoughts and feelings in clear way
   a. tune into verbal cues to increase expression
   b. use nonverbal techniques
   c. use open-ended statements
   d. clarify misinterpretations or misconceptions of feelings by client
3. Define expectations of relationship: assist client in developing realistic and attainable goals
4. Help client define problem
   a. explore alternative solutions to problem with client
   b. encourage client to test out one of solutions in safe, supportive environment
   c. reinforce client's growth-producing behaviors
5. At start of relationship, plan, with client, for termination of relationship
   a. encourage expression of feelings during this time
   b. help client work through any negative reactions

F. Evaluation

1. Client able to initiate contact on own
2. Client interacted and expressed self more clearly
3. Client took active part in goal setting
4. Client explored alternative solutions to problems
5. Client demonstrated greater self-confidence by functioning more independently

Patterns of Behavior

I. WITHDRAWAL PATTERN OF BEHAVIOR

A. Assessment

1. Definition: disintegrative behavior pattern characterized by thinking disorder; withdrawal from reality; bizarre, regressive behavior; poor communication; and impaired interpersonal relationships; this pattern of behavior seen in persons suffering from schizophrenic disorders
2. Classifications of schizophrenia
   a. catatonic
      (1) stuporous state: mute, immobile, waxy flexibility, urinary and fecal retention
      (2) excited state: assaultive, aggressive, hyperactive, agitated
   b. disorganized: incoherent, foolish, regressive
   c. paranoid: delusions of persecution and grandeur
   d. undifferentiated: variety of symptoms found in other classifications
   e. residual: includes all schizophrenic symptoms without displaying gross disorganization, incoherence, delusions, and hallucinations
3. Incidence
   a. onset of active disease before age 45 years
   b. mainly affects adolescents and young adults
   c. occurs in about 1% of population; most prevalent of major psychoses
   d. increased incidence in lower socioeconomic classes
   e. accounts for 50% of psychiatric hospital beds
4. Prognosis
   a. 25% recover completely
   b. 50% to 60% retain some residual symptoms
   c. 10% never improve
5. Signs and symptoms
   a. associative looseness, flattened affect, ambivalence, autism
   b. disrupted thought process
   c. inability to express appropriate emotions
   d. hallucinations
   e. unable to relate to others in meaningful way
   f. delusions

B. Planning, Goals, Expected Outcomes

1. Client takes prescribed medications
2. Client maintains social contact with reality
3. Client initiates a social contact independently
4. Client takes care of own physical needs and functions more independently

C. Implementation

1. Establish trusting relationship; open, honest communication
2. Alleviate client's anxiety
3. Maintain client's biologic integrity

4. Give antipsychotic medications as ordered (Table 10–1)
5. Distract client from preoccupation by approaching client in warm, friendly way to take walk
6. Design reality-oriented activities that make external environment more satisfying for client
7. Approach client for short periods at client's level of functioning
8. Accept client where he or she is and realize that, at this time, it is best client can do
9. Provide consistent, honest interaction with client to develop trust
10. Gradually increase social contacts from one-to-one to include other people in environment
11. Initially, supervise and assist client, as needed, in caring for physical needs
12. Gradually encourage client to make decisions and assume responsibility for personal care
13. Praise client when client does things for self and let client know that he or she can trust self to make choices

D. Evaluation

1. Client complied with medication regimen
2. Client realized when he or she distorted reality and verbalized more realistic perception of self

---

TABLE 10-1 Antipsychotic Agents (Major Tranquilizers)

Classification
Antipsychotic agents (Major tranquilizers)

Action
Target symptoms most likely to decrease include: hyperactivity, combativeness, agitation, hostility, hallucinations, irritability, negativism, acute delusions, insomnia, poor self-care, anorexia

Use
Psychotic disorders, such as schizophrenic disorders, paranoid disorders, affective disorders, and organic mental disorders

Common Side Effects
Sedation, extrapyramidal side effects, anticholinergic effects, allergic side effects

Nursing Implications/Teaching
Additive effect when combined with other central nervous system depressants; check tongue regularly for vermiform movements (early sign of tardive dyskinesia); relieve dry mouth by rinsing—sips of water, chewing sugarless gum or "Quench," a saliva-stimulating gum; use paste adhesive for dentures; add chewing time with extra fluid between bites of food; fluids running out of mouth may signal dysphagia; get patient up slowly (dangle), especially after injections; check for urinary retention and constipation; extra tears for contact lens or may not be able to wear contacts because of dryness; red, hot, dry skin is sign of anhydrosis—cool immediately; sunscreen factor is for photosensitivity; dilute liquid medication

Examples
Haldol (haloperidol), Mellaril (thioridazine), Prolixin (fluphenazine), Loxitane (loxapine), Navane (thiothixene), Thorazine (chlorpromazine), Stelazine (trifluoperazine hydrochloride), Trilafon (perphenazine)

---

3. Client related to others in more effective ways
4. Client assumed more self-care responsibility

II. OVERLY SUSPICIOUS PATTERN OF BEHAVIOR

A. Assessment

1. Definition: disruptive lifestyle characterized by extreme suspiciousness, lack of trust, anger, delusions of persecution or jealousy, tendency to blame others, rigidity, and feelings of being mistreated or misjudged; this pattern seen in people suffering from paranoid disorders
2. Signs and symptoms
   a. suspicious of others' behavior
   b. secretiveness
   c. overconcerned with hidden motives and special meanings
   d. feeling of constant persecution
   e. tense, rigid, insecure
   f. clear, elaborate, and lasting delusions
   g. distorted religious beliefs
   h. alienation (basic mistrust of others)
   i. may be hostile and possibly violent

B. Planning, Goals, Expected Outcomes

1. Client takes prescribed medications
2. Client learns to trust self and others
3. Client has needs met in more realistic way
4. Client uses constructive outlets to deal with anger

C. Implementation

1. Give antipsychotic medications as ordered (see Table 10–1)
2. Approach client slowly, one-to-one, allow plenty of personal space
3. Help client learn to trust self by identifying times that trust occurs in behavior; for example, when client makes positive decision about own life, respond by saying,"That was a good choice that you made; see, you can trust yourself to make decisions about your life."
4. Listen to client without agreeing or disagreeing
5. Communicate understanding to client, but explain that what client is presenting is not reality, always in calm and matter-of-fact way
6. Give honest, specific praise for client's accomplishments
7. Provide noncompetitive, solitary tasks, such as puzzles, ceramics, punching bag, or running, as outlets for anger and aggressive drives

8. Move client into group activities after client develops trust in self and environment

D. Evaluation

1. Client complied with medication regimen
2. Overly suspicious behavior decreased through establishment of trusting behavior
3. Client's delusional system subsided as needs met in more realistic way
4. Client has found safe outlets for aggressive drives

III. PATTERNS OF BEHAVIOR INVOLVING MOOD AND AFFECT

A. Assessment

1. Definition: variety of states that include extremes of mood and affect
   a. depression: sense of loss that overwhelms client
   b. mania: denial of loss with temporary improvement in self-esteem; reaction formation to depression; elation
   c. bipolar (manic-depressive disorders): alternating mania and depression
2. Incidence
   a. depression
      (1) any age, both sexes, but women and people over age 65 years more common
      (2) 1.5 million clients diagnosed per year
      (3) almost half recover without treatment
      (4) most common emotional illness
   b. mania
      (1) more common in women
      (2) occurs much more commonly in siblings or family of sufferers
      (3) highest occurrence in Northern Europeans and descendants
   c. bipolar: occurs before age 30 years
3. Signs and symptoms
   a. depression
      (1) sense of worthlessness, hopelessness, and helplessness
      (2) frequent crying
      (3) withdrawal from others
      (4) sleep disturbance
      (5) changes in appetite and weight
      (6) lack of energy
      (7) flat affect, look of sadness
      (8) decreased mental activities
      (9) potential for suicide
   b. mania
      (1) sense of euphoria, excitement, and talkativeness
      (2) hyperactive, talks continuously
      (3) aggressive behavior
      (4) flight of ideas and delusions
      (5) increased energy with infrequent eating or sleeping
      (6) increased productivity
   c. bipolar: shift from depression to mania and back

B. Planning, Goals, Expected Outcomes

1. Depression
   a. client takes prescribed medications
   b. client becomes more involved in simple activities
   c. client talks about things outside of self
   d. client cares for personal needs, eats regular meals, and sleeps through night
   e. client does not harm self
2. Mania
   a. client takes antimanic medications as ordered
   b. client channels energy into constructive outlets
   c. client is able to get involved in social interactions without losing control
   d. client receives adequate nutrition and rest and is able to care for own personal needs

C. Implementation

1. Depression
   a. administer antidepressant medications (Tables 10–2 and 10–3) as ordered; monitor closely for side effects

TABLE 10-2 Antidepressive Agents (Tricyclic)

Classification
Antidepressive agents (tricyclic)

Action
Mood elevator

Use
Tricyclic antidepressants first line of treatment for depression

Common Side Effects
Anticholinergic effects, orthostatic hypotension, sedation

Nursing Implications/Teaching
Take 1–4 weeks for onset of effect; side effects tend to show up rapidly; client experiences depression plus side effects; body adjusts to side effects in a week or two (ways of relieving side effects included on medication write-up for antipsychotic medications); overdose can be lethal; often ordered as a single dose at bedtime (exception, Vivactil)—sedating effect promotes sleep; danger early in therapy is suicide; client is able to channel energy to formulate and implement a plan before depression significantly improves; not given with monoamine oxidase inhibitor antidepressants

Examples
Tofranil (imipramine), Elavil (amitriptyline), Vivactil (protriptyline), Desyrel (trazodone), Asendin (amoxapine), Norpramin (desipramine hydrochloride), Pamelor (nortriptyline hydrochloride), Prozac (fluoxetine)

b. assist with electroconvulsive therapy as ordered

c. design simple routine, including activities and tasks that client can accomplish that do not require deep concentration

d. express appreciation to client for contribution

e. focus client on own strengths

f. sit with client; avoid overcheerfulness; let client know when you are leaving and when you will return

g. assist client with exploring alternative ways of handling feelings, such as anger or guilt

h. assist client with personal hygiene; offer positive reinforcement for what client accomplishes

i. encourage eating by offering small, attractive portions; use supplemental feedings as needed

j. establish sleep routine; warm milk and relaxation techniques helpful in inducing sleep; avoid use of sleeping pills, which are depressants

2. Mania

a. give client prescribed antimanic medications, lithium carbonate and lithium citrate (Table 10–4), and monitor closely for side effects

b. provide quiet, nonstimulating environment

TABLE 10-3 Antidepressive Agents (Monoamine Oxidase Inhibitors)

Classification
Antidepressive agents (MAOIs)

Action
MAOIs inhibit the oxidase enzyme that breaks down monoamine transmitters at many places in the body, including the intestine; results in greater availability of these transmitters for improved message transmission in the brain

Use
Reserved for symptomatic relief of depression in clients who have failed to respond to other antidepressant therapy

Common Side Effects
Similar to those of tricyclic antidepressants

Toxic Side Effects
Hypertensive crisis resulting in a cerebrovascular accident if foods or medication containing tyramine, a monoamine, is ingested

Nursing Implications/Teaching
Antidepressant effect experienced in 48 hours to 3 weeks
Instruct client about foods to avoid
Tell client what medications to avoid
Warn client how to recognize danger signs of impending hypertensive crisis
Monitor blood pressure regularly at onset of medication therapy

Examples
Marplan (isocarboxazid), Nardil (phenelzine), Parnate (tranylcypromine)

Abbreviation: MAOIs, monoamine oxidase inhibitors.

TABLE 10-4 Antimanic Agents

Classification
Antimanic agents

Action
Decrease hyperactivity, verbalism, agitation, irritability, insomnia, anorexia

Use
Drug of choice for clients with mania and for long-term maintenance to prevent both depressive and manic episodes in bipolar disorder

Common Side Effects
Nausea and fatigue early in therapy; tremor, thirst, edema, and weight gain throughout therapy

Toxic Side Effects
Confusion (often missed), ataxia, impaired coordination, dizziness, headaches, blurred vision, muscle weakness, gastrointestinal symptoms; if untreated, can lead to coma and *death*

Nursing Implications/Teaching
Serum lithium level monitored; 12-hour sample; blood drawn (usually) 12 hours after last dose of medication:
1.2–1.6 mEq/L: therapeutic for most clients
2 mEq/L: risk of toxicity
0.8–1.2 mEq/L: maintenance
Takes 2–3 weeks for therapeutic effect; client receives temporary treatment with antipsychotic medication until therapeutic blood level of lithium obtained; impaired renal function, decreased sodium intake, and diuretic therapy provide risk of toxicity; teach client relationship of sodium and lithium; as long as sodium intake and output is stable, lithium absorption and excretion will be stable; client needs help to adjust to new feeling state

Examples
Eskalith, Lithane, Lithonate, Lithobid (lithium carbonate)

c. set limits on behavior harmful to self or others as well as on behavior interfering with others' rights

d. use client's poor attention span and easy distractibility to avoid difficult situations

e. provide constructive outlets for client's excess energy: jogging, swimming, walking, or noncompetitive sports

f. maintain calm, matter-of-fact, nonjudgmental attitude when client is sarcastic or critical; do not take client's remarks personally

g. protect client from humiliating self in front of others when grandiose

h. laugh with, not at, client; set limits on client's playful, joking behavior

i. encourage client to express negative feelings that may underlie overactivity

j. provide high-carbohydrate, high-protein diet with vitamin supplements; use finger foods and high-calorie liquids if client cannot sit still

k. provide extra rest periods, soothing warm baths, quiet music, and nonstimulating environment

l. encourage acceptable hygiene and clothing

m. monitor elimination; may be too busy to go to bathroom

D. Evaluation

1. Depression
   a. client complied with medication regimen
   b. client became more involved in simple activities
   c. client talked about things outside of self
   d. client cared for personal needs, ate regular meals, and slept through night
   e. client did not harm self
2. Mania
   a. client took antimanic medication as ordered
   b. client channeled energy into constructive outlets
   c. client able to get involved in social interactions without losing control
   d. client received adequate nutrition and rest and became able to care for own personal needs

IV. SUICIDAL PATTERN OF BEHAVIOR

A. Assessment

1. Definition: deliberate action to end one's life
2. Predisposing factors
   a. pathologic depression most common factor
   b. alcoholism next most common factor
   c. inability to deal with unexpected outcomes, so that individual feels overwhelmed
   d. need to control significant others
   e. inability to deal with intolerable emotional pain
3. Signs and symptoms
   a. previous suicide attempts, suicide threats, or extreme depression
   b. giving away prized possessions, especially in young
   c. putting affairs in order after depression
   d. asking questions, such as "How many pills would it take to kill someone?"
   e. cries easily
   f. hears voices telling person to kill self
   g. talks about seeing again people who have died
   h. talks about plan for suicide
   i. sudden euphoria after severe depression

B. Planning, Goals, Expected Outcomes

1. Client uses positive ways of solving problems instead of attempting suicide
2. Client forms relationship with significant other(s) for support during difficult times
3. Client's physical status returns to pre-illness pattern
4. Client focuses on more positive aspects of living
5. Client does not commit suicide

C. Implementation

1. Maintain safe, unchallenging environment; if needed, provide constant supervision during suicide crisis
2. Monitor client's medication usage closely
3. Take every complaint and feeling client expresses seriously
4. Talk openly about client's ideas of suicide
5. Build on client's strengths; previous positive coping mechanisms might be used
6. Be affirmative, but supportive
7. Provide emotional strength by communicating that you know what you are doing and that everything possible will be done for client
8. Contact persons in client's life who are significant and can be supportive, such as ministers, relatives, and friends
9. Pay attention to more subtle and hidden clues that client is self-destructive, such as not eating or caring for personal needs
10. Supervise client when eating and performing hygienic measures
11. Give reassurance that client's feelings of despair and pain are temporary and will pass
12. Mention that as long as life exists, there is a chance for help; death is final
13. Encourage change of pace, such as exercise or relaxation techniques
14. Remove objects that could be used in a suicide attempt

D. Evaluation

1. Client used positive ways of solving problems instead of attempting suicide
2. Client formed relationship with significant other(s) for support during difficult times
3. Client's physical status returned to pre-illness pattern
4. Client focused on more positive aspects of living
5. Client did not commit suicide

V. BEHAVIOR PATTERNS OF YOUNG, CHRONICALLY MENTALLY ILL

A. Assessment

1. Definition: population of previously institutionalized clients, who experience repeated hospitalizations; little or no improvement

2. Behaviors include
   a. developmental disorders
   b. disruptive behavior disorders
   c. anxiety disorders of childhood
   d. eating disorders
   e. gender-identity disorders
3. Signs and symptoms
   a. denial of need for treatment
   b. refusal to take prescribed antipsychotic medications
   c. use of street drugs
   d. may exhibit violent behavior toward self or others
   e. ability to perform activities of daily living may be impaired

B. Planning, Goals, Expected Outcomes

1. Client admits that mental illness exists
2. Client participates in developing *realistic, short-term* goals for self
3. Client uses *rationalization* to explain why not ready to take on too large a task (failure would further deflate ego and evoke guilt about having failed you after all you did for client)
4. Client works with more than one therapist on scheduled basis

C. Implementation

1. Involve client in interests outside self; projects, people, and structured activities
2. Discuss possibility of sheltered employment
3. Encourage involvement with support system
   a. stable one-to-one relationship
   b. ongoing group therapy
   c. follow-up home visits
4. Support use of coping or mental mechanism, rationalization, when client plans tasks that would lead to failure
5. Introduce client to co-therapist relationship during hospitalization to prevent client from feeling abandoned when one therapist is not available
6. Respond to age-related needs; attitude important
7. Administer antipsychotic medications (see Table 10–1) as ordered

D. Evaluation

1. Client involved in structured activity, project, or relationship that can be continued after hospitalization
2. Client consented to testing for sheltered employment

3. Client exhibited beginning trust in self and others
   a. took medications from staff
   b. participated marginally in group therapy
   c. indicated willingness to talk to follow-up home visit staff
4. Client offered rationalization for why client cannot pursue goal at this time, such as go to college
5. Client agreed to see two separate therapists

VI. ANXIOUS PATTERNS OF BEHAVIOR

A. Anxiety

1. Assessment
   a. definition: normal function; diffuse subjective feeling of dread; apprehension or unexplained discomfort; subjectively painful warning of impending danger
   b. Characteristics
      (1) mild
         (a) normal sensation
         (b) motivates person to action
      (2) severe
         (a) disabling
         (b) requires outside intervention
      (3) unrelated to specific object; unable to identify source
   c. incidence
      (1) all people experience mild-to-moderate anxiety
      (2) severe anxiety to panic state affects about 5% of population
   d. signs and symptoms
      (1) mild
         (a) increased perception and alertness
         (b) observations clearer
      (2) moderate
         (a) decreased perception
         (b) increased alertness
         (c) concentration centered; irrelevant tasks ignored
      (3) severe
         (a) decreased, narrowed perception
         (b) poor communication
      (4) generalized
         (a) muscle tension, hyperactivity
         (b) vigilant behavior
      (5) panic state
         (a) sudden, intense periods of extreme fear
         (b) accompanied by physical symptoms of palpitations, dyspnea, chest pain, sensation of choking, dizziness, hot and cold flashes, sweating, trembling
         (c) fear of impending doom

(d) nonpurposeful behavior
(e) unable to fight or take flight
2. Planning, goals, expected outcomes
   a. client learns constructive ways of dealing with anxiety
   b. client recognizes symptoms of onset of anxiety and intervenes before reaching panic state
   c. client cares for personal needs, such as bathing, oral hygiene, nutrition, and sleep
3. Implementation
   a. assist client to recognize feelings of anxiety when they arise and to connect these feelings to relief behaviors, such as use of relaxation, imagery, humor, and other coping behaviors
   b. try to interest client in things outside of self, such as simple concrete task or game, walking, physical activity, sweeping, clearing table, and washing dishes
   c. remind client to care for own physical needs
   d. monitor client's weight
   e. administer antianxiety medications (Table 10–5) as ordered
   f. provide calm, quiet, safe environment
   g. reinforce effective and constructive coping behaviors
   h. reassure client of safety and security
4. Evaluation
   a. client learned constructive ways of dealing with anxiety
   b. client recognized symptoms of onset of anxiety and intervened before reaching panic state
   c. client cared for personal needs, such as bathing, oral hygiene, nutrition, and sleep

B. Phobias

1. Assessment
   a. definition: intense irrational fear of object or situation; may interfere with normal function of client
   b. types
      (1) xenophobia: fear of strangers
      (2) agoraphobia: fear of open or public places from which escape is difficult
      (3) claustrophobia: fear of enclosed or small places
      (4) acrophobia: fear of heights
      (5) post-traumatic stress disorder: frequently reliving psychologically traumatic event
   c. signs and symptoms
      (1) panic attack when exposed to phobic object or situation
      (2) refusal to leave home or face exposure to phobic situation or object
      (3) apprehension, diffuse anxiety
      (4) uses avoidance coping style
      (5) fight-or-flight behaviors when exposed to phobia
2. Planning, goals, expected outcomes
   a. client becomes desensitized to phobic object or situation and no longer experiences phobic response
   b. client acknowledges and discusses fear
   c. client accepts and participates in treatment program aimed at reducing phobic response
3. Implementation
   a. assist in desensitization
   b. administer antidepressant drugs (see Table 10–2), antianxiety drugs, and tranquilizers (see Tables 10–1 and 10–5)
   c. help client understand that facing phobia can lead to adaptive coping behaviors
   d. identify and reinforce positive coping by client
   e. encourage client to identify life situations that generate anxiety and conflict
   f. offer hope that treatment will reduce phobic response
4. Evaluation
   a. client became desensitized to phobic object or situation and no longer experienced phobic response
   b. client acknowledged and discussed fear

TABLE 10–5 Antianxiety Agents (Minor Tranquilizers)

Classification
Antianxiety agents (minor tranquilizers)

Action
Relieve anxiety and muscle tension, anticonvulsant (*no antipsychotic activity*)

Use
Relieve uncomfortable anxiety and muscular tension; leave client with sufficient anxiety to motivate client to seek solution to actual problem; have anticonvulsive action; useful during alcohol detoxification in preventing or decreasing intensity of end-stage withdrawal symptoms (anxiety disorders, somatoform disorders, alcohol detoxification)

Common Side Effects
Additive effect with other central nervous system depressants; drowsiness, fatigue, ataxia most common, confusion especially in the elderly; drug dependence with chronic use; withdrawal symptoms if abruptly withdrawn

Nursing Implications/Teaching
Have client set treatment goals; avoid use with other central nervous system depressants (alcohol, barbiturates); use only as prescribed to avoid psychic or physical dependence; withdrawal symptoms of long-acting drugs such as Valium may be delayed for days and then may be confused with anxiety

Examples
Ativan (lorazepam), Valium (diazepam), Librium (chlordiazepoxide), Xanax (alprazolam), Tranxene (clorazepate dipotassium), Serax (oxazepam)

    c. client accepted and participated in treatment program aimed at reducing phobic response

C. Obsessive-Compulsive Behaviors

1. Assessment
   a. definition: involuntary, recurring thoughts or images that cannot be ignored or treated logically; recurring impulses to perform seemingly purposeless activities
   b. signs and symptoms
      (1) excessive conformity and conscientiousness
      (2) perfectionist, overly meticulous
      (3) rigidity, difficulty making decisions
      (4) selective inattention to new ideas
      (5) concentration on insignificant details
      (6) lack of personal convictions
      (7) when severe, worry borders on delusion
      (8) when anxious, performs repetitive behavior to relieve stress
2. Planning, goals, expected outcomes
   a. client copes effectively with activities of daily living without resorting to obsessive-compulsive behaviors
   b. client accepts limits on repetitive behaviors and participates in alternative adaptive activities
3. Implementation
   a. develop affirming, dependable relationship
   b. determine situations that precipitate repetitive behavior
   c. show acceptance of person without showing disapproval of behavior
   d. provide structure and time so that rituals can be completed without increased anxiety
   e. provide environment so that client can decrease rituals and increase other activities
   f. positively reinforce nonritualistic behaviors
   g. teach client to recognize and anticipate situations that might precipitate rituals
   h. teach techniques to allow client to stop thoughts that precipitate rituals, such as relaxation techniques, constructive activity, and exercise
   i. assist client with dependency conflict
   j. help client find initial source of anxiety
4. Evaluation
   a. client coped effectively with activities of daily living without resorting to obsessive-compulsive behaviors
   b. client accepted limits on repetitive behaviors and participated in alternative adaptive activities

VII. BEHAVIOR PATTERN RELATED TO ORGANIC MENTAL DISORDERS

A. Assessment

1. Description: pattern of behavior characterized by changes in organic functioning because of injury or disease, substance abuse, aging, or medication; can produce either temporary or permanent brain damage
2. Types
   a. delirium: usually stable or self-limiting
   b. dementia: progressive, static, or remitting
   c. primary, degenerative dementia of Alzheimer type, the most common dementia
3. Signs and symptoms
   a. memory impairment
   b. impairment of abstract thinking
   c. impaired judgment and impulse control
   d. loss of other higher cortical functions
   e. personality changes
   f. altered state of consciousness
   g. perceptual disturbances
   h. altered sleep-wakefulness cycle
   i. decreased psychomotor activity
   j. emotional disturbances
   k. sundown syndrome—okay during day and confused at night

B. Planning, Goals, Expected Outcomes

1. Client does as much as possible for self in caring for own physical needs
2. Client maintains sense of self-control by doing for self within modified environment
3. Client maintains human dignity through interaction with staff, other clients, and significant others

C. Implementation

1. Establish structured, consistent, daily routine
   a. supervise health habits, including eating, personal hygiene, exercise, and toileting
   b. have client assist with personal care as much as possible
2. Patiently answer questions in short, simple sentences; repeat answers when needed
   a. demonstrate nonverbally and concretely what you are trying to convey to client
   b. try to help client, whenever necessary, to become oriented through use of clocks, calendars, signs, and written and verbal reminders
   c. modify environment for safety according to individual needs

3. Tell client when you do not understand what he or she is talking about
   a. use client's past memory to bring client to present through reminiscing during one-to-one encounters and reminiscing group
   b. assist family members in their contact with client
4. Administer antipsychotic medications (see Table 10–1) as ordered

D. Evaluation

1. Client did as much as possible for self in caring for own physical needs
2. Client maintained sense of self-control by doing for self within modified environment
3. Client maintained human dignity through interaction with staff, other clients, and significant others

? QUESTIONS

1. A 23-year-old woman was brought to the mental health center by her parents. They are concerned because she does not want to come out of her room, makes up words, and spends hours "decoding" messages that she hears being transmitted to her through television. When you arrive on the unit, you find her sitting in her room, her face expressionless. She does not raise her head or answer when you call her by name. What is her major pattern of behavior?

   ① Overly suspicious
   ② Withdrawal
   ③ Depressive
   ④ Manic

2. A client with overly suspicious pattern of behavior would be diagnosed with which of the following disorders?

   ① Schizophrenia
   ② Reactive depression
   ③ Paranoid state
   ④ Borderline personality

3. What is a core problem for a client with schizophrenia?

   ① Inability to deal with hostile feelings
   ② Inability to adjust to personal confrontation
   ③ Inability to develop relationships outside of self
   ④ Inability to accept decreasing intelligence

4. What is the major defense mechanism used by a client with schizophrenia?

   ① Denial
   ② Reaction formation
   ③ Projection
   ④ Regression

5. How do you respond if a schizophrenic woman asks if you believe that she hears secret messages through television?

   ① "It's probably the Russians; ignore them!"
   ② "No, but I know the 'so-called voices' are real to you."
   ③ "Why do you think you hear messages over the TV?"
   ④ "What do you think? Do you think I hear them?"

6. Which of these reflects positive improvement for a woman diagnosed with schizophrenia?

   ① Rejects you after spending time with her
   ② Is no longer verbally explosive when approached
   ③ No longer believes that she is terminally ill
   ④ Eats and sleeps regularly without special arrangements

7. A young man was brought to the hospital by the police. Neighbors became concerned because they saw him looking out his window with a shotgun in his hand. When people walked by, he shouted, "You can't take my property away! Get away or I will shoot!" On admission, he tells you of his neighbors' plot to take his property away. What is his major pattern of behavior?

   ① Compulsive
   ② Overly suspicious
   ③ Withdrawal
   ④ Anxious

8. What does an overly suspicious behavior pattern tell you about a male client?

   ① His compulsive behavior relieves tension
   ② He needs group interaction and stimulation
   ③ He uses sublimation to deal with anxiety
   ④ He has not learned to trust himself

9. What is an idea not supported by logic called?

   ① Hallucination
   ② Illusion
   ③ Delusion
   ④ Blocking

10. Why would you address a client with overly suspicious behavior as "Mr." during your contact with him?

    ① Casualness may lead him to think you are incompetent
    ② All clients need to be addressed formally
    ③ His use of introjection lowers his self-esteem
    ④ It supports his use of symptoms for now

11. What will you do if your overly suspicious client refuses to eat because of his fear of being poisoned?

    ① Have his family bring him food
    ② Remind him that this is crazy behavior
    ③ Tell him that no one poisoned his food
    ④ Offer to let him serve himself and taste his food for him

12. How would you advise someone regarding use of touch with an overly suspicious client?

① Touch is comforting to him
② A back rub will help him sleep
③ He may misinterpret someone's touching him
④ Touch is a way to reorient him

13. What is a desired response if you are alone and a physically assaultive client tells you to open the door?

① Open the door without resistance
② Block the door with your body
③ Use body language; roll your eyes
④ Attempt to flirt with the client

14. What is meant by "Images go directly to the nervous system"?

① Images can cause damage to the central nervous system
② You become what you imagine you will become
③ Fantasizing is considered unhealthy
④ Imaging is done under supervision

15. Your client, a female nurse, has been calling in sick to the unit where she works. She is always tired, complains of not sleeping well, and has lost 10 pounds within the last 2 weeks owing to loss of appetite. Three months ago, the administration announced that some staff may expect a "layoff" within the next 6 months. Yesterday, she called her mother to say goodbye: "I couldn't take this any longer." When you meet her, you note a deeply sad expression. What is her major pattern of behavior?

① Depression
② Overly suspicious
③ Antisocial personality
④ Withdrawal

16. Which of the following will help you in planning the care of a depressed young woman?

① Your cheerfulness will help elevate her mood
② Sharing your problems will help her focus on others
③ Depression often lifts slightly in the late afternoon
④ Telling her that she is angry increases insight

17. What is the major coping/mental mechanism for a woman suffering from depression?

① Symbolism
② Projection
③ Denial
④ Introjection

18. What would you suggest as a way of dealing with the suicidal feelings of a young woman?

① Encourage her to talk about her suicidal feelings
② Maintain detailed notes concerning her actions
③ Tell her you will keep her from killing herself
④ Remind her that other employees are facing the same problem

19. What approach will you use to get a depressed young woman involved in her care?

① "Do you want to take a bath now?"
② "Stop feeling sorry for yourself."
③ "It's time for us to have our breakfast."
④ "I want you to brush your teeth now."

20. Why might a depressed young woman experience constipation?

① An expression of anger toward you
② A way of manipulating you
③ Emotional needs expressed physically
④ A lack of activity and intake

21. What will you stress as a nursing intervention for a client who is receiving monoamine oxidase inhibitors?

① Set treatment goals
② Avoid tyramine-rich foods
③ Plan for drug holidays
④ Avoid central nervous system depressants

22. A 50-year-old man was admitted this afternoon. He was previously hospitalized with a similar episode 10 years ago. During the past 2 weeks, he has become increasingly agitated and excitable. Both verbalization and physical activity have increased. His wife notes that he "goes from topic to topic and has hardly slept at all." Two days ago, he went on a buying spree and gave all his purchases away. What diagnosis best describes this behavior?

① Panic attack
② Schizophreniform
③ Manic episode
④ Paranoid state

23. Which of the following is a helpful nursing intervention when the manic client is agitated?

① Include him in a card game with other clients
② Set firm, fixed limits on his behavior
③ Separate him from others in a quiet area
④ Encourage him to organize a baseball game

24. What is the core problem for manic behavior?

① An attempt to increase self-esteem
② Inability to develop relationships
③ Overwhelming desire to be liked
④ Exaggeration of basic personality traits

25. How will you respond if the client calls you a "fat, gum-chewing, dumb nurse"?

① Ask him for clarification of his statement
② Be nondefensive and avoid arousing guilt
③ Tell him he is inappropriate; send him to his room
④ Join Weight Watchers, throw out your gum, and go back to school

26. What is the major coping or mental mechanism for a client with mania?

① Regression
② Projection
③ Sublimation
④ Conversion

27. Which of the following is an example of an assertive response?

① "Yes, I'd be willing to go along with your second idea but not with the first one."
② "You make me so angry! You always act as if you know all the answers."
③ "Well, if you really think I should, I'll go along with the suggestion."
④ "You are so critical! Why don't you evaluate your own behavior?"

28. Which of the following statements is an example of assuming responsibility for content of personal conversation?

① "We decided that we want to continue with group meetings."
② "You know that the group meetings benefit all of us together."
③ "Most guys, me included, feel that it's a good idea to continue."
④ "I feel that it's important for me to continue with the group."

29. A 22-year-old woman has experienced repeated hospitalizations because of chronic mental illness. Although she has been stabilized on medication several times, she discontinues the medications on her own shortly after she leaves the hospital. What is a major consideration in developing her care plan?

① Natural rebelliousness of this age group
② The staffing pattern on the unit at night
③ Age range of the present unit staff
④ Age of the parents

30. What coping or mental mechanism may be helpful in dealing with unrealized expectations?

① Denial
② Projection
③ Repression
④ Rationalization

31. A 36-year-old woman was admitted to the center last night because her repetitive hand washing has increased to the point where she is no longer able to complete her work on the job and at home. What is her major pattern of behavior?

① Depression
② Aggression
③ Suspiciousness
④ Compulsion

32. What is the major coping or mental mechanism for a client with compulsive behavior?

① Repression
② Projection
③ Introjection
④ Reaction formation

33. Why does a compulsive woman wash her hands repeatedly?

① To be clean
② To get attention from others
③ For temporary relief of anxiety
④ To sublimate her aggressiveness

34. Why is it important for staff to deal with personal feelings evoked by a compulsive client's behavior?

① Prevent support of negative coping methods
② Interpret meaning of the client's ritual to her
③ Clearly tell her how to stop hand washing
④ Share personal solution to problems with the client

35. What classification of medications will the physician order for relief of the manifestations of compulsive behavior?

   ① Antipsychotic
   ② Antianxiety
   ③ Antidepressant
   ④ Antimanic

36. Which of the following statements is true about use of relaxation techniques?

   ① Everyone benefits from practicing relaxation.
   ② Relaxation techniques are desirable for psychotic clients.
   ③ Relaxation has no known effect on medication.
   ④ A small percentage of the population experiences an opposite effect.

37. How can you direct a compulsive client to use humor to deal with a present situation?

   ① Help her see the humor in other clients' behavior
   ② Have her draw a cartoon that exaggerates the situation
   ③ Point out what is funny about her problem
   ④ Tease her when she gets "too serious"

38. What is empathy?

   ① Respectful, detached concern
   ② Experiencing the client's emotion
   ③ Identifying with the client
   ④ Focusing on client's condition

39. Electroconvulsive therapy is used as a treatment for which of the following conditions?

   ① Primary dementia
   ② Schizophrenia
   ③ Paranoid disorder
   ④ Severe depression

ANSWERS AND RATIONALES

Guide to item identification (see pp. 4–5 for further details about each category):

I, II, II, or IV for the phase of the nursing process
1, 2, 3, or 4 for the category of client needs
A, B, C, D, E, F, or G for the category of human functioning
Specific content category by name; i.e., cholecystectomy

1. Withdrawal is a pattern of behavior usually seen
② in people suffering from schizophrenic disorders.
I, 3, G, Schizophrenia

2. The behavior is suggestive of a client with the
① diagnosis of schizophrenia.
I, 3, G, Schizophrenia

3. Clients with schizophrenia find it difficult to
③ relate to others in a meaningful way. To avoid rejection, they set up barriers that make it difficult for persons to establish contact.
I, 3, G, Schizophrenia

4. Clients experiencing withdrawal patterns of be-
④ havior may have been exposed to a great deal of conflict and turmoil during their early developmental periods. As a result of these early experiences, they never fully develop a basic sense of trust. They continue throughout life to search for acceptance and approval. After numerous rejections, they eventually give up and, using the coping or mental mechanism of *regression*, retreat to a simpler form of existence in a world of their own. In this world, they turn their attention to themselves and relate to their imaginary environment as if it were real.
I, 3, G, Defense mechanisms

5. The nurse should discuss real events with client
② to focus on reality. Refer to voices as "so-called voices." Do not act attentive to discussion regarding hallucinations, which helps to decrease the importance of the hallucinations.
III, 3, G, Schizophrenia

6. Rejection from a client who has previously
① shown acceptance is often a clue that the client has allowed the nurse to enter the client's world. This is not necessarily a permanent rejection but means the nurse should move more slowly.
IV, 3, G, Schizophrenia

7. Clients experiencing the overly suspicious pat-
② tern of behavior are usually diagnosed with a paranoid disorder.
I, 3, G, Overly suspicious behavior

8. Clients suffering from paranoid disorder have
④ usually had a childhood in which distrust, hate, and poor interpersonal relationships developed.
I, 3, G, Overly suspicious behavior

9. A delusion is a belief or idea that is not sup-
③ ported by logic.
I, 3, G, Overly suspicious behavior

10. The nurse must be professional at all times with
① the client to decrease use of projection. Projection is a way the client denies shortcomings and uses the coping or mental mechanism of projection to attribute internal feelings to objects and people outside. This helps the client feel more comfortable and superior to others, while remaining a lonely person, frightened of being exposed as inadequate.
III, 3, G, Overly suspicious behavior

11. If the client thinks food is poisoned, it may be
④ necessary to serve food in closed containers and to allow the client to open the containers. Sometimes the client may want the nurse to taste the food first.
III, 3, G, Overly suspicious behavior

12. Paranoid behavior may cause the client to misin-
③ terpret this type of behavior.
III, 3, G, Overly suspicious behavior

13. The nurse should never try to stop an assaultive
① client alone. Get out of the way and get help, if possible.
III, 3, G, Overly suspicious behavior

14. People often become what they think they can
② become.
I, 3, G, Coping behaviors

15. Clients suffering from depression often express
① feelings of deep sadness and a hopeless expression, loss of energy, fatigability or tiredness, sleeping difficulty, recurrent thoughts of death or suicide or any suicidal behavior including thoughts of wishing to be dead, and poor appetite or weight loss.
I, 3, G, Depression

16. There is usually a time in the late afternoon
③ when depression lifts slightly. This is a good time to reach the client, sharing simple activities.
II, 3, G, Depression

17. Clients who are clinically depressed often deal
④ with anger through the coping technique of *introjection*. By turning the anger inward—intra-aggression—it no longer poses an external threat to the client as an individual.
I, 3, G, Depression

18. Do not be afraid to ask the client directly if the
① client has suicidal thoughts. Talking about it frankly can help prevent the client from carrying out the idea. The client usually welcomes the opportunity to open up and discuss it.
III, 3, G, Depression

19. Often the client's illness limits problem-solving
④ abilities. This client needs the nurse to communicate in simple, clear "I" statements.
III & IV, 3, A & C, Depression

20. Depression slows all internal body functions,
④ so constipation can become a problem for the client.
IV, 3, F & G, Depression

21. Clients taking monoamine oxidase inhibitors
② need to be cautioned about ingesting products that would cause a significant additional supply of monoamines. Some foods contain significant amounts of tyramine, a monoamine that affects blood pressure. Large amounts of tyramine can lead to a hypertensive crisis (an extreme elevation in blood pressure), leading to rupture of blood vessels that results in a cerebrovascular accident (stroke).
III, 3, F & G, Antipsychotic medications

22. When a client is experiencing mania, all pro-
③ cesses speed up.
I, 3, G, Mania

23. During mania, the client needs protection from
③ overstimulation. A quiet area removed from the center of activity is often helpful.
III, 3, G, Mania

24. The client's increase in activity is an attempt to
① increase self-esteem.
I, 3, G, Mania

25. A client suffering from mania needs a nonchal-
② lenging atmosphere, and the nurse should ac-cept verbal abuse calmly and matter-of-factly.
III, 3, G, Mania

26. The client suffering from mania uses projection
② to turn the anger outward toward objects and people in the environment.
IV, 3, G, Mania

27. "I" messages are much more direct and a better
① example of a therapeutic response.
IV, 1 & 3, G, Therapeutic communication

28. It is important for the nurse to allow individuals
④ to own their problems.
IV, 1 & 3, G, Therapeutic communication

29. Clients this age often exhibit natural rebellious-
① ness. This is combined with the client's view that admission of mental illness is equal to failure.
II, 3, G, Chronic mental illness

30. Rationalization is the usual coping mechanism
④ used when a client is unable to meet unrealized expectations.
I, 3, G, Chronic mental illness

31. Clients trying to cope with the overwhelming
④ anxiety may separate (dissociate) the anxiety from the rest of the personality. The resulting manifestations give clues (symbolism) to the underlying problem, of which the client is not consciously aware. Compulsive behavior helps to decrease anxiety.
I, 3, G, Compulsive behavior

32. The client uses repression to attempt to keep the
① threatening experiences and thoughts hidden.
I, 3, G, Compulsive behavior

33. Anxiety is relieved through the repetition of an
③ act, a compulsion, such as hand washing. The compulsion gives the client an increased sense of security.
IV, 3, G, Compulsive behavior

34. Health care workers can find that client behav-
① iors can unleash unresolved personal problems with which the health care provider has not come to terms.
II & IV, 3, G, Compulsive behavior

35. Because compulsive behaviors are engaged in
② to decrease anxiety, the primary medications used to treat this disorder are antianxiety agents.
III, 3, G, Compulsive behavior

36. Approximately 3% of clients respond to relaxation training by actually increasing arousal (e.g., increasing blood pressure instead of decreasing).
④ IV, 3, G, Compulsive behavior

37. Have the client draw or visualize the present situation as a cartoon, exaggerating it so it is ridiculous. By injecting some humor into the situation, the client may be able to deal with it more effectively.
② III, 3, G, Compulsive behavior

38. Empathy can be defined as respectful, detached concern. The nurse understands what the client is experiencing but does not experience the emotion with the client.
① IV, 3, G, Mental health

39. Electroconvulsive therapy is most helpful in clients experiencing severe depression or who are compulsively suicidal.
④ IV, 3, G, Depression

EMOTIONS, BEHAVIOR, AND MENTAL HEALTH

The way people deal with emotions (feelings such as ambivalence, love, hate, and so on) has a significant relationship to how mentally healthy they are; mental health is a state of being defined as:

1. Feeling comfortable about yourself.
2. Feeling right about others.
3. Meeting demands of life.
4. Coping and adjusting to recurrent stresses of everyday living.
5. Dealing with anxiety by the healthy use of defense mechanisms.

Coping or Mental Mechanisms

I. DEFENSE MECHANISMS

A. Assessment

1. Definition: unconscious, automatic ways of dealing with discomfort
2. May develop in childhood when individual is placed in difficult situations person cannot handle
3. Can have healthy or unhealthy effect on individual; depends on degree of use
4. Use of mechanism continues throughout person's life, even when original stress no longer exists

B. Types*

1. Compensation
   a. definition: covering for real or imagined inadequacy by developing or exaggerating desirable trait
   b. example: undersized boy develops intellectual ability instead of participating in sports
2. Conversion
   a. definition: channeling of anxiety into physical symptoms
   b. example: Mrs. Smith develops headache on evening she is scheduled to present paper at convention and is unable to make presentation because of illness
3. Denial
   a. definition: rejection of things, events, or feelings as they actually exist, thus eliminating need for anxiety
   b. example: alcoholic denies alcoholism; "I am a social drinker and can quit anytime."
4. Displacement
   a. definition: occurs when feelings toward object are distorted and transferred to less threatening, more socially acceptable object
   b. example: person who loves to eat collects recipes
5. Dissociation
   a. definition: occurs when painful ideas, situations, or feelings are separated from awareness
   b. example: Carol has forgotten details of accident in which loved one was killed
6. Fantasy
   a. definition: using imagination to solve problems; on conscious level, fantasy used to reduce stress through relaxation; on unconscious level, fantasy used as retreat from threatening environment
   b. example: children work through situations they will encounter in adult life by assuming parental roles in play and using pets or dolls as their children
7. Identification
   a. definition: occurs when persons take on characteristics and values of someone they ad-

---

* Bauer & Hill (1986), pp. 15–21.

mire, recognizing that they are not that person

b. example: teenager dresses like favorite "rock" star

8. Introjection
   a. definition: incorporating or internalizing of conflicting values, standards, persons, objects, or attitudes so that they are no longer external threats
   b. example: political candidate professes to represent every interest group so that none attack platform

9. Projection
   a. definition: attributing to other people or objects motives and emotions that are unacceptable to oneself
   b. example: overweight woman blames her 2-year-old son for her condition, saying that he makes her nervous

10. Rationalization
    a. definition: logical-sounding excuses that conceal real reason for actions, thoughts, or feelings
    b. example: young boy explains why he left for school without feeding dog—"I did it because Johnny came over and told me we had to leave right away"

11. Reaction formation
    a. definition: sometimes viewed as an overcompensation, means of disguising from self an unacceptable desire or drive by developing its exact opposite to an exaggerated degree
    b. example: wife angry at husband for attention he gives dog but reacts by being overly sweet

12. Regression
    a. definition: retreat to an earlier, less stressful time of development
    b. example: adult is faced with stress that cannot be tolerated and throws a tantrum

13. Repression
    a. definition: unconscious withholding of unpleasant thoughts, feelings, or experiences
    b. example: woman cannot remember name of demanding neighbor when she meets neighbor at market

14. Sublimation
    a. definition: substituting socially acceptable behavior for unacceptable or unattainable desire
    b. example: person channels his or her paternal or maternal feelings into caring and loving interest in plants or animals

15. Symbolization
    a. definition: representation of an internal feeling, wish, attitude, or idea through external object or quality (e.g., color)

b. example: diamond ring and its presentation symbolize love and commitment

16. Undoing
    a. definition: attempt to conceal negative action by other positive action
    b. example: father offers his son an allowance after punishing him

17. Conversion reaction
    a. definition: psychologic or emotional problems unconsciously cause physical symptoms
    b. example: person becomes blind after seeing a tragic accident

Crisis Intervention

Short-term therapy that focuses on solving immediate problem.

I. DEALING WITH LOSS (GRIEF AND GRIEVING)

A. Loss

1. Includes both physical and biologic loss; involves total human experiencing grieving process

B. Stages of Grief

1. Shock and disbelief
2. Development of awareness
3. Restitution
4. Resolution of loss

C. Grieving Process

1. Assessment
   a. assess for presence of psychologic symptoms, such as anger, guilt, or depression
   b. assess for presence of physiologic symptoms, such as insomnia, exhaustion, or digestive disturbances
   c. determine stage of grief process that client is experiencing
   d. observe for abnormal reactions to loss, such as absence of grieving or illness

2. Planning, goals, expected outcomes
   a. client is able to express feelings of loss openly
   b. client moves through stages of grieving process at own pace

3. Implementation
   a. encourage client to talk about loss
   b. explore what loss means to client
   c. find out how client feels about loss

    d. be aware of own feelings of sadness so that they do not get mixed up with client's feelings

    e. assist and support client through grief process

4. Evaluation

    a. client verbalized feelings about loss

    b. client accepted loss and found healing process helpful experience

II. CRISIS/CRISIS INTERVENTION

A. Assessment

1. Definition: response to situation perceived as threat or problem when usual problem-solving or decision-making methods no longer adequate; state of psychologic disequilibrium

2. Characteristics

    a. subjective, internal feeling

    b. usually self-limited

    c. may prove to be opportunity for personal growth if successfully resolved

    d. duration usually short, weeks to months

    e. client has high motivation for change because crisis intolerable

3. Types

    a. developmental crisis: results from predictable life change, such as graduation, starting school, starting work, marriage

    b. situational crisis: result of sudden, unanticipated change in life events, such as death, loss of job, natural disaster

4. Signs and symptoms

    a. fight-or-flight response

    b. difficulty thinking clearly

    c. severe anxiety or panic

    d. disorganized behavior

    e. energy directed toward relieving emotional distress

    f. avoids responsibility

    g. increased dependence on others

    h. unable to carry out activities of daily living

B. Planning, Goals, Expected Outcomes

1. Client seeks help to resolve crisis
2. Client returns to previous level of coping
3. Client has decreased level of stress
4. Client recovers without lasting psychologic problems

C. Implementation

1. Assess client's level of stress and coping
2. Encourage client to express emotional response
3. Explore meaning of crisis to client
4. Help client see that others have had similar experiences
5. Use problem-solving skills to help client develop new coping skills
6. Encourage client to use support systems
7. Reinforce use of new coping mechanisms
8. Provide anticipatory guidance

D. Evaluation

1. Patient sought help to resolve crisis
2. Patient returned to previous level of coping
3. Patient has decreased level of stress
4. Patient recovers without lasting psychologic problems

III. PERSON ABUSE (TRAUMA)

A. Spouse Abuse

1. Definition: deliberate and repeated physical or verbal assault on mate

2. Assessment

    a. beginning of violent behaviors

    b. types of violence and frequency

    c. coping techniques that spouse used to deal with violence

    d. resources available in community

    e. effects of violence on family

    f. assess background of abusive mate

    g. assess physical condition of abused mate

3. Planning, goals, expected outcomes

    a. client seeks professional help when violence occurs

    b. client explores alternative situations available to alter cycle of abuse

    c. client increases independent functioning, focusing on strengths and other roles available

4. Implementation

    a. provide safety for client and treat any existing physical injuries

    b. encourage client to get out of dangerous situations

    c. assist client with problem solving, allowing client to make own decisions

        (1) provide needed information on available resources

        (2) assist client, as needed, in initial contacts with resource agencies

    d. assist client in identifying personal strengths, resources, goals

        (1) support use of assertive skills

        (2) encourage client to join support group of

persons who have had similar experiences

5. Evaluation
   a. client used professional resources when abused
   b. client demonstrated decision-making skills and developed plan of action to break abuse cycle
   c. client secured employment and pursued additional vocational training to develop skills further
   d. client joined support group, if available

B. Child Abuse

1. Definition: physical, mental, or sexual assault on child; often occurs within family
2. Assessment
   a. physical condition of child: burns; bruises; abrasions; multiple, old, poorly healed fractures
   b. need for child to be removed from harmful situation
   c. assess behavior of child
      (1) relationship to parents; often seems closest to abusive parent
      (2) functioning at school
         (a) truancy
         (b) fatigue at school
      (3) somatic complaints
      (4) acting-out types of behavior: running away, promiscuity, hurting other children, destructive behaviors
   d. assess behavior of parents
      (1) anger or contradictions in discussing child's injury
      (2) deny involvement in child's injury
      (3) elaborate stories about child's "clumsiness" and how child hurt self
      (4) parents who were abused as children are more likely to abuse their own children
3. Planning, goals, expected outcomes
   a. child is protected from further harm; if necessary, is removed from home
   b. child's physical condition is stabilized, as evidenced by relief of discomfort
   c. child's parents become involved in ongoing treatment program
   d. child's family uses effective problem-solving techniques, providing safe environment for child
4. Implementation
   a. provide protection for child; follow procedure for reporting suspicions of child abuse to proper authorities
   b. provide care for child's injury

c. inform child's parents of resources available, such as Parents Anonymous and parenting classes
   d. support child's family in their use of effective problem-solving techniques to deal with their feelings; use positive reinforcement
5. Evaluation
   a. abused child now in safe environment as determined by legal authorities and demonstrated by more positive behaviors
   b. abused child's physical condition stabilized
   c. child's parents participated in treatment groups and applied positive parenting skills
   d. child's family demonstrated use of effective problem-solving skills in dealing with their anger and frustrations

C. Sexual Abuse

1. Definition: involves sex acts without consent of victim except for child who may be too young to give consent or understand actions
2. Assessment
   a. assess emotional status of client: fear, shame, anger, suspiciousness, panic
   b. assess clients who come in with vague problems; be suspicious of abuse
   c. with children, assess for suspicious signs, such as rectal pain, itching, or bleeding; unexplained bruises; bladder infections; edema around rectum or genitalia
3. Planning, goals, expected outcomes
   a. client is able to give accurate and complete information about sexual assault
   b. client's physical condition is stabilized
   c. client's emotional state is improved, as evidenced by decrease of fear, panic, anger, and shame
   d. client participates in support groups, counseling, and legal proceedings, if necessary
   e. child is removed from abusive situation
4. Implementation
   a. note date and time of assault and what measures client took before examination
   b. assist with physical examination of client
   c. label all specimens and chart clearly; may be part of legal proceeding
   d. identify resources that client has for support
   e. encourage client to use services, such as Rape Crisis Centers, emergency shelters, and so on
   f. care of physical injuries and follow through with laboratory tests ordered
   g. communicate caring and concerned attitude; encourage client to talk about sexual assault and feelings associated with it

h. contact social services for abused children who may need to be removed from dangerous situation

5. Evaluation
   a. client gave accurate and complete information about sexual assault
   b. client recovered from any physical injuries related to sexual assault
   c. client verbalized feelings associated with sexual assault
   d. client participated in support groups and other follow-up treatment, if necessary
   e. child removed from abusive situation

D. Elder Abuse

1. Definition: includes acts of physical, mental, sexual, material (including financial) abuse, and violation of rights of older person, usually age 65 years or older
2. Assessment
   a. assess needs of client being abused: physical, emotional, or material
   b. determine if client is aware of alternatives to remaining in abusive situation
   c. assess if client is fearful of abusive situation or is unaware of being abused
   d. note physical or emotional disability of client
3. Planning, goals, expected outcomes
   a. client is protected from physical, emotional, or material abuse
   b. client is aware of support systems for dealing with abusive situations
   c. client verbalizes fears of being harmed and talks about abusive situation
   d. client increases independent functioning within physical and emotional capabilities
4. Implementation
   a. care for physical injuries, if present
   b. provide for alternate living arrangements for client to avoid fear of abuse
   c. discuss abusive situation(s) with client and encourage client to express fears
   d. encourage client to use strengths to explore activities to provide interest outside self
5. Evaluation
   a. abuse of client ceased
   b. client identified available options other than remaining in abusive situation
   c. client verbalized feelings about abusive situation
   d. client made decisions about life according to ability, so that client's rights were respected

Substance Abuse and Dependence

I. ABUSE AND DEPENDENCE

A. Definitions

1. Substance abuse: pathologic use of substance, although individual aware of harm to self
   a. category includes substances that alter mood or depress or stimulate central nervous system and substances that are abused or that cause dependence
   b. repeated use results in problems with interpersonal relationships, job functioning, poor judgment and impulse control, changes in behavior, and, for some, involvement in criminal activity
   c. abusing individual deteriorates in both physical and psychologic functioning
2. Substance dependence: user experiences physiologic and often psychologic dependence, evidenced by tolerance or withdrawal
   a. tolerance: increasing amounts of drugs needed to achieve desired effect
   b. withdrawal: syndrome experienced by user when amount of drug decreased or discontinued; course of withdrawal varies depending on drug

B. Classes of Substances Associated with Both Abuse and Dependence

1. Alcohol: abrupt withdrawal can result in death
2. Barbiturates (plus antianxiety agents and sedative-hypnotic drugs, all central nervous system depressants)
   a. withdrawal or overdose: medical emergency
   b. abrupt withdrawal without detoxification can result in death
3. Opiates (including opium, morphine, codeine, heroin, hydromorphone [Dilaudid], oxycodone [Percodan], and meperidine [Demerol])
   a. risks for intravenous addicts include hepatitis, overdose, acquired immunodeficiency syndrome (AIDS), and infection
   b. overdose: medical emergency, often fatal
4. Amphetamines (includes benzphetamine, and dextroamphetamine [Dexedrine, Biphetamine], central nervous system stimulants)
   a. risk of amphetamine psychosis (mimics paranoid schizophrenia)
   b. medical complaints: cardiac arrhythmias, hyperthermia, hypertension, and malnutrition
   c. withdrawal: depression, fatigue, disturbed sleep, and potential suicide risk
5. Cannabis (includes marijuana, hashish, hash oil, dope, grass, joint, reefer, roach, weed)

a. intoxication can lead to bizarre, aggressive behavior
b. harmful changes in respiratory, reproductive, and nervous systems

C. Classes of Substances Associated with Abuse Only

1. Cocaine, coke, snow, blow, crack
   a. total preoccupation with drug
   b. reluctant to give it up
   c. stimulant
   d. usually no physical withdrawal symptoms, but produces psychologic dependence
2. PCP (phencyclidine, angel dust, crystal dust, KJ killer, peace pill)
   a. hallucinogenic and central nervous system depressant effect
   b. central nervous system depression in high-dose intoxication; can lead to coma and death
   c. violent outbursts and psychosis
3. Hallucinogens (peyote, magic mushrooms, psilocybin, psilocin, LSD—acid, micro-dots, window pane, purple haze, barrels, blotters, ant domes)
   a. sensory illusions
   b. hallucinations and delusions rare

D. Class of Substance Associated with Dependence Only: Tobacco

1. Nicotine: an alkaloid found in tobacco
   a. rapidly absorbed by the lungs
   b. mild central stimulatory effect
   c. decreased skeletal muscle tone, reduced appetite, occasional nausea, vomiting, dizziness, and irritability
   d. withdrawal: nausea, diarrhea, increased appetite, headache, drowsiness, insomnia, irritability, and poor concentration
2. Risk factors associated with cigarette smoking: bronchogenic carcinoma, coronary artery disease, emphysema, and chronic pulmonary disease
3. Abrupt withdrawal more effective

E. Behavior Patterns Related to Other Substance Abuse or Dependence

1. As with alcohol abuse, all assessment, planning, goals, expected outcomes, implementation, and evaluation relate to:
   a. pattern of pathologic use, how much, and how often
   b. problems in social or occupational functioning caused by drug abuse

c. length of time pathologic use of drug has created problems with social or occupational functioning
   d. history of withdrawal symptoms (limited to drugs that cause physical dependence)
   e. history of drug-related medical complications
2. All abused substances require client to go through stages similar to those with alcohol (detoxification, rehabilitation, and follow-up)

II. CESSATION OF USE

A. Behavior Pattern Related to Use of Alcohol (Detoxification)

1. Assessment
   a. symptoms of alcohol withdrawal: coarse tremors of hands, tongue, and eyelids; nausea and vomiting; malaise; tachycardia; diaphoresis; hypertension; anxiety; depressed mood; irritability; orthostatic hypotension; grand mal seizures may occur
   b. alcohol withdrawal delirium (delirium tremens): symptoms of delirium plus tachycardia, diaphoresis, and hypertension; also, delusions, vivid visual hallucinations, and agitated behavior
   c. hydration
   d. nutritional intake
   e. signs of physical illness
   f. liver function
2. Planning, goals, expected outcomes
   a. client improves physically and is able to care for self in 1 to 3 days
   b. client does not suffer injury during withdrawal
3. Implementation
   a. close observation of symptoms for 1 to 3 days
   b. position on side to prevent aspiration from possible vomiting; reposition frequently
   c. visual check of client every 15 minutes, especially restrained client; monitor for signs of impending delirium tremens
   d. monitor and record vital signs every 2 hours for first 12 hours, then four times per day for next 3 days (unless abnormal), and every day for next 4 days
   e. administer medications as ordered for one or more of following symptoms
      (1) elevated blood pressure (i.e., above 140/90)
      (2) elevated pulse (i.e., above 90)
      (3) diaphoresis
      (4) hallucinations
      (5) seizures or history of seizures during withdrawal
      (6) agitation

f. administer intravenous fluids with B vitamins as ordered

g. check vital signs every 2 hours after each dose of medication given

h. contact physician for further direction if vital signs do not stabilize after usual dose of medication

i. reorient client as needed

j. offer cup of juice every hour

4. Evaluation

a. client moved through detoxification without developing symptoms of end-stage alcohol withdrawal delirium (delirium tremens): convulsions, coma, and death

b. client able to care for self in 1 to 3 days after withdrawal

B. Behavior Pattern Related to Use of Alcohol (Rehabilitation)

1. Assessment

a. use of denial as coping or mental mechanism

b. willingness to participate in developing personal goal

c. willingness to participate in structured daily activities

d. willingness to participate in planned therapeutic activities

2. Planning, goals, expected outcomes

a. client moves through denial phase

b. client learns alternate ways of dealing with stress other than alcohol, ways that produce "natural highs," such as running, meditation, and swimming

3. Implementation

a. involve client in developing own plan of care so that client assumes responsibility and accountability for own care

b. structure daily living and leisure activities; provide consistency

(1) set and maintain limits; minimize manipulative behavior

(2) provide various group experiences: alcohol education, Alcoholics Anonymous (AA) lessons and meetings, work opportunities, social interactions, family sessions, gripe sessions, values clarification sessions, relaxation techniques, nutritional groups, leisure counseling, job interviews, and community living skills

4. Evaluation

a. client admitted inability to control own drinking

b. client involves self in ways of dealing with stress other than alcohol

C. Behavior Pattern Related to Use of Alcohol (Follow-up Care)

1. Assessment: support systems needed by client to maintain sobriety

2. Planning, goals, expected outcomes: client maintains sobriety in home and work setting on continuing basis with help of support systems

3. Implementation

a. attend weekly community AA meetings with other clients and staff before discharge

b. attend closed AA meetings after discharge, starting with day of discharge

c. continue weekly counseling sessions with family members

d. encourage continuation of hobbies and recreational activities that client participated in during inpatient stay

e. practice relaxation techniques daily to lower anxiety level

f. administer tranquilizers (see Table 10–5) as ordered

(1) chemical taken daily to discourage client from drinking

(2) disulfiram (Antabuse) plus alcohol results in violent physical reaction

4. Evaluation: after discharge, client maintained sobriety in home and work settings on continuing basis with help from support systems

Eating Disorders

I. BULIMIA

A. Assessment

1. Definition: pathologic process of binge eating (rapid eating of large amount of food) followed by self-induced vomiting; may be affective disorder

2. Incidence

a. most common in white women who are of average weight or slightly overweight

b. single, late teens to early 20s

3. Signs and symptoms

a. many have symptoms of depression and decreased self-worth

b. overeating and purging usually secretive, solitary events

c. binging may occur daily or weekly

d. binge lasts between 1 and 2 hours—can eat 3000 to 4000 calories before vomiting

e. dental erosion from gastric acid, parotid swelling, stomach ulcers, sore throats

f. low serum potassium, arrhythmias, cardiac arrest may occur

g. feelings of guilt, shame, and self-loathing

h. fear of loss of control and not being able to stop eating

B. Planning, goals, expected outcomes

1. Client verbalizes increased sense of self-esteem
2. Client identifies other ways to deal with stress rather than eating
3. Client begins to eat more appropriately

C. Implementation

1. Administer antidepressant (especially monoamine oxidase inhibitors) as ordered
2. Help client make appropriate food choices
3. Help client find other ways of dealing with stress rather than eating behavior
4. Set limits on client's eating behavior
5. Refer client to Overeaters Anonymous as a source of support
6. Weigh client as ordered and make sure he or she eats with others in dining room

D. Evaluation

1. Client verbalized increased sense of self-esteem
2. Client identified other ways to deal with stress rather than eating
3. Client began to eat more appropriately

II. ANOREXIA NERVOSA

A. Assessment

1. Definition: weight loss of at least 25% of original body weight without physical illness; intense fear of becoming obese with compulsive resistance to eating
2. Incidence
   a. female predominantly
   b. increasing incidence in United States
3. Signs and symptoms
   a. resistance to help
   b. denies that problem exists
   c. feelings of loneliness and isolation, unable to accept nurturance
   d. perfectionist, hard working, and tries to please others
   e. weight loss
   f. amenorrhea
   g. slowing of body functions such as bradycardia, hypotension, constipation, hypothermia
   h. leukopenia, hypoglycemia
   i. reduced metabolism and hormonal function
   j. may die from malnutrition or suicide

B. Planning, Goals, Expected Outcomes

1. Client has nutritional intake improved
2. Client establishes more adequate eating pattern
3. Client participates in care
4. Client possesses more realistic body image
5. Client gains weight

C. Implementation

1. May need to be hospitalized for intravenous or oral feedings
2. Provide for caring and nurturance when possible
3. Use empathic listening
4. Use limit setting to help client gain weight
5. Use behavior modification techniques to help client gain weight
6. Watch client closely during meals to be sure all food eaten and not purged
7. Weigh at least three times a week
8. Provide good skin care
9. Encourage client to discuss feelings appropriately

D. Evaluation

1. Client had nutritional intake improved
2. Client established more adequate eating pattern
3. Client participated in care
4. Client possessed more realistic body image
5. Client gained weight

❓UESTIONS

1. What is the coping or mental mechanism used by someone who experiences many aggressive fantasies and channels these feelings into playing football?

   ① Identification
   ② Sublimation
   ③ Reaction formation
   ④ Projection

2. A 38-year-old man is experiencing his fourth admission to the chemical dependency unit. He has signed himself out before completing the treatment program during each of his other admissions. He has insisted that it is his wife who causes him to drink because of her behavior. This time she has threatened to follow through with a divorce if he does not complete the program; she is tired of being abused by him. On this admission, he is actively involved in treatment, which is based on the Alcoholics Anonymous format. What is his major coping or mental mechanism?

   ① Regression
   ② Denial
   ③ Reaction formation
   ④ Undoing

3. Why are fluids increased during detoxification?

   ① They wash the alcohol from the body
   ② Alcohol has a diuretic effect
   ③ They counteract the constipating effect
   ④ It is a way of preventing cirrhosis

4. What are clinical manifestations of alcohol withdrawal delirium (delirium tremens)?

   ① Elevated temperature, catatonia, convulsions, tremors
   ② Decreased vital signs, increased agitation, hallucinations
   ③ Hypertension, diaphoresis, tachycardia, delusions
   ④ Hypotension, psychomotor retardation, visual hallucinations

5. Which classification of medication is useful in controlling alcohol withdrawal delirium manifestations?

   ① Antipsychotic
   ② Antianxiety
   ③ Antidepressant
   ④ Antimanic

6. What problem will you anticipate when working with a client suffering from long-term alcohol abuse?

   ① Orienting the client
   ② Controlling depression
   ③ Managing guilt
   ④ Setting limits

7. What disease directly related to alcohol consumption can be treated by thiamine?

   ① Wernicke's
   ② Alzheimer's
   ③ Pick's
   ④ Subdural hematoma

8. Why is work therapy a part of psychiatric care, especially associated with substance abuse?

   ① Helps pay for hospitalization fees
   ② Provides a setting for adjusting medications
   ③ Provides for a sense of self-worth
   ④ Keeps the client from focusing on own problems

9. Which of the following is appropriate occupational therapy for the client with alcoholism?

   ① Noncompetitive, solitary, meaningful tasks
   ② Group activities that use the client's talents
   ③ Simple, concrete, repetitive tasks
   ④ Activities that take concentration

10. What option is available to the wife of an alcoholic to deal with feelings about being abused?

    ① Focus on her husband; he needs her, and it is her duty to stand by her man.
    ② Focus on the children; her husband is her only means of support for the children.
    ③ Focus on herself; getting help for herself will influence her husband's behavior.
    ④ Focus on their marriage; he really loves her, because he is so considerate when sober.

11. Which of the following is an essential tool to teach the client in doing crisis intervention?

    ① Giving advice
    ② Interpreting behavior
    ③ Problem solving
    ④ Anticipatory grieving

12. Abrupt withdrawal from which of the following drugs can lead to death?

① Heroin
② Cocaine
③ Barbiturates
④ Morphine

13. Developing trust and cooperation results from:

① Alleviating fears by joking about client's concerns
② Selecting the diet for the client, to eliminate unnecessary decisions
③ Giving involved nursing care until discharge
④ Involving the clients in meeting their own needs

ANSWERS AND RATIONALES

Guide to item identification (see pp. 4–5 for further details about each category):

    I, II, III, or IV for the phase of the nursing process

    1, 2, 3, or 4 for the category of client needs

    A, B, C, D, E, F, or G for the category of human functioning

    Specific content category by name; i.e., cholecystectomy

1. ② The behavior described is sublimation, which is taking an unacceptable behavior and changing it into a socially acceptable behavior.
IV, 3, G, Coping

2. ② Clients suffering from alcohol abuse use denial to perpetuate a continuous cycle of low self-concept, guilt over behavior connected with drinking, and drinking again to deal with feelings of guilt.
IV, 3, G, Alcoholism

3. ② Alcohol exerts a diuretic effect on the body so adequate hydration is important when dealing with the alcoholic client.
III, 3, F & G, Alcoholism

4. ③ The major manifestations of alcohol withdrawal delirium are tachycardia, diaphoresis, hypertension, and delirium. Other manifestations that usually occur include delusions; vivid, visual hallucinations, and agitation.
I, 3, G, Alcoholism

5. ② Antianxiety agents also have an anticonvulsive action and are useful during alcohol detoxification in preventing or decreasing the intensity of end-stage withdrawal symptoms.
I & III, 3, G, Alcoholism

6. ④ When working with a client suffering from alcohol abuse, it is important to set and maintain limits to minimize manipulative behavior.
III, 3, G, Alcoholism

7. ① Wernicke's disease is a neurologic disease manifested by confusion, ataxia, eye movement abnormalities, and other neurologic symptoms. If Wernicke's disease is treated early with large doses of thiamine, alcohol amnestic disorder may not develop.
IV, 3, C & G, Alcoholism

8. ③ When clients take part in work therapy, the result is productivity, and productivity conveys a sense of self-worth and self-dignity to the clients.
III, 3, G, Alcoholism

9. ② The client suffering from alcohol abuse can work with group activities in which the client uses talents and assets. For example, involve client in planning social activities; encourage interaction with others.
III, 3, G, Alcoholism

10. ③ There is a need to get in touch with personal feelings and to understand the reaction to those feelings and how they influence others' behavior.
II, 3, G, Alcoholism

11. ③ Learning the problem-solving process provides people with a conscious growth-producing method of dealing with stressful situations. By confronting the felt anxiety, the person is able to move through the stressful situation.
III, 3, G, Crisis intervention

12. ③ In severe cases, coma and death occur
IV, 3, G, Addictive behaviors

13. ④ Encouraging clients to take responsibility for as many aspects of their own care as possible proves genuine interest on the part of the nurse and results in trust and cooperation from clients.
III, 1, G, Mental health

BIBLIOGRAPHY

Arnold, E., & Boggs, K.U. (1995). *Interpersonal relationships: Professional communication skills for nurses,* 2nd ed. Philadelphia: W.B. Saunders Co.

Bauer, B., & Hill, S. (1986). *Essentials of mental health care: Planning and interventions.* Philadelphia: W.B. Saunders Co.

Betz, C.L., Hunsberger, M., & Wright, S. (1994). *Family-centered nursing care of children,* 2nd ed. Philadelphia: W.B. Saunders Co.

Bolander, V.R. (1994). *Sorensen and Luckmann's basic nursing: A psychophysiologic approach,* 3rd ed. Philadelphia: W.B. Saunders Co.

Cook, J.S., & Fonntaine, K.L. (1991). *Essentials of mental health nursing,* 2nd ed. Redwood City, CA: Addison-Wesley.

Davis, J., & Sherer, K. (1994). *Applied nutrition and diet therapy for nurses,* 2nd ed. Philadelphia: W.B. Saunders Co.

Fortinash, K.M., & Holoday, P.A. (1991). *Psychiatric nursing care plans.* St. Louis: Mosby–Year Book.

Lehne, R.A., Moore, L., Crosby, L., & Hamilton, D. (1994). *Pharmacology for nursing care,* 2nd ed. Philadelphia: W.B. Saunders Co.

Linton, A.D., Matteson, M.A., & Maebius, N.K. (1995). *Introductory nursing care of adults.* Philadelphia: W.B. Saunders Co.

Matassarin-Jacobs, E. (1994). *Saunders review for NCLEX-RN,* 2nd ed. Philadelphia: W.B. Saunders Co.

Varcarolis, E.M. (1994). *Foundations of psychiatric mental health nursing,* 2nd ed. Philadelphia: W.B. Saunders Co.

Wilson, H.S., & Kneisel, C.R. (1992). *Psychiatric nursing,* 2nd ed. Redwood City, CA: Addison-Wesley.

PRACTICE TEST 2

QUESTIONS

1. The nurse would expect the client with hypertension to be prescribed a diet low in:

   ① Potassium
   ② Magnesium
   ③ Sodium
   ④ Folic acid

2. Which of the following actions by the nurse would be *most appropriate* to encourage a pediatric client to eat meals while hospitalized?

   ① Provide a nutritious meal regardless of the child's food preferences
   ② Provide a dessert as an incentive to eat
   ③ Insist that the child eat everything on the tray
   ④ Avoid painful or upsetting procedures immediately before mealtime

3. The nurse would expect a protein-restricted diet to be prescribed for the client with which of the following conditions?

   ① Hepatic coma
   ② Gallbladder disease
   ③ Iron deficiency anemia
   ④ Alcoholism

4. Which of the following nutrient deficiencies would the nurse be alert for in the client with lactose intolerance?

   ① Iron
   ② Calcium
   ③ Potassium
   ④ Sodium

5. Which of the following interventions would the nurse include in the care plan for a client experiencing the "dumping syndrome"?

   ① Provide 1 to 2 glasses of water with meals
   ② Increase fluids to prevent constipation
   ③ Limit fluids between meals
   ④ Limit fluids during mealtimes

6. To increase absorption, the nurse should administer iron with which of the following fluids?

   ① Water
   ② Orange juice
   ③ A carbonated beverage
   ④ Milk

7. Ms. Martin is experiencing tetany. The nurse monitors for low blood levels of:

   ① Iron
   ② Calcium
   ③ Potassium
   ④ Zinc

8. For a diagnosis of pernicious anemia, the nurse would *most likely* be prepared to administer:

   ① Injections of vitamin K
   ② Vitamin B complex orally
   ③ Injections of vitamin B_{12}
   ④ Injections of iron

9. Which of the following foods would the nurse include when teaching the client about good sources of vitamin A?

   ① Lettuce, corn, and vegetable oils
   ② Dark green or deep yellow vegetables
   ③ Citrus fruits and watermelon
   ④ Apples, cranberries, and bananas

10. A 76-year-old client who had surgery for a fractured hip will be discharged soon. Which of the following would be the *greatest* safety hazard in the home environment?

    ① A 6-year-old poodle
    ② Scatter rugs
    ③ Snack tables
    ④ A recliner

11. Constipation is a common complaint of the elderly. An appropriate nursing intervention to suggest to the elderly client is:

    ① Use enemas frequently
    ② Use stool softeners daily
    ③ Add prunes or bran cereal to the diet
    ④ Take milk of magnesia before bed

12. A nurse working with geriatric clients should understand that older people are most frequently abused by a:

    ① Health care worker in a nursing home
    ② Sibling living in the elder's home
    ③ Family member providing care at home
    ④ Home health aide providing home care

13. The profile of the older adult most at risk for abuse is:

   ① A 68-year-old man living in an apartment
   ② A disabled woman, aged 79, living with relatives
   ③ An 81-year-old man living in a congregate housing arrangement
   ④ A woman, aged 85, living with her spouse in a mobile home park

14. A middle-aged worker sustained thoracic injuries. Assessment reveals asymmetric chest movement, dyspnea, and absent breath sounds to the lower right lung lobe. The physician suspects a hemopneumothorax. The nurse should anticipate management to include:

   ① Setup of underwater drainage system to assist with decompression of the lung
   ② Preparation of the client for a thoracotomy
   ③ Setup for pneumonectomy
   ④ Setup for a thoracentesis procedure

15. A client with a diagnosis of asthma is admitted to the hospital with bronchospasms. The physician orders aminophylline to be administered slowly, intravenously. A common adverse reaction associated with this medication is:

   ① Gingival hyperplasia
   ② Hypotension
   ③ Tinnitus
   ④ Rainbow halos around lights

16. A 66-year-old client suspected of having an abdominal aortic aneurysm is admitted to your unit. The physician orders a test to help determine the extent of the aneurysm and its relation to arterial branches and organs. The nurse should plan to provide client teaching about:

   ① Aortic angiography
   ② Computed tomography (CT)
   ③ Magnetic resonance imaging (MRI)
   ④ Positron emission tomography (PET)

17. A man is admitted with possible skull fracture and cerebrospinal fluid leak. Which of the following should the nurse institute *immediately*?

   ① Elevate the head of the bed
   ② Assess and record vital signs, watching closely for a drop in blood pressure
   ③ Have the client blow his nose and test the nasal drainage for glucose presence
   ④ Obtain an order for antibiotic therapy

18. An elderly woman is admitted for hypokalemia. Which of the following would be the nurse's *primary* concern in the assessment of this client?

   ① Hyperthermia
   ② Cardiac dysrhythmias
   ③ Seizures
   ④ Hypotension

19. A 16-year-old insulin-dependent diabetic client is admitted with a diagnosis of ketoacidosis. Which of the following changes is the nurse likely to see while assessing this client?

   ① Slow, shallow respirations with possible apnea
   ② Flushed cheeks and dry mucous membranes
   ③ A widening pulse pressure
   ④ An elevated serum potassium level

20. For a client with Raynaud's disease, which of the following care instructions is *inappropriate*?

   ① Avoiding over-the-counter nasal decongestant cold remedies
   ② Warming a client's hands in warm water
   ③ Elevating the extremities above the heart to promote venous return and prevent swelling
   ④ Wearing warm gloves during cold weather

21. The client you are caring for has just had a tympanoplasty. He is to be released today. Before discharge, he asks you about activity limitations. Which of the following, if planned within the next 2 weeks, is contraindicated?

   ① Warm, relaxing bubble baths
   ② Plans to fly to an annual marketing convention
   ③ An hour nap at least once a day
   ④ Plans to have his wife assist him in getting out of bed

22. A middle-aged man is admitted for diagnostic workup. Test results indicate he has acquired immunodeficiency syndrome (AIDS). He states he has had a relationship with Marcus for 5 years. The client asks the nurse whether he should tell Marcus that he has AIDS. The nurse's best response would be:

   ① "Do you think you contracted AIDS from Marcus?"
   ② "What do you think you should do?"
   ③ "No, I don't think you should tell him."
   ④ "Perhaps you should discuss this with your physician."

23. A 60-year-old woman was admitted after an acute myocardial infarction. Her blood pressure has been unstable, and the physician suspects that she may go into cardiogenic shock. Which of the following would be the most *appropriate* intervention for the nurse to take?

① Elevate the head of the bed to facilitate expansion
② Increase the intravenous nitroglycerine drip rate to prevent onset of chest pain
③ Place the client in Trendelenburg position
④ Lower the head of the bed and elevate the client's lower extremities

24. The client you are caring for is an elderly man admitted following persistent bouts of diarrhea. Which of the following physician orders should the nurse question?

① Collection of a stool specimen
② Administration of *Lactobacillus acidophilus* capsules
③ Administration of lactulose (Cephulac)
④ Administration of intravenous vitamin supplement

25. The client you are caring for is to have a Miller-Abbott tube inserted. The nurse explains that the purpose of this tube is to:

① Examine the upper esophagus
② Examine the sigmoid and descending colon
③ Decompress the stomach
④ Assist in decompressing and correcting intestinal obstruction

26. The client you are caring for has a diagnosis of chronic myelocytic leukemia. He is to undergo a course of chemotherapy. Which of the following interventions would be *inappropriate* in his care?

① Offering small, frequent feedings of bland foods in an effort to meet nutritional needs
② Encouraging a high fluid intake to prevent crystallization of uric acid during chemotherapy
③ Administering aspirin for joint and body aches
④ Monitoring of vital signs every 4 hours for elevated temperature throughout his hospital stay

27. The nurse reviews the plan of care for a premature infant and notes that feedings are scheduled every 2 hours, with the amount not to exceed 5 mL at any one time. It is particularly important that the premature infant not be overfed because:

① Calorie requirements are low
② Overfeeding may cause abdominal distention and may compromise respiratory status
③ The gastrointestinal system absorbs nutrients erratically
④ The majority of nutrients should be given intravenously

28. The nurse is assisting with the care of the newborn immediately after delivery. The mouth and then the nose are gently suctioned with a bulb aspirator. This action is done to meet which of the primary needs of the neonate?

① Assessment of cranium
② Establishment of respiration
③ Protection from infection
④ Thermoregulation

29. A 25-year old single woman is planning to give up her baby for adoption. Before the birth, she had insisted that she did not want to see the child. Now she is requesting to visit and hold the baby for a little while. The *best* response by the nurse is:

① "Maybe you should wait until tomorrow, because you might change your mind again."
② "If you see the baby, it is just going to be harder for you to deal with."
③ "I will notify the nursery of your request. Would it be helpful for me to accompany you?"
④ "First I must check with your physician. We need her authorization before you can see the baby."

30. The nurse assists in collecting information for the history of a pregnant woman at a prenatal clinic. The nurse recognizes that obtaining an accurate history is an important part of prenatal care because this assessment enables the health care provider to:

① Assess reproductive risk and anticipate the special needs of the client
② Control the outcome of the pregnancy
③ Determine whether prenatal visits are necessary
④ Recognize the discomforts of pregnancy the client is likely to experience

31. A 28-year-old gravida 2 with type I diabetes mellitus whose first baby was stillborn is at the prenatal clinic for a check-up at 28 weeks' gestation. Which of the following topics would be a *priority* for the nurse to discuss with this client?

① The high probability that she will experience a cesarean birth
② The importance of a vigorous exercise program for fetal well-being
③ The necessity of reducing calories and fat in the diet
④ The need for increased frequency of prenatal visits and daily fetal movement counts

32. In the care of a client with hyperthyroidism, the nurse takes measures to provide for:

① A restful, cool environment
② A stimulating, warm environment
③ An increase in the metabolic rate
④ Vigorous exercise and relief of constipation

33. The nurse teaches a client how to move to a sitting position after a thyroidectomy by supporting her head with her hands. The rationale for this instruction is to:

① Decrease laryngeal edema and stridor
② Help relieve the symptoms of tetany
③ Minimize strain to neck muscles and the surgical incision
④ Prevent damage to the recurrent laryngeal nerve

34. When developing a care plan for a client with Cushing's syndrome, the nurse includes the diagnosis:

① Altered nutrition: Less than body requirements related to anorexia and nausea
② Fluid volume deficit related to hyponatremia
③ Risk for injury related to osteoporosis and muscle wasting
④ Ineffective airway clearance related to laryngeal spasm

35. When anticoagulant therapy is begun, heparin is administered in conjunction with warfarin (Coumadin) because:

① Heparin has a rapid peak action and a short duration of 6 hours
② Coumadin has a rapid peak and a short duration of 6 hours

③ Heparin has a long peak and a long duration of 2 to 3 days
④ Coumadin has a rapid onset and a long duration of 3 to 5 days

36. When teaching a client about the action of amantadine (Symmetrel), the nurse explains it is:

① To relieve the drooling and difficulty swallowing with myasthenia gravis
② A preoperative relaxation for muscles
③ To relieve muscle rigidity and bradykinesia in Parkinson's disease
④ To relieve muscle spasm in low back injury

37. Side effects of haloperidol (Haldol) include:

① Extrapyramidal reactions and tardive dyskinesia
② Hypertension
③ Diarrhea
④ Nervousness

38. Client teaching for amitriptyline (Elavil) does not include the following measures:

① Avoiding alcohol and central nervous system depressants
② Making position changes slowly
③ Decreasing fluid intake
④ Rinsing mouth frequently and using hard candy

39. Which of the following evaluation criteria indicate that ciprofloxacin (Cipro) is effective?

① Tympanic temperature 99.60° F
② White blood cell count is 8000/mm³
③ Large amount of purulent wound drainage
④ Skin warm, red, and edematous at the wound site

40. During administration of prednisone, which assessment would be *inappropriate*?

① Assessing for hyperglycemia
② Assessing for thin skin and skin tears
③ Assessing for fluid deficit because of steroid therapy
④ Assessing for increased ecchymosis

41. When teaching a client taking an antianemic agent, ferrous sulfate, which of the following side effects would be *incorrect* to include?

① Constipation
② Staining of teeth
③ Abdominal cramps
④ Clay-colored stools

42. Which of the following drugs is *not* an antiarrhythmic?

① Procainamide (Pronestyl)
② Diltiazem (Cardizem)
③ Nifedipine (Procardia)
④ Isosorbide dinitrate (Isordil)

43. When giving client instructions on potassium chloride 20 mEq b.i.d., the nurse states that it is best taken:

① On an empty stomach
② With antacids
③ With breakfast and supper
④ One hour after meals

44. The best time to administer prazosin hydrochloride (Minipress) 1 mg orally daily, is:

① Early in the day
② With the noon meal
③ In mid afternoon
④ At bedtime

45. A client exhibits extreme fatigue, muscle weakness, and an irregular pulse at 45; blood pressure is 90/50. The client is taking digoxin, 0.25 mg, and furosemide (Lasix), 20 mg/day. What would the nurse suspect is the cause?

① Hyperkalemia
② Hypokalemia
③ Hypocalcemia
④ Hypercalcemia

46. On the third day of administration of amoxicillin (Amoxil), the client complains of a rash and itchiness. This would indicate a:

① Hypersensitivity
② Potentiation reaction
③ Idiosyncratic reaction
④ Toxic effect

47. Ototoxicity may occur with gentamicin (Garamycin). Symptoms of this adverse reaction include:

① Increased nasal drainage
② Dizziness, nausea, difficulty in swallowing
③ Tinnitus, mild-to-severe hearing loss
④ Dyspnea, hives, swelling in throat

48. The classification of glycopyrrolate (Robinul) is:

① Cholinergic blocker or anticholinergic
② Cholinergic

③ Narcotic antagonist
④ Adrenergic blocker

49. The health care the client receives during her pregnancy is called:

① Postpartal care
② Antepartal care
③ Parapartal care
④ Intrapartal care

50. To ensure adequate medical supervision during pregnancy, the client should visit her physician at least:

① Every 2 weeks until the seventh month, then every week until the baby is born
② Every 2 months until the seventh month, then every month until the baby is born
③ Every month until the eighth month, then every 2 weeks until the baby is born
④ Every month until the seventh month, then every 2 weeks until the last month, and then every week until the baby is born

51. Which of these vitamins is obtained by the breast-fed infant through the colostrum and breast milk?

① A
② C
③ D
④ E

52. An *inappropriate* wardrobe choice for the pregnant client would be a:

① Girdle
② Tent dress
③ Bra with wide straps
④ Pair of maternity pantyhose

53. One of the best exercises for the pregnant client is:

① Jogging
② Swimming
③ Brisk walking
④ Playing tennis

54. Which of the following is an *inappropriate* reason for a physician to advise against sexual intercourse during the last month of pregnancy?

① To lessen the possibility of abortion
② To lessen the danger of causing infection
③ To lessen the danger of rupturing membranes
④ To lessen the possibility of starting labor prematurely

55. An *inappropriate* way for a nurse to show concern for the pregnant client's feelings is to:

   ① Provide privacy
   ② Explain procedures
   ③ Avoid unnecessary exposure of her body
   ④ Leave the room while the physician examines her

56. While assisting the physician during an examination, the nurse can *best* help the pregnant client to relax by:

   ① Telling her to relax
   ② Holding her hand and telling her to lift her back off the table
   ③ Telling her to hold her breath and to lift her back off the table
   ④ Telling her to breathe normally and to keep her back flat against the table

57. Labor clients needing the *most* emotional support by the nurse would be those who:

   ① Have had previous positive labor experiences
   ② Have obtained information about childbirth from reading
   ③ Have consistently practiced relaxation and breathing techniques
   ④ Are laboring alone or have had an unhappy experience with a previous labor

58. At which of the following centimeters of dilation would the client receive the *most* benefit from pain medication?

   ① 3 to 4
   ② 4 to 5
   ③ 8 to 9
   ④ 9 to 10

59. If RhoGAM is indicated for the Rh-sensitized mother, it should be administered within how many hours of delivery to be effective?

   ① 10
   ② 52
   ③ 72
   ④ 92

60. The nurse is assigned to a client in the prenatal clinic who is in premature labor. Which of the following medications would be given to accelerate fetal lung maturation?

   ① Ritodrine (Yutopar)
   ② Acetaminophen (Tylenol)
   ③ Diazepam
   ④ Betamethasone

61. The nurse is caring for a 1-day postpartum client. Which of the following medications would be given to suppress lactation?

   ① Chlorotrianisene (Tace)
   ② Clomiphene citrate (Clomid)
   ③ Ritodrine (Yutopar)
   ④ Hydromorphone (Dilaudid)

62. The main action of oral contraceptives is to:

   ① Cause abortion
   ② Develop the follicle
   ③ Inhibit ovulation
   ④ Prevent menstruation

63. The first substance secreted from the breast of the postpartum client is:

   ① Estrogen
   ② Prolactin
   ③ Milk
   ④ Colostrum

64. The postpartum, breast-feeding client can anticipate that her milk will flow in about how many days?

   ① 1 to 2
   ② 3 to 4
   ③ 5 to 6
   ④ 7 to 8

65. Which of the following indicates a return of the uterus to its prepregnancy state?

   ① Diuresis
   ② Diaphoresis
   ③ Involution
   ④ Engorgement

66. What would be the expected appearance of the vaginal discharge from a client who delivered vaginally 5 days previously?

   ① White and frothy
   ② Thick and pink-tinged
   ③ Thick and yellow
   ④ Sticky and green

67. Which of the following amounts of vaginal drainage from a 2-day postpartum client would a nurse report immediately to the physician?

① A nickel-sized, light red, superficially saturated drainage over 2 hours
② A 2 × 2 inch superficially saturated, bright red drainage over 3 hours
③ Two completely saturated sanitary napkins over 30 minutes
④ A 4 × 4 inch completely saturated light red drainage over 8 hours

68. When the nurse answered the pregnant client's call light, she found her lying on her back. The client said she felt lightheaded and dizzy, as if she was going to pass out. The *most appropriate* action by the nurse would be to:

① Suspect that she is hemorrhaging and notify the physician
② Suspect that delivery is imminent and notify the physician
③ Suspect that her blood glucose level is low and give her some sweetened orange juice
④ Suspect that she has supine hypotensive syndrome and position her on her side

69. Most infants are able to lift their heads by the age of:

① 2 weeks
② 2 months
③ 3 months
④ 1 month

70. At which age does the anterior fontanel close?

① 2 weeks of age
② 2 to 3 months of age
③ 6 months of age
④ 15 to 18 months of age

71. At birth, James weighed 7 pounds. At his 12-month check-up, the nurse would expect his weight to be approximately:

① 14 pounds
② 21 pounds
③ 28 pounds
④ Cannot be determined; weight gain varies widely

72. The child has a complete set of deciduous teeth at age:

① 1 1/2 years
② 2 years
③ 2 1/2 to 3 years
④ 3 1/2 to 4 years

73. The first permanent teeth appear approximately at age:

① 2 1/2 to 3 years
② 4 to 5 years
③ 6 to 7 years
④ 8 to 9 years

74. Mr. Ford, age 67 years, is admitted to the hospital for surgical treatment of benign prostatic hyperplasia. The type of prostatic surgery that poses the lowest risk for Mr. Ford is:

① Suprapubic
② Retropubic
③ Perineal
④ Transurethral resection

75. If a transurethral resection prostatectomy is done, a three-way Foley catheter will be inserted for continuous irrigation in order to:

① Prevent clots from obstructing the catheter
② Reduce the possibility of postoperative bladder infection
③ Control the pain
④ Monitor intake and output

76. Following a transurethral resection prostatectomy for benign prostatic hyperplasia, the nurse assesses that Mr. Ford's Foley catheter is not draining urine. Which of the following nursing actions is appropriate?

① Increase the rate of the irrigation
② Irrigate the catheter with 30 mL sterile saline solution
③ Notify the physician
④ Increase oral intake

77. Otosclerosis produces loss of hearing because the:

① Auditory nerve is permanently damaged
② External canal of the ear is obstructed
③ Small bones of the middle ear cannot vibrate
④ Auditory nerve is inflamed

78. Following surgery to correct the otosclerosis, the nurse should caution the client against blowing the nose suddenly or violently because this could:

① Rupture the tympanic membrane–malleus junction
② Decrease pressure in the middle ear and thus interfere with the healing process
③ Increase drainage from the external canal
④ Dislodge the prosthesis

79. Gene Ray, 76 years old, has experienced leg cramps for several years. He recently began to have severe headaches, syncope, and short memory lapses. He is admitted to the hospital with a diagnosis of atherosclerosis-arteriosclerosis. His current signs and symptoms may indicate that the condition now includes:

① Pulmonary dysfunction
② Coronary occlusion
③ Cerebral involvement
④ Impending renal failure

80. Gene Ray, 76 years old, has experienced leg cramps for several years. He recently began to have severe headaches, syncope, and short memory lapses. He is admitted to the hospital with a diagnosis of atherosclerosis-arteriosclerosis. The physician orders a low-fat diet. Mr. Ray says that he always has bacon, scrambled eggs, and toast for breakfast. The nurse suggests that a better breakfast would be:

① Poached egg and fresh fruit
② Cooked cereal and orange juice
③ Pancakes and 2% milk
④ French toast and coffee

81. Gene Ray, 76 years old, has experienced leg cramps for several years. He recently began to have severe headaches, syncope, and short memory lapses. He is admitted to the hospital with a diagnosis of atherosclerosis-arteriosclerosis. During the initial assessment of Mr. Ray's lower extremities, the nurse might expect to find:

① Moist, warm skin and regular pulses
② Edema, pain when touched, and bounding pulses
③ Tingling, numbness, and slowed pulses
④ Pale, cool skin and diminished pulses

82. Gene Ray, 76 years old, has experienced leg cramps for several years. He recently began to have severe headaches, syncope, and short memory lapses. He is admitted to the hospital with a diagnosis of atherosclerosis-arteriosclerosis. The physician orders cyclandelate (Cyclospasmol), a peripheral vasodilator. The nurse should observe Mr. Ray for signs and symptoms of:

① Orthostatic hypotension
② Bradycardia
③ Nervousness
④ Lethargy

83. Gene Ray, 76 years old, has experienced leg cramps for several years. He recently began to have severe headaches, syncope, and short memory lapses. He is admitted to the hospital with a diagnosis of atherosclerosis-arteriosclerosis. Mr. Ray was found to have a gangrenous ulcer in his right little toe. Which of the following would the nurse include in his care plan?

① Maintain strict bed rest until ulcer heals
② Apply hot compresses to increase blood flow
③ Keep a bed cradle in place to keep the covers off
④ Elevate the legs whenever sitting

84. A client is admitted to the medical unit with a diagnosis of angina pectoris. Characteristic signs and symptoms of angina pectoris include:

① Substernal chest pain radiating down left arm
② Epigastric pain radiating to the back
③ Nausea, epigastric pain, and anorexia
④ Fatigue, shortness of breath, and dyspnea

85. A client comes into the emergency department exhibiting signs of an acute myocardial infarction. Laboratory data consistent with a diagnosis of acute myocardial infarction are:

① Elevated levels of SGOT (AST), CPK, LDH
② Decreased levels of SGOT (AST), CPK, LDH
③ Elevated levels of SGOT (AST), decreased levels of CPK and LDH
④ Decreased levels of SGOT (AST), increased levels of CPK and LDH

86. When developing a teaching plan for a client with congestive heart failure, you tell your client that he or she is likely to sleep more restfully in which of the following positions?

① Trendelenburg
② Supine
③ Prone
④ Fowler's

87. In teaching a client with a diagnosis of pernicious anemia, you should stress which of the following statements before discharge?

① A diet high in vitamin B_{12} is necessary.
② Oral vitamin B_{12} must be taken once a week.
③ Intramuscular vitamin B_{12} must be taken for life.
④ Iron therapy is necessary for life.

88. Which of the following characteristics of sputum would be assessed in a client with a diagnosis of pulmonary edema?

① Salmon-colored and copious
② Blood-tinged and frothy
③ White and watery
④ Green and copious

89. Your client has peripheral edema resulting from congestive heart failure. Instruct your client to:

① Elevate the head of the bed
② Apply cold compresses to the extremities
③ Elevate affected extremities
④ Apply moist heat to affected extremities

90. Your client has been admitted to the hospital with chronic obstructive pulmonary disease. Which of the following assessments indicate an acute episode?

① Cough, dyspnea, and bradycardia
② Wheezing, restlessness, and tachycardia
③ Tachycardia, barrel chest, and hypertension
④ Confusion, weight gain, and hypotension

91. Your client has just returned from a bronchoscopy. The client should remain on nothing-by-mouth (NPO) status until:

① The gag reflex returns
② The charge nurse gives the order
③ There is no evidence of blood-streaked sputum
④ The respiratory rate is 20 to 22/minute.

92. Your client is admitted to the hospital with the diagnosis of hepatitis B. This type of hepatitis is contracted by:

① Direct contact
② Blood and body fluids
③ Fecal-oral route
④ Contaminated water

93. Your client is scheduled to undergo an upper gastrointestinal endoscopy in the morning. Which of the following nursing interventions will help reduce the client's fears?

① Discuss the procedure with the client
② Arrange for the client to observe the procedure
③ Sedate the client
④ Discuss the possible complications of the procedure

94. When developing a care plan for a client with a neurogenic bladder, the nurse includes:

① Forcing fluids
② Taking the temperature every 4 hours
③ Intermittent catheterization
④ A bladder training program

95. Your client is admitted to a medical unit with a diagnosis of benign prostatic hyperplasia. Which of the following assessments are consistent with this diagnosis?

① Frequent urination, nocturia, difficulty starting a stream
② Bone pain, weight loss, anemia
③ Shortness of breath, enlarged lymph nodes, acute urinary retention
④ Painless hematuria, palpable mass in flank area

96. Your client has just returned from surgery for a subtotal thyroidectomy. Which of the following would be the *most* necessary piece of equipment to be placed at the bedside?

① Pleur-Evac drainage system
② Tracheostomy tray
③ Incentive spirometer
④ Suction setup

97. Which of the following interventions is appropriate in the recovery room for the client who had spinal anesthesia?

① Monitor for the possibility of hypotension
② Maintain semi-Fowler's position
③ Never give medication if the client is unable to move his or her legs
④ High Fowler's position is best for these clients

98. An early sign or symptom of a transfusion reaction is:

① Hypertension
② Flank pain
③ Cyanosis
④ Bradycardia

99. Which of the following findings is considered abnormal for the first postoperative day after upper abdominal surgery?

① Nausea
② Pain over the incision site when coughing
③ Drainage on dressing the size of a half dollar
④ Frequently voiding in small amounts

100. Propranolol (Inderal) has been ordered for an atrial arrhythmia. A note should be made on the nursing care plan to assess the client frequently for:

1. Increased blood pressure
2. Restlessness and anxiety
3. Bradycardia
4. Decreased level of consciousness

101. A client who has had a myocardial infarction is given heparin sodium intravenously. Considering the side effects of this drug, nursing care should include monitoring the client for:

1. Diarrhea
2. Hematuria
3. Increased white blood cell count
4. Shortness of breath

102. A client has been receiving intravenous heparin. The heparin has been changed to subcutaneous injections. Injections should be:

1. Massaged to promote absorption
2. Limited to the upper arms and anterior thigh
3. Given in the lower abdomen
4. Rotated between the arms, thighs, gluteal area, and abdomen

103. Ms. Cohen becomes depressed 2 days after admission for an acute myocardial infarction. The nurse should:

1. Remind her that she is fortunate to be alive after her heart attack
2. Show her a tape of what happens during a myocardial infarction
3. Encourage her to get more exercise to take her mind off her problems
4. Encourage her to express her fears and answer her questions

104. As a nurse, you realize that long-term treatment for the person suffering from chemical dependency should *ideally* include:

1. Withdrawal of the person's driver's license
2. Employment reeducation
3. Family treatment
4. Only individual treatment to maintain confidentiality

105. In caring for a client who is in an acute manic phase, the *most appropriate* diet and meal plan would be which of the following?

1. Three large meals per day
2. Three meals plus a bedtime snack per day
3. A low-calorie diet
4. Nutritious high-calorie finger foods

106. A hospitalized client who has recently been suicidal and now seems elated is:

1. Over the risk of suicide
2. No longer in need of mental health care
3. Now at higher risk of suicide
4. Ready for outpatient services

107. Your client has told you that he does not want to live. The *best* nursing response is to:

1. Reassure him that things will get better
2. Let him have some time alone
3. Maintain his confidentiality
4. Ask him if he has a plan

108. Your client has told you that he plans to end his life. He asks you to keep this information a secret. The *most appropriate* nursing response is to:

1. Call the physician
2. Report this to the RN
3. Maintain the client's spoken request
4. Tell the client there is nothing to be that depressed about

109. Dietary restrictions for the client taking monoamine oxidase inhibitors include restricting:

1. Apples and apple juice
2. Cottage cheese
3. Decaffeinated coffee
4. Cheddar cheese

110. A lithium level of 2.1 mEq/L is:

1. A normal body amount of lithium
2. The therapeutic range of lithium
3. A toxic range of lithium
4. Not something the PN needs to be concerned about

111. The *most appropriate* activity for a client who is experiencing mania would be:

1. Detailed painting
2. Activities that include cutting and pasting
3. A walk
4. Repetitive exercises

112. Benztropine mesylate (Cogentin) may be prescribed for a client who is taking antipsychotic medication because:

1. Many psychotic clients develop Parkinson's disease

② Antipsychotic medication works better with Cogentin

③ Cogentin decreases possible side effects of antipsychotic medication

④ Cogentin enhances the client's nutritional status

113. Early indications of potential neuroleptic malignant syndrome are:

① Decreased blood pressure and pulse
② Elevated temperature and blood pressure
③ Flaccid muscles and weakness
④ Coma and death

114. A child who is brought into the emergency department for accidental injuries should:

① Remain with the mother or caregiver at all times
② Let the mother or caregiver explain the cause of the injury
③ Immediately be given pain medication
④ Be separated from the mother or caregiver to explain the cause of injury

115. The client you are caring for is taking an iron supplement. The client should be instructed to:

① Decrease citrus foods
② Decrease fluids
③ Take the medication with milk
④ Take the medication with orange juice

116. The client you are caring for is receiving radiation therapy. You notice that a first degree burn has developed around the radiated area. The best intervention is to:

① Apply a petroleum-based lotion
② Apply mineral oil
③ Keep the area clean with soap and a mild astringent
④ Inform the radiation department

117. A sprain is best treated within the first 24 hours with:

① Dry heat
② Ice
③ Moist heat
④ Range of motion

118. The client you are caring for has a nasogastric feeding tube. Before administering medications through the tube, you should:

① Flush the tube
② Place the client in the supine position

③ Check the tube for placement
④ Have the client cough and deep breathe

119. An intervention to prevent an ileus includes:

① Strict bed rest
② Assessment of bowel sounds
③ Obtaining of abdominal measurements
④ Ambulation of the client

120. Your client begins to complain of severe right lower quadrant pain. You notice that your client has an elevated temperature. The best nursing response is to:

① Apply a warm blanket or heating pad over the area
② Apply ice to the area
③ Administer pain medication
④ Notify the RN

121. A client receiving chemotherapy for cancer treatment should be instructed to:

① Take stool softeners to avoid constipation
② Use strong mouthwashes to avoid oral infections
③ Decrease fluids to prevent overhydration
④ Use a soft toothbrush

122. Mrs. Arnold has had an abdominal-perineal resection and a colostomy as a result of rectal cancer. Your immediate postoperative nursing care includes:

① Checking for incisional infection
② Teaching the client colostomy care
③ Placing the permanent colostomy appliance
④ Checking for color, size, and patency of stoma

123. Mrs. Arnold has had an abdominal-perineal resection and a colostomy as a result of rectal cancer. Within the first week after surgery, you would expect Mrs. Arnold to experience:

① A change in body image
② A change in social role
③ Guilt feelings due to cancer
④ Regression

124. A client with leukopenia is most susceptible to:

① Infection
② Bleeding
③ Hyperuricemia
④ Hypercalcemia

125. Which of the following assessments would be *unlikely* to occur if your client is hypocalcemic?

① Laryngeal spasms
② Difficulty talking
③ Carpopedal spasms
④ Hyperpnea

126. Local care of irritated skin resulting from radiation treatments should include:

① Applying oil-based cream three times a day
② Washing the area with water only
③ Exposing the area to sunlight at least 1 hour/day
④ Keeping the area covered with a clean, dry dressing

127. The PN is caring for a client receiving radiation therapy. Which of the following should be reported immediately to the physician?

① Platelet count of 50,000
② Increasing fatigue
③ Nausea and vomiting
④ White blood cell count of 2000

128. Which of the following would predispose a person to immunosuppression?

① Diabetes mellitus
② Obesity
③ Hormone imbalances
④ Maladaptive behavior

129. An optimal preventive measure against AIDS is:

① Protective isolation
② Meticulous skin care
③ Respiratory isolation
④ Blood and body fluid precaution

130. Which of the following is not a characteristic of a phobia?

① Anxiety is attributed to an external source
② Displacement keeps the source of anxiety out of consciousness
③ Insight-oriented therapy can help
④ Secondary gains may be important to the client

131. Mr. Applegate is afraid of heights. A term used to describe this type of phobia is:

① Agoraphobia
② Acrophobia

③ Claustrophobia
④ Xenophobia

132. Which of the following nursing interventions would be useful in helping a client overcome a phobia?

① Placing the client in phobic situations to desensitize the client
② Pointing out adaptive coping mechanisms and reinforcing them
③ Helping the client avoid anxiety-producing situations
④ Never administering tranquilizers

133. Your surgical client is to receive nothing by mouth (NPO status) after midnight the night before surgery. The rationale for this is to prevent:

① Fluid overload postoperatively
② Urinary incontinence during surgery
③ Vomiting and aspiration during surgery
④ Pneumonia postoperatively

134. Which of the following laboratory data would be necessary to report to the surgeon before any client undergoes major surgery?

① Serum potassium level of 2.5 mEq/L
② Hematocrit of 42 mL/100 mL
③ Platelet count of 300,000 mm³
④ Total serum protein level of 8 g/100 mL

135. Intravenous fluids are given after major surgery. If the order reads "1000 mL D5W to infuse over 8 hours" and the drip factor is 15, the correct rate of the infusion would be:

① 22 gtt/minute
② 51 gtt/minute
③ 42 gtt/minute
④ 31 gtt/minute

136. A 6-month-old suspected of having cerebral palsy would most likely exhibit:

① Delay or failure to control head and roll over
② Frequent episodes of seizure activity
③ Visual or hearing deficits
④ Frequent respiratory infections

137. The parents of an infant diagnosed with cerebral palsy ask the nurse how severe a handicap their child will have. The best response by the nurse is:

① "With early and vigorous therapy, he may have only mild problems."

② "It's hard to tell so early; some mental retardation is expected."

③ "Children with cerebral palsy vary in symptoms and severity but can be helped with treatment."

④ "No one can really tell how much disability there will be until the child starts school."

138. Children with cerebral palsy are often at risk for nutritional deficits because they have:

① Difficulties controlling the muscles of chewing and swallowing

② Restricted sense of taste and are picky eaters

③ Gastrointestinal impairment, which decreases absorption of nutrients

④ Frequent episodes of vomiting related to muscle spasticity

139. Shirley, a high school sophomore, has not been selected for a favored school team. She is suddenly neglecting her studies and appearance and is uninterested in the world around her. As the nurse in her school, your best action would be to:

① Establish regular appointments for Shirley to talk over problems.

② Encourage Shirley not to discuss her problems with her peer group.

③ Recommend mental health intervention if Shirley's withdrawal continues.

④ Allow Shirley to find her own time to talk about her feelings.

140. After exhibiting depressive behavior, Shirley, a high school sophomore, suddenly becomes more active and begins to give away her prized pictures and audio cassettes, among other things. What might you suspect from her behavior?

① That she has begun to abuse illicit drugs

② That her behavior is more typically adolescent now

③ That she may be pregnant

④ That she is considering suicide

141. Mrs. Ruth Lamb, age 68 years, has had a stroke that left her unable to help herself. She is primarily bedridden. Which of the following *best* describes the psychologic effect of inactivity experienced by many older patients such as Mrs. Lamb?

① Abnormal talkativeness

② Hallucinations

③ Lack of normal initiative

④ Lack of normal inhibition

142. After Mrs. Lamb has had a stroke that left her bedridden and unable to care for herself, the nurse encourages Mr. Lamb to make a footboard for Mrs. Lamb's bed. She explains that the *primary* purpose for using a footboard for Mrs. Lamb is to help prevent:

① Bedsores

② Footdrop

③ Knee contractures

④ Edema in the feet

143. Mrs. Lamb is recovering from a stroke that has left her weak. The nurse moves Mrs. Lamb's knee through range of motion, but the client begins to complain of *considerable* discomfort. Which of the following courses of action should the nurse take?

① Stop the exercise and inform the physician

② Continue with the exercise but at a slower pace

③ Stop the exercise and begin again after the client has had a few minutes of rest

④ Explain to the client that she will experience discomfort when the exercise is done properly

144. The nurse uses trochanter rolls for a post-stroke client on bed rest while the client is in bed. Trochanter rolls are used *primarily* to help prevent:

① Flexion of the knees

② Extension of the hips

③ Hyperextension of the feet

④ External rotation of the legs

145. Because Mrs. Lamb is on bed rest after a stroke, the nurse is teaching Mr. and Mrs. Lamb about the possible complications of inactivity. She explains that each system of the body may be affected. A danger affecting the circulatory system when a client is immobile is:

① The formation of blood clots

② The development of air emboli

③ An increased alkalinity of the blood

④ An excessive white blood cell formation

146. To prevent the effects of immobility on the gastrointestinal system, the nurse suggests that the client:

① Be given daily enemas
② Decrease her fluid intake
③ Increase roughage in her diet
④ Avoid stool softeners

147. A result *least likely* to develop from muscle disuse is:

① Contractures
② Muscular weakness
③ Decreased stamina
④ Hyperactive muscular responses

148. Which of the following electrolyes is lost in the *largest* amount when the client requires a long period of bed rest?

① Sodium
② Calcium
③ Potassium
④ Bicarbonate

149. The *primary* cause of a decubitus ulcer is:

① Excessive perspiration
② Pressure on a body area
③ Poor nutrition and inadequate fluid intake
④ Inability to control voiding and defecating

150. The nurse knows that when a client is on bed rest, the client's position should be changed every:

① 1 to 2 hours
② 3 to 4 hours
③ 6 hours
④ 8 hours

151. Marie is a 14-year-old single, primigravida high school student who has received no prenatal care. Which of the following behaviors indicates that Marie may have been denying her pregnancy?

① Obtaining no prenatal care
② Considering adoption as an alternative
③ Making plans to finish high school
④ Not telling her parents about the pregnancy

152. When Marie, a 14-year-old single, primigravida high school student who has received no prenatal care, is admitted in active labor, the nurse knows that:

① It is too late to teach breathing and relaxation exercises
② If teaching is to be done, Marie should be medicated first so that she will be more relaxed
③ Teaching should begin immediately with short, simple instructions
④ Teaching should be extensive to make up for the lack of prenatal care

153. Marie, a 14-year-old single, primigravida high school student who has received no prenatal care, notices that the fetal monitor indicates that her baby's heart rate is 148 beats per minute and asks you whether that rate is too fast. Your best response would be:

① "Yes, that is too fast. It is because you are so tense."
② "No, that is not too fast. The normal fetal heart beat is 120 to 160 beats every minute."
③ "It's okay because the normal heart rate goes up to 200 beats every minute."
④ "That's great! It means that your baby is a girl."

154. Marie is a 14-year-old single, primigravida high school student who has received no prenatal care. Marie's pregnancy is considered "high risk" because of:

① Lack of prenatal care
② Her age
③ Her educational and marital status
④ All of the above

155. To monitor the frequency of contractions for a woman in labor, the nurse should count the time from the:

① Beginning of one contraction to the beginning of the next contraction
② End of one contraction to the beginning of the next contraction
③ Beginning of the contraction to the end of the same contraction
④ Peak of one contraction to the peak of the next contraction

156. When a client is in labor and her cervix is dilated 6 to 7 cm, she is given meperidine (Demerol) 50 mg intramuscularly. The PN knows that Demerol will:

① Increase the intensity and durations of the contractions
② Prevent nausea during labor

③ Relieve discomfort and promote relaxation

④ Cause the cervix to dilate more rapidly

157. During the delivery of a baby, an episiotomy is performed. An episiotomy is an incision into the:

① Abdomen to facilitate the delivery of the infant

② Cervix to prevent lacerations

③ Perineum to facilitate the delivery of the infant

④ Vagina to prevent lacerations of the reproductive tract

158. Which of the following indicates that Marie, a 14-year-old single, primigravida high school student who has received no prenatal care, understands her postpartum teaching? She:

① Washes hands, does perineal care, and applies a clean perineal pad back to front

② Washes hands, does perineal care, and applies a clean perineal pad front to back

③ Washes hands and changes perineal pad four times a day

④ Showers twice a day and applies a clean perineal pad

159. Marie, a 14-year-old single, primigravida high school student who has received no prenatal care, tells you that she plans to bottle-feed her infant. Your best response would be:

① "Your baby would do much better if you would breast-feed."

② "Holding and cuddling your baby during feeding are very important."

③ "That's a good idea. That way anyone can feed the baby."

④ "That's a good idea because you cannot breast-feed and go to school or have a job."

160. Marie, a 14-year-old single, primigravida high school student who has received no prenatal care, is concerned about her ability to lose weight after the baby is born. Which of the following statements indicates that Marie understands her nutritional needs?

① "I won't eat any food between meals."

② "I won't eat any bread, potatoes, cereal, or pasta."

③ "I guess I'd better not eat any pizza or fast food."

④ "Drinking milk with my pizza and salad will be a real change."

161. Before Marie, a 14-year-old single, primigravida high school student who received no prenatal care, is discharged, it will be important to discuss with her:

① Plans for the future and her support system

② Who got her pregnant and why

③ How unrealistic her ideas are about caring for her baby

④ The rules of society and morality so she will not get pregnant again

162. Mr. Zimmer, a patient with congestive heart failure, has an order for digoxin, 0.25 mg, to be administered intravenously. Before administering this medication, the nurse will:

① Check his apical pulse

② Take his temperature

③ Recount his respirations

④ Take his blood pressure

163. Mr. Zimmer is a patient with congestive heart failure who has just started a digoxin regimen. He asks what effect digoxin has on his body. He is instructed that it will:

① Slow and strengthen the action of his heart muscle

② Dilate the blood vessels of his heart

③ Cause fluid to drain out of his lungs by dilating the alveoli

④ Improve the function of the heart valves

164. Mr. Zimmer has congestive heart failure and has started a digoxin regimen. Until his heart has compensated, he will probably be more comfortable in which of the following positions?

① Supine

② Prone

③ Sims'

④ Fowler's

165. A common intervention for patients with congestive heart failure is to check the pulse pressure every 8 hours. This is done by:

① Checking the blood pressure lying and standing

② Assessing the amplitude of the pulse

③ Subtracting the diastolic blood pressure from the systolic

④ Describing the character and rate of the pulse

166. Clients with congestive heart failure often must restrict their fluid intake until their edema has subsided. This restriction usually involves:

① Cooperation between dietary and nursing personnel when planning all fluids
② Limiting intake of between-meal beverages only
③ Limiting all fluids except those needed for oral medications
④ Limiting the intake of water only

167. Mr. Zimmer, who has congestive heart failure, is instructed that in following his low-sodium diet, he can season his food with:

① Lemon juice
② Steak sauce
③ Catsup
④ Prepared mustard

168. Mr. Zimmer, who has congestive heart failure, asks how long he will need to continue taking digoxin. He is instructed that it will probably be necessary to continue this drug:

① Until his pulse rate returns to normal
② Until all the edema is gone
③ Until after the physician does a stress test to prove that his heart has compensated
④ For the rest of his life

169. Mary Love is admitted to the hospital with acute exacerbation of chronic obstructive pulmonary disease (COPD). An early sign or symptom of COPD is:

① Dyspnea on mild exertion
② Barrel chest
③ Clubbing of the distal ends of fingers and toes
④ Cyanosis

170. Ms. Love has a history of COPD. She is admitted with an acute exacerbation of the condition. She is receiving oxygen at 1 L/minute by nasal prongs. High concentrations of oxygen can cause:

① Decreased respiratory rate
② Increased secretions in the respiratory tract
③ Increased episodes of coughing
④ Respiratory alkalosis

171. Aminophylline, 500 mg intravenously, in normal saline is ordered for your client with COPD. This drug is given to:

① Liquefy bronchial secretions
② Reduce anxiety
③ Relax bronchial muscles
④ Depress the cough reflex

172. Emphysema is a condition:

① Manifested by scar tissue of the bronchi and bronchioles
② Characterized by distention of the bronchioles and destruction of the alveolar walls
③ Caused only by smoking and air pollution
④ Affecting the cilia of the respiratory passage

173. Discharge instructions for a client who has had an acute exacerbation of COPD would *not* include which of the following?

① Avoiding people with infections
② Not taking any over-the-counter drugs without physician approval
③ Avoiding large meals
④ Attending an exercise class at least three times a week

174. Ms. Love, a patient with COPD, is taught to use pursed-lip and diaphragmatic breathing to:

① Increase air space within the lungs
② Assist in eliminating carbon dioxide
③ Improve respiratory muscle tone
④ Conserve energy needed to breathe

175. Nerve receptors for thirst are located in the:

① Hypothalamus
② Adrenal glands
③ Brainstem
④ Cerebral cortex

176. Intracellular fluid is contained:

① Between the cells
② In the blood stream
③ Outside the cells
④ Inside the cells

177. A situation that would *not* result in edema is:

① Congestive heart failure
② Hyponatremia
③ Cirrhosis of the liver
④ Renal failure

178. A nursing intervention that would *not* be appropriate for a client with edema is:

① Monitoring intake and output
② Weighing daily

③ Encouraging oral fluids
④ Reducing high-sodium foods

179. When thiazide diuretics are ordered to correct edema, the nurse should observe the client for signs and symptoms of:

① Hypernatremia
② Hypokalemia
③ Elevated blood glucose levels
④ Lowered blood glucose levels

180. Mr. Elliot is dehydrated. Which of the following signs and symptoms indicates the presence of dehydration?

① Loss of skin turgor
② Increased blood pressure
③ Lowered body temperature
④ Restlessness

181. Mr. Jay's serum sodium level is 155 mEq. The nurse should assess him for:

① Poor skin turgor
② Hypotension
③ Bradycardia
④ Pitting edema

182. One common cause of a decreased sodium level in cardiac clients is:

① Administration of diuretics
② Inadequate fluid intake
③ Poor dietary intake
④ Decreased renal function

183. Your client has severe hyperkalemia. The nurse expects that the physician will order:

① Intravenous Ringer's lactate solution
② Kayexalate enemas
③ A low-sodium diet
④ Increased use of salt substitutes

184. An *early* symptom of hypokalemia is:

① Muscle cramping
② Cardiac irritability
③ Fatigue
④ Tetany

185. A disorder brought on by prolonged immobility is:

① Hyperkalemia
② Hyponatremia
③ Hypokalemia
④ Hypercalcemia

186. The nurse should observe a client for signs and symptoms of hypocalcemia following a:

① Cholecystectomy
② Thoracotomy
③ Thyroidectomy
④ Hysterectomy

187. An example of a hypotonic solution is:

① Ringer's lactate solution
② 5% dextrose in water
③ 0.45% saline solution
④ Dextran solution

188. A symptom of fluid overload is:

① Increased urinary output
② Decreased blood pressure
③ Increased body temperature
④ Increased heart rate

189. The nurse should assess the site of intravenous insertion:

① At least once a shift
② Every 2 hours
③ Every time the tubing is changed
④ After each new solution is started

190. Jason Kane is brought to the emergency department with dyspnea and severe abdominal pain. He has a history of sickle cell disease. A common precipitating factor of sickle cell crisis is:

① Tension
② Dehydration
③ Decreased food intake
④ Depression

191. The pain associated with sickle cell disease is due to:

① Muscle spasms in the affected area
② Pressure from the edema caused by fluid retention
③ Irritation of nerve endings of the mucus-secreting glands
④ Occlusion of small blood vessels

192. The diagnostic test that differentiates between sickle cell trait and sickle cell disease is a:

① Hemoglobin electrophoresis
② Sickle cell preparation
③ Sickledex
④ Blood smear

193. Jason, a young man with a history of sickle cell disease, should be instructed to:

  ① Limit fluid intake
  ② Avoid wearing tight clothes
  ③ Keep his room cool at all times
  ④ Not take any immunizations

194. In discharge planning, Jason, a young man with sickle cell disease, is taught that management of a mild crisis would not include which of the following?

  ① Increasing fluid intake
  ② Controlling fever with antipyretic medications
  ③ Getting adequate rest
  ④ Checking for blood in the urine

195. The most critical assessment of Jason, a young man with sickle cell disease, is his abdomen for:

  ① Signs of splenomegaly
  ② Active bowel sounds
  ③ Generalized tenderness
  ④ Changes in skin color

196. The nurse assesses for signs and symptoms of ketoacidosis, which include:

  ① Odor of acetone on breath
  ② Oliguria
  ③ Hypoglycemia
  ④ Absence of acetone in the urine

197. The nurse knows that initial treatment of diabetic ketosis usually includes administration of:

  ① Regular insulin
  ② Intravenous glucose
  ③ Long-acting insulin
  ④ Intravenous diuretics

198. John, a 63-year-old insulin-dependent diabetic client, is able to give himself insulin, but because he has not been compliant in the past, it might be of value if:

  ① He is given the phone numbers of the health department and nearest hospital
  ② Someone checks his urine daily to make sure that he is taking his insulin
  ③ Someone else in his family also learns to give insulin
  ④ The physician changes him to oral medications

199. Elaine, age 30 years, has had symptoms of Graves' disease for 4 years. She is admitted to the hospital for surgery. Symptoms of Graves' disease include:

  ① Weight loss
  ② Decreased energy
  ③ Bradycardia
  ④ Intolerance to cold

200. When Elaine, a 30-year-old with a 4 year history of Graves' disease, is admitted, the nurse's assessment would most likely reveal:

  ① Swollen ankles
  ② A fine tremor of the hands
  ③ Ascites
  ④ Low blood pressure

201. Elaine is a 30-year-old with a 4-year history of Graves' disease. Elaine's previous medical treatment for Graves' disease may have included:

  ① A low-sodium diet
  ② A high-sodium diet
  ③ Drugs that block production of thyroid hormones
  ④ Administration of synthetic thyroid hormones

202. Preoperatively, Elaine, a 30-year-old with a 4-year history of Graves' disease, is given drugs in an attempt to establish a euthyroid state to decrease the risk of postoperative:

  ① Hypothyroidism
  ② Iodine intoxication
  ③ Loss of pituitary activity
  ④ Thyroid crisis

203. Elaine returns from the operating room following a thyroidectomy for Graves' disease. Once she is fully awake, the nurse should position her:

  ① With head of the bed elevated
  ② Flat in bed
  ③ Turned on her side
  ④ In any position she desires

204. Following a thyroidectomy for Graves' disease, Elaine is observed for signs and symptoms of respiratory obstruction, which would most likely be due to:

  ① Bronchoconstriction owing to decrease in thyroid hormones
  ② Constriction of the airway by the surgical dressing

③ Enlargement of the remaining part of the thyroid gland
④ Edema in or near the operative area

205. Following a thyroidectomy for Graves' disease, a sudden temperature elevation to 106°F accompanied by restlessness, tachycardia, and delirium would lead the PN to suspect:

① Pneumonitis
② Thyroid crisis
③ Atelectasis
④ Hemorrhage

ANSWERS AND RATIONALES

1. The client with hypertension will have a
③ sodium-restricted diet. Sodium restriction improves the effectiveness of diuretic therapy. If diuretics are used, the client may have decreased potassium levels and potassium-rich foods may be needed. Folic acid and magnesium are not related to hypertension.
II, 2, Hypertension

2. Painful or upsetting procedures performed be-
④ fore meals may produce anxiety and decrease appetite. The child's food preferences are always considered. Desserts should not be used as an incentive to bribe the child to eat. Children should not be forced to eat everything on their plate.
II, 1, Providing for the nutritional needs of the child

3. Protein intake is restricted in hepatic coma
① to help reduce high ammonia levels that accumulate in the blood because of the inability of the diseased liver to remove the excess ammonia released during the metabolism of protein. Diets for gallbladder disease, iron deficiency anemia, and alcoholism do not restrict protein.
II, 1 & 2, Liver disease

4. Lactose intolerance is the inability to digest
② milk sugar (lactose) caused by a deficiency of the enzyme lactase. Because the body cannot tolerate milk or milk products, a calcium deficiency may occur. Deficiencies of iron, potassium, and sodium are not related to lactose intolerance.
I, 2, Lactose intolerance

5. Shortly after meals, clients who have had a
④ gastric resection may experience a "dumping" of the gastric contents directly into the small intestine, causing weakness, fainting, and possibly diarrhea. To minimize these symptoms, fluids are limited during mealtimes. No other fluid restrictions are necessary.
II, 2, Gastric resection

6. The absorption of iron is enhanced by the
② presence of vitamin C. Of the beverages listed orange juice has the highest vitamin C content.
III, 1 & 2, Mineral absorption

7. Tetany is a condition resulting in muscular
② spasms or twitching and is generally related to low blood levels of calcium. Low blood levels of iron, potassium, and zinc are not related to tetany.
II, 2, Calcium deficiency

8. The cause of pernicious anemia is the inability
③ of the body to absorb vitamin B_{12} because of a lack of the intrinsic factor in the gastric secretions. Injections of vitamin B_{12} are necessary to bypass this absorption problem.
II, 1, Pernicious anemia

9. Of the foods listed, dark green or deep yellow
② vegetables are the highest in vitamin A.
III, 4, Sources of vitamin A

10. The greatest hazard in most homes of older
② adults who are unsteady in walking are throw rugs or scatter rugs because they can get caught with canes, crutches, and walkers.
I, 1, Fractured hip

11. It is preferable to treat constipation with di-
③ etary changes instead of medications.
III, 2, Constipation

12. Most abuse stems from stressful caregiving
③ situations in which frustration and exhaustion prevail when there is no respite from the care.
I, 3, Elder abuse

13. The typical profile of an older adult at risk is
② a disabled woman over 75 years of age, dependent physically, socially, or financially.
I, 3, Elder abuse

14. A thoracentesis is the insertion of a large-
④ bore needle or trocar into the pleural space of the chest for the purpose of removing air or fluid. A thoracentesis precedes a chest tube insertion. Although an underwater seal system is required after a chest tube insertion, the lung is reexpanded, not decompressed. A thoracotomy generally refers to a surgical procedure likely to be done during lung or open heart surgery, and a pneumonectomy is the removal of a diseased portion of the lung or a lobe.
II, 1, Respiratory

15.
② Adverse reactions of aminophylline, a potent bronchodilator known for its effectiveness in reducing bronchospasms, include hypotension, dizziness, faintness, palpitations, and headaches. Toxicity can lead to seizures. The therapeutic range is between 15 and 20 $\mu g/$ mL. Gingival hyperplasia is commonly seen with prolonged use of phenytoin (Dilantin) for seizure control. Tinnitus is associated with furosemide (Lasix), aspirin, and ototoxic drugs. Rainbow halos are a symptom often reported by clients who suffer from angle-closure glaucoma.
IV, 2, Respiratory

16.
② Computed tomography provides information about the extent of the aneurysm and can even identify the presence of retroperitoneal hemorrhage. All the other mentioned diagnostic studies may be used but are not as effective as computed tomography.
III, 1, Cardiovascular

17.
① As with all head injuries, the nurse should anticipate the possibility of increased intracranial pressure from yet to be identified injuries. Until a thorough assessment and skull x-ray studies have ruled out major injuries, the head of the bed is elevated in an effort to prevent increased intracranial pressure from occurring. Continued assessment is essential. The nurse would anticipate an elevated blood pressure in early shock and should assess the pulse rate and rhythm as well. Blowing of the nose should never be encouraged. The client may inadvertently blow infectious pathogens into the brain. Antibiotic therapy is likely to be initiated but is not the nurse's top priority.
III, 2, Neurologic

18.
② Hypokalemia (a low potassium level) is associated with flattened T waves and depressed ST segments and can lead to dysrhythmia, especially in clients receiving cardiac glycosides. Hyperthermia is seen in hypernatremia, and seizures are most likely to be seen with hypocalcemia. Hypotension is a common clinical manifestation of hypomagnesemia.
I, 2, Fluids and electrolytes

19.
② Flushed cheeks and dry mucous membranes are associated with the dehydrated state that typically accompanies ketoacidosis. The excess glucose in the blood stream increases the concentration of the intravascular fluid, raising its osmotic pressure, and pulls water from the cells and interstitial fluid, leading to cellular dehydration and excessive loss of water via urine. Slow, shallow respirations with possible apnea are typically seen in metabolic alkalosis. A widening pulse pressure is most likely to be seen with increased intracranial pressure. Sodium and potassium levels are likely to be decreased during ketoacidosis, as glucose and electrolytes tend to be lost with the diuresis of ketoacidosis.
I, 1, Endocrine system

20.
③ Raynaud's disease is associated with occlusive arterial disease, and symptoms tend to mimic those of clients with peripheral vascular disease. Elevation of the extremities is not recommended because this would further decrease the blood supply to the affected area. Choices 1, 2, and 4 are appropriate for this client. Over-the-counter medications should be avoided because many contain vasoconstrictors. Avoiding extremes in temperature is highly recommended because such action decreases the chance of an attack or alleviates the symptoms.
III, 1, Cardiovascular

21.
② Airplane travel and high altitudes are contraindicated because increased pressure within the middle ear can lead to tympanic membrane rupture or to dislodgment of any prosthesis that may have been placed during surgery. Baths are encouraged because this decreases the risk of water getting into the ear. Rest is an important basic physiologic need. Assistance from the client's partner ensures added protection against sudden jarring of the head or dislodgment of the prosthesis.
III, 2, Special senses

22.
② In a therapeutic relationship, clients are supported in making decisions. The nurse should avoid giving an opinion because this takes decision making away for the client. The nurse should avoid prying into a client's personal life or blocking communication by putting the client off with such statements as used in choice 4.
I, 3, Communication skills

23. Proper positioning in cardiogenic shock is low
④ Fowler's with lower extremity elevation. Until
the blood pressure is stabilized, do not elevate
the head of the bed. Trendelenburg positioning
of the client is contraindicated, and a nurse
must have a physician's order or standing protocol to adjust intravenous rates. Keep in mind,
however, that nitroglycerine is a vasodilator
and causes a further drop of the blood pressure.
III, 2, Shock

24. Lactulose is a laxative and at best is used to
③ lower ammonium blood levels in clients with
hepatic encephalopathy. Persistent diarrhea
can lead to electrolyte imbalance, dehydration, and vitamin deficiencies as well as skin
breakdown. Thus, vitamin supplements and
identification of the causative agents via stool
analysis are essential. *Lactobacillus acidophilus*
is administered to help recolonize the bowel.
III, 1, Malabsorption

25. The Miller-Abbott and Cantor tubes, similar
④ to the Harris tube, contain a mercury-filled bag
at the end that propels the tip of the tube beyond the stomach and into the small intestine.
These tubes are used to stimulate peristalsis
and are left in place until the intestinal lumen
is patent. An endoscopy tube is used during
a sigmoidoscopy; it differs from the others, in
that it contains a lighted scope at one end.
Nasogastric tubes (Levin and Salem sump) are
used in partial obstruction or when the problem is high in the small intestine.
III, 3, Gastrointestinal decompression

26. As with other leukemias, anemia caused by
③ inadequate erythrocyte production and bleeding tendencies secondary to inadequate platelet counts may be seen in these patients.
Thus, aspirin administration is contraindicated. Small frequent feedings are strongly
recommended because chemotherapy often
leads to immunosuppression, decreased nutritional intake, and increased uric acid levels,
given the massive cell destruction of chemotherapy.
III, 2, Hematopoietic

27. The dangers of overfeeding a premature in-
② fant are real. Overdistention of the stomach
crowds the diaphragm, which interferes with
a normal breathing pattern, can trigger vomit-

ing, and can predispose to aspiration of stomach contents. A preterm infant has high
energy requirements and needs frequent
feedings of calorie-rich formulas. The other
statements do not describe the unique needs
of prematurity.
II, 1 & 2, Infants with special needs (prematurity)

28. Suctioning the mouth and nose immediately
② after delivery helps to clear the airway of secretions and is necessary to promote the establishment of a normal respiratory pattern. The other
primary needs of the newborn are best met by
other actions.
III, 2, Newborn care

29. The mother who is relinquishing her infant
③ grieves and needs acceptance and emotional
support. The nurse should be responsive to
her needs and desires regarding seeing and
interacting with the infant. The other responses
by the nurse do not convey acceptance.
III, 3, Special situations associated with childbirth (adoption)

30. Assessing for risk factors in order to plan
① care is an integral part of effective prenatal
care. An adequate history reveals reproductive risk factors and guides the practitioner in
planning care. The outcome of the pregnancy
cannot always be controlled; however, risk
factors can be minimized. Regular prenatal
visits are essential for every pregnancy. Pregnancy is characterized by minor discomforts,
but these are not generally threatening to life
or health.
I, 4, Prenatal care

31. The pregnant client with diabetes is at in-
④ creased risk for fetal demise in the last trimester, particularly if she has a history of previous
stillbirth. Frequent monitoring of fetal well-
being through close supervision and maternal
awareness of fetal activity levels is critical for
this client. A cesarean delivery is not indicated
at this point. Vigorous exercise is often contraindicated for a pregnant woman with type I
diabetes because it may contribute to placental
ischemia. The client's overall caloric intake
should *increase* by approximately 300 calories
per day, not decrease.
II, 2 & 4, Complications associated with childbearing (diabetes mellitus)

32. Hyperthyroidism increases the metabolism, causing the client to be sensitive to heat and excessive stimulation. Calming measures and efforts to keep the client cool are indicated. The other measures would be helpful for a client with hypothyroidism because those measures tend to stimulate the metabolism.
①
III, 2, Hyperthyroidism

33. The client who has had a thyroidectomy should be taught measures to reduce strain to the incision; supporting her head while she is changing positions is one method to accomplish this goal. Laryngeal edema, stridor, and tetany are symptoms of hypocalcemia associated with accidental removal of the parathyroids during surgery. Damage to the laryngeal nerve is assessed for by checking the voice for hoarseness periodically; supporting the head would not prevent this complication.
③
III, 2 & 4, Thyroidectomy

34. Cushing's syndrome predisposes to osteoporosis and muscle wasting, which can lead to injury. Anorexia and nausea are not direct signs and symptoms of Cushing's syndrome. The fluid and electrolyte balance likely to be associated with this disorder is hypernatremia with water retention. Laryngeal spasm is not related to Cushing's syndrome.
③
I, 1, Cushing's syndrome

35. Intravenous heparin has an immediate onset and peaks within 5 to 10 minutes. The duration of heparin is 6 hours. With Coumadin, the peak of action is 2 to 3 days, and duration of drug is 2 to 5 days. For immediate anticoagulation effects, intravenous heparin is begun, and oral therapy with Coumadin is started after the client's condition stabilizes. If the partial thromboplastin time is not in therapeutic range, the heparin can be regulated and completely excreted in 6 hours. If the prothrombin time is abnormal, it may take up to 5 days for Coumadin to be excreted.
①
II, 2, Anticoagulation therapy

36. Symmetrel is based in the treatment of Parkinson's disease. It potentiates the action of dopamine in the central nervous system, which reduces tremors and rigidity of muscles. Bradykinesia is slow voluntary movement and speech.
③
III, 4, Symmetrel

37. Haldol is used in the treatment of acute and chronic psychosis. It alters the central nervous system and has an anticholinergic effect (drying). Extrapyramidal reactions and tardive dyskinesia are drooling; tremors; uncontrolled movement of the face, mouth, and tongue; and uncontrolled movement of the extremities. Hypotension, constipation, respiratory depression, and sedation are other side effects.
①
I, 2, Haldol

38. Fluids should be increased because of the side effects of dry mouth and constipation with antidepressants. Alcohol and central nervous system depressants work against the intended action (mood elevation). Hypotension is a common side effect, and changing position slowly lessens the possibility of falling.
③
III, 4, Elavil

39. Normal values for white blood cells are 5000/mm^3 to 10,000/mm^3. This value of 8000 is within the normal range and indicates resolution of an infection. The antibiotic Cipro is effective against the type of organism the patient has in his wound. Normal tympanic/ear temperature is 98.60°F. Purulent drainage indicates that the wound is still infected and should be becoming more serosanguineous and in lesser amounts. The skin should be returning to pink, and no edema or hot spots should be present.
②
IV, 1, Antibiotic/infection

40. Prednisone is a corticosteroid and affects the adrenal gland by disturbing the natural balance of hormone secretion. Steroids affect the 3 S's (sugar, salt, and sex balance in the body). Steroids increase retention of salt/sodium, which retains fluids, and fluid volume excess should be assessed. Hyperglycemia is caused by decreased carbohydrate tolerance. Thin skin, skin tears, and ecchymosis are caused by inhibition of fibroblast formation and collagen deposition in decreased wound healing.
③
I, 1, Steroid therapy

41. Stools become dark, black, or tarry with iron. Liquid preparations should be given with a straw to prevent staining of teeth. Nausea and vomiting and abdominal cramps are common side effects.
④
I, 2, Ferrous sulfate/iron

42.
④
Diltiazem and nifedipine are calcium channel blockers, antianginal agents, and coronary vasodilators and are used to treat hypertension. Procainamide is an antiarrhythmic drug. Isosorbide dinitrate is an antianginal drug.
I, 2, Antiarrhythmic

43.
③
Potassium is irritating to the lining of the stomach. To prevent gastrointestinal upset, give with a full glass of water or juice or with meals.
III, 2, Potassium chloride

44.
①
All diuretics are best taken in the morning to prevent frequent urination in the night.
III, 2, Minipress/diuretic

45.
②
Furosemide (Lasix) is a potassium-depleting diuretic. There is an increased risk of digoxin toxicity with hypokalemia. These are signs and symptoms of hypokalemia and digoxin toxicity; withhold the medication and notify the physician.
IV, 2, Digoxin and Lasix.

46.
①
Hypersensitivity or an allergic reaction is caused by the drug reacting to the antibodies, causing cell damage and release of histamines. Symptoms can range from mild rashes, hives, or pruritus to anaphylactic shock. Potentiation occurs when two drugs with different mechanisms of action produce greater effects when taken together. Idiosyncratic reaction is an unexpected reaction to a drug (e.g., a sedative causing anxiety in a client). Toxicity occurs when the drug level exceeds the therapeutic range and/or when the liver or kidneys cannot metabolize or excrete the drug at the proper rate.
I, 2, Drug reactions

47.
③
Gentamicin is an aminoglycoside that may cause permanent ototoxic effects on the eighth cranial acoustic nerve. Signs and symptoms are headache, dizziness, vertigo, nausea and vomiting, tinnitus, and hearing impairment.
I, 2, Gentamicin

48.
①
Glycopyrrolate is a cholinergic blocker or agent used with preoperative medications. The action is to dry respiratory secretions and saliva. Cholinergic drugs are used in urinary retention and myasthenia gravis to increase the tone in the genitourinary tract and skeletal muscles. Narcotic antagonists reverse the effects of narcotics. Adrenergic blockers block the sympathetic effects of epinephrine and norepinephrine in hypertensive crisis.
I, 2, Robinul, anticholinergic

49.
②
Antepartal care is the care a woman receives before the birth of a child. Antepartal care is also called prenatal care. Postpartal care is the care received after the child's birth. Parapartal care is the care received by the pregnant client both during her pregnancy and after the birth of the child. Intrapartal care is care received during the birthing process itself.
III, 4, Maternity nursing

50.
④
As the pregnancy progresses, the client should see the physician more frequently because of the increasing possibility of maternal complications relating to increased size and weight of the baby. Also, the chance of dilatation and effacement and the onset of labor increases as the pregnancy progresses. The other answers allow either too little or too much time between examinations.
I, 4, Maternity nursing

51.
①
Vitamin A is the only vitamin obtained through the colostrum and breast milk. All the other vitamins must be obtained from the diet.
I, 4, Maternity nursing

52.
①
Clothing worn by the pregnant woman should be supportive but loose and should allow for growth. A girdle restricts blood flow to and from the legs and also is uncomfortable.
I, 4, Maternity nursing

53.
③
Swimming, jogging, and playing tennis may be too strenuous for most pregnant clients, especially if these activities were not part of their prepregnancy routine. Brisk walking is not too strenuous, and it allows for deep breathing and clearing of the mind.
I, 4, Maternity nursing

54.
①
An abortion occurs only before the age of viability, not during the last month of pregnancy. All the other answers are appropriate reasons for the physician to advise against sexual intercourse during the last month of pregnancy.
II, 4, Maternity nursing

55.
④ The nurse should remain with the client, especially while the physician is examining her. This not only shows concern for the client's feelings but also protects the physician from any false accusations of a sexual nature. All other answers do show concern for the client's feelings.
III, 4, Maternity nursing

56.
④ When the client breathes normally and keeps her back flat against the table, it makes it more difficult to contract pelvic muscles. Therefore, the client is more relaxed and the examination is easier. It is fine to tell her to relax, but whenever the client lifts her back off the table, she is contracting pelvic muscles, which makes the examination more difficult and more uncomfortable, leading to increased anxiety instead of relaxation.
III, 2, Maternity nursing

57.
④ Whenever a client has had a positive experience, is well read about childbirth, and has practiced relaxation techniques, her labor will probably go more smoothly than the client who has had an unhappy experience or is alone. Therefore, the client who is alone needs more emotional support from the nurse.
II, 4, Maternity nursing

58.
② The progress of labor is less likely to be affected when medication for pain relief is given at 4 to 5 cm of dilation. When given too early, at 3 to 4 cm, the progress of labor may stop. If given too late, at 8 to 9 or 9 to 10 cm of dilation, delivery may soon be accomplished and the baby's respiratory efforts may be depressed.
II, 4, Maternity nursing

59.
③ RhoGam can be given within 10 or 52 hours after delivery and still be effective, but 72 hours may elapse before RhoGam is given to the Rh-sensitized woman and it will still be effective. If RhoGam is not given until 92 hours after delivery, the Rh-sensitized woman will already have antibodies against Rh-positive blood cells and the medication will be ineffective.
II, 4, Maternity nursing

60.
④ Betamethasone is used to accelerate fetal lung maturation. Yutopar is a smooth muscle relaxant and is used to stop uterine contractions in premature onset of labor. Tylenol is an analgesic-antipyretic. Diazepam is an anti-anxiety agent.
III, 4, Maternity nursing

61.
① Tace suppresses lactation. Clomid is a fertility drug used to stimulate ovulation. Yutopar is a smooth muscle relaxant used to stop premature labor. Dilaudid is an analgesic.
III, 4, Maternity nursing

62.
③ Oral contraceptives are used to inhibit ovulation and thereby prevent pregnancy. Oral contraceptives do not cause abortion, develop the ovarian follicle, or prevent menstruation.
I, 4, Maternity nursing

63.
④ Colostrum is the first substance produced by a postpartum client's breasts. Milk appears in the breasts about 3 to 4 days after birth (after colostrum). Estrogen is a female sex hormone, and prolactin is a hormone that increases blood supply to the breasts and increases glandular activity of the breasts.
IV, 4, Maternity nursing

64.
② Milk replaces colostrum in the breasts of a breast-feeding postpartum client about 3 to 4 days after birth and continues until suckling stops.
II, 1, Maternity nursing

65.
③ Involution is the return of the uterus to its prepregnancy size and position within the pelvis. Diuresis is a marked increase in the daily output of urine. Diaphoresis is excessive perspiration. Engorgement is the congestion of the breasts caused by an increased blood supply and glandular activity in preparation for lactation.
IV, 4, Maternity nursing

66.
② Thin pink-tinged drainage from the vagina, called lochia serosa, is what you would expect to find from a client on the fifth postpartum day. Vaginal discharge that is white and frothy, thick and yellow, or sticky and green at any time may indicate a vaginal infection.
IV, 4, Maternity nursing

67.
③ Bleeding that would completely saturate two sanitary napkins in a 30-minute period of time is entirely too much bleeding at any time postpartum. This is an indication that the client is experiencing a postpartum hemorrhage. All the other amounts of drainage are acceptable for the amount of time that had elapsed on the second postpartum day.
IV, 4, Maternity nursing

68.
④ Even though dizziness and lightheadedness may be present with hemorrhaging, imminent delivery, and low blood glucose, the fact that it occurs while lying flat on the back indicates that it may be due to decreased return blood flow to the brain. Positioning the client on her side takes pressure off the aorta, allowing more blood flow to the body and brain.
I, 4, Maternity nursing

69.
③ Normally, at 3 months, most infants can lift their heads. Some infants may perform this earlier. Premature infants may do so later.
I, 4, Pediatric growth and development

70.
④ The anterior fontanel closes and becomes useless as an assessment tool after age 15 to 18 months. The posterior fontanel closes much earlier.
I, 4, Pediatric growth and development

71.
② By 12 months, the child usually triples the birth weight.
I, 4, Pediatric growth and development

72.
③ All 20 deciduous teeth are in by 30 to 36 months of age.
I, 4, Pediatric growth and development

73.
③ Although the child will lose the first tooth just before this age, the first permanent tooth, normally a bottom incisor, presents itself at about 6 to 7 years of age. Choice 1 is the age at which all deciduous teeth are in. Choices 2 and 4 are incorrect.
I, 4, Pediatric growth and development

74.
④ A transurethral resection presents the lowest risk for the client because there is no abdominal or perineal incision and, therefore, fewer postoperative complications and shorter hospitalization. It can also be done easily with spinal anesthesia.
II, 1 & 2, Benign prostatic hyperplasia

75.
① The prostate is vascular, and some bleeding is expected postoperatively. The continuous flow of irrigating solution prevents clots from obstructing the catheter.
II, 1 & 2, Benign prostatic hyperplasia

76.
③ The Foley catheter may be blocked with clots. This is an abnormal finding that should be reported immediately.
I & III, 1 & 2, Benign prostatic hyperplasia

77.
③ The ossicles or bones of the middle ear are fused together and unable to vibrate to transmit the sound waves to the inner ear. This disease does not involve obstruction or nerve damage.
I, 2 & 4, Otosclerosis

78.
④ Sudden or violent blowing of the nose causes increased pressure in the middle ear and may dislodge the prosthesis that replaces the stapes. Choices 1, 2, and 3 represent incorrect theoretical concepts.
III, 2 & 4, Otosclerosis

79.
③ The symptoms that the client is exhibiting are of decreased cerebral blood flow owing to narrowing of the cerebral vessels.
I, 2, Atherosclerosis

80.
② The diet that the client usually follows is high in fat and cholesterol. Eggs are high in cholesterol. Cereal and juice provide the lowest amounts of fat and cholesterol for his breakfast.
III, 4, Atherosclerosis/nutrition

81.
④ The signs and symptoms that the nurse is observing are typical signs of peripheral vascular disease. When a client has atherosclerosis in one area of the body, it is also likely to be present in other parts of the body.
II, 2, Peripheral arterial disease

82.
① A vasodilator causes dilation of all vessels, not just those affected by disease. When generalized vasodilation occurs, the client's blood pressure can drop, resulting in lightheadedness and faintness.
I, 1 & 2, Peripheral vascular disease

83.
③ Peripheral venous disease can result in venous stasis with ulcer formation. It is important to prevent injury or trauma, even from the weight of the bed covers.
II, 1 & 2, Peripheral vascular disease

84.
① Substernal chest pain is a classic symptom of angina resulting from lack of oxygen and blood supply to the heart. Fatigue, shortness of breath, and dyspnea are symptoms of congestive heart failure. Nausea, epigastric pain, and anorexia are symptoms of acute gastritis, and epigastric pain radiating to the back is a symptom of pancreatitis.
I, 2, Cardiovascular disease

85. Elevation of LDH, CPK, and SGOT (AST) levels in the serum is indicative of a myocardial infarction. Elevated levels of SGOT (AST) indicate congestive heart failure, and increased levels of CPK and LDH, although indicative of cardiac involvement, are not clearly signs of a myocardial infarction.
① II, 1, Cardiovascular disease

86. Fowler's position relieves pulmonary congestion by lowering venous return, and dyspnea becomes less prevalent. The Trendelenburg position is used for a client who is going into shock. Lying supine or prone increases the pressure on the cardiopulmonary system by the diaphragm, thus increasing cardiac workload and oxygen requirements.
④ IV, 4, Cardiovascular disease

87. Vitamin B_{12} must be given intramuscularly every 2 months for the rest of the client's life to keep the client free of signs and symptoms because of the inability of the gastric mucosa to produce the intrinsic factor necessary for absorption of the vitamin B_{12}. Although a diet high in vitamin B_{12} is of importance, the B_{12} is not absorbed because of the lack of the intrinsic factor. Oral vitamin B_{12} supplements are not as readily absorbed as the intramuscular form. Iron therapy is used in conjunction with vitamin B_{12} injections, not alone.
③ III, 4, Cardiovascular disease

88. Frothy sputum is produced from air mixing with the fluid in the alveoli and is blood-tinged from blood cells that have exuded into the alveoli. Copious green sputum is produced in a client who has a *Pseudomonas*-type respiratory infection. Sputum that is copious and salmon-colored is characteristic of staphylococcal pneumonia. White and watery sputum is common in a client with normal sputum production.
② I, 2, Respiratory disease

89. The affected extremity is elevated periodically above heart level to prevent venous stasis and reduce edema. Elevating the head of the bed to Fowler's position relieves pulmonary congestion by lowering venous return to the cardiopulmonary system. The client with acute congestive heart failure should remain on complete bed rest. Applying moist heat to the extremities is an intervention used for clients with a diagnosis of thrombophlebitis. Application of cold compresses is inappropriate.
③ III, 4, Cardiovascular disease

90. Expiration of air against a collapsed airway causes wheezing, cerebral hypoxia results in restlessness, and hypoxia causes tachycardia. Clients with chronic obstructive pulmonary disease exhibit chronic weight loss. Bradycardia and hypertension are more cardiac-related.
② I, 2, Respiratory disease

91. The gag reflex is anesthetized during the bronchoscopic procedure; until the ability to swallow returns, there is an increased risk for aspiration. If there is an order for NPO status after the procedure, it is given by the physician, not the charge nurse. The respiratory rate of 20 to 22/minute is normal. Blood-streaked sputum can be expected for a few days after a biopsy.
① III, 1, Respiratory disease

92. Hepatitis B is spread by blood transfusions and direct contact with body fluids from infected persons, such as breast milk and sexual contact. Hepatitis A is spread by direct contact, usually by food and water contaminated with feces. Hepatitis E is spread through the fecal contamination of water.
② I, 4, Gastrointestinal disease

93. Explaining the procedure allows clients to ask the appropriate questions, thus alleviating their concerns. Arranging for clients to view the procedure only adds to their concerns.
① III, 3, Gastrointestinal disease

94. The goal of management of the client with neurogenic bladder is to establish urinary elimination and prevent complications. With a diagnosis of cystitis, the client should be encouraged to drink 2000 mL of fluid per day. When continence is established, intermittent catheterization is used to determine whether the bladder is emptying in a client with urinary retention. Monitoring body temperature every 4 hours is a nursing intervention used for a client with chills and fever associated with pyelonephritis.
④ II, 2, Urinary disease

95. Pressure on the urethra from the prostate gland causes frequent urination, nocturia, and difficulty starting a stream, which are all symptoms of benign prostatic hyperplasia. Hematuria, dysuria, urinary retention, bone pain, and weight loss are symptoms of cancer of the prostate. Painless hematuria and a palpable mass in the flank area are symptoms of renal tumors.
① I, 2, Urinary disease

96.
② A tracheostomy tray is the most important piece of necessary equipment after a thyroidectomy because of the possibility of neck swelling resulting in respiratory distress. A Pleur-Evac drainage system is connected to a chest tube after thoracic surgery. A suction setup is at the bedside for emergency use should the client have difficulty mobilizing secretions postoperatively. An incentive spirometer is not used because coughing, resulting from the use of the apparatus, puts a strain on the suture line.
III, 1, Endocrine disease

97.
① Hypotension is the major complication of spinal anesthesia because it causes peripheral vasodilation.
III, ,1 Surgical intervention

98.
② An early clinical manifestation of a transfusion reaction is flank pain and low back pain because of the renal involvement.
I, 1 & 2, Surgical Intervention

99.
④ Frequent voiding of small amounts of urine can be a sign of bladder distention. Nausea can occur after surgery but should be reported if it persists. Pain at the incision site and drainage are to be expected.
IV, 1, Surgical intervention

100.
③ Inderal lowers the blood pressure and pulse rate; it does not raise it. Inderal sometimes causes depression in older clients.
III & IV, 2, Myocardial infarction/medication

101.
② Heparin can cause bleeding from mucous membranes if the level is too high. It is important to evaluate the urine for the presence of blood.
I & IV, 2, Myocardial infarction

102.
③ Subcutaneous heparin should be given in the fat of the abdomen. This area is less prone to trauma and bleeding. Do not massage the area because this increases bruising.
III, 2, Myocardial infarction/medication

103.
④ Depression is common after a myocardial infarction. It is important for clients to be able to express what is concerning them and have their questions answered fully.
III, 3, Myocardial infarction

104.
③ Substance abuse is generally an illness that affects the family; the family can unknowingly encourage substance abuse. It is ideal to provide family treatment. It is not just ideal but mandatory that confidentiality is maintained; the client needs to agree to family involvement. There is no evidence that driving is a problem for this client. There is no suggestion that employment reeducation is necessary.
II, 3, Mental health

105.
④ Clients experiencing mania burn an increased amount of calories. These clients usually do not have the attention span to sit down for a meal; high-calorie finger foods are something they can eat as they move.
II, 4, Mental health

106.
③ Elation may signal that the client now has a suicide plan. Elation may give the client energy to carry out that plan. A suicidal client needs ongoing treatment. It would be premature to discharge this client without further assessment.
I, 3, Mental health

107.
④ Whenever a death wish is expressed, the nurse needs to assess whether the client has a plan with intent. Reassurance can be perceived as nongenuine and false assurance. Time alone increases the client's sense of loneliness and does not provide the client the observation needed. Confidentiality is not appropriate in this situation; it would not get the client the help he or she wants and needs.
III, 3, Mental health

108.
② It is the responsibility of the PN to report to the RN. The RN is responsible for informing the physician. Usually, verbalization of suicide is a cry for help; remaining silent is not appropriate and would not get the client the help he or she needs. A client does not necessarily need a reason to be depressed.
III, 3, Mental health

109.
④ Cheddar cheese, aged products, and many legumes are some of the foods that are restricted for the client taking monoamine oxidase inhibitors. Consumption of these foods sometimes leads to a hypertensive crisis. The other foods listed are not contraindicated for people taking monoamine oxidase inhibitors.
II, 4, Mental health

110.
③ The therapeutic range of lithium is 0.8 to 1.5 mEq/L. Imminent toxicity can occur at 1.5 to 2.0 mEq/L. Actual toxicity can occur over 2.0 mEq/L.
I, 2, Mental health

111.
③ A walk would be in line with the client's current need to move. A client with mania can be impulsive and impatient; activities with scissors can be dangerous if the client has suicidal or homicidal impulses. Clients usually do not have the attention span for detailed or repetitive activities while they are in the manic phase.
II, 3, Mental health

112.
③ Extrapyramidal effects are side effects of many antipsychotic medications. These effects resemble Parkinson's disease. Cogentin decreases these side effects. Cogentin does not increase the effects of antipsychotic medications, and it does not directly affect nutritional status.
III, 2, Mental health

113.
② Neuroleptic malignant syndrome is a life-threatening condition initiated by neuroleptic (antipsychotic) medications. Elevation of temperature and blood pressure are early signals of this syndrome. The muscles become rigid as this syndrome progresses. Coma and death are late signs of this disorder.
I, 2, Mental health

114.
④ It is important to allow the child to tell what happened without the mother or caregiver present. It is also important to compare the stories of the caregiver and the child. Stories that are contrasting may indicate child abuse. Pain medication is not always indicated.
I, 3, Mental health

115.
④ Taking iron with a food containing vitamin C increases absorption of the iron; orange juice contains a high amount of vitamin C. Decreasing fluids leads to an increased potential of constipation. Taking the iron with milk offers no special benefit. Decreasing citrus foods decreases vitamin C–containing foods, which decreases the absorption of iron.
II, 2, Pharmacology

116.
④ Radiation burns should be reported to the radiation department, which may provide topical medication for the burn. Astringents contain alcohol, which leads to further tissue damage. Oil-based products are absorbed into the skin and cause more intense burning with future radiation treatments.
III, 2, Cancer

117.
② Ice reduces swelling, which is likely to occur within the first 24 hours. Heat increases swelling. Range of motion is contraindicated at this time; rest and elevation of the involved area lead to decreased swelling and decreased pain.
II, 2, Musculoskeletal

118.
③ To prevent aspiration, the nurse should check the tube for proper placement. The supine position increases the risk of aspiration; the head of the bed should be elevated to at least 45 degrees. Flushing the tube before checking the tube for placement increases the risk of aspiration. Coughing and deep breathing do not decrease the risk of aspiration.
III, 1, Respiratory/gastrointestinal

119.
④ Ambulating the client increases peristalsis, which decreases the risk of an ileus. Strict bed rest increases the likelihood of an ileus because of the decrease in peristalsis associated with bed rest. Assessing bowel sounds and obtaining abdominal measurements are not direct interventions.
III, 2, Gastrointestinal

120.
④ These are signs and symptoms of appendicitis requiring immediate attention. As a PN, you have the responsibility of reporting these signs and symptoms to the RN. Applying heat to the area increases the risk of rupture. Administering pain medication without further medical evaluation may mask symptoms and lead to more serious complications. Ice to the area can increase spasms and increase risk of rupture.
III, 2, Gastrointestinal

121.
④ Chemotherapy causes changes in the red blood cells and white blood cells of clients undergoing this therapy. These clients are at high risk for bleeding disorders; use of a soft toothbrush prevents bleeding of the gums. Clients undergoing chemotherapy should generally increase their fluid intake. Constipation is generally not a side effect of chemotherapy. Strong mouthwashes may increase risk of oral tissue damage.
III, 2, Cancer

122.
④ Immediate postoperative care of the colostomy client must include close observation of the stoma for possible circulatory impairment. This is the most significant observation.
I, 2, Colostomies

123.
① Change in body image is a reality within the first week after a colostomy is performed. Change in social role and regression are not expected, and guilt feelings about cancer are only a conjecture.
I, 3, Colostomies

124.
① Clients with leukopenia are most susceptible to infections. Bleeding may occur because of thrombocytopenia or because of chemical toxicity on fragile blood vessels. Hyperuricemia may occur because of massive cell destruction as a result of cancer or because of effects of chemotherapeutic drugs or radiation therapy. Hypercalcemia may result from cancer, not leukopenia.
IV, 1 & 2, Chemotherapy

125.
④ Hypocalcemic tetany is manifested by laryngeal spasms, difficulty talking, and carpopedal spasms.
I, 2, Chemotherapy

126.
② Irradiated skin is fragile and susceptible to injury. Protection from the sun and other irritants is necessary. Care of the skin includes washing gently with warm water, patting gently dry, and applying lanolin or A&D ointment to dry areas with physician's orders. A dressing is not necessary.
III, 1, Radiation therapy

127.
① A platelet count of less than 100,000 should be reported because bleeding can result. Nausea, vomiting, and fatigue do occur with radiation therapy. White blood cell counts less than 1000 should be reported.
III, 1, Radiation therapy

128.
① Immunosuppression may be linked to diabetes mellitus but not to obesity, maladaptive behaviors, or hormone imbalances.
I, 1, Immunosuppression

129.
④ Preventing direct contact with body fluids and secretions is the best safeguard against AIDS. The other options are required for other infectious conditions.
III, 1 & 2, AIDS

130.
③ A phobia cannot be treated by insight-oriented therapy. Desensitization is the most common form of therapy. The other options are common characteristics associated with phobias.
I, 3, Phobias

131.
② Xenophobia is fear of strangers, agoraphobia is fear of outdoors, acrophobia is fear of heights, and claustrophobia is fear of closed spaces.
I, 3, Phobias

132.
② When attempting to help the client overcome a phobia, the nurse should help the client recognize and strengthen any adaptive coping mechanisms that the client develops. The client cannot be placed directly into situations that confront the phobia but must be helped to face anxiety-producing situations gradually. Tranquilizers are commonly used to help control the anxiety the client is feeling.
III, 3, Phobias

133.
③ Keeping the client on nothing-by-mouth (NPO) status prevents aspiration of gastric contents during or after the surgery.
IV, 1, Surgical intervention

134.
① The normal serum potassium level is 3.5 to 5.0 mEq/L. A low potassium level can lead to cardiac abnormalities and death. The other values are within normal limits.
III & IV, 1 & 2, Surgical intervention

135.
④ 1000/480 × 15 = gtt/min, 100/48 × 15 = 1500/48 = 31 gtt/min.
III,2, Medication administration

136.
① The delayed acquisition of gross motor milestones is usually the primary complaint in the history of infants with cerebral palsy.
I, 2, Cerebral palsy

137.
③ When talking to parents, the nurse must remember that cerebral palsy varies from mild to severe.
III, 2 & 3, Cerebral palsy

138.
① Persistent oral reflexes, poor breathing patterns, tongue thrust, excessive opening of the mouth, and drooling make it difficult for the child to obtain adequate nutrition.
II, 4, Cerebral palsy

139.
③ A major part of the nurse's role in working with adolescents who are depressed is to make appropriate referral when necessary.
III, 3, Suicidal behavior

140.
④ Depression is found in two thirds of the cases of suicide. The nurse should be alert for any changes in behavior as well as the giving away of personal belongings, which may signal a suicide attempt.
I, 3, Suicidal behavior

141.
③ Being inactive tends to perpetuate itself, causing the client to lose the initiative to do what she is capable of doing.
I, 2, Immobility/older adults

142.
② Footdrop is a common result of immobility. A footboard keeps the foot in proper alignment and prevents footdrop.
III, 4, Immobility

143.
① Range-of-motion exercises should not cause considerable pain. The physician should be notified before the exercises are continued.
IV, 2, Immobility

144.
④ Trochanter rolls are placed on the outside of the hips and legs and prevent them from rolling outwardly.
III, 2, Immobility

145.
① Without muscle movement, blood becomes static in the venous system; in turn, this increases the likelihood of thrombi or emboli.
I, 4, Immobility

146.
③ Immobility can lead to constipation related to decreased peristalsis. Increased bulk and roughage in the diet can help prevent this problem. Enemas should be avoided. Stool softeners along with increased fluid intake are suggested.
III, 4, Immobility

147.
④ Hyperactivity is not normally an effect of immobility. The other choices are normally caused by immobility.
II, 2 & 4, Immobility

148.
② Calcium is lost in large amounts from the bones, leading to disuse osteoporosis.
II, 2 & 4, Immobility/fluid and electrolytes

149.
② Pressure on an area decreases circulation, resulting in cell death. Choices 1, 3, and 4 are contributing factors, but not the primary cause.
I, 2 & 4, Immobility

150.
① This interval is usually adequate to prevent breakdown. In choices 2, 3, and 4, the time intervals are too long.
III, 2 & 4, Immobility

151.
① Denial is a primary defense mechanism, especially among younger adolescents. Denial is characterized by the inability or unwillingness to acknowledge pertinent information.
I, 3 & 4, Labor and delivery

152.
③ In anxiety-producing situations, concentration is diminished, so communication should be short and simple. Medication would simply further interfere with concentration.
III, 3 & 4, Labor and delivery

153.
② The normal fetal heart rate is 120 to 160 bpm. It is important to give the client correct information so that she will not be so anxious. The other answers are untrue and would not be therapeutic.
III, 3 & 4, Labor and delivery

154.
④ The teenager is at risk for all of these reasons. Teenage pregnancy is always a higher risk.
I & II, 4, Labor and delivery

155.
① Contractions are measured from the beginning of one contraction to the beginning of the next contraction.
I, 4, Labor and delivery

156.
③ Demerol is a narcotic analgesic that can be given for pain during the active phases of labor.
III & IV, 2 & 4, Labor and delivery

157.
③ An episiotomy is an incision made into the perineum before delivery. It is done to facilitate the delivery of the baby and to prevent tearing when the baby is delivered.
I, 4, Labor and delivery

158.
② Hand washing is imperative; it is the most basic form of hygiene and infection prevention. All perineal care should be done from front to back.
IV, 4, Postpartum

159.
② The client's decision should be supported. Bonding and attachment are encouraged by frequent, loving contact with the parent. It is not necessary to breast-feed the infant in order to bond.
III, 3 & 4, Postpartum

160.
④ Answers 1, 2, and 3 indicate a lack of nutritional knowledge. Nutritional intake must provide sufficient calories and a wide variety of nutrients to meet the adolescent's own growth needs.
IV, 4, Postpartum

161.
① Consideration must be given to identifying and supporting the adolescent's need for a lifestyle that is both realistic and satisfying.
II, 4, Postpartum

162.
① Digoxin slows the heart rate and increases the force of contractions. A possible side effect is that the heart rate may slow down too much. To prevent this, the nurse should check the apical pulse before administering digoxin. If the pulse is below 60, the medication is withheld and the physician is notified.
III, 1 & 2, Congestive heart failure

163.
① Digoxin slows the heart rate and strengthens the contractions.
III, 2 & 4, Congestive heart failure

164.
④ With congestive heart failure, breathing can be difficult as the lungs fill with fluid. The client will be much more comfortable sitting up to breathe.
III, 1 & 2, Congestive heart failure

165.
③ The pulse pressure is the difference between the systolic and diastolic blood pressure. This can reflect a number of different changes in cardiac function and even in intracranial pressure.
III, 1 & 2, Congestive heart failure

166.
① The fluid restrictions associated with congestive heart failure can be quite severe, as low as 1000 mL/day. To maximize client comfort, the dietary and nursing staffs must collaborate in planning care for a fluid restriction of this severity so that the client has maximum comfort.
II, 1 & 2, Congestive heart failure

167.
① Lemon juice is a good seasoning substitute for salt because it adds a great deal of flavor to food while adding no sodium. The other options are all high in sodium.
III, 4, Congestive heart failure

168.
④ Treatment for congestive heart failure is continued for the rest of the client's life because the heart can never be cured of its failure. Congestive heart failure is controllable as the heart compensates.
III, 4, Congestive heart failure

169.
① Dyspnea with mild exertion is an early symptom of the hypoxia associated with COPD. The other options listed are late symptoms of COPD.
I, 2, COPD

170.
① The COPD client has a chronically high carbon dioxide level, so that this is no longer a stimulus for respiration. The COPD client's stimulus for breathing is hypoxia. If the client receives too much oxygen, the stimulus for respiration is lost and the respiratory rate drops.
IV, 2, COPD

171.
③ Aminophylline is a smooth muscle relaxant that promotes relaxation of the bronchial smooth muscles. As COPD becomes worse, the medication becomes less effective.
IV, 2, COPD

172.
② Emphysema is characterized by air trapping. As the air is trapped in the alveoli, the bronchioles and alveoli become distended and blebs, or air pockets, are formed.
IV, 2, COPD

173.
④ Once the client has symptomatic COPD, exercise must be limited. The other options are instructions that are important for the client to follow.
III, 2 & 4, COPD

174.
② With COPD, the air becomes trapped in the alveoli; therefore, an increase in carbon dioxide occurs. Pursed lip and diaphragmatic breathing increase the outflow of air, helping to remove some of the air trapped in the alveoli.
III, 2 & 4, COPD

175.
① One of the functions of the hypothalamus is to control thirst.
I, 2, Fluid and electrolytes

176. The intracellular fluid is contained within the
④ cells. The fluid outside the cells is referred to
as extracellular fluid.
I, 2, Fluid and electrolytes

177. A low serum sodium level, unless it is dilu-
② tional hyponatremia, is not associated with
edema. Usually, when sodium levels are low,
so are water levels. All the other options cause
edema.
IV, 2, Fluid and electrolytes

178. Edema is a condition in which the client has
③ too much fluid in the body, usually in the third
space. The client with edema is usually on a
fluid restriction regimen, so that further water
retention can be limited. Sodium intake is reduced because sodium holds water in the
body.
III, 2, Fluid and electrolytes

179. Thiazide diuretics work by causing potassium
② to be lost through the kidneys along with the
excessive water. When these diuretics are used,
the client is usually directed to increase potassium content in the diet.
I, 2, Fluid and electrolytes

180. Dehydration is characterized by loss of skin
① turgor, hypotension, conservation of urine,
and an elevated temperature.
I, 2, Fluid and electrolytes

181. An increased serum sodium level leads to the
④ retention of water in the body to dilute it.
When the client has hypernatremia, he or she
also exhibits edema. With a high serum sodium level, pitting edema is seen.
I, 2, Fluid and electrolytes

182. Diuretics act by causing loss of potassium or
① sodium. As these electrolytes are lost, loss of
water also occurs. Because cardiac clients often
exhibit hypertension or congestive heart failure, they typically receive diuretic medications.
I, 2, Fluid and electrolytes

183. A severely increased serum potassium level
② predisposes the client to potentially fatal cardiac arrhythmias. It is important, therefore,
to lower the serum potassium level rapidly.
Kayexalate can be given either orally or by
enema. It acts to bind the excessive potassium
and causes it to be excreted through the feces.
II, 2, Fluid and electrolytes

184. A low serum potassium level produces muscle
③ weakness and accompanying fatigue.
I, 2, Fluid and electrolytes

185. When a client is immobilized for any pro-
④ longed period of time, calcium is released from
the bone, leading to hypercalcemia.
IV, 2, Fluid and electrolytes

186. The parathyroid glands lie directly posterior
③ to the thyroid gland. The parathyroids control
calcium metabolism. When a thyroidectomy is
performed, the parathyroids are often inciden-
tally removed, damaged or, at least, trauma-
tized and edematous from the surgery. This
leads to altered calcium metabolism, usually
reversible after healing occurs.
I, 2, Fluid and electrolytes

187. 0.9% or normal saline is an isotonic solution,
③ which means that it is the same concentration
as blood, used intravenously. Hypotonic
means that the solution is less concentrated
than the blood; 0.45% saline is less concentrated.
III, 2, Fluid and electrolytes

188. When there is a fluid overload, the workload
④ of the heart and circulatory system is dramatically increased. To compensate for this problem, the heart rate increases.
I, 2, Fluid and electrolytes

189. The intravenous site should be assessed every
① shift for problems such as infiltration and inflammation. The dressing over the site is usually changed every 48 to 72 hours.
I, 1, Fluid and electrolytes

190. Dehydration leads to hemoconcentration,
② which can precipitate sickle cell crisis because
of the abnormal shape of the red blood cells.
I, 2, Sickle cell anemia

191. The abnormally shaped, sickled red blood cells
④ clog small vessels, leading to occlusion and
ischemia.
I, 2, Sickle cell anemia

192. To differentiate the sickle cell trait from the
① disease, hemoglobin electrophoresis is necessary. The other tests are not as specific.
I, 2, Sickle cell anemia

193.
② Because occlusion of vessels is a common problem with this disorder, nothing that increases the risk of this should be done.
III, 2 & 4, Sickle cell anemia

194.
④ This is not a problem of mild crisis. The other actions are appropriate.
III, 2 & 4, Sickle cell anemia

195.
① The abnormal-shaped cells can become trapped in the spleen, causing enlargement. As the spleen becomes enlarged, even more red blood cells and platelets are destroyed.
I, 2, Sickle cell anemia

196.
① Symptoms of ketoacidosis include acetone on the breath and in urine, polyuria, and hyperglycemia. Other choices are incorrect theoretical concepts.
I, 2, Endocrine/diabetes

197.
① Initial treatment is usually regular insulin, which has a rapid action and helps to improve symptoms quickly. Intravenous glucose or diuretics will worsen the symptoms. Long-acting insulin acts too slowly to treat diabetic ketosis initially.
III, 2, Endocrine/diabetes

198.
③ Others in the family may be able to assist John or administer his insulin to him if he neglects to do so. Phone numbers would be valuable in an emergency but do not prevent one; checking urine does not ensure that he is taking his insulin because diet and exercise also influence his metabolism. Oral medications are effective only if the client has some functional pancreatic tissue, and they do not necessarily increase compliance.
III, 4, Endocrine/diabetes

199.
① Increased metabolism causes weight loss despite normal or increased calorie intake. Clients have high levels of energy, rapid pulse, increased appetite, and increased heat production owing to the increased metabolic rate.
I, 2, Endocrine/thyroid

200.
② The increased metabolism increases muscle stimulation and interferes with fine muscle coordination. Choices 1, 3, and 4 do not occur.
I, 2, Endocrine/thyroid

201.
③ If the production of thyroid hormones is blocked, the symptoms of Graves' disease decrease or are eliminated. Sodium levels are not relevant to this disease. Thyroid hormones increase symptoms.
I, 2 & 4, Endocrine/thyroid

202.
④ Handling of the thyroid gland in surgery may cause release of more hormones, causing extreme life-threatening hyperthyroid symptoms known as thyroid crisis. Decreasing production of hormones preoperatively is usually an effective preventive measure. Other choices represent incorrect theoretical concepts.
III, 2, Endocrine/thyroid

203.
① Elevation of the head decreases pressure to the head and neck, which prevents edema and hemorrhage. The other choices may promote edema or hemorrhage.
III, 2, Endocrine/thyroid

204.
④ Some edema is normal owing to the trauma of surgery. Because of the small size of the neck area, this edema can compress the trachea and is the most likely cause of respiratory obstruction. The other choices are incorrect theoretical concepts.
I, 2, Endocrine/thyroid

205.
② Increased and exaggerated postoperative symptoms of Graves' disease is the complication known as thyroid crisis. The other choices represent incorrect theoretical concepts.
I, 2, Endocrine/thyroid

Appendix

STATE BOARDS OF NURSING

Board of Nursing
One/East Building
Suite 203
500 East Boulevard
Montgomery, AL 36117

Board of Nursing
Department of Commerce and
    Economic Development
Division of Occupational Licensing
PO Box D-LIC
Juneau, AK 99811–0800

Board of Nursing
1123 S. University Avenue
Suite 800
Little Rock, AR 72204

State Board of Nursing
2001 W. Camelback Road
Suite 350
Phoenix, AZ 85015

Board of Registered Nursing
1030 13th Street
Suite 200
Sacramento, CA 94244–2100

Board of Nursing
1560 Broadway
Suite 760
Denver, CO 80202

Department of Health Services, Nurse Licensure
150 Washington Street
Hartford, CT 06106

Board of Nursing
PO Box 1401
Dover, DE 19901

Nurses' Examining Board
614 H Street NW
Room 904
Washington, DC 20001

Board of Nursing
111 E. Coastline Drive
Suite 504
Jacksonville, FL 32202

Board of Nursing
166 Pryor Street SW
Suite 400
Atlanta, GA 30303

Board of Nursing
PO Box 3469
Honolulu, HI 96801

Board of Nursing
500 S. 10th Street
Suite 102
Boise, ID 83720

Nursing Committee
Department of Registration and Education
320 W. Washington Street
Springfield, IL 62786

State Board of Nursing
One American Square
Suite 1020
Indianapolis, IN 46282–0001

Board of Nursing
State Office Building
1223 E. Court
Des Moines, IA 50319

Board of Nursing
900 S.W. Jackson
Suite 551-S
Topeka, KS 66612–1256

Board of Nursing
4010 Dupont Circle
Suite 430
Louisville, KY 40207

State Board of Nursing
150 Baronne Street
Room 907
New Orleans, LA 70112

Board of Nursing
295 Water Street
Augusta, ME 04330–2240

Board of Examiners of Nurses
4201 Patterson Avenue
Baltimore, MD 21215–2299

Board of Registration in Nursing
100 Cambridge Street
Room 1519
Boston, MA 02202

Board of Nursing
611 N. Otiana
Lansing, MI 48909

Board of Nursing
2700 University Avenue W
Suite 108
St. Paul, MN 55114

Board of Nursing
239 N. Lamar Street
Suite 401
Jackson, MS 39201

Board of Nursing
3524 N. Ten Mile Drive
Jefferson City, MO 65102

Board of Nurses
Department of Commerce
1424 Ninth Avenue
Helena, MT 59620–0407

Board of Nursing
Department of Health
Bureau of Examining Boards
PO Box 95007
Lincoln, NE 68509

Board of Nursing
1281 Terminal Way
Suite 116
Reno, NV 89502

Board of Nursing
Education and Registration
6 Hazen Drive
Concord, NH 03301

New Jersey Board of Nursing
1101 Raymond Boulevard
Room 508
Newark, NJ 07102

Board of Nursing
4253 Montgomery NE
Suite 130
Albuquerque, NM 87109

Board of Nursing
State Education Department
Cultural Education Center
Albany, NY 12230

Board of Nursing
PO Box 2129
Raleigh, NC 27602

Board of Nursing
Kirkwood Office Tower
7th and Arbor Avenue
Suite 504
Bismarck, ND 58504

Board of Nursing
Education and Registration
77 S. High Street
Columbus, OH 43266–0316

Board of Nurse Registration and Nursing Education
2915 N. Classen Boulevard
Suite 524
Oklahoma City, OK 73106

Board of Nursing
1400 S.W. 5th Avenue
Suite 904
Portland, OR 97201

Board of Nurse Examiners
PO Box 2649
Harrisburg, PA 17105–2649

Board of Nurse Education and Registration
Cannon Health Building
75 Davis Street
Suite 104
Providence, RI 02908

Board of Nursing
1777 St. Julian Pl.
Suite 102
Columbia, SC 29204

Board of Nursing
304 S. Phillips Avenue
Suite 205
Sioux Falls, SD 57102

Board of Nursing
283 Plus Park Boulevard
Nashville, TN 37219–5407

Board of Nurse Examiners
9101 Burnet Road
Suite 104
Austin, TX 78758

Board of Nursing
160 E. 300 South Street
Salt Lake City, UT 84145

Board of Nursing
26 Terrace Street
Montpelier, VT 05602

Board of Nursing
1601 Rolling Hills Drive
Richmond, VA 23229

Board of Nursing
Division of Professional Licensing
PO Box 9649
Olympia, WA 98504

Board of Examiners
922 Quarrier Street
Suite 309
Charleston, WV 25301

Board of Nursing
PO Box 8935
Room 174
Madison, WI 53708

Board of Nursing
Barrett Building, 3rd Floor
2301 Central Avenue
Cheyenne, WY 82002

Index

Note: Page numbers in *italics* refer to illustrations.
Page numbers followed by the letter c refer to charts,
and t to tables.

Abdomen, cancer of, radiation therapy for, 237t
Abdominal binder(s), 53
Abortion, spontaneous, 369
Abruptio placentae, 370, *371*
Absence seizure(s), 71, 312
Abuse, 424–426
  of children, 327–328
  of elderly patient, 106, 426
  spousal, 424–425
Accident(s), automobile, prevention of, 323t–324t
  in adolescents, 325t
  in children, 322, 323t–325t
  in infants, 323t
  in preschoolers, 324t
  in toddlers, 324t
Ace bandage, application of, 48
ACE (angiotensin-converting enzyme) inhibitor(s), 133t
Acetaminophen (Tylenol), 72, 135t
Acetaminophen with codeine (Tylenol #3), 70, 345t
Acetazolamide (Diamox), 72
Acetohexamide (Dymelor), 75, 224t
Acetone test(s), 58
Achromycin (tetracycline), 144t, 295, 296t
Acid-base imbalance(s), 158–161. See also individual type(s)
Acidosis, lactic, 161
  metabolic, 160–161
  respiratory, 158–159
Acne vulgaris, 331
Acquired immunodeficiency syndrome (AIDS), 191t, 193–194, 333
ACTH (adrenocorticotropic hormone), excess of, 122–123
  insufficiency of, 123–124
Active listening, 405–406
Active transport, 153
Acyanotic heart defect(s), in pediatric patient, 84–87
Acyclovir (Zovirax), 86, 325
Addison's disease, 112–113, 333–334
Adenoiditis, in pediatric patient, 306
ADH (antidiuretic hormone), in fluid balance, 153
Adolescent(s), 288–290, 289t
  accidents in, 325t
  development of, nursing interventions for, 289t
    physical, 288–289
    social, 290
  developmental stages in, Eriksonian, 290
    Piaget's, 289

Adolescent(s) (*Continued*)
  nutrition for, 90, 289
  perioperative care of, 332
Adrenal disorder(s), 227–229
Adrenergic agent(s), 146t
Adrenocorticotropic hormone (ACTH), excess of, 122–123
  insufficiency of, 123–124
Adriamycin (doxorubicin), 73, 198t
Adsorbent agent(s), 131t
Adult patient(s), 117–275. See also under specific disorder(s).
  autoimmune disorders in, 199–200, *201–202*, 203–204
  cardiovascular disorders in, 130–138
  central nervous system disorders in, 169–174
  female, menopause in, 121–122
    reproductive disorders in, 119–122
    reproductive system of, 151
  growth and development of, 117–119
  immune disorders in, 199–200, *201–202*, 203–204
  infectious conditions in, 170–171
  life stages of, 117–118
  male, reproductive disorders in, 122–124. See also individual disorder(s).
    reproductive system of, 151–152
  metabolic disorders in, 221–266
  middle-aged, cardiovascular function in, 117
    cognitive changes in, 117
    common health problems of, 118
    emotional development of, 117–118
    generativity vs. self-absorption in, 118
    hearing in, 117
    hormonal changes in, 117
    metabolism in, 117
    midlife crisis in, 118
    musculoskeletal system of, 117
    skin of, 117
    vision in, 117
  older. See *Elderly patient(s)*.
  oxygenation in, 130–161
  perioperative care of, 195–199
  postoperative care of, 197–199, 198t
  protective functions in, 5, 190–204
  pulmonary disorders in, 146–152
  renal disorders in, 151–163
  sensory/perceptual alterations in, 169–183
  urinary disorders in, 151–163
  young, as mental health client, 411–412
    development of, 361–362
Advil (ibuprofen), 73t, 74

Affect, behavior patterns and, 409t–410t, 409–411
Age, and drug action, 67
AIDS (acquired immunodeficiency syndrome), 191t, 193–194, 333
Airway, neonatal, 397
Alcohol, abuse of, 426–428
  and cirrhosis, 250
  and pregnancy, 367
Alcoholics Anonymous, 428
Aldactone (spironolactone), 69, 133t
Aldomet (methyldopa), 69, 133t
Aldosterone, in fluid balance, 153
Alkaloid(s), plant, 198t
  vinca, 74
Alkalosis, metabolic, 161
  respiratory, 159–160
Alkylating agent(s), 73, 198t
Allergic rhinitis, in pediatric patient, 307–308
Alpha-fetoprotein level(s), 367
Aluminum, as antacid, 76
Alzheimer's disease, 414–415
Amblyopia, in pediatric patient, 317
Ambu bag(s), 49
Aminoglycoside(s), 70, 144t
Amniocentesis, 367
Amniotic fluid, complications involving, 382–383
Amniotic sac, development of, 364
Amoxicillin, 144t
Amphetamine(s), abuse of, 426
Amphojel, 76
Ampicillin (Polycillin), 70, 144t, 150t
Amputation(s), in peripheral vascular disorders, 141–142
Analgesia, during labor, 375–381
  for postoperative pediatric patient, 333t
Analgesic(s), 72, 130t, 135t
Anastomosis, colon resection with, for colorectal cancer, 246
  end-to-end, colon resection with, for Crohn's disease, 243
Androgen(s), 68
  as antineoplastic agents, 201t
Anesthesia, during labor, 375–381
Angina pectoris, 131t, 135–136
Angiography, cerebral, in head trauma, 171
  in coronary artery disease, 134
Angiotensin-converting enzyme (ACE) inhibitor(s), 133t
Anorexia nervosa, 349, 429
Antacid(s), 76, 235t

Antiandrogen(s), as antineoplastic agents, 201t
Antianginal drug(s), 131t
Antianxiety drug(s), 73, 413t
Antiarrhythmic drug(s), 134t
Antibiotic(s), 70–71, 73, 144t, 201t. See also specific drugs, e.g., *Penicillin(s)*.
Anticholinergic drug(s), 76, 235t
  for Parkinson's disease, 72t
Anticoagulant(s), 69, 135t
Anticoagulant antagonist(s), 69–70
Anticonvulsant(s), 74–75, 312t
Antidepressant(s), 409t–410t
Antidiarrheal drug(s), 75, 231t
Antidiuretic hormone (ADH), in fluid balance, 153
Antiemetic(s), 75, 131t, 251t
Antiestrogen drug(s), as antineoplastic agents, 199t
Antihyperlipidemic drug(s), 70
Antihypertensive drug(s), 68–69, 132, 133t
Anti-inflammatory drug(s), 73t, 74, 214
Antimanic drug(s), 410t
Antimetabolite(s), 73, 199t
Antimicrobial drug(s), in bowel, 135t
Antineoplastic drug(s), 73, 200, 201t–202t
Antiparkinsonian drug(s), 72t, 75, 177t
Antipsychotic drug(s), 73, 408t
Antiretroviral drug(s), 71, 144t
Antispasmodic drug(s), 135t
Antithyroid drug(s), 76
Antitubercular drug(s), 71–72, 147t
Antitumor drug(s), 73, 200, 201t–202t
Antitussive(s), 70
Anus, imperforate, 350
Anxiety, as behavior pattern, 412–414, 413t
  in respiratory alkalosis, 160
Aorta, coarctation of, *295*, 296–297
Apgar score(s), 397
Appendicitis, 351–352
Apresoline (hydralazine), 133t
AquaMEPHYTON (oral vitamin K), 69
Arterial peripheral vascular disorder(s), 138, 139c, 140
Arteriosclerosis, 130–131, 131t
Arteriovenous shunt(s), for dialysis, *264*
Arthritis, 214, *215*, 216
  anti-inflammatory drugs for, 73t, 214
  rheumatoid, juvenile, 340
    vs. osteoarthritis, *215*
Ascites, in cirrhosis, 137
Aspiration, of meconium, 397
Aspirin, 72, 135t
Assessment, in nursing process, 4, 8, 47
Asthma, in pediatric patient, 307
Astringent(s), 131t
Atherosclerosis, 130–131, 131t
Atherosclerosis obliterans, 138–140, 139c
Atonic seizure(s), 71, 312
Atrial septal defect(s), 84, *85*
Atropine, 72t, 75
  diphenoxylate hydrochloride with (Lomotil), 75, 131t
Auditory disorder(s), 77–78. See also individual disorder(s), e.g., *Otitis media*.
Auditory function, normal, 77
Autoimmune disorder(s), in adult patient, 199–200, *201–202*, 203–204
  in pediatric patient, 333–334
Automobile accident(s), prevention of, 323t–324t
Autonomy, vs. shame and doubt, in toddlers, 282

Azactam (aztreonam), 71, 134t
AZT (zidovudine), 71, 144t, 191, 193

Baclofen (Lioresal), 74
Bacterial disease(s), in pediatric patient, 326t, 326–327
Bactrim (trimethoprim-sulfamethoxazole), 76, 143t
Baking soda, 340t
Bandage(s), application of, 48, 53
Barbiturate(s), 72–73, 75
  abuse of, 426
Barium enema, for ulcerative colitis, 231
Barium swallow, in peptic ulcer disease, 231, 233
Barron's ligation, for hemorrhoids, 131
Bath(s), bed, 51
Bed making, 51–52
Behavior, of mental health client, 405–415
  patterns of, 407–415
    anxious, 412–414, 413t
    mood and affect and, 409t–410t, 409–411
    obsessive-compulsive, 414
    suicidal, 411
    suspicious, 408t, 408–409
    withdrawal, 407–408
Benadryl (diphenhydramine), 115, 120
Bentyl (dicyclomine), 135t
Benzodiazepine(s), 73
Benzquinamide (Emete-con), 146t
Beta-receptor antagonist(s), 68
Bethanechol (Urecholine), 72
Bicarbonate of soda, 235t
Bile acid sequestrant(s), 70
Biliary disorder(s), 143–145, 144t, 146t
Binder(s), application of, 53
Biopsy, gastroscopy with, in gastric cancer, 237
  of breast tumors, 119
  of liver, in hepatitis, 145
Bipolar disorder, 409–411, 410t
Bisacodyl sodium (Dulcolax), 75, 135t
Bladder, irrigation of, 58
  tumors of, 266–268, *267*
Blind spot, in pediatric patient, 317
Blood, diseases of, 142–146. See also individual disorder(s), e.g., *Hemophilia*.
  in pediatric patient, 300–304
Blood vessel(s), immobility and, 103
Blow bottle(s), use of, 48
Body alignment, 53
Body fluid(s). See *Fluid(s), body*.
Body image, of elderly patients, 105
Body mechanic(s), nursing skills related to, 55
Body temperature, assessment of, postpartum, 389
Body weight, maintenance of, calories required for, calculation of, 90
Bonding, parent-infant, 390, 397
Bordetella pertussis, 327
Bowel, antimicrobial drugs in, 135t
  function of, nursing skills related to, 56
  impaction of, manual extraction of, 56–57
Brain scan, in head trauma, 171
Brain tumor(s), 174–175
  in pediatric patient, 316–317
  radiation therapy for, 203t
Breast(s), benign tumors of, 119
  carcinoma of, 119–120
  self-examination of, 48

Breastfeeding, 390
Breathing, deep, assistance with, 48
Bronchiolitis, in pediatric patient, 304–305
Bronchitis, in pediatric patient, 305
Bronchodilator(s), 70, 149t
Bronchoscopy, in lung cancer, 149
Bryant's traction, 340
Buccal route, for administration of drugs, 78
Buck's extension, 211, *212*
Buerger-Allen exercise(s), in peripheral vascular disorders, 138
Bulimia, 428–429
  in pediatric patient, 349
Burn(s), 194–195
  in pediatric patient, 328–329
  prevention of, 323t–324t
  rule of nines in, 194, 328

CAD (coronary artery disease). See *Coronary artery disease (CAD)*.
Calan (verapamil), 69, 131t
Calcium, disorders involving. See also *Hypercalcemia*; *Hypocalcemia*.
  foods high in, 93, 93t
Calcium channel blocker(s), 69, 131t
Calculi, urinary, 155–156, 156t
Calorie(s), calculation of, for body weight, 90
Cancer, 199t, 199–201, 201t–203t. See also specific site(s).
  chemotherapy for, 200, 201t–202t
  radiation therapy for, 200, 203t
  risk factors for, 199, 199t
Cannabis, abuse of, 426–427
Capsule(s), definition of, 66
Carbapenem, 71, 144t
Carbidopa (Sinemet), 72t, 75
Carbohydrate(s), and wound healing, 93t
Carbonic anhydrase inhibitor(s), 72
Carcinoma. See *Cancer* and specific site(s).
Cardiac disease, during pregnancy, 371
Cardiac glycoside(s), 69, 134t
Cardiac surgery, in pediatric patient, 298–299, 361
Cardiopulmonary resuscitation (CPR), 152
  in pediatric patient, 300
Cardiovascular disorder(s). See also individual disorder(s), e.g., *Congestive heart failure (CHF)*.
  in adult patient, 130–142
  in pediatric patient, 294–300
Cardiovascular function, during pregnancy, 363
  immobility and, 208
  in elderly patient, 104, 108, 118
  in middle-aged patient, 117
  in neonate, 395
Care environment, safety in, client need for, 4, 8–9
Cast(s), 211
  for pediatric patient, 338–340, *339*, 339t
Castor oil, 341t
Cataract(s), 75–76
Catatonic schizophrenia, 407
Catheter(s), care of, 57
Ceftriaxone, 86t, 87
Celiac disease, in pediatric patient, 346–347
Central nervous system (CNS), disorders of. See also individual disorder(s), e.g., *Seizure(s)*.
  in adult patient, 169–175
  in pediatric patient, 312–317
  infection of, clinical presentation in, 326t

Cephalosporin(s), 70–71
Cephalothin (Keflin), 71
Cerebral angiography, in coronary artery disease, 134
in head trauma, 171
Cerebral palsy, 313
Cerebral vasodilator(s), 69
Cerebrovascular accident (CVA), 172–174
Cervical traction, 211, 212
Cervix, cancer of, 120
Cesarean section, 383
Chadwick's sign, 364
Chemolysis, of ruptured intervertebral disc, 111
Chemotherapy, agents for, 200, 201t–202t
for leukemia, 142–143, 144t, 201t–202t
for lymphoma, 143, 201t–202t
Chest, binders for, 53
cancer of, radiation therapy for, 203t
surgery on, 150, 151
Chest tube(s), drainage systems for, 151
CHF (congestive heart failure). See Congestive heart failure (CHF).
Chickenpox (varicella zoster), 325–326
Child(ren). See also Adolescent(s); Infant(s); Pediatric patient(s); Preschooler(s); School-age child(ren); Toddler(s).
abuse of, 327–328, 425
accidents in, 322, 323t–325t
administration of drugs to, 79
mentally handicapped, 313–315
Childbearing family, 361–400. See also Delivery; Labor; Neonate(s); Postpartum period; Pregnancy.
Chlamydial infection(s), 190, 191t
during pregnancy, 365–366
Chloride, loss of, in metabolic alkalosis, 161
Chlorpromazine (Thorazine), 73
Chlorpropamide (Diabinese), 124t
Cholecystitis, 148–149, 150t
Cholecystography, 148–149
Cholelithiasis, 148–149, 150t
Cholesterol, foods low in, 92, 92t
Cholestyramine (Questran), 70
Cholinergic agent(s), 74t
Cholinomimetic(s), 72
Chorionic villus sampling (CVS), 367
Choroid, 74
Chronic obstructive pulmonary disease (COPD), 144t, 148–149, 149t
Cigarette smoking, dependence on, 427
during pregnancy, 367
Cilastatin/imipenem (Primaxin), 71, 144t
Cimetidine (Tagamet), 76, 130t
Ciprofloxacin (Cipro), 76, 153t
Circulation, fetal, 366
Circulatory system, infection in, clinical presentation of, 326
Cirrhosis, 249t, 250–253, 252t–253t
Cisplatin (Platinol), 201t
Cleft lip, 347–348
Cleft palate, 347–348
Clidinium bromide (Quarzan), 130t
Client(s), needs of, 4–5, 8–10
Clonazepam (Klonopin), 312t
Closed fracture(s), 316, 318
Closed-angle glaucoma, 76
Clubfoot (talipes equinovarus), 338, 338
CNS (central nervous system). See Central nervous system (CNS).
Coarctation of aorta, 295, 296–297
Cobalamin, 89
Cocaine, abuse of, 427
Codeine with acetaminophen (Tylenol #3), 70, 135t

Cognitive function, in elderly patient, 105
in middle-aged patient, 117
Colace (docusate sodium), 75, 104t, 135t
Cold, application of, 48
Colitis, ulcerative, 72t–73t, 144t, 240t, 241
barium enema for, 241
diet in, 242t
in pediatric patient, 353
pharmacologic treatment of, 72t–73t, 242t
Colon, resection of, for colorectal cancer, 247
with end-to-end anastomosis, for Crohn's disease, 243
Colonoscopy, in diverticulosis/ diverticulitis, 239
Colorectal cancer, 201t–203t, 246–248
Colostomy, care of, 247
"double barrel," for diverticulosis/ diverticulitis, 239
for colorectal cancer, 247
irrigation of, 57
permanent, for Crohn's disease, 243–244
Coma, in cirrhosis, 147
Communicable disease(s), in pediatric patient, 322, 324–327, 326t
Communication, process of, 405–406
with mental health client, 405–415
Compazine (prochlorperazine), 75, 236t
Compensation, as defense mechanism, 422
Complete fracture(s), 211
Comprehensive Drug Abuse Prevention and Control Act of 1970, 65–66
Compression stockings, application of, 48
Computed tomography (CT), in head trauma, 171
Computer(s), testing on, 1, 2
Conception, 364
Concrete operation(s), Piaget's stage of, in school-aged child, 287–288
Confusion, in elderly patient, 105
Congestive heart failure (CHF), 133t, 137–138
in pediatric patient, 133t–134t, 299, 302t
medications for, 133t–134t, 137
Conjunctivitis, 75
Contraceptive(s), oral, 68
Contraction(s), hypertonic, 381
hypotonic, 381
Controlled Substances Act, 65–66
Conversion, as defense mechanism, 422
Conversion reaction, 423
COPD (chronic obstructive pulmonary disease), 144t, 148–149, 149t
Coping mechanism(s), 422–423
Coronary artery disease (CAD), 132–135, 134t–136t
diet for, 134, 136t
medications for, 134, 134t–135t
Cortisone (prednisone), 73t, 74
Corynebacterium diptheriae, 326
Cough preparation(s), 70
Coughing, assistance with, 48
Coumadin (warfarin), 69, 135t
CPR (cardiopulmonary resuscitation), 152
in pediatric patient, 300
Cretinism, 76–77, 346
Crisis intervention, 423–424
Crohn's disease, 242t, 243–244
diet in, 242t
ileostomy care in, 244
treatment of, pharmacologic, 242t
surgical, 243–245
Cross-eye, in pediatric patient, 317–318
Croup, 305–306
Cryptorchidism, 354

CT (computed tomography), in head trauma, 171
Cultural/psychosocial function(s), 5
Culture specimen(s), collection of, 51
Cushing's syndrome, 227–228
CVA (cerebrovascular accident), 172–174
CVS (chorionic villus sampling), 367
Cyanotic heart defect(s), congenital, 297–298
Cyanotic heart disease, congenital, 297–298
Cyclophosphamide (Cytoxan), 73, 202t
Cystectomy, 266
Cystic fibrosis, in pediatric patient, 306–307
Cystitis, 256–258, 258t
during pregnancy, 370–371
Cystoscopy, in urinary calculi, 260–261
Cytomegalovirus infection(s), during pregnancy, 371
Cytoxan (cyclophosphamide), 73, 202t

Dalmane (flurazepam), 73
Decadron (dexamethasone), 74
Decubitus ulcer(s), from immobility, 104
Deep breathing, assistance with, 48
Defense mechanism(s), 422–423
Degenerative disorder(s), in pediatric patient, 317
Dehydration, 154–155
Delivery, normal, 380
operative procedures for, 383
with HIV-positive mother, 383–384
Delta agent (hepatitis D), 143–145, 144t, 146t
Dementia, 414–415
Demerol (meperidine), 73, 135t, 153t
Demulcent(s), 131t
Denial, as defense mechanism, 422
Depakene (valproic acid), 312t
Depression, 409t–410t, 409–411
in elderly patient, 105
DES (diethylstilbestrol), 68, 202t
Despair vs. ego integrity, in elderly patient, 105, 119
Detoxification, 427–428
Developmental stage(s). See Adolescent(s); Adult patient(s); Infant(s); Piaget's developmental stage(s); Preschooler(s); School-aged child(ren); Toddler(s).
Dexamethasone (Decadron), 74
DiaBeta (glyburide), 229t
Diabetes mellitus, 229t, 229–231, 230–231
diet modifications for, 93t–96t, 94
during pregnancy, 371
hypoglycemic reaction in, vs. hyperglycemia, 232c–233c
in pediatric patient, 336, 337c–338c, 347
insulin for, dosage of, 229t
injection sites for, 231
oral hypoglycemics for, 229t
type I, insulin-dependent, 229
type II, non-insulin-dependent, 229
Diabetic ketoacidosis, 161
Diabinese (chlorpropamide), 229t
Dialysis, arteriovenous shunt for, 264
peritoneal, 263, 263
Diamox (acetazolamide), 72
Diazepam (Valium), 73, 135t
Dicyclomine (Bentyl), 135t
Diet, 87–97
and drug action, 67
food groups in, 87–88, 88
for arteriosclerosis, 131t
for cholethiasis/cholecystitis, 255t
for cirrhosis, 253t

Diet (*Continued*)
  for congestive heart failure, 133t, 138
  for coronary artery disease, 134, 136t
  for Crohn's disease, 242t
  for diabetes, 93t–96t, 94
  for diverticulosis/diverticulitis, 94, 95t
  for hyperkalemia/hypokalemia, 96t, 156
  for hypernatremia, 93t–94t, 155
  for hypertension, 131t, 132, 133t
  for immobile patient, 209
  for peptic ulcer disease, 235t
  for pyelonephritis, 260t
  for ulcerative colitis, 242t
  high- or low-potassium, 92, 92t, 241t
  high-calcium, 93, 93t
  high-protein, 242t, 260t
  low-calorie, 93t, 94
  low-cholesterol, 92, 92t
  low-fat, 92, 92t, 255t
  low-protein, 96, 96t, 253t
  low-residue, 242t
  low-sodium, 9t, 91–92
  nutritional requirements in, 87–91, *88*, 90t
  postsurgical, 91
  vitamins in, 88–89
Diethylstilbestrol (DES), 68, 202t
Diffusion, 153
Digestion, immobility and, 103
Digestive disorder(s), 126–150. See also
    under individual disorder(s), e.g.,
    Colitis, ulcerative.
Digoxin (Lanoxin), 69, 134t
Dilantin (phenytoin), 71, 75, 312t
Diphenhydramine (Benadryl), 120, 135
Diphenoxylate (Lomotil), 75, 236t
Diphtheria, 322t, 326–327
Dipyridamole (Persantine), 69
Disc(s), intervetebral, ruptured, 216t, 216–217
Discharge, from hospital, procedures for,
    54–55
Displacement, as defense mechanism, 422
Dissociation, 422
Diuretic(s), 147t
  loop, 69, 133t
  potassium-sparing, 69, 133t
  thiazide, 69, 133t
Diverticulosis/diverticulitis, 239–241, 240t
  colonoscopy in, 239
  diet in, 239, 240t
  treatment of, pharmacologic, 240t
    surgical, 239
Docusate sodium (Colace), 75, 209t, 240t
Domestic violence, 424–425
Dopamine, 146t
Dorsal recumbent position, 52, *52*
"Double-barrel" colostomy, for
    diverticulosis/diverticulitis, 239
Douche, vaginal, 47
Down's syndrome, 314
Doxorubicin (Adriamycin), 73, 201t
Doxycycline, 85, 86t
Drainage secretion precaution(s), 53
Drainage system(s), for chest tubes, *151*
Dressing(s), for wound care, 53
Drowning, prevention of, 323t–324t
Drug(s), absorption of, 66
  action of, factors affecting, 67
  administration of, five rights of, 77
    in elderly patient, 79
    routes of, 77–79
  adverse effects of, 67
  affecting elimination, 75–77
    antidiarrheal agents as, 75
    laxatives as, 75
    quinolones as, 76, 153t
    sulfonamides as, 75–76

Drug(s) (*Continued*)
  affecting metabolism, 75–77
    anticholinergic, 72t, 76, 235t
    for thyroid, 76–77
    hypoglycemic, 75
  affecting mobility, 74–75
  affecting nutrition, 75–77
    antacids as, 76, 235t
    antiemetics as, 75, 236t, 251t
    histamine receptor antagonists as, 76,
      235t
  affecting oxygenation, 68–72
    antibiotics as, 70–71, 144t, 201t, 258t
    anticoagulant antagonists as, 69–70
    anticoagulants as, 69, 135t
    antihyperlipidemics as, 70
    antihypertensives as, 68–69, 132, 133t
    antitubercular agents as, 71–72, 147t
    bronchodilators as, 70, 149t
    cardiac glycosides as, 69, 134t
    cough preparations as, 70
    iron preparations as, 72
    vasodilators as, 69, 131t
  affecting perception, 72–74
    analgesics as, 72, 135t, 235t
    anti-anxiety agents as, 73, 413t
    antipsychotic agents as, 74, 408t
    barbiturates as, 72–73, 75
    carbonic anhydrase inhibitors as, 72
    miotic-cholinergics as, 72
    nonbarbiturates as, 73
  affecting protective functions, 73–74
  affecting sexuality, 67–68
    beta-receptor antagonists as, 68
    hormones as, 68
    uterine smooth muscle stimulants as,
      67–68
  categories of, 67–77
  chemical names of, 65
  controlled, categories of, 65–66
  distribution of, 66
  effects of, local vs. systemic, 67
  excretion of, 67
  forms of, 66
  generic names of, 65
  legislation concerning, 65–67
  metabolism of, 66–67
  pharmacokinetics of, 66–67
    in elderly patient, 106–107
  reactions to, 67
  regulation of, 65–66
  side effects of, 67
  sources of, 66
  sources of information on, 65
  suppository, 66, 78–79, 240t
  tolerance to, 67
  trade names of, 65
Drug abuse, 426–428
Drug therapy, in elderly patient, 79,
    106–107, 109
  nursing process and, 67
Dubowitz evaluation, 397
Dulcolax (bisacodyl sodium), 75, 240t
Duodenal peptic ulcer disease, 231
Dwarfism, hypopituitary, 345–346
Dying patient(s), care of, 54
Dymelor (acetohexamide), 75, 229t
Dystocia, 381–382, *382*

Ear(s), irrigation of, 49
  medications for, administration of, 78
  middle, infections of, 78
  physiology of, 77
Eating disorder(s), 428–429

ECF (extracellular fluid), deficit of, 154–155
ECG (electrocardiography), in coronary
    artery disease, 133–134
Echocardiography, in coronary artery
    disease, 134
Eclampsia, 368
Ectopic pregnancy, 369
Eczema, infantile, 329
Edema, 133t, 154
Educable mentally handicapped, 314
EEG (electroencephalography), in head
    trauma, 171
EES (erythromycin ethylsuccinate), 71, 144t
Ego integrity vs. despair, in elderly patient,
    105, 119
Elderly patient(s), abuse of, 106, 426
  administration of drugs to, 79
  body image of, 105
  cardiovascular function in, 104, 108
  cognitive function in, 105
  common health problems of, 106
  confusion in, 105
  depression in, 105
  drug therapy in, 106–107, 109
  ego integrity vs. despair in, 105, 119
  environment for, 105
  finances of, 105
  gastrointestinal function in, 104
  genitourinary function in, 104, 108, 118
  hearing in, 103–104, 118
  hematopoietic system in, 104
  legal concerns of, 106
  loss in, 105
  metabolism in, 104, 108
  musculoskeletal function in, 104–105,
    108, 118
  nervous system of, 103, 118
  nursing process and, 107–109
  nutritional requirements of, 91
  pharmacokinetics in, 106–107
  postural hypotension in, 104
  proprioception in, 103
  psychosocial alterations in, 108–109,
    118–119
  respiratory function in, 104, 108, 118
  retirement and, 105
  role changes in, 105
  self-medication in, 107
  sensory function in, 103–104
  sexuality in, 105–106
  skin of, 105, 108
  smell in, 104
  societal attitudes toward, 106
  taste in, 104
  touch in, 104
  vision in, 103, 118
Electrocardiography (ECG), in coronary
    artery disease, 133–134
Electroencephalography (EEG), in head
    trauma, 171
Electrolyte(s), imbalances of, 155–158. See
    also individual type(s), e.g.,
    Hyperkalemia.
Elimination, components of, 5
  disorders of, 221–266
    in pediatric patient, 345–355
  drugs affecting, 75–77
  immobility and, 208–209
  neonatal, 396
  nursing skills related to, 55–58
  postpartum, 389–390
Elixir(s), definition of, 66
Embolism, peripheral, 140–141
  medications for, 135t
  patient information about, 139c
Embryonic stage, 364–365

Emete-con (benzquinamide), 146t
Emotion(s), in mental health client, 423–428
Emotional development, in middle-aged patient, 117–118
Emotional support, of preoperative pediatric patient, 332t
Emulsion(s), definition of, 66
Enalapril (Vasotec), 133t
Encephalitis, 170–171
Encephalopathy, hepatic, in cirrhosis, 252
Endocrine system, disorders of, 221–231
    in pediatric patient, 345–346
    during pregnancy, 362
    functions of, 222c–224c
Endometriosis, 121
Endometritis, postpartum, 390
Endoscopy, in peptic ulcer disease, 233
End-to-end anastomosis, with colon resection, for Crohn's disease, 243
Enema(s), administration of, 56
    barium, for ulcerative colitis, 241
Enteric precaution(s), 53–54
Enteritis, regional, 242t, 243–245. See also Crohn's disease.
Environment, for care. See Care environment.
    for elderly patient, 105
    hazards in, during pregnancy, 365–367
Epidural anesthesia, during labor, 375
Epilepsy, 70–71
    in pediatric patient, 312–313
Episiotomy, 383
Epispadias, 354
Eriksonian stage(s), of autonomy vs. shame and doubt, in toddlers, 282
    of ego integrity vs. despair, in elderly patient, 105, 119
    of generativity vs. self-absorption and stagnation, in middle-aged patient, 118
    of identity formation vs. identity diffusion, in adolescent, 288
    of industry vs. inferiority, in school-aged child, 287
    of initiative vs. guilt, in preschooler, 284
    of intimacy vs. isolation, 362
    of trust vs. mistrust, in infant, 279
Erythema, from immobility, 104
Erythromycin, 71, 144t
Eserine (physostigmine), 72
Esophageal atresia, 138
Essential hypertension, 131
Estrogen(s), 68
    as antineoplastic agents, 202t
    functions of, 361–362
Ethambutol (Myambutol), 71–72, 147t
Eulexin (flutamide), 201t
Evacuant(s), suppositories as, 235t
Evaluation, in nursing process, 4, 8, 47
Evisceration, postpartum, 392
Exanthema subitum (roseola), 324–325
Excretion, of drugs, 67
Exercise(s), Buerger-Allen, in peripheral vascular disorders, 138
    range-of-motion, 55, 209
Exercise stress test, in coronary artery disease, 134
Expectorant(s), 70
External fixation, of fractured bones, 108
Extracellular fluid (ECF), deficit of, 154–155
Eye(s), function of, 74–75
    irrigation of, 49
    medication for, administration of, 78

Failure to thrive, in pediatric patient, 308
Family(ies), childbearing, 361–401. See also Delivery; Labor; Neonate(s); Postpartum period; Pregnancy.
Fantasy, as defense mechanism, 422
Fat(s), and wound healing, 93t
    in food, 92t
Fat-soluble vitamin(s), 88–89
Febrile seizure(s), 313
Feeding patient(s), skills related to, 55–56
Female(s). See Adult patient(s), female.
Femoral hernia, 244
Ferrous sulfate (Feosol), 72
Fetal stage, 365, 366
Fetus, assessment of, during labor, 378
    circulation of, 366
    delivery of, 380
    presentation of, 376, 376, 376t
Fibric acid drug(s), 70
Filtration, 153
Finance(s), of elderly patient, 105
Fixation, of fractured bones, 108
Fluid(s), body, imbalances of, 153–154. See also under individual disorder(s).
    extracellular, deficit of, 154–155
    universal precautions for, 53, 174t
    volume of, regulation of, 68–69
Fluid and electrolyte balance, 153–154
    antidiuretic hormone in, 153
    dynamics of, 153–154
    fluid intake in, 153
    fluid output in, 153
    in pediatric patient, 308
Flurazepam (Dalmane), 73
Flutamide (Eulexin), 201t
Folic acid, 89
Food(s), calcium content of, 93, 93t
    and urinary calculi, 261t
    cholesterol content of, 92, 92t
    fat content of, 92t
    potassium content of, 92, 92t, 241t
    protein content of, 96, 96t, 253t
    sodium content of, 91t, 91–92, 238t
Food, Drug, and Cosmetic Act, 65
Food group(s), 87–88, 88
Food pyramid, 87–88, 88
Forceps delivery, 383
Fowler's position, high, 52
Fracture(s), 211, 213, 213–214
    in pediatric patient, 338
Freud, developmental stages of, in preschoolers, 283t
Full-thickness burn(s), 195
Functioning, categories of, 5
Furosemide (Lasix), 69, 133t, 147t

Gantrisin (sulfisoxazole), 76
Garamycin (gentamicin), 70, 144t
Gastrectomy, for gastric cancer, 238
Gastric. See also entries under Stomach.
Gastric cancer, 201t–202t, 237t, 237–239
Gastric peptic ulcer disease, 231
Gastric resection, subtotal, for peptic ulcer, 239
Gastrointestinal function, during pregnancy, 363
    in elderly patient, 104
Gastrointestinal system, immobility and, 208–209
Gastrointestinal tract, disorders of, 231–255
    in pediatric patient, 347–353
    lower, 239–248
    infection in, clinical presentation of, 221t

Gastroscopy, with biopsy, in gastric cancer, 237
Gelucil, 76
Gemfibrozil (Lopid), 70
Generativity, vs. self-absorption and stagnation, in middle age, 118
Genital herpes, 191t
Genitourinary function, in elderly patient, 104, 108, 118
Gentamicin (Garamycin), 70, 144t
German measles, during pregnancy, 365, 371
Gestational age, assessment of, 397
Gestational trophoblastic disease, 369–370, 370
Glands, in endocrine system, functions of, 222c–224c
Glaucoma, 76
Glipizide (Glucotrol), 229t
Glomerulonephritis, acute, in pediatric patient, 343t, 355
Glucose test(s), 58
Glucotrol (glipizide), 229t
Glyburide (DiaBeta, Micronase, Glynase, PresTab), 229t
Glycoside(s), cardiac, 69, 134t
Gonorrhea, 295, 296t, 297
    during pregnancy, 366
Goodell's sign, 363
Grafting, skin, for burns, 195
Grand mal seizure(s), 312
Granulomatous colitis. See Colitis, ulcerative.
Great vessel(s), transposition of, 296, 298
Greenstick fracture(s), 211
Grieving, 423–424
Growth and development, components of, 5
    in pediatric patient, 279–290. See also Adolescent(s); Preschooler(s); School-age child(ren); Toddler(s).
Guaifenesin (Robitussin), 70
Guilt vs. initiative, in preschoolers, 284

Haemophilus b vaccine, administration of, 322t
Hair care, 51
Harrison Narcotic Act, 65
HAV (hepatitis A), 143–145, 144t, 146t
Hay fever, in pediatric patient, 307–308
HBV (hepatitis B), 143–145, 144t, 146t
HCV (hepatitis C), 143–145, 144t, 146t
Head, cancer of, radiation therapy for, 203t
    circumference of, in neonate, 395
Head trauma, 171–172, 173c–174c
    home care instructions after, 173c
Health, maintenance of, client need for, 4–5, 9–10
    promotion of, client need for, 4–5, 9–10
Hearing, in elderly patient, 103–104, 118
    in middle-aged patient, 117
    neonatal, 396–397
    normal, 77
Heart, immobility and, 103
Heart defect(s), congenital, acyanotic, 294–297
    cyanotic, 297–298
Heart failure, congestive. See Congestive heart failure (CHF).
Heat, application of, 48
Hegar's sign, 363
Helicobacter pylori, in gastric cancer, 237
    in peptic ulcer disease, 231
HELLP syndrome, 368–369

Hematopoietic system, in elderly patient, 104
  infection in, clinical presentation of, 326t
Hemodialysis, 263, *264*
Hemophilia, 302–303
Hemorrhage, during pregnancy, 369–370, *370–371*
  postpartum, 390
Hemorrhoid(s), 245–246
Hemorrhoidectomy, 246
Heparin, 69, 135t
Hepatic encephalopathy, in cirrhosis, 252
Hepatitis, 248–250, 249t, 251t
  diagnostic tests for, 249–250
  pharmacologic treatment of, 251t
  vaccine for, 251t
Hernia, 245–246
  femoral, 245
  hiatal, 235, 237
  incisional, 244
  irreducible, 245
  reducible, 245
  strangulated, 245
  surgical intervention for, 245
  umbilical, 246
Herpes simplex virus (HSV), 296t
Herpes virus infection(s), during pregnancy, 366, 371
Hiatal hernia, 235, 237
High-calcium diet, 93, 93t
High-calorie diet, for ulcerative colitis, 242t
High-cholesterol food(s), 92t
High-potassium diet, 92, 92t, 241t
High-protein diet, for pyelonephritis, 260t
  for ulcerative colitis, 242t
High-residue diet, for diverticulosis/diverticulitis, 239, 240t
Hip, congenital dislocation of, 338
Hip replacement, for arthritis, 214, 216
Hirschsprung's disease (megacolon), 245
Histamine receptor antagonist(s), 76, 235t
HIV (human immunodeficiency virus) infection. See *Acquired immunodeficiency syndrome (AIDS); Human immunodeficiency virus (HIV) infection.*
Hives (urticaria), 330–331
HMC-CoA reductase inhibitor(s), 70
Hodgkin's disease, in pediatric patient, 302
Home care, after head trauma, 173c
Hormone(s), and sexual function, 278
  as antineoplastic drugs, 74, 201t
  in middle age, 117
Hospital, discharge from, procedures for, 54–55
  play in, for pediatric patient, 334t
HSV (herpes simplex virus), 29t
Human functioning, categories of, 5
Human immune globulin, action of, 251t
Human immunodeficiency virus (HIV) infection, during pregnancy, 366–367
  in pediatric patient, 333–334
  maternal, delivery with, 383–384
Hydantoin, 75
Hydatiform mole, 369–370, *370*
Hydralazine (Apresoline), 133t
Hydramnios, 382
Hydrocephalus, 313–314
Hydrochlorothiazide (HydroDIURIL), 69, 133t
Hydronephrosis, 240t, 249t, 258t, 261–262
Hydroxychloroquine (Plaquenil), for systemic lupus erythematosus, 203
Hygiene, nursing skills related to, 51

Hypercalcemia, 157–158
Hyperemesis gravidarum, 369
Hyperglycemia, vs. hypoglycemic reaction, 232c–233c
Hyperkalemia, 136t, 156–157
Hypernatremia, 133t–134t, 155
Hyperparathyroidism, 133t, 227
Hypertension, 131t, 131–132, 133t
  diet for, 131t, 132, 133t
  during pregnancy, 368
  essential, 131
  medications for, 132, 133t
  portal, in cirrhosis, 252
  primary, 131
  secondary, 132
Hyperthyroidism, 221, 225, 225t
Hypertonic contraction(s), 381
Hypocalcemia, 158
Hypoglycemic agent(s), 75, 229t
Hypoglycemic reaction, vs. hyperglycemia, 232c–233c
Hypokalemia, 136t, 156–157
Hyponatremia, 156
Hypoparathyroidism, 226
Hypopituitary dwarfism, 345–346
Hypospadias, 354
Hypotension, postural, in elderly patient, 104
Hypothyroidism, 225–226
  congenital, 286–287, 346
Hypotonic contraction(s), 381

Ibuprofen (Advil, Motrin), 73t, 74
IDDM (insulin-dependent diabetes mellitus), 229
  diet for, 93t–96t, 99
Identification, as defense mechanism, 422–423
Identity formation vs. identity diffusion, in adolescent, 289
Ileal conduit, 256–257, *257*
Ileostomy, care of, 245
  in pediatric patient, 353
Imferon (iron dextran), 72
Imipenem/cilastatin (Primaxin), 71, 144t
Immobility, 208–210
  and cardiovascular system, 208
  and gastrointestinal system, 313–314
  and integumentary system, 209–210
  and musculoskeletal system, 209
  and positioning, *210*
  and respiratory system, 208
  and urinary system, 210
  diet for, 209
  psychological aspects of, 210
Immune disorder(s). See also specific disorders.
  in adult patient, 199–200, 201t–202t, 203–204
  in pediatric patient, 333–334
Immunization(s), administration of, 322t
Impaction, bowel, manual extraction of, 56–57
Imperforate anus, 245
Impetigo, 329–330
Implementation, in nursing process, 4, 8, 47
Incentive spirometer(s), use of, 48
Incisional hernia, 244
Incomplete fracture(s), 211
Inderal (propranolol), 134t
Indiana pouch, 267
Indomethacin, in ventral septal defect, 294
Industry vs. inferiority, in school-age child, 287

Infant(s), 279–281
  accidents in, 323t
  bonding with, 390, 397
  development of, Eriksonian stages of, trust vs. mistrust as, 279
    physical, 279
    Piaget's stages of, 280
    psychosocial, 279–280
    social, 280–281
  eczema in, 329
  nutritional requirements of, 270, 300
  perioperative care of, 331
  play in, 279
  sleep in, 279
  spasms in, 312
  speech in, 280
Infection(s). See also under individual disease(s).
  clinical presentation of, 326t
  during pregnancy, 370–371
Infectious mononucleosis, 303–304
Inferiority vs. industry, in school-age child, 287
Inflammatory bowel disease. See *Colitis, ulcerative.*
Influenza, *Haemophilus b,* vaccine for, 322t
INH (isoniazid), 71–72, 147t
Initiative vs. guilt, in preschoolers, 284
Injection(s), administration of, in children, 289
  intramuscular, for administration of drugs, 77–78
  intravenous, for administration of drugs, 78
Insulin, 75
  dosage of, 229t
  injection sites for, *231*
Insulin-dependent diabetes mellitus (IDDM), 229
  diet for, 93t–96t, 99
Intake, monitoring of, 49
Integumentary system. See *Skin.*
Intermittent positive-pressure breathing (IPPB), administration of, 48–49
Internal fixation, of fractured bones, 213
Interpersonal relationship(s), therapeutic, 406–407
Intervertebral disc(s), ruptured, 216t, 216–217
Intimacy, vs. isolation, Eriksonian stage of, 362
Intracranial pressure, increased, 169t, 169–170, 172c
  signs of, 172c
Intradermal route, for administration of drugs, 78
Intramuscular injection, administration of drugs by, 77–78
Intravenous route, for administration of drugs, 78
Introjection, 423
Intussusception, 246, *246*
IPPB (intermittent positive-pressure breathing), administration of, 48–49
Iron dextran (Imferon), 72
Iron preparation(s), 72
Islet of Langerhans, function of, 224c
Isolation precaution(s), 53–54
Isolation vs. intimacy, Eriksonian stage of, 362
Isoniazid (INH), 71–72, 147t
Isopto Carpine (pilocarpine), 72
Isoxsuprine (Vasodilan), 69

Juvenile rheumatoid arthritis, 340

Kanamycin (Kantrex), 144t
Kaolin, with pectin, 76
Keflin (cephalothin), 71
Ketoacidosis, diabetic, 161
    vs. hypoglycemic reaction, 232c–233c
Kidney(s). See also entries under *Renal*.
    infections of. See *Pyelonephritis*.
Kidney tumor(s), 201t–203t, 265–266
Klonopin (clonazepam), 312t
Knee-chest position, 52, *52*

Labor, anesthesia/analgesia during,
    375–381
    assessment during, 377–378
    difficult, 381–382, *382*
    normal, *376*, 376t, 376–377
    precipitate, 381
    preterm, 381
    rupture of membranes during, 378
    rupture of uterus during, 381
    stages of, 378–380
Lactation, 390
    nutrition during, 90
Lactic acidosis, 161
Laminectomy, 216
Lanoxin (digoxin), 69, 134t
Laryngeal cancer, 150–152
Lasix (furosemide), 69, 133t, 147t
Lateral position, 52
    immobility and, *210*
Laxative(s), 75, 131t
Lazy eye, in pediatric patient, 317
Lead poisoning, in pediatric patient, 317
Legal right(s), of elderly patient, 106
Legg-Calvé-Perthes disease (osteochronditis
    deformans juvenilis), 341
Legislation, concerning drugs, 65–67
Leukemia, 142–143
    chemotherapy for, 144t, 201t–202t
    in pediatric patient, 201t–203t, 301–302
Leuprolide (Lupron), 202t
Level of consciousness (LOC), assessment
    of, 49
    in increased intracranial pressure, 169,
    172c
Levodopa, 72t, 75
Levothyroxine (Synthroid), 76–77
Lice, 330
Lifting patient(s), skills related to, 55
Liniment(s), definition of, 66
Lioresal (baclofen), 74
Liquid drug(s), forms of, 66
Listening, active, 405–406
Lithotomy position, 52, *52*
Liver, biopsy of, for hepatitis, 250
Liver disorder(s), 248–250, 249t, 251t
LOC (level of consciousness), assessment
    of, 49
    in increased intracranial pressure, 169,
    172c
Lochia, assessment of, 389
Lomotil (diphenoxylate), 75, 236t
Loop diuretic(s), 69, 133t
Lopid (gemfibrozil), 70
Loss, in elderly patient, 105
    process of, 423–424
Lotion(s), definition of, 66
Low-calorie diet, 93t, 94
Low-cholesterol diet, 92, 92t
Low-fat diet, 92, 92t, 255t
Low-potassium diet, 92, 92t
Low-protein diet, 96, 96t, 253t
Low-residue diet, 242t
Low-sodium diet, 91t, 91–92

Lozenge(s), definition of, 66
Luminal (phenobarbital), 71, 75, 312t
Lung(s), aeration of, immobility and, 208
Lung cancer, 149–150
Lung disease, chronic obstructive, 144t,
    148–149, 149t
Lupron (leuprolide), 202t
Lupus erythematosus, systemic, 200,
    203–204
Luteal phase, of menstrual cycle, 361
Luteinizing hormone, synthetic, as
    antineoplastic agent, 202t
Lymphangiography, in lymphoma, 143
Lymphoma, 143, 145, 201t–202t

Maalox, 76
Macrolide(s), 71, 144t
Magnesium, as antacid, 76
Male(s), reproductive system of, 361–362
Mammography, 329
Manic-depressive disorder, 409–411, 410t
Many-tailed binder(s), application of, 53
MAO (monoamine oxidase) inhibitor(s),
    410t
Marijuana, abuse of, 426–427
Mastitis, postpartum, 390
Measles, 322, 322t, 324
    German, during pregnancy, 365, 371
Mechanical ventilation, in respiratory
    alkalosis, 160
Meconium aspiration, 397
Medication(s). See *Drug(s)*; individual
    types, e.g., *Antibiotic(s)*.
Megacolon (Hirschsprung's disease), 245
Membrane(s), rupture of, during labor, 378
Meningitis, 170, 315–316
Meningocele, 315
Menopause, 331–332
Menstrual cycle, 361
Mental disorder(s), organic, 414–415
Mental health client. See also under
    specific disorder, e.g., *Depression*.
Mental health client(s), 405–429
    behavior of, 405–415
    chronically ill, 411–412
    communication with, 405–415
    emotions of, 423–425
    with organic disorders, 414–415
    young, 411–412
Mentally handicapped child(ren), 313–315
Meperidine (Demerol), 72, 135t
Mestinon (pyridostigmine bromide), 74t
Metabolic acidosis, 160–161
Metabolic alkalosis, 161
Metabolism, basic nursing skills related to,
    55–58
    components of, 5
    disorders of, 153–163
      in adult patient, 153–163. See also
        under individual disorder(s).
      in pediatric patient, 345–355
    drugs affecting, 75–77
    in elderly patient, 104, 108, 118
    in middle-aged patient, 117
Metamucil (psyllium), 75, 104
Methocarbamol (Robaxin), 74, 111
Methotrexate (Mexate), 73, 201t
Methyldopa (Aldomet), 69, 133t
MgOH (milk of magnesia), 75–76
MI (myocardial infarction), 134t–135t,
    136–137
Micronase (nonmicronized glyburide), 229t
Midlife crisis, 118
Milk of magnesia (MgOH), 75–76

Mineral(s), and wound healing, 93t
Mineral oil, as laxative, 75
Miotic-cholinergic(s), 72
Miscarriage, 369
Mistrust vs. trust, in infants, 279
Mobility, basic nursing skills associated
    with, 55
    drugs affecting, 74–75
    in pediatric patient, 338–341
    lack of. See *Immobility*.
Mobility/activity/comfort, 5, 208–217
    musculoskeletal disorders and, 211–217,
      212–215. See also *Musculoskeletal
      system, disorders of.*
Molar pregnancy, 369–370, *370*
Monoamine oxidase (MAO) inhibitor(s),
    410t
Monobactam(s), 71, 144t
Mononucleosis, infectious, 303–304
Montgomery strap(s), application of, 53
Mood disorder(s), 409t–410t, 409–411
Morphine sulfate, 72, 135t
Mother-infant bonding, 390, 397
Motor vehicle accident(s), prevention of,
    323t–324t
Motrin (ibuprofen), 73t, 74
Mouth care, 51
Moving patient(s), skills related to, 55
Multiple sclerosis (MS), 72–73, 73t
Mumps, 322t, 326
Muscle relaxant(s), 74, 321t
Muscular dystrophy, in pediatric patient,
    341
Musculoskeletal system, disorders of,
    211–217, *212–215*
    chronic, 214, *215*, 216–217
    from trauma, 211, *212*, 213–214
      casts for, 211
      fractures as, 211, *213*, 213–214
      traction in, 211, *212*
    in pediatric patient, 338
    function of, in elderly patient, 104–105,
      108, 118
      in middle-aged patient, 117
    immobility and, 209
Myambutol (ethambutol), 71–72, 147t
Myasthenia gravis, 73t–74t, 73–74
Myelogram, in ruptured intervetebral disc,
    216
Myelomeningocele, 315
Mylanta, 235t, 251t
Myocardial infarction (MI), 134t–135t,
    136–137
Myoclonic seizure(s), 71, 312
Myringotomy, for otitis media, 288
Mysoline (primidone), 312t

Nägele's rule, 365
Nail care, 51
Nalidixic acid (NegGram), 153t
Narcotic analgesic(s), 72, 135t
Nasogastric (NG) tubes, care of, 56
National Formulary (NF), 65
NCLEX-PN, format of, 3–5
    practice tests for, 11–46, 435–469
    preparation for, 1–2
    retaking of, 10
    scoring of, 1
    studying for, 2–3
    test-taking strategies for, 7–10. See also
      Test-taking.
Nebulizer(s), use of, 48
NegGram (nalidixic acid), 153t

Neomycin, 135t, 147t
Neonate(s), airway of, 397
  appearance of, 395
  cardiovascular system of, 395
  care of, 397–398
  elimination in, 396
  head circumference of, 395
  reflexes of, 396
  screening tests for, 397
  sensory development of, 396–397
  skin of, 396
  vital signs of, 396
  weight of, 396
Nephroblastoma (Wilms' tumor), 249–250
Nephrolithiasis, 260–261, 261t
Nephrolithotomy, 261
Nephrosis, 259
Nephrostomy, care of, 262t
Nephrostomy tube(s), in renal failure, 267
Nephrotic syndrome (nephrosis), in
      pediatric patient, 355
Neurologic function, assessment of, 50
  in elderly patient, 103, 118
NF (National Formulary), 65
NG (nasogastric) tubes, care of, 56
Niacin, 98
Nicotine, dependence on, 427
Nitroglycerin (Nitro-Bid), 69, 131t
Nolvadex (tamoxifen), 74, 202t
Nonbarbiturate(s), 73
Nonnarcotic analgesic(s), 72, 135t
Nonsteroidal anti-inflammatory drugs
      (NSAIDs), 73t, 74
Non–stress test, 367
Nonverbal communication, 405
Norfloxacin (Noroxin), 76, 258t
Norgestrol, 68
NPH (intermediate acting insulin), 75
NSAIDs (non-steroidal anti-inflammatory
      drugs), 73t, 74
Nursing mother(s), nutritional
      requirements of, 90
Nursing process, and drug therapy, 67
  and elderly patient, 107–109
  assessment in, 4, 8, 47
  evaluation in, 4, 8, 47
  implementation in, 4, 8, 47
  phases of, 3–4, 8
  planning in, 4, 8, 47
Nursing skill(s), related to elimination,
      55–58
  related to feeding, 55–56
  related to hygiene, 51
  related to metabolism, 55–58
  related to mobility, 55
  related to oxygenation, 48–49, 50
  related to protective functions, 51–55, 52.
      See also Protective function(s).
  related to sensory/perceptual alterations,
      49–51
  related to sexuality, 47–48
Nutrient(s), classes of, 87
Nutrition, age and, 90–91
  and wound healing, 198, 198t
  drugs affecting, 75–77
    antacids as, 76
    antiemetics as, 75, 131t, 146t
    histamine receptor antagonists as, 76,
        130t
  during pregnancy, 90, 365
  in adolescents, 79
  in infants, 90, 279
  in nursing mothers, 90
  in preschoolers, 90, 283t
  in school-age children, 77, 77t
  principles of, 87–91

Obesity, in pediatric patient, 349–350
Obsessive-compulsive disorder, 414
Ocular medication(s), administration of, 78
Ointment(s), definition of, 66
Oligohydramnios, 382–383
Omphalocele, 350–351
Oncovin (vincristine), 74, 202t
Open reduction, 213
Open-angle glaucoma, 76
Opiate(s), 131t
  abuse of, 426
Oral care, 51
Oral contraceptive(s), 68
Organic mental disorder(s), 414–415
Orinase (tolbutamide), 229t
Orphan Drug Act, 66
Orthopneic position, 52, 52
Osmolality, 154
Osmosis, 153
Osteoarthritis, 214, 215, 216
Osteochondritis deformans juvenile
      (Legg-Calvé-Perthes disease), 341
Osteoporosis, immobility and, 209
Otic medication(s), administration of, 78
Otitis media, acute, 78
  in pediatric patient, 304
Otosclerosis, 77–78
Output, monitoring of, 49
Ovary(ies), endocrine function of, 118c
Ovrette (norgestrel), 68
Oxacillin, 258t
Oxycodone (Percodan), 130t
Oxygen, administration of, 49, 50
Oxygenation, 130–161
  components of, 5
  drugs affecting, 68–72. See also Drug(s),
      affecting oxygenation.
  in pediatric patient, 294–308
  nursing skills related to, 48–49, 50
Oxytocin (Pitocin), 68
Oxytocin challenge test, 367

Pain management, 51
Pancreas, Islets of Langerhans of, function
      of, 224c
Pancreatin (Viokase), 257t
Pancreatitis, 255–256, 257t
Pancreatography, 256
Panic disorder, 412–413
Pantothenic acid, 89
Pap smear, 47–48
Para-aminophenol(s), 72
Para-aminosalicylic acid (PAS), 72
Paracervical block, during labor, 380
Paranoid schizophrenia, 407
Parathyroid, disorders of, 226–227
  function of, 224c
Parent-infant bonding, 390, 397
Parkinson's disease, 72, 72t
Partial-thickness burn(s), 195
PAS (para-aminosalicylic acid), 72
Patent ductus arteriosus, 294, 295, 296
Patient(s), discharge of, procedures for,
      54–55
  needs of, 4–5, 8–10
  positioning of, 10, 52, 52–53
PCP (phencyclidine), abuse of, 427
PDR (Physicians' Desk Reference), 65
Pectin, kaolin with, 76
Pediatric patient(s). See also Adolescent(s);
      Infant(s); Preschooler(s); School-age
      child(ren); Toddler(s).
  blood disease in, 300–304
  burns in, 328–329
    prevention of, 323t–324t

Pediatric patient(s) (Continued)
  cardiac surgery in, 298–299
  cardiovascular disorders in, 294–300. See
      also under individual disorder(s).
  casts for, 338–340, 339, 339t
  central nervous system disorders in,
      312–317
  communicable diseases in, 322, 324–327,
      326t
  degenerative disorders in, 317
  diabetes mellitus in, 336, 337c–338c, 347
  endocrine disorders in, 345–346
  epilepsy in, 312–313
  failure to thrive in, 308
  fluid and electrolyte balance in, 308
  gastrointestinal disorders in, 347–353
  Hodgkin's disease in, 302
  ileostomy care in, 353
  immune/autoimmune disorders in,
      333–334
  immunizations for, 322t
  leukemia in, 301–302
  metabolism/elimination in, 343t, 345–355
  mobility in, 338–341
  nephrotic syndrome in, 355
  obesity in, 349–350
  otitis media in, 304
  oxygenation in, 294–308
  perioperative care of, 331–334
  pinworms in, 352
  poisoning in, 323t–325t, 328
    lead, 317
    prevention of, 323t–324t
  postoperative care of, 332–333, 333t–334t
  preoperative care of, 332–333, 333t–334t
  protective functions in, 322–334
  sensory/perceptual alterations in,
      312–318
  skin disorders in, 328–331
  trauma in, 322, 323t–324t, 338–340
  upper respiratory infections in, 304
  urinary disorders in, 354–355
  viral diseases in, 322, 324–326, 326t
  visual disorders in, 317–318
Pediculosis, 330
Pelvic traction, 211, 212
Pelvis, cancer of, radiation therapy for, 203t
Penicillin(s), 70, 86t, 88, 144t
Peptic ulcer disease, 231–235, 234, 236
  barium swallow in, 231
  diet for, 235t
  duodenal, 231
  endoscopy in, 233
  gastric, 231
  pharmacologic treatment of, 235t–236t
  surgical intervention for, 234, 236
Perception, drugs affecting, 72–73. See also
      Drug(s), affecting perception.
Percodan (oxycodone hydrochloride), 130t
Perineal care, 47
Perineal prostatectomy, 122
Perioperative care, of adolescent, 332
  of adult patient, 195–199
  of infant, 331
  of pediatric patient, 331–334
Peripheral embolism, 140–141
  drugs for, 135t
  patient information about, 139c
Peripheral vascular disorder(s), 138–142,
      139c
  amputations in, 141–142
  arterial, 138–140, 139c
  atherosclerosis obliterans as, 138–140,
      139c
  Buerger-Allen exercises in, 138
  medications for, 131t, 138

Peripheral vascular disorder(s) (*Continued*)
  patient information in, 139c
  thrombophlebitis as, 140
  varicose veins as, 141
  venous, 139c, 140–141
  venous stasis ulcers as, 141
Peripheral vasodilator(s), 69
Peritoneal dialysis, 263, *263*
Persantine (dipyridamole), 69
Pertussis (whooping cough), 322t, 327
Petit mal seizure(s), 71, 312
Pharmacokinetics, 66–67
  in elderly patient, 106–107
Pharmacology, 65–67
Phenazopyridine (Pyridium), 258t
Phencyclidine (PCP), abuse of, 427
Phenobarbital (Luminal), 71, 75, 312t
Phenothiazine, 131t
Phenylketonuria, 346
Phenytoin (Dilantin), 71, 75, 312t
Phobia(s), 413–414
Physician's Desk Reference (PDR), 65
Physiologic integrity, client need for, 4, 9
Physostigmine (Eserine), 72
Piaget's developmental stage(s), in
    adolescent, 289
  in infants, 280
  in preschoolers, 284
  in school-age children, 287–288
  in toddlers, 282
PIH (pregnancy-induced hypertension), 368
Pilocarpine (Isopto Carpine), 72
Pinworm(s), in pediatric patient, 352
Pitocin (oxytocin), 68
Pitting edema, 154
Pituitary gland, function of, 117c
Placenta, development of, 364
  endocrine function of, 328c
Placenta previa, 370, *370*
Planning, in nursing process, 4, 8, 47
Plant alkaloid(s), 201t
Plaquenil (hydroxychloroquine), for
    systemic lupus erythematosus, 203
Platinol (Cisplatin), 201t
Play, in hospitalized children, 334t
  in infants, 279
  in preschoolers, 283t, 284
  in school-age children, 287, 287t
  in toddlers, 28, 281t
Pleura-Evac, in chest surgery, 150, *151*
Pneumonia, 144t, 146–147
  in pediatric patient, 305
Poisoning, in pediatric patient, 323t–325t,
    328
  lead, 317
  prevention of, 323t–324t
Poliomyelitis, 322t, 326
Polycillin (ampicillin), 70, 144t, 255t
Polyhydramnios, 382
Portal hypertension, in cirrhosis, 252
Positioning, 10, 52, 52–53, 56
  immobility and, 208, *210*
Postmortem care, 54
Postoperative care, diet in, 91
  of adult patient, 197–199, 198t
  of pediatric patient, 332–333, 333t–334t
Postpartum period, hemorrhage during,
    390
  infections during, 390–391
  normal, 390–391
  thrombophlebitis during, 391
  wound separations during, 391–392
Postural drainage, 49
Postural hypotension, in elderly patient,
    104

Potassium. See also *Hyperkalemia;*
    Hypokalemia.
  deficit of, in metabolic alkalosis, 161
  foods high in, 92, 92t, 241t
Potassium-sparing diuretic(s), 69, 238t
Povan (pyrvinium), 247
Practice test(s), for NCLEX-PN, 11–46,
    435–469
Pravastatin (Pravachol), 70
Precipitate labor, 381
Prednisone (cortisone), 73t, 74, 257t
Preeclampsia, 368
Pregnancy, 364–372
  alcohol and, 367
  cardiac disease during, 371
  cardiovascular function during, 363
  complications of, 368–372, 369t,
    370–371
  cystitis during, 370–371
  diabetes mellitus during, 371
  diagnostic tests during, 367
  discomforts of, 367–368
  ectopic, 369
  embryonic stage of, 364–365
  endocrine function during, 362
  environmental risks to, 365–367
  fetal stage of, 365, *366*
  gastrointestinal function during, 363
  gynecologic disorders during, 362
  hemorrhage during, 369–370, *370–371*
  infections during, 370–371
    chlamydial, 365–366
    cytomegalovirus, 371
    German measles, 365, 371
    gonococcal, 366
    herpes virus, 366, 371
    human immunodeficiency virus,
      366–367
    of kidney, 371
    rubella, 365, 371
    syphilis, 366
  molar, 369–370, *370*
  nutrition during, 90, 365
  prenatal care during, 365
  psychologic changes during, 362–363
  radiation during, 367
  sexually transmitted diseases during,
    365–367
  signs of, 363–364
  ultrasonography during, 367
  weight gain during, 365
Pregnancy-induced hypertension (PIH), 368
Preoperative care, of adult patient, 195–197
  of pediatric patient, 332–333, 333t–334t
Preschooler(s), 283t–285t, 284
  accidents in, 324t
  developmental stages in, Erikson's, 284
  developmental stages of, Freud's, 283t
    Piaget's, 284
  emotional-social competency in, 283t
  intellectual competency in, 283t
  nutrition in, 73t, 90
  perioperative care of, 331–332
  physical competency in, 283t
  physical development in, 284
  play in, 283t, 284
  safety of, 283t
  sleep in, 284
Presentation, fetal, 376, *376,* 376t
Preterm labor, 381
Primaxin (imipenem/cilastatin), 71, 144t
Primidone (Mysoline), 312t
Privacy, nursing skills for, 47
Pro-Banthine (propantheline), 76
Procainamide (Procan), 134t
Prochlorperazine (Compazine), 75, 236t

Progesterone, functions of, 361
  during pregnancy, 362–363
Projection, 423
Prone position, 52, *52*
  immobility and, *210*
Propantheline (Pro-Banthine), 76
Propranolol (Inderal), 134t
Proprioception, in elderly patient, 103
Propylthiouracil (PTU), 76
Prostate, cancer of, 123–124
Prostate-specific antigen (PSA), 123
Prostatic hyperplasia, benign, 122–123
Protamine sulfate, 69
Protamine zinc insulin (PZI), 75
Protective device(s), use of, 50–51
Protective functions, 5, 190–204
  basic nursing skill(s) related to, 51–55, *52*
    bandages and binders as, 53
    bed making as, 51–52
    care of dying as, 54
    culture and sensitivity specimens
      as, 51
    hygiene needs as, 51
    isolation precautions as, 53–54
    wound care as, 53
  drugs affecting, 73–74
  in pediatric patient, 322–334
Protein(s), and wound healing, 93t
  in food, 96, 96t, 253t
PSA (prostate-specific antigen), 222
Psychiatric client(s). See *Mental health
    client(s).*
Psychological alteration(s), from
    immobility, 210
Psychological development, during
    pregnancy, 362–363
  in adults, 117–118
  in infants, 279–280
  in preschoolers, 283t, 283–284
  in school-age children, 286t–288t, 287
  in young adult, 362
Psychosocial alteration(s), in elderly
    patient, 105, 108–109
Psychosocial integrity, client need for,
    4–5, 9
Psychosocial need(s), of dying patient, 54
Psychosocial/cultural function(s), 5
Psyllium (Metamucil), 75, 209
PTU (propylthiouracil), 76
Pudendal block, during labor, 380
Puerperal infection(s), 390
Pulmonary disorder(s). See also under
    individual disorder(s).
  in adult patient, 146–152
  in pediatric patient, 304–308
Pulmonary stasis, immobility and, 208
Pupillary response(s), assessment of, 50
  with increased intracranial pressure, 169,
    172c
Pyelolithotomy, 261
Pyelonephritis, 257t, 259–260, 260t
  diet for, 260t
  during pregnancy, 371
  medications for, 257t
Pyloric stenosis, 243, 243–244
Pyloroplasty, for peptic ulcer disease, 234
Pyridium (phenazopyridine), 258t
Pyridostigmine bromide (Mestinon), 74t
Pyridoxine, 72, 299
Pyrvinium (Povan), 247
PZI (protamine zinc insulin), 75

Quarzan (clidinium bromide), 130t
Questran (cholestyramine), 70

Quinidine gluconate (Quinaglute), 134t
Quinolone(s), 76, 153t

Radiation, during pregnancy, 367
Radiation therapy, 200, 203t
Range of motion (ROM), exercises for, 55
    immobility and, 209
Ranitidine (Zantac), 76, 235t
Rationalization, 423
Reaction formation, 423
Rectal tube(s), care of, 56
Reduction, of fractured bones, 213
Reflex(es), in increased intracranial
    pressure, 169
    neonatal, 396
Regional anesthesia, during labor, 375–381
Regional enteritis, 242t, 243–244. See also
    Crohn's disease.
Regression, 423
Rehabilitation, after substance abuse, 428
Relationship(s), therapeutic, 406–407
Renal. See also entries under Kidney(s).
Renal calculi, 260–261, 261t
Renal disorder(s). See also under
    individual disorder(s).
    in adult patient, 256–258
    in pediatric patient, 354–355
Renal failure, 262–265, 263–265
    treatment of, 263, 264
Renal tubular disease, in metabolic
    acidosis, 161
Reproductive system, disorders of, female,
    119–122. See also under individual
    disorder(s).
    in men, 122–124
    during pregnancy, 362
    female, 361
    male, 361–362
Respiratory acidosis, 158–159
Respiratory alkalosis, 159–160
Respiratory function, in elderly patient,
    104, 108, 118
Respiratory infection(s), upper, in pediatric
    patient, 304
Respiratory isolation, 53
Respiratory system, during pregnancy, 363
    immobility and, 208
    infection in, clinical presentation of, 326t
Rest/activity, skills related to, 55
Restraint(s), use of, 50–51
Retina, 75
    detached, 76–77
Retirement, in elderly patient, 105
Retropubic prostatectomy, 123
Retrovir (zidovudine), 71, 144t, 296
Retroviral infections(s), treatment of, 144t
Reverse isolation, skills related to, 54
Reye's syndrome, 316
Rh incompatibility, 372
Rheumatic fever, 299–300
Rheumatoid arthritis, 214, 215, 216
    juvenile, 340
Rhinitis, allergic, in pediatric patient,
    307–308
Riboflavin, 89
Rifampin (Rifadin), 71–72, 147t
Ringworm, 330
Riopan, 235t
Ritodrine (Yutopar), 68
Robaxin (methocarbamol), 74, 216
Robitussin (guaifenesin), 70
Role change(s), in elderly patient, 105
ROM (range of motion), exercises for, 55,
    209

Roseola (exanthema subitum), 324–325
Rubber band ligation, for hemorrhoids, 246
Rubella, during pregnancy, 365, 371
    vaccination for, 390
Rubeola (measles), 322, 322t, 324
Rule of nines, 194
Rupture of membranes, during labor, 378
Russell's traction, 211, 212

Saddle block, during labor, 380
Safety, in care environment, client need for,
    4, 8–9
    of preschoolers, 283t
    of school-age children, 287, 287t
Salicylate(s), 72, 135t
    abuse of, and respiratory alkalosis, 160
Scarlet fever, 327
Schizophrenia, 407–408
    antipsychotic agents for, 408t
School-age child(ren), 284, 286t–288t,
    286–288
    development of, physical, 284, 286–287
    developmental needs of, nursing
        strategies for, 288t
    developmental stages in, Eriksonian, 287
        Piaget's, 287–288
    emotional-social competency in, 286t
    intellectual competency in, 286t
    nutrition for, 90, 287, 287t
    perioperative care of, 332
    physical competency of, 286t
    play in, 287, 287t
    safety of, 287, 287t
Sclera, 74
Scoliosis, 340–341
Screening test(s), for neonates, 397
Scultetus binder(s), application of, 53
Secobarbital (Seconal), 73
Secretory phase, of menstrual cycle, 361
Seizure(s), anticonvulsants for, 312t
    classification of, 71, 312
    febrile, 313
    in pediatric patient, 312–313
Self-absorption, vs. generativity, in middle
    age, 118
Self-medication, in elderly patient, 107
Semi-Fowler's position, 52, 52
Semisolid(s), drugs in form of, 66
Sensitivity specimen(s), collection of, 51
Sensory function, in elderly patient,
    103–104, 107–108
    in neonate, 396–397
Sensory/perceptual alteration(s), 5
    in adult patient, 169–185
    in pediatric patient, 312–318
    nursing skills related to, 49–51
Septra (trimethoprim), 76
Sexual abuse, 425–426
Sexuality, drugs affecting, 67–68
    in elderly patient, 105–106
    nursing skills related to, 47–48
Sexually transmitted diseases (STDs),
    190–194, 191t, 295–299, 296t
    during pregnancy, 365–367
Shame and doubt vs. autonomy, in
    toddlers, 282
Shock, 145–146, 146t
Shunt(s), arteriovenous, for dialysis, 264
Sickle cell anemia, 145
    in pediatric patient, 300–301, 301
SIDS (sudden infant death syndrome), 306
Sigmoidoscopy, in diverticulosis/
    diverticulitis, 239
Simple fracture(s), 211

Sims position, 52, 52, 56
Sinemet (carbidopa), 72t, 75
Sitting position, immobility and, 210
Skeletal muscle relaxant(s), 74
Skeletal traction, 211, 212, 340
Skin, breakdown of, classification of, 104,
    105
    care of, 51
    changes in, during pregnancy, 364
    disorders of, 194–195
        in pediatric patient, 328–331
    immobility and, 209–210
    infection of, clinical presentation in, 326t
    of elderly patient, 105, 108
    of middle-aged patient, 117
    of neonate, 396
    traction of, 211, 212, 340
    ulcers of, prevention of, 104–105
SLE (systemic lupus erythematosus), 73t,
    200, 203–204, 362
Sleep, in infants, 280
    in toddlers, 282, 282t
    nursing skills related to, 55
Smell, in elderly patient, 104
Smoking, dependence on, 427
    during pregnancy, 367
Smooth muscle relaxant(s), uterine, 369t
Societal attitude(s), toward elderly person,
    106
Sodium. See also Hypernatremia;
    Hyponatremia.
    in fluid and electrolyte balance, 153
    in foods, 91t, 91–92, 133t
Sodium bicarbonate, in metabolic alkalosis,
    161
Solid(s), drugs in form of, 66
Solution(s), definition of, 66
Speech, in infants, 280
    in toddlers, 282, 282t
Spica cast(s), 211
Spina bifida, 315
Spinal cord injury(ies), 69
Spinal fusion, 216
Spinal tap, in meningitis, 380
Spiritual need(s), of dying patient, 54
Spirometer(s), incentive, use of, 48
Spironolactone (Aldactone), 69, 133t
Spontaneous abortion, 369
Spousal abuse, 424–425
Sputum specimen(s), collection of, 48
Stagnation, vs. generativity, in middle age,
    118
STDs (sexually transmitted diseases),
    190–194, 191t, 295–299, 296t
    during pregnancy, 365–367
Steroid(s), 73t, 74, 362t, 363t
Stockings, compression, application of, 48
Stomach. See also entries under Gastric.
    anatomy of, 129
    cancer of, 236t, 237–239
Stool, examination of, in hepatitis, 250
Stool softener(s), 92t, 131t
Stool specimen(s), collection of, 57
Strabismus, in pediatric patient, 317–318
Streptomycin, 72, 147t
Stress test, during pregnancy, 367
    in coronary artery disease, 134
Strict isolation, nursing skills related to, 53
Stroke, 172–174
Subarachnoid block, during labor, 380
Subcutaneous route, for injection of
    drugs, 78
Sublimation, 423
Sublingual route, for administration of
    drugs, 78
Substance abuse, 426–428

Suctioning, 49
Sudden infant death syndrome (SIDS), 306
Suicidal behavior pattern, 411
Sulfamethoxazole-trimethoprim (Bactrim), 258t
Sulfisoxazole (Gantrisin), 76
Sulfonamide(s), 75–76
Supine position, 52, 52
  immobility and, 210
Suppository(ies), 135t
  administration of, 78–79
  definition of, 66
Suprapubic prostatectomy, 123
Suspension(s), definition of, 66
Suspiciousness, as behavior pattern, 408t, 408–409
Symbolization, 423
Sympathetic inhibitor(s), 69, 133t
Synthroid (levothyroxine sodium), 76–77
Syphilis, 296t, 297–298
  during pregnancy, 366
Systemic lupus erythematosus (SLE), 73t, 200, 203–204, 362

Tablet(s), definition of, 66
Tagamet (cimetidine), 76, 130t
Talipes equinovarus (clubfoot), 338, 338
Tamoxifen (Nolvadex), 74, 202t
Taste, in elderly patient, 104
T-binder(s), application of, 53
TED hose, application of, 48
Temperature, assessment of, postpartum, 389
Terminally ill patient(s), care of, 54
Testes, function of, 119c
  self-examination of, 48
Testosterone, functions of, 361–362
Testosterone propionate(s), 68, 201t
Test-taking, 7–10
  on computers, 1, 2
  reading questions in, 7
  repeat, 10
  time management in, 7
Tetracycline (Achromycin), 71, 144t, 295, 296t
Tetralogy of Fallot, 296, 297
Theophylline (Theo-Dur), 70, 149t
Therapeutic relationship, 406–407
Thiamine, 89
Thiazide diuretic(s), 69, 238t
Thoracentesis, 149
Thorazine (chlorpromazine), 73
Thrombophlebitis, 135t, 139c, 140–141
  postpartum, 391
Thymus, function of, 119c
Thyroid, disorders of, 221–226
  drugs for, 76–77
  function of, 222c
Tigan (trimethobenzamide), 75
Time management, in test-taking, 7
Tincture, definition of, 66
Tinea, 330
Tobacco, dependence on, 427
Toddler(s), 280t–282t, 281–282
  accidents in, 324t
  developmental needs of, nursing strategies for, 282t
  developmental stages in, Eriksonian, 282
    Piaget's, 282
  emotional-social competency in, 280t

Toddler(s) (Continued)
  intellectual competency in, 280t
  nutrition for, 71, 71t
  perioperative care of, 331
  physical competency in, 280t
  physical development of, 281
  play in, 281, 281t
  safety of, 281t
  sleep in, 281
  speech in, 282, 282t
Tolazamide (Tolinase), 229t
Tolbutamide (Orinase), 229t
Tolerance, to drugs, 67
Tonic-clonic seizure(s), 71, 312
Tonsillitis, in pediatric patient, 306
Topical preparation(s), administration of, in children, 79
TORCH (Toxoplasmosis, Other infections, Rubella, Cytomegalovirus, Herpes), 371
Touch, in elderly patient, 104
Toxoplasmosis, Other infections, Rubella, Cytomegalovirus, Herpes (TORCH), 371
Tracheostomy, care of, 48
Traction, 211, 212
  in pediatric patient, 340
Trainable mentally handicapped client, 315
Tranquilizer(s), 135t
  major, 408t
  minor, 413t
Transdermal route, for administration of drugs, 66, 78
Transferring patient(s), skills related to, 55
Transurethral prostatectomy, 122
Trauma, and musculoskeletal disorders. See Musculoskeletal system, disorders of, from trauma.
  from abuse, 424–426
  in pediatric patient, 322, 323t–324t, 338–340
Trendelenburg position, 52, 52
  reverse, 53
Tricyclic antidepressant(s), 409t
Trimethobenzamide (Tigan), 75
Trimethoprim (Bactrim, Septra), 76
Trisomy 21, 314
Troche(s), definition of, 66
Trust vs. mistrust, in infants, 279
Tube feeding(s), 56
Tuberculosis, 147t, 147–148
Tumor(s). See under specific site(s).
Turning patient(s), skills related to, 55
Tylenol (acetaminophen), 72, 135t
Tylenol #3 (acetaminophen with codeine), 70, 135t

Ulcer(s), decubitus, from immobility, 104
  prevention of, 104–105
  peptic, 231, 233–235, 234, 235t–236t, 236. See Peptic ulcer disease.
  venous stasis, 246
Ulcerative colitis. See Colitis, ulcerative.
Ultrasonography, during pregnancy, 367
Umbilical cord, development of, 364
  prolapsed, 381–382, 382
Umbilical hernia, 244
United States Pharmacopeia (USP), 65
Universal precautions, 53, 174t
Upper respiratory infection (URI), in pediatric patient, 304
Urecholine (bethanechol), 72
Ureterolithotomy, 261
Ureterosigmoidostomy, 267, 267

Ureterostomy, 267, 267
Urethritis, 258–259
URI (upper respiratory infection), in pediatric patient, 304
Urinalysis, in hepatitis, 249
Urinary calculi, 260–261, 261t
Urinary diversion, 266–267, 267
Urinary elimination, nursing skills related to, 57
Urinary tract, disorders of, 256–260
  in adult patient, 256–268
  in pediatric patient, 354–355
  during pregnancy, 363
  immobility and, 210
  infections of, postpartum, 391
Urine, production of, 258
Urine specimen(s), collection of, 57–58
Urticaria (hives), 330–331
USDA Food Guide Pyramid, 87–88, 88
USP (United States Pharmacopeia), 65
Uterine smooth muscle relaxant(s), 369t
Uterine smooth muscle stimulant(s), 67–68
Uterus, fundus of, postpartum assessment of, 389
  rupture of, during labor, 381
  tumors of, 120

Vaccination, for Haemophilus b influenza, 322t
  for rubella, 390
Vaginal delivery, after cesarean section, 383
Vaginal douche, 47
Vagotomy, for peptic ulcer, 234
Valium (diazepam), 73, 312t
Valproic acid (Depakene), 312t
Vaporizer(s), use of, 48
Varicella zoster (chickenpox), 325–326
Varicose vein(s), 246
Vasodilan (isoxsuprine), 69
Vasodilator(s), 69, 131t
Vasopressor(s), 146t
Vasotec (enalapril), 133t
Veneral Disease Research Laboratory (VDRL) test, 296t, 297
Venous peripheral vascular disorder(s), 244c, 245–246
Venous stasis ulcer(s), 246
Ventilation, mechanical, in respiratory alkalosis, 160
Ventricular septal defect(s), 294, 295
Verapamil (Calan), 69, 131t
Verbal communication, 405
Vinca alkaloid(s), 74
Vincristine (Oncovin), 74, 201t
Viokase (pancreatin), 257t
Violence, domestic, 424–425
Viral disease(s), in pediatric patient, 322, 324–326, 326t
Vision, disorders of, 75–77
  in pediatric patient, 317–318
  in elderly patient, 103, 118
  in middle-aged patient, 117
  neonatal, 396
Vital sign(s), assessment of, postpartum, 389
  neonatal, 396
Vitamin(s), 88–89
  and wound healing, 198t
Vitamin B_6 (pyridoxine), 72, 89
Vitamin K, 251t, 252t
  oral (AquaMEPHYTON), 69

von Recklinghausen's disease, 133t, 332

Walking cast(s), 211
Warfarin (Coumadin), 69–70, 135t
Water. See under *Fluid*.
Water-soluble vitamin(s), 89
Weight, maintenance of, calculation of calories for, 90
  neonatal, 396
Weight gain, during pregnancy, 365

Weight loss, postpartum, 390
Whooping cough (pertussis), 322t, 327
Wilms' tumor (nephroblastoma), 249–250
Withdrawal, as behavior pattern, 407–408
Wound(s), care of, 53
  healing of, nutrition and, 198, 198t
  separation of, postpartum, 391–392
  surgical, care of, 198

Xanthine derivative(s), as bronchodilators, 70

Young adult(s), as mental health client, 411–412
  development of, 361–362
Yutopar (ritodrine), 68

Zantac (ranitidine), 76, 235t
Zidovudine (AZT, Retrovir), 71, 144t, 191, 193
Zovirax (acyclovir), 296, 325

Common Questions about the NCLEX-RN Software Program to Accompany
Saunders Review of Practical Nursing for NCLEX-PN, Third Edition

1. How do I install the program onto my computer?

DOS Version

- Go to your DOS or command prompt on the hard drive of your computer.
- Type "A:INSTALL".
- Answer the questions presented by the install program. If you use the suggested directory, the install program will put the program "NCLEXPN.EXE" in a directory called "REVIEW" on your hard drive.
- To start up the review software, switch to the directory you chose during the installation and type "NCLEXPN".

> EXAMPLE: "C:"
> "cd\review"
> "nclexpn"

WINDOWS 3.1 Version

- From the Program Manager, pick "File", "Run", and then enter "A:INSTALL".
- Answer the questions presented by the install program. If you use the suggested directory, the install program will put the program "NCLEXPN.EXE" in a directory called "REVIEW" on your hard drive.
- To start up the review software, double click on the "NCLEX-PN" icon created during the installation.

WINDOWS 95 Version

- Select "Start", then "Run", and then enter "A:INSTALL".
- Answer the questions presented by the install program. If you use the suggested directory, the install program will put the program "NCLEXPN.EXE" in a directory called "REVIEW" on your hard drive.
- To start up the review software, choose "START", followed by "PROGRAMS", then "NCLEX Review", and finally "NCLEX-PN".

2. How do I obtain a MAC version of this software?

If you need to obtain a disk that will be compatible with your MAC computer, please complete the attached business reply card bound into this book. W.B. Saunders Company will fulfill your request for the MAC version of the NCLEX review software immediately.

To install the MAC version onto your computer, please follow these instructions:

- To run the software from the disk, double click on the "NCLEXPN" icon.
- If you are installing the software on a hard drive, be sure to copy all the files to the same folder.

3. How can I print the results in DOS?

The review software prints to the standard printer port (LPT1). It does not use any special control characters specific to any particular printer. If you have trouble printing out the results of your tests, exit the review software and type "CONFIG" at the command prompt and press ENTER. This will allow you to customize some of the printer settings. If you have any further difficulty with our software, please call our Customer Support line toll free at (800) 523-1649, extension 5038.

4. Is a network version of this software available?

Institutions wishing to install this software on networks in their computer labs can purchase a site license for the software. Please contact your local W.B. Saunders Company Sales Representative or call our Sales Support Team at (215) 238-8406. In Canada, please call W.B. Saunders Canada at (800) 387-7278. The ISBN for the network version is 0-7216-6996-4.

5. Where can I call for help?

Call our Customer Support line toll free at (800) 523-1649, extension 5038.